Pesticide, veterinary and other residues in food

Related titles from Woodhead's food science, technology and nutrition list:

Detecting allergens in food (ISBN 1 85573 728 0)
Allergens pose a serious risk to consumers, making effective detection methods a priority for the food industry. Bringing together key experts in the field, this important collection both reviews the range of analytical techniques available and their use to detect specific allergens such as nuts, dairy and wheat products.

Detecting pathogens in food (ISBN 1 85573 670 5)
Methods for detecting pathogens need to balance accuracy, specificity and speed. There have been major advances in techniques in all these areas. *Detecting pathogens in food* sums up the wealth of recent research, the range of techniques available and their applications. The first part of the book looks at general issues such as the role of microbiological analysis in food safety management, sampling techniques and ways of validating individual detection methods. The second part of the book examines individual techniques, including microscopy, immunological and genetic methods.

Detecting foreign bodies in food (ISBN 1 85573 729 9)
A foreign body is any undesirable solid object in a food. Foreign bodies range from external matter such as metal fragments or insects to internal matter such as bones or stalks. Foreign bodies in food remain a significant risk to consumers and to a company's reputation. They can also be difficult to detect, particularly if they are part of the raw material used in food processing. This collection discusses ways of preventing and managing incidents involving foreign bodies. It also reviews the range of technologies available for effective detection and control of foreign bodies from both external and internal sources.

Details of these books and a complete list of Woodhead's food science, technology and nutrition titles can be obtained by:

- visiting our web site at www.woodhead-publishing.com
- contacting Customer Services (email: sales@woodhead-publishing.com; fax: +44 (0) 1223 893694; tel.: +44 (0) 1223 891358 ext. 30; address: Woodhead Publishing Limited, Abington Hall, Abington, Cambridge CB1 6AH, UK)

Selected food science and technology titles are also available in electronic form. Visit our web site (www.woodhead-publishing.com) to find out more.

If you would like to receive information on forthcoming titles in this area, please send your address details to: Francis Dodds (address, tel. and fax as above; e-mail: francisd@woodhead-publishing.com). Please confirm which subject areas you are interested in.

Pesticide, veterinary and other residues in food

Edited by
David H. Watson

CRC Press
Boca Raton Boston New York Washington, DC

WOODHEAD PUBLISHING LIMITED
Cambridge England

Published by Woodhead Publishing Limited
Abington Hall, Abington
Cambridge CB1 6AH
England
www.woodhead-publishing.com

Published in North America by CRC Press LLC
2000 Corporate Blvd, NW
Boca Raton FL 33431
USA

First published 2004, Woodhead Publishing Limited and CRC Press LLC

British Library Cataloguing in Publication Data
A catalogue record for this book is available from the British Library.

Library of Congress Cataloging-in-Publication Data
A catalog record for this book is available from the Library of Congress.

Woodhead Publishing Limited ISBN 1 85573 734 5 (book); 1 85573 910 0 (e-book)
CRC Press ISBN 0-8493-2558-7
CRC Press order number: WP2558

The publisher's policy is to use permanent paper from mills that operate a sustainable forestry policy, and which have been manufactured from pulp which is processed using acid-free and elementary chlorine-free practices. Furthermore, the publisher ensures that the text paper and cover board used have met acceptable environmental accreditation standards.

Project managed by Macfarlane Production Services, Markyate, Hertfordshire
(e-mail: macfarl@aol.com)
Typeset by MHL Typesetting Limited, Coventry, Warwickshire
Printed by TJ International Limited, Padstow, Cornwall, England

Contents

Contributor contact details

Chapter 1

Dr S. Omaye
University of Nevada
Department of Nutrition
Room 215B
142 Fleischmann Building
Reno NV 89557
USA

E-mail: omaye@unr.edu

Chapter 2

Professor D. Eaton, Dr S. Peterson and Dr J. Lampe
School of Public Health
University of Washington and Fred Hutchinson Cancer Research Center
4225 Roosevelt Way NE, Suite 100
Seattle
WA 98105-6099
USA

Fax: +1 206 685-4696
E-mail: deaton@u.washington.edu

Chapter 3

Professor J. Parry
School of Biological Sciences
University of Wales – Swansea
Singleton Park
Swansea SA2 8PP
UK

E-mail: jmp@swansea.ac.uk

Chapter 4

Professor C. Regan, Dr I. de Souza and Dr H. Gallagher
Conway Institute
University College Dublin
Ireland

E-mail: ciaran.regan@ucd.ie

Chapter 5

Dr E. Meulenberg
ELTI Support
The Netherlands

Dr M. Remrev-Boom
ResQ Lab
The Netherlands

Dr K. Koopal
Sensor Technology Department
TNO Nutrition and Food Research
PO Box 360
3700 AJ Zeist
The Netherlands

Tel: +31 30 6944636
Fax: +31 30 6944901
E-mail: koopal@voeding.tno.nl

Chapter 6

R. Early
Harper Adams University College
Newport
Shropshire TF10 8NB
UK

E-mail: rearly@harper-adams.ac.uk

Chapters 7 and 8

Dr K. Woodward
International Federation for Animal Health
Rue Defacqz 1
1000 Brussels
Belgium

E-mail: kevin.woodward@spcorp.com

Chapter 9

Dr N. van Hoof, Dr K. de Wasch, Dr H. Noppe, Dr S. Poelmans and Dr H. de Brabender,
Department of Veterinary Public Health and Food Safety
University of Ghent
Salisburylaan 133
B-9820 Merelbeke
Belgium

E-mail: Katia.DeWasch@UGent.be

Chapter 10

Dr E. Magner and Dr M. Jamal
Materials and Surface Science Institute
Department of Chemical and Environmental Sciences
University of Limerick
Limerick
Ireland

E-mail: edmond.magner@ul.ie
mamun.jamal@ul.ie

Chapter 11

Dr M. Tuomola and Professor T. Lövgren
University of Turku
FIN 20014 Turku
Finland

Email: timo.lovgren@utu.fi

Chapter 12

Professor C. Winter
Department of Food Science and Technology
University of California
One Shields Avenue
Davis
CA 95616-8598
USA

E-mail: ckwinter@ucdavis.edu

Chapter 13

Dr R. Luxton and Dr J. Hart
Faculty of Applied Sciences
University of the West of England
Frenchay Campus
Coldharbour Lane
Bristol BS16 1QY
UK

E-mail: Richard.Luxton@uwe.ac.uk
John.Hart@uwe.ac.uk

Chapter 14

Dr Y. Picó, Dr G. Font and Dr J. Mañes
University of Valencia
Departament de Medicina Preventiva
Av. Vicent Andres Estelles s/n
46100 Burjasot
Valencia
Spain

Tel: 963544288
Fax: 963544954
E-mail: jordi.manes@uv.es

Chapter 15

Dr M. Sheehan, Dr H. Berney and Dr A. Matthewson
University College
Lee Maltings
Prospect Row
Cork
Ireland

Tel: 353 21 4904177
Fax: 353 21 4270271
E-mail: alan.mathewson@nmrc.ie

Chapter 16

Dr J. L. Tadeo, Dr C. Sánchez-Brunete and Dr B. Albero
INIA
Carretera de la Coruña pk7
Madrid E28040
Spain

E-mail: tadeo@inia.es

Chapter 17

Professor I. Shaw
Pro Vice-Chancellor (Science)
University of Canterbury
Private Bag 4800
Christchurch
New Zealand

Tel: 64 3364 2351
Fax: 64 3364 2490

E-mail: ian.shaw@canterbury.ac.nz

B. Thompson and P. Cressey
Institute of Environmental Science & Research
New Zealand

Chapter 18

Professor S. Hendrich
Department of Food Science and Human Nutrition
College of Family and Consumer Services
124 MacKay
Iowa State University
Ames, IA 50011
USA

Tel: 515 294 0859
Fax: 515 294 0190
E-mail: shendric@iastate.edu

Chapter 19

Dr K. Tamakawa
Sendai City Institute of Public Health
2-5-10 Oroshimachi-higashi
Wakabayishi Ward
Sendai City
Japan

E-mail: Katsutam44171@mni.ne.jp

Chapter 20

Dr L. Hoogenboom
Department of Food Safety and Health
RIKILT Institute of Food Safety
PO Box 230
6700 AE Wageningen
The Netherlands

E-mail:
l.a.p.hoogenboom@rikilt.dlo.nl

Chapter 21

S. Van Leeuwen,
RIVO
PO Box 68
NL-1970 Ijmuiden
The Netherlands

Email: stefan.vanleeuwen@wuc.nl

Chapter 22

Dr C. Mills, Dr J. Jenkins and Dr J. Robertson
Institute of Food Research
Norwich Research Park
Colney
Norwich NR4 7UA
UK

Tel: 44 1603 255000
Fax: 44 1603 255000
E-mail: clare.mills@bbsrc.ac.uk

Dr S. Griffiths-Jones
Wellcome Trust Sanger Institute
UK

Dr P. Shewry
Institute of Arable Crops Research
UK

Chapter 23

Professor A. von Wright
Institute of Applied Biotechnology
University of Kuopio
PO Box 1627
Kuopio FIN-70211
Finland

E-mail: wright@mail.uku.fi

Chapter 24

Dr R Montoro
Poligono La Coma s/n
46980 Paterna
Valencia
Spain

E-mail: rmontoro@iata.csic.es

Chapter 25

M. Miraglia, F. Debegnach and C. Brera
Italian National Institute for Health
Via Regina Elena 299
I-00161 Rome
Italy
E-mail: miraglia@iss.it

1

Introduction to food toxicology

S. T. Omaye, University of Nevada, USA

1.1 Introduction: defining food toxicology

Food toxicology can be defined as the science that deals with toxicants in food (Shibamoto and Bjeldanes, 1993). Food toxicology is a heterogeneous field and spans many scientific disciplines. It may be considered as a branch of food science, nutrition, or toxicology. As a branch of food science, food toxicology evolved from the disciplines of food safety, pesticide chemistry, risk assessment, toxicokinetics, and legal fields emphasizing the presence of toxicants in foods.

Toxicology is defined as the science dealing with poisons or toxicants (Klaassen *et al.*, 1996). Nutritional toxicology can be considered as a parallel branch to food toxicology and although the two are related and overlap, they are not synonymous. Overall, scientists working in the area of food toxicology investigate the impact of natural and synthetic compounds present in food on human health, taking into account dangerous effects such as carcinogenicity, allergic reactions, immunotoxicity, and neurotoxicity on the one side, and the potential for the prevention of disease on the other. On the other hand, nutritional toxicology tends to be concerned with toxicants in the diet and their interrelations with nutrition (Hathcock, 1976, 1982). Nutritional toxicology is concerned with the diet as a source of toxicants, the effects of toxicants on nutrients and nutritional metabolism of toxicants. It is also concerned with nutrients in foods when they are consumed in excess and can become toxicants, for example vitamins A and D and essential minerals. Toxicants may alter nutrient intake, digestion, absorption, transport, activation, function, metabolism, or elimination. The detoxification of toxicants may be affected by food, food consumption patterns, and nutritional status. In addition, both food and nutritional toxicology are concerned with the scientific basis and consequences of regulatory decisions relating to control of toxicant residues in foods, which involve setting legal tolerances or maximum permissible levels of natural toxicants such as mycotoxins.

The purpose of this chapter is provide a brief review of the scope of food toxicology and highlight some current concerns facing the field. No attempt has been made to provide an exhaustive review of this enormous subject area.

The range of toxicants found in food is varied but can be broadly subdivided into:

- Contaminants or those substances that inadvertently get into our food as by-products of industrial manufacturing or waste or as residues from intentional food chemicals, such as pesticides.
- Naturally-occurring toxicants or those substances that are found naturally in our food because they are products of plants, animals, and other organisms.
- Food processing toxicants or those substances that incidentally become part of our food as byproducts of various processing situations. Also, other substances added intentionally to the food for some benefit could potentially, if added in excess, adversely affect the consumer. However, chemicals added intentionally are under strict regulatory control and will not be discussed.

1.2 Types of toxicant: contaminants

Contaminating substances may enter the food chain at many different stages. Through various constituents like fertilizer ingredients and contaminants, irrigation water, contaminants and pesticides can enter food crops through plant roots. Contaminants in forages and other feeds can be transmitted to animal products. Veterinary drugs can leave residues in animal products. Environmental chemicals such as heavy metals (e.g., lead and mercury) from many sources have sometimes been found as food contaminants. We will focus on a few selected pesticide residues, metals, and industrial contaminants for illustrative purposes.

1.2.1 Pesticides

Pesticides play an important role in food production by controlling insects, weeds, organisms responsible for plant diseases, and other pests. In protecting food plants, pesticides assist in ensuring substantial yield and providing consumers with a wide variety of foods at inexpensive prices. Pests are living organisms that occur where they are not wanted or that cause damage to crops, humans, or other animals. Most pesticides create some degree of risk of harm to humans, animals, or the environment because they are inherently designed to kill or otherwise adversely affect living organisms but be selective with regard to target species (Albert, 1979). At the same time, pesticides are useful to society, destroying potential disease-causing organisms and control insects, weeds, and other pests. Understanding the modes of action of pesticides is important to the food toxicologist both for the design of compounds to be specific for the targeted species and for understanding potential adverse human health effects.

Pesticides have several modes of action. They may physically alter the organism in a mechanical way which blocks their cellular processes. Examples include oil (petroleum products) that are used as sprays, which clog the respiratory mechanism of insects, or compounds like bypyridylium herbicides, which act by destroying the cell membranes of plants causing desiccation. Petroleum oils can also deter feeding or egg laying in some insects. Some pesticides are metabolic system inhibitors and restrict the transfer of energy within the target organisms. Inhibitory pesticides in this category are many, such as rotenone and cyanide, which disrupt respiratory functions in animals, or herbicides that inhibit seed germination or plant growth, and various fungicides that inhibit germination of spores. Some pesticides require metabolic activation into the toxic form before they become toxic to the target pest. For example, sodium monofluoroacetate is converted to fluorocitrate before it becomes toxic to vertebrates.

Other pesticides owe their effectiveness to the alteration of protein synthesis or enzyme disruption. Proteins, as the basic building blocks of all cell components, are crucial and substances made up of proteins, such as enzymes, control many important cell functions. Pesticides can disrupt enzyme processes or denature proteins. Examples include inorganic copper compounds, dithiocarbamate fungicides, phosphoro amino acid herbicides, such as glyphosate and organophosphate insecticides. Other pesticides alter hormone actions that control many of the biological functions of organisms, including growth and reproductive cycles. Several pesticides simulate or otherwise interfere with hormones to disrupt these cycles, for example phenoxy herbicides that interfere with plant growth hormones, and insect growth regulators that interfere with cuticle formation in insects during molting. Nervous system disruptor pesticides affect mainly animal groups such as insects, nematodes, and rodents. Some pesticides, such as some fumigant pesticides, are narcotics. Others disrupt the movement of nerve impulses, such as the organophosphate, carbamate, and pyrethroid pesticides. Some pesticides affect photosynthesis, the process of using sunlight energy to create carbohydrates from carbon dioxide and water. Pesticides that disrupt photosynthesis prevent the plant from producing or storing energy and ultimately kill the plant, for example triazine, substituted urea and uracil herbicides. Finally, some pesticides work in more than one way and fall into more than one of these categories. The modes of action of many pesticides are not fully understood. Some pesticides are residual in action and continue to be effective for days, weeks, or months after their application. Examples are the triazine herbicides that persist in the soil and kill emerging weeds over the lifetime of a crop, or insecticides that remain active for several years as a barrier to termites entering buildings.

Modern pesticides are designed not to persist for long in the environment, which was a problem associated with organochlorines like dichloro-diphenyltrichloroethane (DDT). Modern pesticides act quickly and are then degraded to innoxious substances by chemical or microbial processes. This helps prevent their build-up in crops or other organisms. Pesticide breakdown depends on the compound's chemical properties, how much is applied, and how it is distributed, as well as environmental factors such as temperature, moisture, soil pH, and the availability of microorganisms.

1.2.2 Metals

Many metals, including heavy metals which have particular concerns for health problems, end up in our food supply and can be traced back to industry via effluent, sewage, dumps, and dust into the environment, and eventually into the food chain. Not all the traces of heavy metals in plants and animals are subsequent to human activity. Metals arise through absorption processes of naturally-occurring soil components. Arsenic, cadmium, lead, mercury, and nickel are the most prevalent heavy metals with health concerns. The definition of a heavy metal is one that has a specific gravity of more than $5\,g/cm^3$. By definition this would account for 60 metals, several of which are biologically essential, and many others lack sufficient information regarding toxicity, including platinum, silver, and gold.

Arsenic

Arsenic is found in the environment and originates from both natural and industrial sources. Sources of arsenic exposure include air pollution, antibiotics given to commercial livestock, certain marine plants, chemical processing, coal-fired power plants, defoliants, drinking water, drying agents for cotton, fish, herbicides, insecticides, meats (from commercially raised poultry and cattle), metal ore smelting, pesticides, seafood (fish, mussels, oysters), specialty glass, and wood preservatives.

Chronic arsenic poisoning occurs throughout the world because of high arsenic content in drinking water (greater than $1000\,\mu g/L$), in such places as Taiwan, Hungary, Chile, Inner Mongolia, Mexico and Bangladesh. In some Western United States, such as New Mexico, Arizona, Nevada, Utah, and Southern California, arsenic levels are in the $50–100\,\mu g/L$ range and the health effects may be less pronounced. Epidemiological evidence implicates arsenic as an inducer of skin and bladder cancer and affecting heart disease, neurological, vascular, and cognitive function.

Cadmium

Cadmium is ubiquitous and is actively extracted from ores for commercial purposes. Contributions to residues include industrial processes such as metal refining, coal and oil industry, and electroplating plants. Other sources of cadmium exposure include air pollution, art supplies, bone meal, cigarette smoke, food (coffee, fruits, grains, and vegetables grown in cadmium-laden soil, meats [kidneys, liver, poultry], or refined foods), freshwater fish, fungicides, highway dusts, incinerators, mining, nickel-cadmium batteries, oxide dusts, paints, phosphate fertilizers, power plants, seafood (crab, flounder, mussels, oysters, scallops), sewage sludge, softened water, smelting plants, tobacco and tobacco smoke, and welding fumes.

Cadmium is concentrated in the kidneys, liver, lungs, and in blood-forming organs. Ingestion of cadmium can lead to kidney damage and metabolic anomalies usually through enzyme inhibition. Itai-itai (ouch-ouch) disease in Japan is an example of an illness caused by a food, namely rice, highly contaminated with cadmium. Cadmium is a cumulative poison but unlike lead, the definition of an exact toxicity limit has been difficult to determine because of bioavailabiliity questions.

Lead

The main sources of lead pollution in the environment are industrial production processes and their emissions, road traffic with leaded petroleum, the smoke and dust emission of coal and gas. Other sources of lead exposure include air pollution, ammunition (shot and bullets), bathtubs (cast iron, porcelain, steel), batteries, canned foods, ceramics, chemical fertilizers, cosmetics, dolomite, dust, foods grown around industrial areas, gasoline, hair dyes and rinses, leaded glass, newsprint and colored advertisements, paints, pesticides, pewter, pottery, rubber toys, soft coal, soil, solder, tap water, tobacco smoke, and vinyl mini-blinds.

Both the acute and chronic forms of lead poisoning occur. Acute toxicity occurs by the consumption of large single doses of soluble lead salts. Chronic toxicity can occur through the regular consumption of foodstuffs which may be only slightly contaminated with lead and represent the greater problem of cumulative poisoning. The mode of action of lead is related to the metal's high affinity for proteins, such as hemoglobin, plasma proteins, and the subsequent inhibition of protein-mediated processes. Lead ingestion leads to inhibition of the synthesis of red blood cells, which in turn compromises oxygen transport. When the binding capacity of blood proteins are exceeded, lead affects other organs, such as bone-marrow, liver, nervous system, reproductive tissues, and kidney. Organic lead compounds are particularly troublesome and likely lead to injuries to mental development with reduction in intelligence, growth, and cognitive function.

Although lead has been largely eliminated from gasoline and the lead content of populations has fallen sharply, lead in water continues to be a problem in many countries, such as some parts of the United Kingdom. Thus, foodstuffs contribute to the lead burden, particularly, lead found in vegetables, fruits, drinking water, beverages (wine), and cereal products. Fruits and vegetables mostly acquire their lead contamination through impurities in the air, which can be greatly reduced by washing.

Mercury

Mercury (from cinnabar, quicksilver, in pure form) has been extracted since ancient times and is used in electrical devices, catalysts, thermometers, and pigments. Other sources of mercury exposure include air pollution, batteries, cosmetics, dental amalgams, diuretics (mercurial), electrical devices and relays, explosives, foods (grains), fungicides, fluorescent lights, freshwater fish (especially large bass, pike, and trout), insecticides, mining, paints, pesticides, petroleum products, saltwater fish (especially large halibut, shrimp, snapper, and swordfish), shellfish, and tap water.

Mercury passes into the environment through emissions from chemical plants, power stations, often as effluents and sludge. Mercury becomes concentrated in shellfish, crustaceans, and fish, and passes on in the food chain in its highly toxic form, methylated mercury. The Minamata sickness in Japan in 1965 was the result of consumption of fish taken from regions of the sea contaminated by industrial effluent.

Methyl mercury compounds are the most toxic of heavy metals. Ingestion of organic mercury results in distribution to the liver, kidneys, and brain. Salts of mercury cause tiredness, loss of appetite, weight loss, muscular weakness, perhaps paralysis, and eventually kidney failure. Methyl mercury damages the central nervous system and the immune system, and has been shown to produce teratogenic effects.

Nickel

Sources of nickel exposure include appliances, buttons, ceramics, cocoa, cold-wave hair permanent, cooking utensils, cosmetics, coins, dental materials, food (chocolate, hydrogenated oils, nuts, food grown near industrial areas), hair spray, industrial waste, jewelry, medical implants, metal refineries, metal tools, nickel-cadmium batteries, orthodontic appliances, shampoo, solid-waste incinerators, stainless steel kitchen utensils, tap water, tobacco and tobacco smoke, water faucets and pipes, and zippers.

High nickel concentrations in tissues has been associated with depression of prolactin secretion, and inhibition of insulin secretion. Nickel has carcinogenic effects when inhaled, producing lung and nasal cancers.

1.2.3 Industrial byproducts and waste

As noted above, many of the metals may find their way into our food as industrial byproducts or waste. Since the Industrial Revolution, industrial and mining operations have been accompanied by industrial waste, which may be toxic, ignitable, corrosive, or reactive. Obviously, proper management is the key and improperly managed waste can pose dangerous health and environmental risks. It is estimated that, in the United States, the amount of hazardous waste generated by manufacturing industries has increased from 4.5 million tons annually after World War II to some 265 million tons by 1990 (Council on Environmental Quality, 1981) Waste is generated at every stage in the production process, use, and disposal of manufactured products. The introduction of many new technologies for the home and office (computers, drugs, textiles, paints and dyes, plastics) in recent times has introduced more hazardous waste, including toxic chemicals, into the environment. The EPA estimated in 1980 that more than 70,000 different chemicals were being manufactured in the United States, with some 1,000 new chemicals being added each year (Petulla, 1988). The human health and environmental impacts of many of these chemicals are largely unknown. Industrial waste may be solid, liquid, or gaseous and is divided into hazardous and non-hazardous waste. Hazardous waste may result from manufacturing or other industrial processes. Certain commercial products such as cleaning fluids, paints, or pesticides discarded by commercial establishments or individuals can also be defined as hazardous waste. The definition of hazardous waste has been further refined through regulations. Non-hazardous industrial waste is that which does not meet the EPA's definition of hazardous waste and is not municipal waste.

1.3 Types of toxicant: naturally-occurring toxicants

Natural or raw foods contain an array of chemicals and only a few of these chemicals actually possess nutritional importance. Most of the chemicals found in food neither enhance nor detract from the wholesomeness and nutrient quality of the food. They move through the gastrointestinal tract unchanged and exert little to no effect on surrounding tissues or other nutrients they pass. However, there is a group of chemicals found in foods that can affect health by impairing nutrient absorption, inhibiting or destroying nutrients (antinutrients), or acting as mutagens, teratogens or carcinogens. Such chemicals occur in food in small quantities and if the diet is nutritionally adequate and widely varied, these minute amounts of otherwise toxic compounds can be tolerated or rendered harmless.

1.3.1 Plant and animal toxicants

Many plant and animal foods contain natural or processing-induced constituents with biological activity in mammals. Among the plant family these are glycoalkaloids, amines, glucosinolates, cyanogenic glycosides, protease inhibitors, oxalates, coumarins, polyphenols, cyclopropenoid fatty acids, phytates, xanthines, and essential oils. Recently, various lines of evidence have suggested that plant-derived constituents may play an important role in determining spontaneous rates of genetic damage and tumor incidence. On the other hand, genotoxic constituents such as certain flavones, anthraquinones, browning products, benzoxazinones, and acetals have been identified in plant-derived foods, and unsaturated oilseed lipids have been found to increase cancers of certain sites, particularly intestine and breast, in laboratory animals. Whether these constituents play a significant quantitative role in human health is a key scientific issue which is at present not adequately resolved.

With the increase in fish consumption for health or other individual preferences, concerns for higher exposures to animal toxins are increased. As will become apparent, whether to classify these as true animal toxins is debatable since they seem to be more microbial in their origin. Ciguatera is a form of poisoning caused by the consumption of finfish (barracudas, snappers, jacks, mackerel, and triggerfish) which have accumulated naturally-occurring toxins that originate from several dinoflagellate (algae) species that are common to ciguatera. Manifestations of ciguatera usually involves a combination of gastrointestinal, neurological, and cardiovascular disorders. Shellfish poisoning is caused by a group of toxins elaborated by planktonic algae, dinoflagellates, upon which the shellfish feed. The toxins are accumulated and metabolized by the shellfish. The 20 toxins responsible for paralytic shellfish poisonings (PSP) are all derivatives of saxitoxin. The effects are predominantly neurological and include tingling, burning, numbness, drowsiness, incoherent speech, and respiratory paralysis. Scombroid poisoning is caused by the ingestion of fish that contain high levels of histamine and other vasoactive amines and compounds. Histamine and other amines are formed by the growth of certain bacteria in the fish or any food that contains the appropriate amino acids. Fish poisoning can also occur by consumption of members of the pufferfish family. Tetrodotoxin has also been isolated from widely differing animal species, including the California newt, parrotfish, frogs of the genus Atelopus, the blue-ringed octopus, starfish, angelfish, and xanthid crabs. Recent reports of the production of tetrodotoxin/anhydrotetrodotoxin by several bacterial species, including strains of the family Vibrionaceae, *Pseudomonas* sp., and *Photobacterium phosphoreum*, point toward a bacterial origin of this family of toxins.

1.3.2 Microbial/fungal toxicants

Microbiological and perhaps fungal contamination of food should cause more concern than any other food safety hazard. Bacteria are by far the most common and are responsible for many diverse foodborne diseases. According to the national FoodNet database, 76 million persons were estimated to have contracted foodborne diseases in the United State in 2001. Because only a small minority of the cases seek medical attention, the number is likely higher. Many people who experience foodborne disease are unaware since the characteristics are similar to those of the 'flu'.

In 2001, the Centers for Disease Control and Prevention (CDC) released a report showing a decline in the major bacterial foodbone illnesses. According to the data, the four major bacterial foodborne illnesses *Campylobacter, Salmonella, Listeria*, and *E. coli O157*, posted a 21% decline in the past six years. *Campylobacter* infections dropped 27%, infections from *Listeria* fell 35%, and *Salmonella* infections decreased by 15%. *E. coli O157* infections dropped 21%, but all of that decline occurred since 2000. These declines signify important progress toward meeting the Healthy People 2010 objectives for reducing the incidence of disease caused by these bacterial infections. Other less common bacterial foodborne illnesses also showed significant declines since

1996. *Yersinia* infections decreased 49% and *Shigella* infections dropped by 35%. CDC notes the data do not show a sustained decline in some infections indicating that increased efforts are needed to further reduce the incidence of foodborne illness.

CDC notes several factors have contributed to the decline in foodborne illnesses. These include enhanced surveillance, the implementation of Pathogen Reduction/Hazard Analysis Critical Control Point (HACCP) regulations in meat and poultry plants, HACCP regulation of fruit and vegetable juices, seafood HACCP, publication and outreach of good agricultural practices for fresh produce, increased regulation of imported food, and last, but certainly not least, extensive food safety education. Food safety education and research have played important roles with consumer educational efforts in this area.

In 1996, the FoodNet surveillance system began collecting information about laboratory-diagnosed cases of foodborne illnesses caused by *Campylobacter, Cryptosporidium, Cyclospora, E. coli O157, Listeria, Salmonella, Shigella, Yersinia,* and *Vibrio*. Each year the surveillance area, has expanded. The total population of the current surveillance area is 38 million persons or 13% of the United States population. Several sites in New York State are part of that surveillance area. USDA issued a release showing that the prevalence of *Salmonella* in raw meat has decreased. USDA compared prevalence levels before and after the implementation of the HACCP system of inspection, which began in 1998. As USDA notes, the decrease in *Salmonella* in raw meat and poultry from 1998 to 2001 correlates with the reports from the CDC indicating a decline in human illness linked to *Salmonella* during the same period.

Problems from molds and mycotoxins have considerable worldwide significance in terms of public health, agriculture, and economics. Examples of molds affecting health include:

- **Aflatoxins**, metabolic products of the molds *Aspergillus flavus* and *A. parasiticus*, may occur in food as a result of mold growth in a number of susceptible commodities including peanuts and corn. Other domestic nuts and grains are susceptible but less prone to contamination with aflatoxins. Because aflatoxins are known carcinogens to laboratory animals and presumably man, the presence of aflatoxins in foods should be restricted to the minimum levels practically attainable using modern processing techniques.
- **Fumonisins** (Fumonisin B_1 and Fumonisin B_2) are natural toxins produced by *Fusarium moniliforme* and other *Fusarium* species; these molds are common natural contaminants of corn. Fumonisins have been linked to fatalities in horses and swine. Recent studies have demonstrated the presence of fumonisins in human foods, including corn meal and breakfast cereals. Epidemiological investigations demonstrating a possible association of *F. moniliforme* with esophageal cancer and recent animal studies indicating the carcinogenicity of fumonisin B_1 have highlighted the need to ensure that foods do not contain excessive amounts of fumonisins.

- **Deoxynivalenol (DON)**, commonly called vomitoxin, is a natural toxin produced by several molds of the genus *Fusarium,* especially *F. graminearum*, which is a common contaminant of several grains, including wheat, corn, barley, and rye. DON has been associated with a number of adverse health effects in humans and animals. Several adverse weather related DON contamination episodes in the United States motivated the FDA to issue advisory levels for food (wheat) and feed in 1982 and updated levels in 1993. FDA is continuing to study the scope and toxicological significance of the DON problem in order to make a determination as to whether further regulatory measures are needed to control DON in food and feed products.
- **Ochratoxin A** is a naturally-occurring nephrotoxic fungal metabolite produced by certain species of the genera *Aspergillus* and *Penicillium*. It is mainly a contaminant of cereals (corn, barley, wheat, and oats) and has been found in edible animal tissues as well as in human blood sera and milk. Studies indicate that this toxin is carcinogenic in mice and rats. It is not completely destroyed during the processing and cooking of food, therefore the implication for risk to human health and safety must be considered.
- **Patulin** is a mycotoxin produced by several species of mold fungi including *Penicillium expansum*, the causal organism of apple rot. Apple juice prepared from apples contaminated with *Penicillium expansum* could be a possible source of patulin in the human diet. The World Health Organization (WHO) has recommended a maximum patulin level of 50 ppb based on a toxicological assessment. At least 12 countries regulate patulin at 30–50 ppb. The United Kingdom's Food Advisory Committee announced recently its intention to establish control measures on patulin. FDA identified patulin as a potential hazard in fruit juice in its juice HACCP proposal. In the Codex Alimentarius, FDA participated in negotiations as to what limitation on patulin in apple juice is appropriate for apple juice and concentrate in international commerce.

1.4 Types of toxicant: food processing toxicants

During the processing of foods, products may be produced that, if present in large amounts, could potentially adversely affect health. For example, cooking certain meats at high temperatures creates chemicals that are not present in uncooked meats. A few of these chemicals may increase cancer risk, such as polycyclic aromatic hydrocarbons and heterocyclic amines. Another example is when nitrates and nitrites react with secondary amines to form nitrosamine. Nitrosamines are mutagens which have been linked to cancers. Nitrates and nitrites are used to preserve meats and contribute to prevention of growth of *Clostridium botulinum*, the bacterium responsible for producing the highly potent botulinum toxin.

1.4.1 Polycyclic aromatic hydrocarbons

Polycyclic aromatic hydrocarbons (PAH) are produced when any incomplete combustion occurs. Thus, they are found in polluted air, cooking oil fumes, tobacco smoke, smoked foods and foods cooked at high temperature.

Most PAHs are not carcinogenic, although a few are, for example benzo(a)pyrene. They appear mainly in meats cooked during high temperature grilling. Microwaving does not produce PAHs, and foods other than meats contain negligible amounts of PAHs. Foods low in fat, or cooked beneath the source of heat, contain many fewer PAHs, so the type of food cooked and the method of cooking are important determinants of PAHs.

Breathing air containing PAHs can occur in the workplace of coking, coal-tar, and asphalt production plants, smokehouses, and municipal trash incineration facilities. Breathing air containing PAHs can also occur from cigarette smoke, wood smoke, vehicle exhausts, asphalt roads, or agricultural burn smoke. Coming in contact with air, water, or soil near hazardous waste sites can also increase exposure to PAHs. Eating grilled or charred meats, contaminated cereals, flour, bread, vegetables, fruits, meats, and processed or pickled foods increases an individual's exposure to PAHs. Drinking PAH-contaminated water or cow's milk can increase an individual's exposure to PAHs. Nursing infants of mothers living near hazardous waste sites may be exposed to PAHs through their mother's milk.

1.4.2 N-nitrosamines

Nitrosamines are a class of chemical compounds that were first described over 100 years ago. In 1956 it was reported that dimethylnitrosamine produced liver tumors in rats. Approximately 300 of these compounds have been tested and 90% of them have been found to be carcinogenic in a wide variety of experimental animals. Dimethylnitrosamine (DMNA) (also called N-nitrosodimethylamine or NDMA) is a member of a group of chemicals known as nitrosamines which are recognized as cancer-causing substances. DMNA is a volatile liquid, which dissolves easily in water and in oil. It can be broken down by light or microorganisms but, in their absence, DMNA can persist in water for a very long time. Even in a sewage treatment plant, DMNA degrades only very slowly. Nitrosamines (including DMNA) are also formed in tobacco smoke. An interesting observation is that the concentration of nitrosamines in side-stream smoke from a cigarette has 20–200 times more nitrosamines than the mainstream smoke. Exposure to very smoky rooms can result in as much DMNA exposure as smoking. Most nitrosamines are mutagens and a number are transplacental carcinogens. Most are organ-specific. For instance, DMNA causes liver cancer in experimental animals, whereas some of the tobacco-specific nitrosamines cause lung cancer. Since nitrosamines are metabolized the same in human and animal tissues, it seems highly likely that humans are susceptible to the carcinogenic properties of nitrosamines.

Foods which contain nitrogen sources and amines have particularly high levels of DMNA and other nitrosamines. Amines occur commonly and sodium nitrite is added to cured meats to prevent toxin production by *Clostridium botulinum*. Such foods are bacon, prepared meats, fish, tomatoes, spinach, beer, and many others. In the body, nitrosamines are formed as a result of these nitrates and nitrites (present in meat and other food and vegetables as preservatives) reacting with saliva in the mouth or with gastric juices in the stomach. DMNA can also be formed naturally as a result of certain biological processes associated with bacteria.

Cured meats can contain nitrosamines because meats contain amines and sodium nitrite, a source of nitrosating agents added to cured meats as a preservative. Of all the cured meats, bacon has received the most attention. It almost always contains detectable levels of nitrosamines, principally nitrosopyrrolidine and, to a lesser extent, DMNA. The very high cooking temperatures used to fry bacon are conducive to nitrosamine formation. In the late 1970s, extensive attention was focused on the issue of nitrosamines in cured meats and the removal of sodium nitrite as a food additive was considered. However, the prospect of sodium nitrite removal presented a formidable dilemma for the regulatory agencies. Removal of sodium nitrite would prevent nitrosamine formation, but it might also increase the risk of botulism poisoning. Sodium nitrite and sodium chloride together are particularly effective against *Clostridium botulinum*. The solution to the dilemma was to limit the addition of sodium nitrite to 120 ppm, the lowest level found to be effective in controlling growth and toxin production by *Clostridium botulinum*.

Ascorbic acid also inhibits nitrosamine formation. The addition of 550 ppm of ascorbic acid is now required in the manufacture of cured meat in the United States. Actually, most cured meat manufacturers add erythorbic acid (a less expensive isomer of ascorbic acid) rather than ascorbic acid. Another antioxidant, alpha-tocopherol (vitamin E), is added to some cured meats to inhibit nitrosamine formation. As a result of these strategies, there are now significantly lower levels of nitrosamines in fried bacon and other cured meats than there were some years ago. Ascorbic acid, erythorbic acid, and alpha-tocopherol inhibit nitrosamine formation due to their oxidation and N reduction properties.

Dimethylnitrosamine has been found in beer, formed by direct-fire drying of barley malt, an ingredient used in making beer. By converting the process from direct-fire drying to indirect-fire drying, the nitrosating agents and the formation of DMNA were markedly reduced. Thus beer now contains only 2% of the DMNA that was present 20 years ago.

Nitrosamines can form in the gastric juice of the human stomach, referred to as endogenous nitrosation. Bacteria in the mouth chemically reduce nitrate, which is prevalent in many vegetables, to nitrite, which in turn can form nitrosating agents. Many foods contain amines that can react with nitrosating agents in the acidic stomach to form nitrosamines.

Nitrosamines are carcinogenic in animals. Current exposure is probably closer to 0.1 μg per day due to successful efforts over the past 20 years to reduce nitrosamine formation in foods and beverages. In contrast, there is an estimated exposure of 17 μg per day from cigarette smoking. An enormous amount of indirect evidence indicates that nitrosamines are human carcinogens. For instance, tobacco-specific nitrosamines are one of the major groups of chemical carcinogens in tobacco products and no doubt remains about the causal link between tobacco use and cancer. But, it is difficult to evaluate the risk of cancer from daily exposure of 1 μg from foods and beverages. The same difficulty applies to the risk assessment of the exposure to minute amounts of aflatoxin, PAHs, and heterocyclic amines in a variety of foods and beverages.

1.4.3 Heterocyclic amines

Heterocyclic amines (HCAs) are the carcinogenic chemicals formed from the cooking of muscle meats such as beef, pork, fowl, and fish (Bjeldanes *et al.*, 1982, 1983; Felton *et al.*, 1994: Sugimura, 2002). HCAs form when amino acids (the building blocks of proteins) and creatine (a chemical found in muscles) react at high cooking temperatures. Some 17 different HCAs have been found, resulting from the cooking of muscle meats, that may pose human cancer risk. Research conducted by the National Cancer Institute (NCI) as well as by Japanese and European scientists indicates that HCAs are created within muscle meats during most types of high temperature cooking. Further evaluation is needed of the relationship between methods of cooking meat and the development of specific types of cancer. One study conducted by researchers from NCI's Division of Cancer Epidemiology and Genetics found a link between individuals with stomach cancer and the consumption of cooked meats. Those who ate their beef medium-well or well-done had more than three times the risk of stomach cancer than those who ate their beef rare or medium-rare. They also found that people who ate beef four or more times a week had more than twice the risk of stomach cancer than those consuming beef less frequently. Additional studies have shown that an increased risk of developing colorectal, pancreatic, and breast cancer is associated with high intakes of well-done, fried, or barbequed meats.

1.5 Current issues: pathogens, genetic variability and antibiotic resistance

Food toxicology is playing a crucial role in the world today in terms of foodborne illnesses/food safety, agricultural fitness, economic survival, and trade. There are many issues in food toxicology but only a few will be discussed in this section. With a growing population and need for more resources, including food security, concerns about the potential threat of foodborne illness persist. In recent times, the added concern of using our food supply as a target of chemical or bioterroism further emphasizes that we need to be diligent of what those versed in food toxicology can do to protect populations from food-related illnesses.

1.5.1 Emerging and re-emerging pathogens

Following World War II, development and availability of pharmaceuticals, particularly antibiotics and vaccines, along with public health measures that resulted in improved sanitation, and eradication of diseases like smallpox, provided the expectation that communicable diseases would no longer pose a major threat to our population's health. However, from the 1980s through the present, the appearance of new agents, such as human immunodeficiency virus (HIV) and severe acute respiratory syndrome (SARS), which have rapidly swept all over the world, has increased our awareness that these agents pose a growing global threat. Also, the threat is not restricted to new agents because there is a re-emergence of old agents which likely are related to development of common pathogens resistant to the old drugs. The reappearance and spread of cholera in South America, Ebola hemorrhagic fever in Uganda and Zaire, and plague in India are just a few examples..

The epidemiology of foodborne diseases is rapidly changing as new pathogens are recognized and old pathogens re-emerge or become associated with new food vehicles (Altekruse *et al.*, 1997; IFT Expert Report, 2000). Emergence of foodborne diseases, particularly those that are due to the growth of microbes is driven by the same factors as emergence of other infectious diseases. The factors are multifaceted (Altekruse *et al.*, 1997) and include changes in demographics, human behavior, industry and technology changes, shift toward global distribution, agent adaptation, and sometimes a breakdown in public health infrastructure. New foodborne disease threats occur for a number of reasons. These include increases in international travel and trade, microbial adaptation and changes in the food production system, as well as human demographics and behavior.

Some foodborne diseases are well recognized but are considered emerging because they have recently been reported more frequently. Outbreaks of salmonellosis have been reported for decades but within the past 25 years, the disease has increased in incidence around the world. Salmonella serotype Enteritidis (SE) has become the predominant strain. Investigations of SE outbreaks indicate that its emergence is largely related to consumption of poultry or eggs.

In 1991 on the South American continent cholera appeared, making it another example of an infectious disease that is both well-recognized and re-emerging. While cholera is often waterborne, many foods also transmit infection. In Latin America, ice and raw or underprocessed seafood are important epidemiological pathways for cholera transmission.

Other foodborne pathogens are considered emerging because they are new microorganisms or because the role of food in their transmission has been recognized only recently. Infection with *Escherichia coli* serotype O157:H7 (*E. coli*) was first described in 1982. Subsequently, it has emerged rapidly as a major cause of bloody diarrhea and acute renal failure. The infection is sometimes fatal, particularly in children. Outbreaks of infection, generally associated with ground beef, have been reported in Australia, Canada, Japan, the

United States, various European countries, and in southern Africa. Outbreaks have also implicated alfalfa sprouts, unpasteurized fruit juice, lettuce, game meat, and cheese curd. Two outbreaks of undercooked hamburgers from a fast-food restaurant chain, in 1982, resulted in the first recognition of *E. coli* O157:H7 as a human pathogen. Subsequently, the pathogen has been linked to as many as 20,000 cases of bloody and nonbloody diarrhea and likely 250 deaths per year in the United States. Outbreaks have occurred in Japan, Africa, the United Kingdom, and Canada. The effects can be devastating in children, causing hemolytic uremic syndrome and responsible as the leading cause of acute kidney failure in children in the United States. In 1996, an outbreak of *Escherichia coli* O157:H7 in Japan affected over 6,300 schoolchildren and resulted in two deaths. This is the largest outbreak ever recorded for this pathogen.

Listeria monocytogenes (Lm) is considered emerging because the role of food in its transmission has only recently been recognized. In pregnant women, infections with Lm can cause abortion and stillbirth, and in infants and persons with a weakened immune system, it may lead to septicemia (blood poisoning) and meningitis. The disease is most often associated with consumption of foods such as soft cheese and processed meat products that are kept refrigerated for a long time because Lm can grow at low temperatures. Outbreaks of listeriosis have been reported from many countries, including Australia, Switzerland, France, and the United States. Two recent outbreaks of *Listeria monocytogenes* in France in 2000 and in the United States in 1999 were caused by contaminated pork tongue and hot dogs, respectively. Listeriosis has been recognized as a foodborne transmitted disease since the 1980s. Listeriosis has been associated with coleslaw, milk, soft cheese made from nonpasteurized milk, and pâté. Fatality rates as high as 40% have been reported during outbreaks.

Foodborne trematodes are also emerging as a serious public health problem, especially in south-east Asia and Latin America, in part due to a combination of increased aquaculture production, often under unsanitary conditions, and consumption of raw and lightly processed freshwater fish and fishery products. Foodborne trematodes can cause acute liver disease, and may lead to liver cancer. An estimated 40 million people worldwide are affected.

Bovine Spongiform Encephalopathy (BSE), a fatal, transmissible, neurodegenerative disease of cattle, was first discovered in the United Kingdom in 1985. The cause of the disease was traced to an agent related to scrapie in sheep, which contaminated recycled bovine carcasses used to make meat and bone meal additives for cattle feed. Recycling of the BSE agent led to a distributed common source epidemic of more than 180,000 diseased animals in the United Kingdom alone. The agent affects the brain and spinal cord of cattle and lesions are characterized by sponge-like changes visible under a microscope. The agent has been identified as prions, which are unique proteinaceous material capable of replication. At this time, 19 countries have reported endemic BSE cases and the disease is no longer confined to the European Union: a case of BSE has been reported in a cattle herd in Japan.

In human populations, exposure to the BSE agent (probably in contaminated bovine-based food products) has been strongly linked to the appearance in 1996 of a new transmissible spongiform encephalopathy of humans called variant Creutzfeldt-Jakob Disease (vCJD). As of January 2002, 119 people have developed vCJD, most are from the UK but five cases have been reported from France.

Noroviruses (genus *Norovirus*, family Caliciviridae) are a group of related, single-stranded RNA, nonenveloped viruses that cause acute gastroenteritis in humans. Norwalk virus is the prototype of a family of unclassified small round structured viruses (SRSVs) which may be related to the caliciviruses. They contain a positive strand RNA genome of 7.5 kb and a single structural protein of about 60 kDa. The 27–32 nm viral particles have a buoyant density of 1.39–1.40 g/ml in CsCl. The family consists of several serologically distinct groups of viruses that have been named after the places where the outbreaks occurred. In the United States, the Norwalk and Montgomery County agents are serologically related but distinct from the Hawaii and Snow Mountain agents. The Taunton, Moorcroft, Barnett, and Amulree agents were identified in the United Kingdom, and the Sapporo and Otofuke agents in Japan. Their serological relationships remain to be determined.

Norovirus was recently approved as the official genus name for the group of viruses provisionally described as 'Norwalk-like viruses' (NLV). Another genus of the calicivirus family that can cause gastroenteritis in humans is Sappovirus formerly described as 'Sapporo-like virus' (SLV) and sometimes referred to as classic or typical calicivirus. Currently, there are at least four norovirus genogroups (GI, GII, GIII, and GIV), which in turn are divided into at least 20 genetic clusters. CDC estimates that 23 million cases of acute gastroenteritis are due to norovirus infection, and it is now thought that at least 50% of all foodborne outbreaks of gastroenteritis can be attributed to noroviruses.

1.5.2 Challenges of special populations – human genetic variability

Foodborne illnesses tend disproportionately to affect the very young, the elderly, and those who are immune compromised. However, individual's susceptibility to foodborne illnesses may vary, and for a healthy individual, genetic polymorphism may play a distinct role. The threats to the food and water supply are numerous and varied, whether it be *Escherichia coli* (*E. coli* O157:H7) in meat and juices, *Salmonella* in eggs or vegetables, *Cyclospora* on fruit, *Cryptosporidium* in drinking water, or hepatitis A virus in frozen berries, and whether an individual becomes sick, might well be mutifactorial.

The ability of humans to biotransform toxicants appears to be related to genetic background, which in turn is related to the presence, amount, and activation of an array of enzyme systems that metabolize ingested toxicants into chemical derivatives that are less or sometimes more toxic than the original toxicant (Daly *et al.*, 1994; Hodgson and Goldstein, 2001). The level of expression for CyP1A3, a cytochrome P-450 (CYP)-dependent monooxygenase is an example of an enzyme where the level of expression varies considerably. CyP1A3 is responsible for the metabolism of aflatoxin B_1 and acts coordinately with microsomal epoxide hydrolase, another enzyme that can vary up to 40-fold in human tissue. It has been suggested that epoxide hydrolase polymorphisms may alter the risk of aflatoxin-associated liver cancer (Eaton *et al.*, 1995; Seidegard and Ekstrom, 1997; McGlynn *et al.*, 1995).

Because of natural selection, different alleles on our genes are more likely to confer a survival advantage in different environments. Cycles of infectious disease prevalence and virulence often reflect natural selection. If natural selection eliminates individuals with detrimental phenotypes from a population, then it seems ironic that harmful mutant alleles persist in a gene pool. A disease can remain prevalent when heterozygotes have some other advantage over individuals who have two copies of the wild type allele. When carriers have advantages that allow a detrimental allele to persist in a population, *balanced polymorphism* is at work. This form of polymorphism often entails heterozygosity for an inherited illness that protects against an infectious illness. Sickle cell disease is one example of an autosomal recessive disorder that causes anemia, joint pain, swollen spleen, and frequent, severe infections. It illustrates balanced polymorphism because carriers are resistant to malaria, an infection by the parasite *Plasmodium falciparum* that causes cycles of chills and fever. The parasite spends the first stage of its life cycle in the salivary glands of the mosquito *Anopheles gambiae.* When an infected mosquito bites a human, the malaria parasite enters the red blood cells, which transport it to the liver. The red blood cells burst, releasing the parasite throughout the body. The frequency of sickle cell carriers in tropical Africa was found to be higher in regions where malaria raged for many years. It was found through blood tests from children hospitalized with malaria, that nearly all were homozygous for the wild type of sickle cell allele. The few sickle cell carriers among them had the mildest cases of malaria. Thus, it is likely that the presence of malaria somehow selected for the sickle cell allele by toppling people who did not inherit it. The fact that sickle cell disease is far less common in the United States, where malaria is rare, supports the idea that sickle cell heterozygosity provides a protective effect.

Balanced polymorphism may explain why cystic fibrosis (CF) is so common and the anatomical defect that underlies CF protects against diarrhea illnesses, such as cholera. Cholera epidemics have left their mark on human populations, causing widespread death in just days. In the summer of 1831, an epidemic killed 10 percent of the population of St Louis, and in 1991, an epidemic swept Peru. Cholera bacteria causes diarrhea, which rapidly dehydrates the body and may lead to shock and kidney and heart failure. The bacterium produces a toxin that opens chloride channels in the small intestine. Water rushing out of intestinal cells leaves the body as diarrhea.

In 1989, when geneticists identified the CF gene and described its protein product as a regulator of a chloride channel in certain secretory cells, a possible explanation for the prevalence of the inherited disorder emerged. Cholera opens chloride channels letting chloride and water leave cells. The CF protein does just the opposite, closing chloride channels and trapping salt and water in cells, which dries out mucus and other secretions. A person with CF cannot contract cholera, because the toxin cannot open the chloride channels in the small intestine.

Carriers of CF enjoy the mixed blessing of a balanced polymorphism. They do not have enough abnormal chloride channels to cause the labored breathing and clogged pancreas of cystic fibrosis, but they do have enough of a defect to prevent cholera from taking hold. During the devastating cholera epidemics that have spotted history, individuals carrying mutant CF alleles had a selective advantage and they disproportionately transmitted those alleles to future generations. However, because CF arose in Western Europe and cholera in Africa, perhaps an initial increase in CF herterozygosity was a response to a different diarrhea infection.

Gut defensins, a family of structurally related antimicrobial molecules, are likely another example of gene-based defense systems that may account for greater or lesser susceptibility to foodborne illnesses. These small protein molecules are often induced by infections and contribute to antimicrobial defense in living mammals. Experiments have shown that genetic transplant of human defensin 5 (HD-5) into mice greatly improved their ability to resist intestinal infection with *Salmonella typhimurium*. When *S. typhimurium* infect normal mice, the bacteria spread from the intestine to other organs and was fatal (Salzman *et al.*, 2003; Ganz, 2003).

Genetic factors that determine gastrointestinal as well systemic disease expression and markers of genetic susceptibility to complications of foodborne disease affect the manifestations of the risk factors for the acquisition, transmission, and expression of foodborne disease particularly in children and the elderly. Eventually, human markers of genetic susceptibility to complications of foodborne disease and the identification and testing of interventions might lead to improved management of gastrointestinal disease as well as extra-gastrointestinal complications. Of prime importance is the development of new diagnostic and therapeutic techniques that would lead to early medical intervention and prevention of complications of foodborne illnesses.

1.5.3 Impact of antibiotic resistance organisms on foods

The increased prevalence of antibiotic resistance is an outcome of microbial evolution. Populations of organisms, such as bacteria, naturally includes subpopulations of variants with anomalous traits. The ability to withstand an antibiotic's attack on a microbe can be one of those anomalous traits. Taking an antibiotic will kill defenseless bacteria, 'selecting' those bacteria that can resist it. These maverick microbes multiply, becoming the predominant micro-organism. The antibiotic does not produce the resistance, however it provides an environment that favors where an already existing subpopulation can flourish. Also, it is known that resistant genes to antibiotics of one bacteria can be transferred to genes of other bacteria.

In clinical situations, a patient can develop a drug-resistant infection either by contracting a resistant bug at the start, or by having a resistant subpopulation of microbes develop in the body following antibiotic treatment. Thus, drug-resistant infections increase risk of death, cause complications, and are often associated with prolonged hospitalizations. Sometimes this involves the extreme where it might necessitate removing part of a damaged tissue, such as a lung or damaged heart valve.

For over a decade, the scientific and medical communities have cautioned consumers about the overuse of antibiotics, particularly for pediatric care and animal production. Antibiotics used as growth promotion agents in the livestock and poultry industries likely contribute significantly to the problem of antibiotic resistance (Hamer and Gill, 2002). It is estimated that more than 11 million kg of antimicrobial agents is sold for nontherapeutic purposes in animals compared to 900,000 kg used for treatment of infections, annually (Hamer and Gill, 2002). Both in Europe and the United States, studies have shown that the transfer of multidrug-resistant pathogens from food animals to humans occurs. A recent survey of meats taken from Washington, DC found *Salmonella* with alarming frequency (White *et al.*, 2001; Fey *et al.*, 2000). When the isolates were tested for resistance to antibiotics, most were resistant to at least one antibiotic and over 50% were resistant to at least three antibiotics, including many common compounds, for example tetracycline, streptomycin, sulfamethoxozole, and ampicillin. Some were resistant to cephalosporins and ceftriaxone, or third-generation antibiotics, which are important analogs of human antibiotics. Avoparcin is a growth promoter used for years in European food animals. Avoparcin-resistant organisms are also cross-resistant to vancomycin and vancomycin-resistant *Enterococcus faecium* in humans has recently been associated with increased hospital stays, costs of care, and patient mortality (Levison and Mallela, 2000). Thus, the European Union banned the use of avoparcin in 1997.

The use of antibiotics in animal feed is associated with the presence of resistant bacteria in animals which can be passed on to humans following consumption of such animals. Also, the resistant isolates can exhibit cross-resistance to antimicrobial agents, some of which are important for the care of infections in humans. Human infections from such organisms are increasing and are a threat to human health. Thus, as noted by the American Veterinary Medical Association (2002), it behooves us to address this situation by at least developing judicious principles for the use of antibiotic agents in food animals. It may, as debated by many, be important to restrict or ban the use of antibiotics (McDermott *et al.*, 2002). However, it is likely that new antibiotic-resistant strains of microbial organisms will contribute emerging foodborne pathogens in the future.

1.6 Current issues: novel foods and natural toxicants

Functional food has been defined as food either natural or formulated, which will enhance physiological performance or prevent or treat diseases and disorders (Wildman, 2001) or as defined by the Food and Nutrition Board of the National Academy of Sciences, any food or food ingredient that may provide a health benefit beyond the traditional nutrients it contains. The functional food market has likely doubled in the past ten years to over $10 billion and many food companies are taking full advantage of the public's growing awareness of food in health. Thus, a natural extension of the functional food area is modifying or cultivating food plants and animals to maximize their ability to produce the desirable compounds that are important to health, for example more vitamin E, vitamin A. Genetic modification (GM) of plants or animals for the purpose of producing more functional foods, is at the cutting edge of food science (Reilly, 2000; Harlander, 2002). Some have claimed that this is a new 'second generation' of GM crops, being developed to be genetically modified to express traits for delivering apparent benefits to the consumer and unlike the 'first generation,' developed for delivering only producer benefits. Others will contend that because the density of nutritive and health-beneficial functional chemicals can vary dramatically among plants and animals, with levels often being quite low or non-existent, there is a need to develop strategies that would improve the composition of such chemicals in certain foods. Conventional breeding techniques can be used to achieve this goal, but GM is an attractive alternative that would enable investigators to overcome the genetic diversity within existing germplasm that limit the extent of improvement that can be achieved through conventional techniques. Examples include the engineering of beta-carotene in rice grains, elevating iron content in rice, enhancing vitamin C content in lettuce, increasing flavonols in tomato. The research is complex because often there is a need not only to understand the biochemical pathway for producing such metabolites, but also a need to appreciate the complexity of the metabolites trafficking through the organism, which likely require the identification of several genes for use in a transgenic improvement strategy.

Safety considerations for a functional food derived by GM should not be treated any differently from the functional food derived by conventional plants or animals. Alterations introduced into the genome are very specific and minor, altering one or a few genes and their gene products. The overall safety evaluation of a GM functional food will be conducted under the concept known as 'substantial equivalence' where GM products with one or a few new introduced traits remain substantially equivalent to their traditional counterparts (Cockburn, 2002; Kuiper *et al.*, 2002). A detailed profile on each step in the GM transformation process from parent to new product can be done to assess whether any differences can be detected, which might affect safety. Over 50 GM crops have undergone such evaluation and been judged safe, via World Health Organization and the Food and Agriculture Organization of the United Nations (FAO/WHO, 2000). Overall, the safety assessment is focused on those genes and their products that are introduced into the new variety. Typically, the emphasis is placed on proteins expressed by the introduced atypical gene. Consumption of DNA, regardless of the source, is considered highly digestible and safe (Beever and Kemp, 2000; Jonas, *et al.*, 2001). For novel organisms not judged substantially equivalent to the traditional counterpart, which might be the situation when a large number of genes are introduced or the nutritional content has been altered substantially, a more thorough safety evaluation will be needed. If the parent plant is known to have antinutrient properties, natural toxicants, or allergenic substances, the novel organism will be tested to determine the concentration of such compounds. Currently, the safety assessment approach for such products is voluntary in the United States; however, a mandatory system is likely to be imposed by the FDA in the near future.

1.6.1 Natural toxicants

Plants have in their arsenal an array of thousands of chemicals noxious or toxic to bacteria, fungi, insects, herbivores, and or other species feeding upon them. Fortunately for humans, this chemical diversity also includes many compounds that are beneficial to health: nutrients, antioxidants, anticarcinogens, and many compounds with medicinal value. Most plant species in the world are not edible, many because of the toxins they produce. Plant domestication has gradually reduced the levels of these compounds so that the plant foods we eat today are far less toxic than their wild parents. However, such domestication has resulted in modern food plants being much more susceptible to disease. Toxins range from known carcinogens to skin irritants. A few lipid-soluble plant toxins are capable of bioaccumulation, for example, solanine from potatoes. Toxin concentrations in a plant can vary tremendously and the concentration can be dictated dramatically by environmental stress on the plant (drought, heat/cold, mineral deficiencies, etc.), and disease. Also, different varieties of plant species can differ in the levels of toxins and nutritional value.

1.6.2 Antinutrients

Antinutrients, although not necessarily toxic *per se*, are plant compounds which decrease the nutritional value of a plant food, usually by making an essential nutrient unavailable or indigestible when consumed by humans/animals, i.e. cause nutritional deficiencies. For example, phytate, a common component of most seeds and cereals, forms a complex with many important minerals, making less of the minerals available or making an antimineral substance. Antinutritives can have important health implications particularly with populations facing malnutrition or in marginal nutritional states (Janssen, 1997).

Several substances are antinutrients because they interfere with protein digestion, or the absorption or utilization of amino acid Phytohaemagglutinin are compounds referred to as lectin or hemagglutinin and have been used by immunologists for years to trigger DNA synthesis in T lymphocytes, and more recently, to activate latent human immunodeficiency virus type 1 (HIV-1, AIDS virus) from human peripheral lymphocytes. In addition to inducing mitosis, lectins are known for their ability to agglutinate many mammalian red blood cell types, alter cell membrane transport systems, alter cell permeability to proteins, and generally interfere with cellular metabolism. Lectins originate from plants, particularly legumes. Bean lectins, extracted from raw beans, bind to intestinal mucosal cells and interfere with absorption of amino acids, thyroxine, and various lipophilic compounds. Ricin, found in the castor bean, is toxic and causes intestinal cell necrosis.

Protease inhibitors are proteins that inhibit proteolytic enzymes usually by binding to the active sites. Ovomucoid and ovoinhibitor are protease inhibitors found in raw eggs, which inactivate trypsins. Elastase is inhibited by protease inhibitors found in soybeans, kidney beans and sand potatoes. Many are heat-labile but some are heat-resistant.

1.6.3 Antiminerals

Besides phytic acid, which can interfere with bivalent and tervalent metal ions, oxalic acid, gossypol, glucosinolates, and dietary fiber are other known substances that can compromise mineral status. Oxalic acid reduces the availability of essential bivalent ions and is rich in rhubarb, spinach, and celery. Foods rich in oxalic acid exhibiting an oxalic acid to calcium ratio higher than 1 may decrease calcium availability. Foods rich in glucosinolates such as cabbage, legumes, rutabaga, and turnips may compromise iodine absorption promoting goiter. Gossypol is found in the cotton plant and forms insoluble chelates with many essential metals, such as iron. However, processing of cotton seed removes up to 99% of the gossypol. Dietary fiber has the capacity to complex with various metals, such as calcium, magnesium, zinc and phosphorus.

1.6.4 Allergenic compounds

Genetic modification of foods ultimately results in alteration of protein products either in quantity or the introduction of new proteins. The synthesis of new proteins into foods may present concerns about safety, particularly allergenicity (Hefle *et al.*, 1996; Taylor, 1997; Wal, 1999). Although all allergens are not proteins, most are and, fortunately, only a few of the many diverse proteins found in foods are allergenic when ingested. It is important that the potential allergenicity of an introduced protein be evaluated because the incidence of food allergies can be traumatic and life-threatening. A task force of the International Food Biotechnology Council (IFBC) and the Allergy and Immunology Institute of the International Life Sciences Institute (ILSI) developed a decision tree approach for the assessment of potential allergenicity of plants produced by GM in 1996. The decision tree approach was modified by the FAO/WHO and focuses on evaluating the source of the gene, the sequence homology of the newly introduced protein to known allergens, the immunoreactivity of the novel protein with serum IgE from individuals with known allergies to the source of the transferred genetic material (Taylor and Hefle, 2001). It is useful to have information regarding various physical and chemical properties of the novel protein, for example heat and digestive stability. It is likely that application of such criteria to GM foods will provide assurance that the novel protein in question will be assessed adequately for safety. However, some consumers and interest groups who are opposed to agricultural biotechnology have repeatedly called for mandatory labeling of such foods. Labeling would be generic and of limited value to consumers with respect to information regarding specific food allergies.

1.6.5 Safety testing of genetically engineered varieties

The FDA maintains a list of many common plant toxins and antinutrients and has guidelines defining 'acceptable toxin levels' that it applies to all new crop varieties. The levels are based partly on toxicology studies and partly on measurements of 'normal' toxin levels in samples of food. But in all likelihood, the standards do not represent the natural range of toxin levels actually present in conventional foods. In some cases, the safety margin between the 'acceptable level' and levels considered 'toxic' are less than a ten-fold difference.

The FDA suggests (but does not *require*) the developers of GM varieties to quantify their levels of common toxins and antinutrients and compare them to conventional varieties. In most cases, the GM variety fell within the range of toxin levels observed in conventional varieties, and differences between the same plant variety grown in different locations were much larger than the differences between GM and non-GM varieties.

1.7 Conclusions

As an applied area of toxicology, food toxicology is playing a predominant role in food science, food safety, and consumer health. Whether it be a concern regarding emerging foodborne illnesses, testing the safety of new foods derived from genetically manipulated organisms or their processed products to the sensitivity of subpopulations to specific chemicals found in foods, food toxicology is at the forefront. Food scientists and technologists can support the responsible introduction of GM techniques provided that issues of product safety, environmental concerns, information, and ethics are satisfactorily addressed. Many consider that they are being addressed by the food toxicologist and need intensively to continue to be addressed. Only in this way may the benefits that this technology can provide become available to help feed the world's escalating population in the coming decades. The study of food toxicology includes an appreciation of contamination of the food chain from drinking water, raw materials, via preservation and processing, and those chemicals that might result from genetic modification. Novel foods and the use of functional ingredients (functional foods) represent other areas where a knowledge of food toxicology would be beneficial. Food toxicology is also concerned with natural toxins in food plants and animals, cancer modulating substances, mycotoxins, and all groups of contaminants such as pesticides, persistent organic pollutants, metals, packaging materials, hormones, and animal drug residues. Also, the role of genetic polymorphisms, gender, and lifestyle factors on the sensitivity of humans for toxic compounds, and biomarkers to assess these effects should be included in future research goals of food toxicology.

1.8 References

ALBERT A. *Selective Toxicity: The Physico-Chemical Basis of Therapy*. Sixth Edition, Chapman and Hall, London, 1979.

ALTEKRUSE, S. F., COHEN, M. L. and SWERDLOW, D. L. Emerging foodborne diseases. *Emerging Infectious Diseases* 3: 285–293, 1997.

AMERICAN VETERINARY MEDICAL ASSOCIATION. *Judicious therapeutic use of antimicrobials* (2002). http: //www.avma.org/scienact/jtua/jtua98

BEEVER, D. E. and KEMP, C. F. Safety issues associated with the DNA in animal feed derived from genetically modified crops. A review of scientific and regulatory procedures. *Nutr Abstract Rev B* 70: 175–182, 2000.

BJELDANES L. F., MORRIS M. M., FELTON J. S., HEALY S., STUERMER D., BERRY P., TIMOURIAN H. and HATCH F. T. Mutagens from the cooking of food. III. Survey by Ames/ Salmonella test of mutagen formation in secondary sources of cooked dietary protein. *Food Chem Toxicol* 20: 357–63, 1982.

BJELDANES L. F, MORRIS M. M, TIMOURIAN H. and HATCH F. T. Effects of meat composition and cooking conditions on mutagen formation in fried ground beef. *J Agric Food Chem* 31: 18–21, 1983.

COCKBURN, A. Assuring the safety of genetically modified (GM) foods; The importance of an holistic, integrative approach. *J Biotechn* 98: 79–106, 2002.

COUNCIL ON ENVIRONMENTAL QUALITY, EXECUTIVE OFFICE OF THE PRESIDENT, *Environmental Trends*. (U.S. Government Printing Office, Washington, DC, July 1981), 84.

DALY, A. K., CHOLERTON, S., ARMSTRONG, M. and IDLE, J. R. Genotyping for polymorphisms in xenobiotic metabolism as predictor of disease susceptibility. *Environ Health Perspect* 102: S44–S61, 1994.

EATON, D. A., GALLAGHER, E. P., BAMMLER, T. K. and KUNZE, K L. Role of cytochrome P4501A2 in chemical carcinogenesis: Implications for human variability in expression and enzyme activity. *Pharmacogen* 5: 259–274, 1995.

FAO/WHO CONSULTATION. Safety aspects of genetically modified foods of plant origin. Report of a joint FAO/WHO consultation. Geneva, Switzerland. World Health Organization, 2000.

FELTON J. S., FULTZ E., DOLBEARE F. A., *et al.* Effect of microwave pretreatment on heterocyclic aromatic amine mutagens/carcinogens in fried beef patties. *Food Chemical Toxology* 32(10): 897–903, 1994.

FEY, P. D., SAFRANEK, T. J., RUPP, M. E., *et al.* Ceftriaxone-resistant Salmonella infection acquired by a child from cattle. *N Engl J Med* 342: 1242–1249, 2000.

GANZ, T. Gut defense. *Nature* 422: 478–479, 2003.

HAMER, D. H. and GILL, C. J. From the farm to the kitchen table: the negative impact of antimicrobial use in animals on humans. *Nutr Rev* 60: 261–264, 2002.

HARLANDER, S. K. The evolution of modern agriculture and its future with biotechnology. *J Am Coll Nutr* 21: 161S–165S, 2002.

HATHCOCK, J. N. Nutrition: Toxicology and pharmacology. *Nutr Rev* 34: 65–70, 1976.

HATHCOCK, J. N. *Nutritional Toxicology*. Academic Press, New York, 1982.

HEFLE, S. L., NORDLEE, J. A. and TAYLOR, S. L. Allergenic foods. *Crit Rev Food Sci Nutr* 36: S69–S89, 1996.

HODGSON, E. and GOLSTEIN. Metabolism of toxicants: Phase I reactions and pharmacogenetics. In: *Introduction to Biochemical Toxicology*. Hodgson, E. and Smart, R. C., (eds), Wiley Inter-Science, New York, 2001. pp. 67–114.

IFT EXPERT REPORT. *Emerging Microbiological Food Safety Issues*. Institute of Food Technologists, 2000.

JANSSEN, M. M. T. Antinutritives. In: *Food Safety and Toxicity*. deVries, J. (ed.), CRC Press, Boca Raton, FL., 1997, pp. 39–54.

JONAS, D. A., ELMADFA, I., ENGEL, K-H, HELLER, K. J., KOZIANOWSKI, G., KONIG, A., MULLER, D., NARBONNE, J. F., WACKERNAGEL, W. and KLEINER, J. Safety considerations of DNA in food. *Annals Nutr Metabol* 45: 235–254, 2001.

KLAASSEN, C. D., AMDUR, M. O. and DOULL, J. *Casarett and Doull's Toxicology: The Basic Science of Poisons*, Fifth Edition, McGraw-Hill, New York, 1996.

KUIPER, H. A., KLETER, G. A., NOTEBORN, H. P. and KOK, E. J. Substantial equivalence – an appropriate paradigm for the safety assessment of genetically modified foods? *Toxicology* 181/182: 427–431, 2002.

LEVISON, M. E. and MALLELA, S. Increasing antimicrobial resistance: therapeutic implications for Enterococcal infections. *Cur Infec Dis Rep* 2: 417–423, 2000.

MCDERMOTT, P. F., ZHAO, S., WAGNER, D. D., SIMJEE, S., WALKER, R. D. and WHITE, D. G. The food safety perspective of antibiotic resistance. *Anim Biotechnol* 13: 71–84, 2002.

MCGLYNN, K. A., ROSVOLD, E. A., LUSTBADER, E. D., HU, Y., CLAPPER, M. L., ZHOUP, T., WILD, C. P., XIA, X. L., BAFTOE-BONNIE, A., OFONI, ADJEL, D., CHEN, G-C., LONDON, W. T., SHEN, F-M. and BUETOW, K. W. Susceptibility to hepatocellular carcinoma is associated with genetic variation in the enzymatic detoxification of aflatoxin B1. *Proc Natl Acad Sci* 92: 2384–2387, 1995.

PETULLA, *J. American Environmental History*. Merrill Publishing Company, Columbus, OH, 1988, p. 428.

REILLY, P. R. Public concern about genetics. *Annu Rev Genomics Hum Genet* 1: 485–506, 2000.

SALZMAN, N. H., GHOSH, D., HUTTNER, K. M., PATERSON, Y. and BEVINS. Protection against enteric salmonellosis in transgenic mice expressing a human intestinal defensin. *Nature* 422: 522–526, 2003.

SEIDEGARD, J. and EKSTROM, G. The role of human glutathione transferases and epoxide hydrolases in the metabolism of xenobiotics. *Environ Health Perspec* 105: 791–799, 1997.

SHIBAMOTO, T. and BJELDANES, L. F. *Introduction to Food Toxicology*. Academic Press, New York, 1993.

SUGIMURA, T. Food and cancer. *Toxicology* 181/182: 17–21, 2002.

TAYLOR, S. L. Food from genetically modified organisms and potential for food allergy. *Environ Toxicol Pharmacol* 4: 121–126, 1997.

TAYLOR, S. L. and HEFLE, S. L. Will genetically modified foods be allergenic? *J Allergy Clin Immunol* 107: 765–771, 2001.

WAL, J. M. Assessment of allergic potential of (novel) foods. *Nahrung* 43: 168–174, 1999.

WHITE, D. G., ZHAO, S., SUDLER, R., *et al.* The isolation of antibiotic-resistant Salmonella from retail ground meats. *N. Engl J Med* 345: 1147–1154, 2001.

WILDMAN, R. E. C., Nutraceuticals: A brief review of historical and teleological aspects. In: *Handbook of Nutraceuticals and Functional Foods*. Wildman, R. E. C. (ed.), CRC Press, Boca Raton, FL, 2001, pp. 1–11.

Part I

Assessing and managing risks

2

Genetic susceptibility to dietary carcinogens

S. Peterson, J. W. Lampe and D. L. Eaton, University of Washington and Fred Hutchinson Research Center, USA

2.1 Introduction: diet and cancer

Diet is often considered to be one of the most important 'risk factors' for cancer, yet the very complexity of the diet makes it difficult to discern what specific components of the diet increase or decrease overall cancer risk[1] There is little question that components of the diet can act as a 'doubled-edged sword.' Chemicals in the diet can act directly or indirectly as carcinogens, thereby increasing cancer risk at select sites; conversely, components of the diet can act in a variety of ways to reduce cancer risk. Layered on top of this complexity is human genetic diversity – there is increasing evidence that genetic polymorphism in the human genome contributes to individual variability in response to specific dietary components (both carcinogenic and 'anti-carcinogenic'). The purpose of this chapter is to summarize briefly the current state of understanding of so-called 'gene–diet' interactions, including a look at both carcinogenic and anticarcinogenic components of the diet.

Dietary behaviors can contribute significantly to carcinogen exposure depending on food choices and preferences in food preparation methods. Typically, carcinogens are biotransformed (metabolized) by a variety of biotransformation enzymes to facilitate excretion. However, in the biotransformation process reactive intermediates may be formed that enhance the carcinogenicity of the chemical. Additional biotransformation pathways usually eliminate the reactive intermediate, although not with 100% efficiency. Thus, the relative carcinogenic potency of a specific chemical is often determined by the relative rates of activation and detoxification. Further influencing the metabolic fate of a carcinogen (and ultimately its mutagenicity) is genetic variability in biotransformation enzymes. Thus, depending on how the genetic variation influences an enzyme's function (i.e., increase or decrease activity depending on the compound), there is the potential that certain genetic variations could result in a higher or lower risk for cancer. At the same time, just as diet can be the source of carcinogens, it can also be the source of a variety of plant compounds that may prevent cancer through manipulation of biotransformation enzyme activity in a manner that also could be genotype-dependent. It should be noted here that there are many other mechanisms – besides alterations of biotransformation enzymes – by which components of the diet might alter cancer risk, including effects on: signal transduction pathways, apoptosis, immune surveillance, hormonal status, modification of oxidative stress, DNA repair processes, and a host of other epigenetic mechanisms. However, the growing field of 'gene–diet' interactions has developed most extensively in the area of dietary modification of carcinogen biotransformation.

This chapter first will focus briefly on exposure and metabolism of four major classes of dietary carcinogens: mycotoxins, heterocyclic amines, polycyclic aromatic hydrocarbons and *N*-nitroso compounds. A discussion of carcinogenic and anticarcinogenic plant compounds will also be included. Next, the influence of genetics on carcinogen-metabolizing enzymes will be addressed and examples given to illustrate the implications for carcinogenesis. Evidence of gene–diet interactions will also be provided. Finally, an overview of the future trends as well as additional sources on the topic of gene–diet interactions and cancer will conclude the chapter.

2.2 Dietary carcinogens and anticarcinogens: mycotoxins, heterocyclic amines, aromatic hydrocarbons, *N*-nitroso compounds and phytochemicals

Mycotoxins, heterocyclic amines, polycyclic aromatic hydrocarbons and *N*-nitroso compounds have been studied for many years. For the purposes of this chapter, the exposure and metabolism of each will be presented briefly. A more in-depth discussion of polycyclic aromatic hydrocarbons is found in Chapter 19. For additional information on heterocyclic amines, please see reviews by Keating *et al.*,[2] Knize *et al.*,[3] and Sinha.[4]

2.2.1 Mycotoxins

Fungi or molds produce mycotoxins, which are secondary metabolites with no known biochemical significance in the growth or development of fungi.[5] Mycotoxin-producing molds of dietary interest are primarily found in cereal grains, forages, corn, rice, peanuts and peanut oil.[6–9]

Of the common dietary mycotoxins, aflatoxins (a group of closely related difuranocoumarin mycotoxins) are classified as carcinogenic to humans, and ochratoxins and fumonisins are classified as possible carcinogens.[6] Aflatoxin B_1

(AFB_1) is not only the most potent of these mycotoxins but it is among the most potent hepatocarcinogens ever identified.

To be carcinogenic, AFB_1 must be activated to a highly reactive intermediate, aflatoxin B_1-8,9-epoxide (AFBO), before adduct formation and DNA damage can occur. Under conditions of the relatively low concentrations encountered in the human diet, it appears that human microsomal cytochrome P450 1A2 (CYP1A2) is the primary biotransformation enzyme that activates AFB_1 to the highly reactive AFBO, with CYP3A4 playing a lesser role in activation.[10] It is interesting to note that CYP1A2 is a liver-specific form of cytochrome P450, and that AFB seems only to cause liver cancer from dietary exposures, perhaps because of this. Once activated, AFBO can covalently bind to the N-7 position of guanine in DNA.[11] This adduct formation renders the DNA susceptible to damage and can proceed to somatic alterations of genes. In mice, and to a lesser extent rats, conjugation of the reactive epoxide with glutathione occurs via a specific alpha class form of glutathione-*S*-transferase (GST). This represents an important detoxification step, such that mice are completely resistant to the carcinogenic effects of even high doses of AFB. Although rats are highly susceptible to the hepatocarcinogenic effects of AFB, inclusion of dithiolthione compounds in the diet can greatly reduce susceptibility of rats to the DNA adduction and subsequent carcinogenic effects of AFB.[12,13] The mechanism of this dietary reduction in carcinogenesis is apparently mediated via the induction of a non-constitutively expressed form of GST in the rat liver, rGSTA5, that is orthologous to the constitutively expressed form in mouse liver, mGSTA3, that confers the resistance of mice.[14] However, in humans alpha class GSTs have little to no activity toward the epoxide, although the mu class of GSTs exhibits slight but measurable activity (in the order of 10,000 times less than mouse GSTA3).[15] Alternative to glutathione conjugation, the reactive epoxide may also be hydrolyzed spontaneously, or possibly by microsomal epoxide hydrolase.[15–17] Both pathways of conjugation with glutathione and hydrolysis result in detoxification of the reactive epoxide. The profound protection of rats from the carcinogenic effects of AFB produced by dietary treatment with the synthetic dithiolthione, Oltipraz, provided the initial rationale to implement exploratory clinical trials in a population in China with a high incidence of hepatocellular carcinoma and high dietary aflatoxin exposures.[18] While the treatment with Oltipraz did appear to have some effect in reducing AFB-DNA adduct formation (as determined by the levels of excretion of the AFB-N7-guanine adduct in urine), the apparent protective effect may have been due to Oltipraz-mediated inhibition of CYP1A2, as well as enhancement of GSH-mediated detoxification.

The animal and human studies on the mechanisms of aflatoxin hepatocarcinogenesis provide an excellent example of how relatively slight differences in the activity and/or level of expression of a single biotransformation enzyme can have profound differences in species' (or individuals') susceptibility to a dietary carcinogen. They further illustrate the potentially important role that diet-related changes in biotransformation enzyme activity and/or expression can have on individual susceptibility to chemical carcinogenesis.

2.2.2 Heterocyclic amines

Intake of heterocyclic amines (HCAs; such as the tryptophan pyrolysis products IQ, MeIQ, MeIQx, PhiP[a]) may be associated with several types of cancer. *In vitro* experiments have shown HCAs to be potent mutagens and their carcinogenicity has been demonstrated repeatedly in laboratory animal studies. Epidemiologic studies have found relationships to pancreatic cancer,[19] breast cancer,[20] and colon cancer.[21–22] There have also been reports to the contrary,[23-27] but it is proposed that the discrepancy is due to lack of specificity when assessing level of exposure.[3,4,19,21] HCAs in the diet are formed during the cooking of meat and are most concentrated in the meat juices.[28] The challenge in classifying degree of exposure stems from the numerous factors determined to influence HCA formation: cooking method, how well the meat is cooked, type of meat, and frequency of consumption (reviewed extensively by Keating *et al.*[2] and Knize *et al.*[3]).

The key first step in bioactivation of HCAs is *N*-hydroxylation by CYP1A2.[29, 30] Subsequent to this, further activation is mediated by sulfotransferases and the *N*-acetyltransferases NAT1 and NAT2, yielding highly reactive esters capable of binding to DNA.[31–33] However, an alternative path after *N*-hydroxylation by CYP1A2 is detoxification through glucuronidation, possibly mediated primarily by the UGT1A class of UDP-glucuronosyltransferases (UGTs).[30]

2.2.3 Polycyclic aromatic hydrocarbons

Polycyclic aromatic hydrocarbons (PAHs; such as benzo[*a*]pyrene, dibenz[*a,h*]anthracene, and various other substituted pyrenes, anthracenes and chrysenes) are the result of incomplete combustion of organic matter, and the primary dietary source is meats. Diets high in PAHs repeatedly cause foregut tumors and lung tumors in animal studies[34–39] and PAHs are suspected to be human carcinogens as well.[40]

Generally, the activation of PAHs is as follows: initial activation by cytochrome P450s to reactive epoxide intermediates, subsequent hydrolysis of the epoxide intermediate by microsomal epoxide hydrolase, and then oxidation again by cytochrome P450s to maximally reactive diol-epoxide PAH metabolites, which can interact with DNA.[41–44] For example, the tumorigenic activity of benzo[*a*]pyrene is due to its reactive metabolite, (+)-anti-7,8-dihydroxy-9,10-epoxy-7,8,9,10-tetrahydrobenzo[*a*]pyrene, which has an electrophilic epoxide center, the site of nucleophilic attack by nucleophilic centers in DNA.[45] (See Chapter 19 for a more detailed discussion of PAH metabolism and carcinogenicity.) The most important cytochrome P450s in the activation of PAHs and PAH dihydrodiols are CYP1A1 and CYP1B1, with CYP1A2, CYP2C9, and CYP3A4 also being able to activate though at much

---

[a] IQ, 2-amino-3-methylimadazo[4,5-*f*]quinoline; MeIQ, 2-amino-3,4-dimethylimadazo[4,5-*f*]quinoline; MeIQx, 2-amino-3,8-dimethylimadazo[4,5-*f*]quinoxaline; PhiP, 2-amino-1-methyl-6-phenylimadazo[4,5-*b*]pyridine

lower rates compared to CYP1A1 and CYP1B1.[46] GSTs can conjugate and detoxify both the epoxide intermediates and final diol-epoxides, but the specific GSTs that are primarily involved in this process have yet to be identified.[44, 45]

2.2.4 *N*-nitroso compounds

N-nitroso compounds (NOCs) are formed when natural amines in protein interact with nitrosating agents (usually nitrite salts) that are added to foods to inhibit bacterial growth and prolong shelf-life. The most likely NOCs to be encountered in the diet are *N*-nitrosamines, which are commonly found in smoked or cured meats (including seafood) and beer (for full review, including discussion of specific NOCs, see Lijinsky[47]). *In vivo*, two additional means of NOC exposure include gastric and salivary gland microflora that may reduce nitrates to nitrites, which can then combine with nitrosatable substances, and macrophage-mediated nitrosation at sites that are inflamed or infected.[48,49]

The carcinogenicity of NOCs has been acknowledged for years. As discussed at length in several reviews dating back to the 1980s, these compounds are known carcinogens in at least 40 species and have multiple target sites for inducing tumors.[47,50–52] Human ecologic studies have found associations between NOC exposure and cancers of the stomach, esophagus, nasopharynx, bladder, and liver.[53] Epidemiologic studies provide further support of the correlation of NOCs with human cancer. Rogers *et al.*[54] observed increased risk of upper aerodigestive tract cancer with frequent consumption of foods containing nitrosodimethylamine (NDMA); De Stefani *et al.*[55] reported a significant dose-response pattern between lung cancer and increasing intake of NDMA.

N-nitrosamines are activated (hydroxylated) by CYP2E1, CYP2A6, and CYP1A1. More specifically, it appears that CYP2A6 is responsible for the activation of those *N*-nitrosamines with longer alkyl chains and found in tobacco smoke while CYP2E1 is responsible for activation of *N*-nitrosamines that have relatively short alkyl chains.[56–59] After *N*-nitrosamines are activated to α-hydroxynitrosamines, they spontaneously decompose sequentially to monoalkylnitrosamines, alkyldiazohydroxides and nitrogen separated ion pairs.[52] The alkyldiazohydroxides alkylate nucleophiles resulting in formation of diazoalkanes, some of which especially alkylate the DNA bases at N-7 and O-6 of guanine and O-4 of thymine. Thus, instead of pairing with cytosine the O^6-alkylguanines pair with thymine resulting in G:C→A:T mutations and initiation of carcinogenesis.[52]

2.2.5 Phytochemicals: anticarcinogenic and carcinogenic activity

Phytochemicals are substances in plant foods that impart the plant's color, flavor, defense against pests, etc., but which may also have some bioactive effect when ingested by humans. They present an interesting case such that in many instances they are toxins to the primary predators and pests of the plant; yet they frequently impart positive effects on human health. Most research focuses on the positive human health effects of various phytochemicals.

Resveratrol is a polyphenolic compound found in grapes and peanuts. It has been shown to inhibit the increase in *CYP1A1* expression caused by aryl hydrocarbons in human hepatoma HepG2 cells.[60] Evidence for multiple roles of resveratrol in cancer prevention have been presented,[61,62] including: growth inhibition, S-phase arrest, induction of apoptosis, inhibition of cell proliferation and sensitization of cancer cells to cytotoxic drugs.

Cruciferous vegetables (the broccoli family) are rich sources of glucosinolates. When the plant undergoes physical damage (crushed, chewed, etc.) the glucosinolates come in contact with a plant enzyme called myrosinase. Myrosinase action on glucosinolates produces a number of metabolites ranging from isothiocyanates to indoles, depending on the glucosinolate precursor. Some of these compounds have been implicated in goitrogenic effects in man, but epidemiologic studies indicate inverse associations with cruciferous intake and cancer risk (reviewed by Talalay and Fahey[63] and Verhoeven *et al.*[64]) and most animal studies with isothiocyanates show protection against cancers at various sites (reviewed by Zhang and Talalay[65] and Hecht[66]). In one controlled human feeding study ($n = 10$), Pantuck *et al.*[67] showed that 500 g of cruciferous vegetables (cabbage and Brussels sprouts) consumed for ten days stimulated formation of acetaminophen glucuronyl conjugates and increased the ratio of acetaminophen glucuronide to free acetaminophen, indicating the vegetables were likely inducing UGTs. Similarly, Hecht *et al.*[68] reported that watercress (a cruciferous vegetable) also induced UGT activity. Focusing on individual compounds, investigation of sulforaphane, an isothiocyanate, has revealed that sulforaphane is a potent inducer of GSTs and UGTs,[69–71] with one possible mechanism of induction being activation of the transcription factor Nrf2.[72] Sulforaphane has also demonstrated inhibitory effects on some cytochrome P450 enzymes, most notably causing a decrease in both CYP3A4 activity and expression.[70]

However, other phytochemicals may also exert a toxic effect in humans. Psoralen, bergapten and xanthotoxin (furanocoumarins found in celery, parsley, and parsnips) can cause photosensitization, and can be photomutagenic and photocarcinogenic.[73,74] Perhaps of greater concern due to its availability in supplement form, is the discovery that indole-3-carbinol (also found in cruciferous vegetables) could enhance tumor development. Using a trout model, Oganesian *et al.*[75] found that indole-3-carbinol (at doses approximating those recommended for human supplementation) promoted AFB_1-initiated liver cancer. Indole-3-carbinol has also been shown to enhance the levels of the heterocyclic amine 2-amino-3-methyl-imidazo[4,5-*f*]quinoline (IQ) in male F344 rats compared with controls when given at low doses; high doses exhibited opposite and more favorable effects.[76] Similarly, chlorophyllin at low doses in male F344 rats increased multiplicity of 1,2-dimethylhydrazine-induced colon tumors while having no effect on IQ-induced colon tumors.[77] The authors of these studies point out that individual plant compounds could have varying effects dependent on the dose or species used for investigation and that caution should be used with regard to human use of phytochemical supplements until more is understood about their effects.

2.3 Genetic influences on carcinogen-metabolizing enzymes

As illustrated above, there are numerous biotransformation enzymes, and thus genes, involved in the metabolism of dietary carcinogens. Further, the expression and activity of several of these enzymes can be influenced by the presence of various phytochemicals in the diet. Adding to the complexity of carcinogen metabolism are the potential effects of genetic mutations or polymorphisms in the genes that code for biotransformation enzymes. (Polymorphism is defined as more than one alternative allele at a genetic locus such that the rare allele has a frequency of at least 1% in the population.)

Depending on the mutation, the kinetic efficiency (measured as the ratio of V_{max} (maximum reaction velocity of K_m (Michaelis constant)) of the enzyme can be either increased or decreased. First, as an example of effects on V_{max}, a gene deletion (null allele) will result in no functional enzyme, loss of activity and a poor-metabolizer phenotype in those homozygous for the null allele. Next, in the opposite direction, gene duplication with multiple copies of a functional gene within a gene locus will result in accumulation of the enzyme and potentially an ultra-rapid metabolizer phenotype. A third possibility affecting V_{max} is alternative splicing and frameshifts in DNA leading to alternatively spliced mRNA and a decrease in synthesis of functional enzyme. There is also the potential for mutations in the promoter (control) regions of the gene, including specific response elements, which could alter the rate of transcription of DNA to RNA and thus either increase or decrease enzyme production. V_{max} can additionally be influenced by altered degradation of the enzyme; a polymorphism that results in changes to the structure of the enzyme that can lead to increased degradation of it while the rate of synthesis remains the same. Lastly alterations in catalysis due to polymorphisms may affect V_{max}, causing amino acid substitutions but which subsequently result in increased or decreased catalytic efficiency. Similarly with K_m, amino acid substitutions can increase or decrease binding affinity and the stability of the enzyme-substrate complex.

In regard to regulation of biotransformation enzymes involved in the metabolism of dietary carcinogens, variance in genes involved in the regulation of gene expression could have a broad effect beyond polymorphisms in the biotransformation enzyme genes themselves. The activity of transcription factors, receptors, and response elements involved in regulating biotransformation enzyme expression and function could all be influenced by polymorphisms in their respective genes and thus provide additional avenues of potential susceptibility to, or protection from, dietary carcinogens.

Polymorphisms have been identified in many of the enzymes involved in the biotransformation of mycotoxins, HCAs, PAHs, and NOCs. Specific examples are polymorphism of cytochrome P450s, *N*-acetyltransferases (NATs), GSTs, UGTs, sulfotransferases, and microsomal epoxide hydrolase. This section will focus on *CYP1A2*, *NAT1*, *NAT2*, and *GSTM1* to illustrate examples of where a genetic polymorphism has a functional effect on activity of the enzyme.

2.3.1 *CYP1A2*

Polymorphisms in all seven exons, in intron 1, and in the 5′-flanking region of *CYP1A2* have been revealed through sequencing of genomic DNA,[78–82] but only two polymorphisms thus far identified have known functional effects. *CYP1A2*1C* (-3858G>A, 5′-flanking region) appears to be associated with decreased induction by smoking via an effect on transcriptional activation.[82] Conversely, *CYP1A2*1F* (-164C>A, intron 1) appears to confer higher inducibility and possibly differential binding of regulatory proteins to the surrounding sequence leading to varied levels of expression.[82]

The impact of these alterations in inducibility is not yet fully identified, but there is evidence that the polymorphisms in *CYP1A2* might lead to altered cancer risk. In a study on permanent hair dye use and bladder cancer, Gago-Dominguez *et al.*[83] found that bladder cancer risk associated with use of permanent hair dye was mainly confined to individuals with slow (versus rapid) *CYP1A2* phenotype. Lang *et al.*[84] found in a case-control study a slightly increased risk for colon cancer and colon polyps among those with higher *CYP1A2* activity. However, studies showing an opposite association[85] and no association[86] with colon cancer also exist.

2.3.2 *NAT1* and *NAT2*

Over 25 alleles have been identified for *NAT1* and *NAT2* each with *NAT1*4* and *NAT2*4* defined as the reference human *NAT1* and *NAT2* alleles. This is due to both being associated with high activity and both being most frequent in the original populations studied.[33] Depending on the polymorphism, or combination of polymorphisms, *NAT1* and *NAT2* catalytic activity can be increased or decreased to produce rapid or slow acetylator phenotypes.

Several investigators have examined the effect of genetic variation in *NAT1* and *NAT2* on risk of lung, bladder, and colon cancer. With regard to lung cancer, Zhou *et al.*[87] reported that *NAT2* rapid acetylator genotypes were protective against lung cancer in non-smokers but were risk factors in heavy smokers. In a recent study on permanent hair dye use among lifelong non-smoking women, those without the *NAT1*10* genotype showed a statistically significant increase in bladder cancer risk associated with hair dye use (odds ratio (OR) = 6.8, confidence interval (CI) = 1.7–27.4), whereas the OR in those with the *NAT1*10* genotype was 1.0.[83] Furthermore, the same study found that all frequency- and duration-related dose-response relationships between hair dye use and bladder cancer were confined to those without the *NAT1*10* genotype while those with the *NAT1*10* genotype showed none of those associations.

2.3.3 *GSTM1*

The most common polymorphism in *GSTM1* (approx. 50–60% of the population) is a gene deletion resulting in no production of *GSTM1* in those homozygous for the null allele. Despite the broad prevalence of this polymorphism in the population, which argues strongly against the physiological importance or necessity of the enzyme, there could be an associated cancer risk to the homozygous *GSTM1*-null genotype. McGlynn *et al.*[88] reported a significant association in a Ghanaian population between *GSTM1* genotype and the presence of AFB_1 adducts and a suggestive association (though not statistically significant) between *GSTM1* genotype and hepatocellular carcinoma (HCC); however the association with HCC was significant with epoxide hydrolase genotype. Other epidemiology studies in China have also suggested that the *GSTM1* null polymorphism is associated with enhanced susceptibility to AFB_1 hepatocarcinogenesis, especially in association with hepatitis B virus antigen positivity.[89,90]

Although the above examples of polymorphisms in *CYP1A2, NAT1, NAT2,* and *GSTM1* do not provide conclusive evidence of significant modification in cancer risk, they do illustrate that the potential exists. The examples also illustrate the potential for the true effects of various exposures to be masked or missed when consideration (and thus investigation) is not given to the possibility of a subgroup being more susceptible due to their genotype. Certainly, more studies that are sufficiently powered to examine various gene interactions with exposures are needed to better understand the effect and associated risk of genetic polymorphisms in biotransformation enzymes. The influence of the varied components of diet also needs to be addressed in study design when investigating genetic response to carcinogens.

2.4 Evidence of gene–diet interactions

As mentioned previously, the diet is not only a source of various carcinogens but also a source of potentially anticarcinogenic compounds, many of which are capable of modulating biotransformation enzymes (their expression and/or their activity). Thus, just as genetic polymorphisms in these enzymes can lead to variation in response to carcinogen exposure it is quite plausible that they can also lead to variation in response to the anticarcinogenic compounds in diet as well. The following discussion presents evidence from epidemiologic and human intervention studies of the impact of gene–diet interactions.

2.4.1 Epidemiologic studies

Selecting a population in the Sudan, Omer *et al.*[91] tested whether there was an association between peanut butter intake (a source of AFB_1 in the Sudan due to improper storage and processing) and *GSTM1* genotype in the etiology of HCC. They found a positive association with peanut butter intake that was essentially limited only to subjects with the *GSTM1*-null genotype (OR for highest vs. lowest quartile of intake = 16.7, 95% CI = 2.7–104.8). In a case-control study on HCA metabolism and colorectal adenomas, a six-fold increase in adenoma risk was observed among *NAT1* rapid acetylators with >27 ng of MeIQx intake per day.[86] As part of the Physicians' Health Study, Chen *et al.*[92] also investigated diet interaction with *NAT* genotypes and risk of colorectal cancer. They observed that consumption of more than one serving of red meat per day, compared to 0.5 servings per day or less, was associated with a relative risk of cancer of 5.82 (95% CI = 1.11–30.6) in men who were rapid acetylators for both *NAT1* and *NAT2*. In another case-control study, Lin *et al.*[93] reported that individuals with the highest quartile of broccoli intake had the lowest risk for colorectal adenomas, compared to individuals who reportedly never ate broccoli. However, this inverse association was observed only in those with the *GSTM1*-null genotype. Corroborating this finding is the study by Slattery *et al.*[94] that found that colon cancer risk was modified by cruciferous vegetables in particular subgroups defined by age, smoking status, and *GSTM1* genotype.

Three studies on lung cancer and isothiocyanate (ITC) intake reported similar significant gene–diet interactions. First, a study by Spitz *et al.*[95] compared newly diagnosed lung cancer patients before treatment with controls and investigated the effects of *GST* genotype and intake of ITCs. Based on 503 cases and 465 controls, their results showed that 49.4% of cases and 48.8% of controls were homozygous *GSTM1*-null, 27.3% of cases and 22.7% of controls were homozygous *GSTT1*-null, and 13.0% of cases and 10.0% of controls were null for both genotypes. They found no evidence of a main effect for the *GSTM1* genotype adjusted for age, gender, smoking status, and ITC intake, but there was some evidence of a main effect for *GSTT1* genotype (OR = 1.41, CI = 1.03–1.93). Stratifying by 'current smoker' vs. 'former smoker' status (too few 'never smoked' subjects were recruited), statistically significant associations were observed among smokers with either the homozygous null genotype or both null genotypes *and* who had a low dietary intake of ITCs.

The second study was part of a larger prospective study of men in Shanghai, China.[96] From their sample 52.6% of cases and 60.1% of controls were homozygous *GSTM1*-null, 57.8% of cases and 60.0% of controls were homozygous *GSTT1*-null, and 36.6% of cases and 38.7% of controls were null for both. When comparisons were made based on ITC intake (based on whether ITCs were detectable in the urine or not) a pattern emerged that was similar to the previous study's results. There was a decreased risk of lung cancer among those with detectable amounts of ITCs in their urine (indicating higher intake of ITCs) *and* who had either or both of the null genotypes. Similar to the previous study, there was no main effect on lung cancer by *GSTM1* or *GSTT1* genotype alone.

The final study, conducted among Chinese women in Singapore by Zhao *et al.*,[97] confirmed the same pattern. They found that 62.7% of cases and 63.6% of controls were homozygous *GSTM1*-null, 56.7% of cases and 54.5% of controls were homozygous *GSTT1*-null, and 35.2% of cases and 35.3% of controls had both null alleles. As with the previous two studies, there was no significant association with lung cancer and *GSTM1* or *GSTT1* genotype, but they did observe an inverse association of dietary ITC intake with lung cancer risk, which was modified by *GSTM1* and *GSTT1* genotypes. Those with the null genotype for either or both enzymes had a somewhat significant reduction in risk with higher intake of ITCs, but the effect was smaller and not statistically significant if either or both genes were present. All three studies provide indication that ITCs play a role in the prevention of lung cancer in humans and suggest that this chemopreventive effect of ITCs may vary between individuals and across populations based on the genetic variation in *GSTM1* and *GSTT1*. Since ITCs are substrates for GSTs, the proposed mechanism to explain the observed effect of null genotypes having higher lung cancer risk with low ITC intake and lower lung cancer risk with high ITC intake is that the ITC compounds are less rapidly metabolized and eliminated from the body in individuals with the null genotypes.

However, not only have epidemiologic studies provided evidence of gene–diet interactions, but they have also provided evidence of gene–gene–diet interactions. MacLeod *et al.*[98] reported that CYP1A2 activity was ~23% higher in individuals with the *GSTM1*-null genotype compared with those who expressed at least one *GSTM1* allele, and Probst-Hensch *et al.*[99] found that among frequent consumers of broccoli, *GSTM1*-null individuals had a 21% higher geometric mean level of CYP1A2 activity relative to *GSTM1*+ individuals. These findings have interesting implications regarding the apparent protective effects of the *GSTM1* and *T1* alleles and susceptibility to aflatoxin hepatocarcinogenesis. As discussed above, several studies[88–90] have suggested that individuals homozygous for either or both *GSTM1* or *GSTT1* null alleles appear to be at increased risk for AFB-induced liver cancer. Although the initial conclusion drawn from these findings is that the GSTs may be involved directly in detoxification of AFB-epoxide, *in vitro* work has found that these forms have little activity toward AFB-exo-epoxide. An alternative explanation might be the following: individuals that are *GSTM1* and/or *T1* null have a lower rate of metabolic clearance of phytochemicals that act as inducers of CYP1A2. The decreased rate of clearance (longer half-life) of the inducing phytochemicals leads to enhanced CYP1A2 activity, which in turn leads to greater activation of AFB to AFB-8,9-*exo*-epoxide and thus enhanced genotoxicity and carcinogenesis. Further research is required to test this hypothesis, but it does illustrate the complexities of interpreting the effects of diet on carcinogenesis in gene–diet interaction studies.

2.4.2 Human intervention studies

Very few human intervention studies have examined gene–diet interactions. In a study conducted in 1995,[100] 66 healthy individuals ate a control diet for seven days that contained lean ground beef cooked at a low temperature. Caffeine phenotyping (an *in vivo* measure of CYP1A2 functional activity) was performed on day eight to determine CYP1A2 activity level of the subjects. After the phenotyping, subjects then consumed lean ground beef (cooked at a high temperature) containing 9.0 ng of MeIQx/g of meat. Each subject ate 3.1–4.0 g of meat/kg of body weight and then MeIQx from urine samples taken every 12 hours was measured by gas chromatography. The authors reported inter-individual variation in CYP1A2 activity and an association between higher CYP1A2 activity and lower levels of total unconjugated MeIQx in the urine. Looking at GSTs and cruciferous vegetable intake, a controlled feeding study tested *a priori* if *GSTM1* genotype affects the response to a diet high in cruciferous vegetables.[101] Men and women were recruited based on their *GSTM1* genotype and given four 1-week controlled diet treatments in a randomized crossover fashion. The four diet treatments were a basal fruit- and vegetable-free diet and the basal diet supplemented with a) cruciferous, b) allium (onion family), or c) apiaceous (carrot family) vegetables. In *GSTM1*-null individuals only, serum GSTα concentration, a surrogate measure of hepatic GSTα and an enzyme increased by ITCs, increased significantly in response to cruciferous vegetable feeding. GSTμ activity in leukocytes was also increased but only among *GSTM1+* individuals in response to both cruciferous and allium feeding.

2.5 Summary and future trends

Many naturally occuring dietary carcinogens, including mycotoxins, HCAs, PAHs, and NOCs, as well as a variety of synthetic chemical carcinogens, are metabolized by a complex mixture of biotransformation enzymes. Human genetic polymorphisms have been identified in many of the genes that code for various biotransformation enzymes. A polymorphism can have functional effects such that enzyme production, efficiency, and stability can be affected. There is a body of work accumulating that indicates that inter-individual variation in response to carcinogens may be dependent on biotransformation enzyme genotype. Furthermore, not only does response to carcinogens appear to be genotype-dependent, but also response to anticarcinogens in the diet as well. This makes for an intriguing challenge in deciphering the risk vs. benefit of various dietary components. It also raises the possibility of moving towards more individualized dietary recommendations.

2.5.1 Future trends

Two major areas gaining attention and momentum for future progress in understanding genetic susceptibility to dietary carcinogens are those of dietary assessment and biological assessment. With regard to dietary assessment, it is generally understood that improvements need to be made with food databases for better accuracy in estimating exposure to dietary carcinogens and anticarcinogens. Data on phytochemical content are lacking as are data on HCA and PAH content. Our tools for collecting dietary intake data from subjects do not always reflect the current state of knowledge. For example, when obtaining data on meat intake, information on preparation, cooking methods, type of meat, and how well the meat is cooked should always be obtained to better assess HCA exposure.

As for biological assessment, there is a concerted effort to continue to use technology to develop better biomarkers. Better means to identify and measure indicators of dietary intake, biochemical and cell activity, and predictive molecular markers of disease are needed in order to determine the effects of genetics on disease risk when factoring in environmental interactions. A particular challenge with biomarkers – especially in this era of '-omics' (genomics, proteomics, metabonomics, etc.) – is interpretation of complex data sets. A single dietary exposure does not result in a single biological change. Much attention is currently focused on determining the best statistical methods to interpret a cascade of multiple perturbations. An additional trend for the future in making biological assessments, is improved methods for investigating human biotransformation processes. Animal models will always play an important role, but great species variation exists in biotransformation efficiency, susceptibility to carcinogens, and response to anticarcinogens. Implementation of yeast expression systems and improved use of human hepatocytes can allow for investigation of human response in ways previously unavailable. Furthermore, with improved understanding of drug metabolism pathways, safe compounds that share metabolic pathways with carcinogens (for example, caffeine and CYP1A2; acetaminophen and aspirin and UGTs) can be used as probes in human intervention studies to test gene–diet interactions. The use of such '*in vivo* phenotyping' measures to evaluate carefully the functional significance, or lack thereof, of putative genetic polymorphisms is desperately needed to ensure that large-scale molecular epidemiology studies are biologically based and focused on truly 'functional' polymorphisms. However, full genome scans that examine thousands of polymorphic markers may ultimately replace the 'target gene' approach in molecular epidemiology studies. Although such studies may have substantial power to identify genomic patterns (multiple allelic variants) associated with disease outcome, the biological interpretation of such associations will be difficult to discern. Nevertheless, such tools will ultimately be of value in understanding the complex interaction between diet, genetics, and cancer risk.

An additional trend in both areas of dietary and biological assessment is greater multidisciplinary involvement. Researchers from numerous disciplines are actively investigating genetic susceptibility to carcinogens and the impact of diet and other environmental factors. Collaboration between disciplines capitalizes on the unique skills, training, and perspectives that are inherent to varied training backgrounds. Thus, a cohesive interdisciplinary team can attack one research question from a variety of directions (for instance toxicology, nutritional science, and epidemiology) and end up with a more complete picture of the answer.

2.6 Sources of further information and advice

For a more in depth review of cytochrome P450s and known polymorphisms, see http://www.imm.ki.se/CYPalleles/[82] and Ingelman-Sundberg;[102] for NATs, see Hein;[33] for GSTs, see Eaton and Bammler;[103] for sulfotransferases, see Glatt *et al.*;[104] for UGTs, see Tukey and Strassburg;[105] and for microsomal epoxide hydrolase, see Omiecinski *et al.*[106]

2.7 References

1. POTTER J D, ed. *Food, Nutrition and the Prevention of Cancer: A Global Perspective*. American World Cancer Res Fund, Institute for Cancer Res, Mesasha, Banta Book Group, 1997.
2. KEATING G A, LAYTON D W, FELTON J S, 'Factors determining dietary intakes of heterocyclic amines in cooked foods,' *Mutat Res*, 1999 **443** 149–156.
3. KNIZE M G, KULP K S, SALMON C P, KEATING G A, FELTON J S, 'Factors affecting human heterocyclic amine intake and the metabolism of PhIP,' *Mutat Res*, 2002 **506–507** 153–162.
4. SINHA R, 'An epidemiologic approach to studying heterocyclic amines,' *Mutat Res*, 2002 **506–507** 197–204.
5. MOSS M O, 'The environmental factors controlling mycotoxin formation,' in Smith J E, Anderson R A, *Mycotoxins and Animal Foods*, Boca Raton, CRC Press, 37–56, 1991.
6. HUSSEIN H S, BRASEL J M, 'Toxicity, metabolism, and impact of mycotoxins on humans and animals,' *Toxicology*, 2001 **167** 101–134.
7. STRESSER D M, WILLIAMS D E, MCLELLAN L I, HARRIS T M, BAILEY G S, 'Indole-3-carbinol induces a rat liver glutathione transferase subunit (Yc2) with high activity toward aflatoxin B1 exo-epoxide. Association with reduced levels of hepatic aflatoxin-DNA adducts in vivo,' *Drug Metab Dispos*, 1994 **22** 392–399.
8. STRESSER D M, BAILEY G S, WILLIAMS D E, 'Indole-3-carbinol and beta-naphthoflavone induction of aflatoxin B1 metabolism and cytochromes P-450 associated with bioactivation and detoxication of aflatoxin B1 in the rat,' *Drug Metab Dispos*, 1994 **22** 383–391.
9. WANG J S, HUANG T, SU J, LIANG F, WEI Z, LIANG Y, LUO H, KUANG S Y, QIAN G S, SUN G, HE X, KENSLER T W, GROOPMAN J D, 'Hepatocellular carcinoma and aflatoxin exposure in Zhuqing Village, Fusui County, People's Republic of China,' *Cancer Epidemiol Biomarkers Prev*, 2001 **10** 143–146.
10. GALLAGHER E P, KUNZE K L, STAPLETON P L, EATON D L, 'The kinetics of aflatoxin B1 oxidation by human cDNA-expressed and human liver microsomal cytochromes P450 1A2 and 3A4,' *Toxicol Appl Pharmacol*, 1996 **141** 595–606.
11. SALBE A D, BJELDANES L F, 'Effect of diet and route of administration on the DNA binding of aflatoxin B1 in the rat,' *Carcinogenesis*, 1989 **10**(4) 629–634.
12. RAMSDELL H S, EATON D L, 'Modification of aflatoxin B1 biotransformation in vitro and DNA binding in vivo by dietary broccoli in rats,' *J Toxicol Environ Health*, 1988 **25** 269–275.
13. KENSLER T W, GROOPMAN J D, EATON D L, CURPHEY T J, ROEBUCK B D, 'Potent inhibition of aflatoxin-induced hepatic tumorigenesis by the monofunctional

enzyme inducer 1,2-dithiole-3-thione,' *Carcinogenesis*, 1992 **13** 95–100.

14. EATON D L, GALLAGHER E P, 'Mechanism of Aflatoxin Carcinogenesis,' *Annu Rev Pharmacol Toxicol*, 1994 **34** 135–172.
15. EATON D L, BAMMLER T K, KELLY E J, 'Interindividual differences in response to chemoprotection against aflatoxin-induced hepatocarcinogenesis: implications for human biotransformation enzyme polymorphisms,' *Adv Exp Med Bio*, 2001 **500** 559–576.
16. EATON D L, RAMSDELL H S, NEAL G E, 'Biotransformation of aflatoxins,' in Eaton D L, Groopman J D, *The Toxicology of Aflatoxin: Human Health, Veterinary, and Agricultural Significance*, San Diego, Academic Press, Inc., 45–71, 1994.
17. GUENGERICH F P, JOHNSON W W, UENG Y F, YAMAZAKI H, SHIMADA T, 'Involvement of cytochrome P450, glutathione S-transferase, and epoxide hydrolase in the metabolism of aflatoxin B1 and relevance to risk of human liver cancer,' *Environ Health Perspect*, 1996 **104**(Suppl. 3) 557–562.
18. KENSLER T W, EGNER P A, WANG J B, ZHU Y R, ZHANG B C, QIAN G S, KUANG S Y, GANGE S J, JACOBSON L P, MUNOZ A, GROOPMAN J D, 'Strategies for chemoprevention of liver cancer,' *Eur J Cancer Prev*, 2002 **Suppl 2** S58–64.
19. ANDERSON K E, SINHA R, KULLDORFF M, GROSS M, LANG N P, BARBER C, HARNACK L, DIMAGNO E, BLISS R, KADLUBAR F F, 'Meat intake and cooking techniques: associations with pancreatic cancer,' *Mutat Res*, 2002 **506–507** 225–231.
20. ZHENG W, GUSTAFSON D R, SINHA R, CERHAN J R, MOORE D, HONG C P, ANDERSON K, KUSHI L H, SELLERS T A, FOLSOM A R, 'Well-done meat intake and the risk of breast cancer,' *J Natl Cancer Inst*, 1998 **90** 1724–1729.
21. BUTLER L M, SINHA R, MILLIKAN R C, MARTIN C F, NEWMAN B, GAMMON M D, AMMERMAN A S, SANDLER R S, 'Heterocyclic amines, meat intake, and association with colon cancer in a population-based study,' *Am J Epidemiol*, 2003 **157** 434–445.
22. SINHA R, KULLDORFF M, CHOW W, DENOBILE J, ROTHMAN N, 'Dietary intake of heterocyclic amines, meat-derived mutagenic activity, and risk of colorectal adenomas,' *Cancer Epidemiol Biomarkers Prev*, 2001 **10** 559–562.
23. AUGUSTSSON K, SKOG K, JäGERSTAD M, DICKMAN P W, STEINECK G, 'Dietary heterocyclic amines and cancer of the colon, rectum, bladder, and kidney: a population-based study,' *Lancet*, 1999 **353** 703–707.
24. MUSCAT J E, WYNDER E L, 'The consumption of well-done, grilled red meat and the risk of colorectal cancer,' *Am J Public Health*, 1994 **84** 856–858.
25. KAMPMAN E, SLATTERY M L, BIGLER J, LEPPERT M, SAMOWITZ W, CAAN B J, POTTER J D, 'Meat consumption, genetic susceptibility, and colon cancer risk: a United States multicenter case-control study,' *Cancer Epidemiol Biomarkers Prev*, 1999 **8** 15–24.
26. DELFINO R J, SINHA R, SMITH C, WEST J, WHITE E, LIN H J, LIAO S Y, GIM J S, MA H L, BUTLER J, ANTON-CULVER H, 'Breast cancer, heterocyclic aromatic amines from meat and N-acetyltransferase genotype,' *Carcinogenesis*, 2000 **21** 607–615.
27. GERTIG D M, HANKINSON S E, HOUGH H, SPIEGELMAN,D, COLDITZ G A, WILLETT W C, KELSEY K T, HUNTER D J, 'N-acetyl transferase 2 genotypes, meat intake and breast cancer risk,' *Int J Cancer*, 1999 **80** 13–17.
28. SINHA R, ROTHMAN N, SALMON C P, KNIZE M G, BROWN E D, SWANSON C A, RHODES D, ROSSI S, FELTON J S, LEVANDER O A, 'Heterocyclic amine content of beef cooked by different methods to varying degrees of doneness and gravy made from meat drippings,' *Food Chem Toxicol*, 1998 **36** 279–287.
29. BOOBIS A R, LYNCH A M, MURRAY S, DE LA TORRE R, SOLANS A, FARRE M, SEGURA J,

GOODERHAM N J, DAVIES D S, 'CYP1A2–catalyzed conversion of dietary heterocyclic amines to their proximate carcinogens is their major route of metabolism in humans,' *Cancer Res*, 1994 **54** 89–94.

30. MALFATTI M A, FELTON J S, 'N-glucuronidation of 2-amino-1-methyl-6-phenylimidazo[4,5-b]pyridine (PhIP) and N-hydroxy-PhIP by specific human UDP-glucuronosyltransferases,' *Carcinogenesis*, 2001 **22** 1087–1093.
31. BUONARATI M H, TRUTELTAUB K W, SHEN N H, FELTON J S, 'Role of sulfation and acetylation in the activation of 2-amino-1-methyl-6-phenyl-midazo[4,5-b]pyridine to intermediates which bind DNA,' *Mutat Res*, 1990 **245** 185–190.
32. OZAWA S, CHOU H, KADLUBAR F F, NAGATA K, YAMAZOE Y, KATO R, 'Activation of 2-hydroxyamino-1-methyl-6-phenylimidazo[4,5-b]pyridine by cDNA-expressed human and rat arylsulfotransferases,' *Jpn J Cancer Res*, 1994 **85** 1220–1228.
33. HEIN D W, 'Molecular genetics and function of NAT1 and NAT2: role in aromatic amine metabolism and carcinogenesis,' *Mutat Res*, 2002 **506–507** 65–77.
34. BENJAMIN H, STORKSON J, NAGAHARA A, PARIZA M W, 'Inhibition of benzo(a)pyrene-induced forestomach neoplasia by dietary soy sauce,' *Cancer Res*, 1991 **51** 2940–2942.
35. WEYAND E H, CHEN Y C, WU Y, KOGANTI A, DUNSFORD H A, RODRIGUEZ L V, 'Differences in the tumorigenic activity of a pure hydrocarbon and a complex mixture following ingestion: benzo[a]pyrene vs manufactured gas plant residue,' *Chem Res Toxicol*, 1995 **8** 949–954.
36. CULP S J, GAYLOR D W, SHELDON W G, GOLDSTEIN L S, BELAND F A, 'A comparison of the tumors induced by coal tar and benzo[a]pyrene in a 2-year bioassay,' *Carcinogenesis*, 1998 **19** 117–124.
37. SINGH S V, BENSON P J, HU X, PAL A, XIA H, SRIVASTAVA S K, AWASTHI S, ZAREN H A, ORCHARD J L, AWASTHI Y C, 'Gender-related differences in susceptibility of A/J mouse to benzo[a]pyrene-induced pulmonary and forestomach tumorigenesis,' *Cancer Lett*, 1998 **128** 197–204.
38. TRIOLO A J, APONTE G E, HERR D L, 'Induction of aryl hydrocarbon hydroxylase and forestomach tumors ben benzo(a)pyrene,' *Cancer Res*, 1977 **37** 3018–3021.
39. STONER G D, GREISIGER E A, SCHUT H A, PEREIRA M A, LEOB T R, KLAUNIG J E, BRANSTETTER D G, 'A comparison of the lung adenoma response in strain A/J mice after intraperitoneal and oral administration of carcinogens,' *Toxicol Appl Pharmacol*, 1984 **72** 313–323.
40. IARC, *IARC monographs on the evaluation of the carcinogenic risk of chemicals to humans. Polynuclear aromatic compounds, Part 1, Chemical, Environmental, and Experimental Data. Vol. 32*, Lyon, International Agency for Research on Cancer, 1983.
41. GELBOIN H V, 'Benzo[a]pyrene metabolism, activation, and carcinogenesis: role and regulation of mixed-function oxidases and related enzymes,' *Physiol Rev*, 1980 **60** 1107–1166.
42. PELKONEN O, NEBERT D W, 'Metabolism of polycyclic aromatic hydrocarbons: etiologic role in carcinogenesis,' *Pharmacol Rev*, 1982 **34** 189–222.
43. CONNEY A H, 'Induction of microsomal enzymes by foreign chemicals and carcinogenesis by polycyclic aromatic hydrocarbons,' *Cancer Res*, 1982 **42** 4875–4917.
44. CORTESSIS V, SIEGMUND K, CHEN Q, ZHOU N, DIEP A, FRANKL H, LEE E, ZHU Q, HAILE R, LEVY D, 'A case-control study of microsomal epoxide hydrolase, smoking, meat consumption, glutathione S-transferase M3, and risk of colorectal adenomas,'

Cancer Res, 2001 **61** 2381–2385.

45. SRIVASTAVA S K, XIA H, PAL A, HU X, GUO J, SING S V, 'Potentiation of benzo[a]pyrene pulmonary and forestomach tumorigenesis in mice by D,L-buthionine-S,R-sulfoximine-mediated tissue glutathione depletion,' *Cancer Lett*, 2000 **153** 35–39.
46. SHIMADA T, ODA Y, GILLAM E M J, GUENGERICH F G, INOUE K, 'Metabolic activation of polycyclic aromatic hydrocarbons and other procarcinogens by cytochromes P450 1A1 and P450 1B1 alellic variants and other human cytochromes P450 in Salmonella typhimurium NM2009,' *Drug Metab Dispos*, 2001 **29** 1176–1182.
47. LIJINSKY W, 'N-nitroso compounds in the diet,' *Mutat Res*, 1999 **443** 129–138.
48. TANNENBAUM S R, 'Endogenous formation of N-nitroso compounds: a current perspective,' in *Relevance of N-nitroso Compounds to Human Cancer: Exposures and Mechanisms*. 1987, Lyon, International Agency for Research on Cancer, 292–296, 1987.
49. MIWA M, STUEHR D J, MARLETTA M A, WISHNOK J S, TANNENBAUM S R, 'Nitrosation of amines by stimulated macrophages,' *Carcinogenesis* (Lond.), 1987 **8** 955–958.
50. BOGOVSKI P, BOGOVSKI S, 'Animal species in which N-nitroso compounds induce cancer,' *Int J Cancer*, 1981 **27** 471–474.
51. SCHMAHL D, HABS M, 'Carcinogenicity of N-nitroso compounds. Species and route differences in regard to organotropism,' *Oncology*, 1980 **37** 237–242.
52. MIRVISH S S, 'Role of N-nitroso compounds (NOC) and N-nitrosation in etiology of gastric, esophageal, nasopharyngeal and bladder cancer and contribution to cancer of known exposures to NOC,' *Cancer Lett*, 1995 **93** 17–48.
53. BARTSCH H, 'N-nitroso compounds and human cancer: where do we stand?,' in *Relevance to human cancer of N-nitroso compounds, tobacco smoke and mycotoxins,* Lyon, International Agency for Research on Cancer, 1–10, 1991.
54. ROGERS M A M, VAUGHAN T L, DAVIS S, THOMAS D B, 'Consumption of nitrate, nitrite, and nitrosodimethylamine and the risk of upper aerodigestive tract cancer,' *Cancer Epidemiol Biomarkers Prev*, 1995 **4** 29–36.
55. DE STEFANI E, DENEO-PELLEGRINI H, CARZOGLIO J C, RONCO A, MENDILAHARSU M, 'Dietary nitrosodimethylamine and the risk of lung cancer: a case-control study from Uruguay,' *Cancer Epidemiol Biomarkers Prev*, 1996 **5** 679–682.
56. KAMATAKI T, NUNOYA K, SAKAI Y, KUSHIDA H, FUJITA K, 'Genetic polymorphism of CYP2A6 in relation to cancer,' *Mutat Res*, 1999 **428** 125–130.
57. FUJITA K, KAMATAKI T, 'Role of human cytochrome P450 (CYP) in the metabolic activation of N-alkylnitrosamines: application of genetically engineered Salmonella typhimurium YG7108 expressing each from of CYP together with human NADPH-cytochrome P450 reductase,' *Mutat Res*, 2001 **483** 35–41.
58. KAMATAKI T, FUJITA K, NAKAYAMA K, YAMAZAKI Y, MIYAMOTO M, ARIYOSHI N, 'Role of human cytochrome P450 (CYP) in the metabolic activation of nitrosamine derivatives: application of genetically engineered Salmonella expressing human CYP,' *Drug Metabolism Reviews*, 2002 **34** 667–676.
59. LIN H L, PARSELS L A, MAYBAUM J, HOLLENBERG P F, 'N-nitrosodimethylamine-mediated cytotoxicity in a cell line expressing P450 2E1: evidence for apoptotic cell death,' *Toxicol Appl Pharmacol*, 1999 **157** 117–124.
60. CIOLINO H P, YEH G C, 'Inhibition of aryl hydrocarbon-induced cytochrome P-450 1A1 enzyme activity and CYP1A1 expression by resveratrol,' *Mol Pharmacol*, 1999 **56** 760–767.
61. JOE A K, LIU H, SUZUI M, VURAL M E, XIAO D, WEINSTEIN I B, 'Resveratrol induces growth inhibition, S-phase arrest, apoptosis, and changes in biomarker expression

in several human cancer cell lines,' *Clin Cancer Res*, 2002 **8** 893–903.

62. CAL C, GARBAN H, JAZIREHI A, YEH C, MIZUTANI Y, BONAVIDA B, 'Resveratrol and cancer: chemoprevention, apoptosis, and chemo-immunosensitizing activities,' *Curr Med Chem Anti-Canc Agents*, 2003 **3** 73–93.
63. TALALAY P, FAHEY J W, 'Phytochemicals from cruciferous plants protect against cancer by modulating carcinogen metabolism,' *J Nutr*, 2001 **131** 3027S–3033S.
64. VERHOEVEN D T, GOLDBOHM R A, VAN POPPEL G, VERHAGEN H, VAN DEN BRANDT P A, 'Epidemiological studies on brassica vegetables and cancer risk,' *Cancer Epidemiol Biomarkers Prev*, 1996 **5**(9) 733–748.
65. ZHANG Y, TALALAY P, 'Anticarcinogenic activities of organic isothiocyanates: chemistry and mechanisms,' *Cancer Res*, 1994 **54 (suppl.)** 1976s-1986s.
66. HECHT S S, 'Chemoprevention by isothiocyanates,' *J Cell Biochem*, 1995 **22** 195–209.
67. PANTUCK E J, PANTUCK C B, ANDERSON K E, WATTENBERG L W, CONNEY A H, KAPPAS A, 'Effect of Brussels sprouts and cabbage on drug conjugation,' *Clin Pharmacol Ther*, 1984 **35** 161–169.
68. HECHT S S, CARMELLA S G, MURPHY S E, 'Effects of watercress consumption on urinary metabolites of nicotine in smokers,' *Cancer Epidemiol Biomarkers Prev*, 1999 **8** 907–913.
69. ZHANG Y, TALALAY P, CHO C, POSNER G H, 'A major inducer of anticarcinogenic protective enzymes from broccoli: isolation and elucidation of structure,' *Proc Natl Acad Sci*, 1992 **89** 2399–2403.
70. MAHÉO K, MOREL F, LANGOUËT S, KRAMER H, LE FERREC E, KETTERER B, GUILLOUZO A, 'Inhibition of cytochromes P-450 and induction of glutathione S-transferases by sulforaphane in primary human and rat hepatocytes,' *Cancer Res,* 1997 **57** 3649–3652.
71. BASTEN G P, BAO Y, WILLIAMSON G, 'Sulforaphane and its glutathione conjugate but not sulforaphane nitrile induce UDP-glucuronosyl transferase (UGT1A1) and glutathione transferase (GSTA1) in cultured cells,' *Carcinogenesis*, 2002 **23** 1399–1404.
72. THIMMULAPPA R K, MAI K H, SRISUMA S, KENSLER T W, YAMAMOTO M, BISWAL S, 'Identification of Nrf2-regulated genes induced by the chemopreventive agent sulforaphane by oligonucleotide microarray,' *Cancer Res*, 2002 **62** 5196–5203.
73. KOCH W H, 'Psoralen photomutagenic specificity in Salmonella typhimurium,' *Mutat Res*, 1986 **160** 195–205.
74. BEIER R C, 'Natural pesticides and bioactive components in foods,' *Rev Environ Contam Toxicol*, 1990 **113** 47–137.
75. OGANESIAN A, HENDRICKS J D, PEREIRA C B, ORNER G A, BAILEY G S, WILLIAMS D E, 'Potency of dietary indole-3-carbinol as a promoter of aflatoxin B1-initiated hepatocarcinogenesis: results from a 9000 animal tumor study,' *Carcinogenesis*, 1999 **20**(3) 453–458.
76. DASHWOOD R H, XU M, 'The disposition and metabolism of 2-amino-3-methylimidazo-[4,5-f]quinoline in the F344 rat at high versus low doses of indole-3-carbinol,' *Food Chem Toxicol*, 2003 **41** 1185–1192.
77. XU M, ORNER G A, BAILEY G S, STONER G D, HORIO D T, DASHWOOD R H, 'Post-initiation effects of chlorophyllin and indole-3-carbinol in rats given 1,2-dimethylhydrazine or 2-amino-3-methyl-imidazo,' *Carcinogenesis*, 2001 **22** 309–314.
78. NAKAJIMA M, ORNER G A, BAILEY G S, STONER G D, HORIO D T, DASHWOOD R H, 'Phenotyping of CYP1A2 in Japanese population by analysis of caffeine urinary

metabolites: absence of mutation prescribing the phenotype in the CYP1A2 gene,' *Cancer Epidemiol Biomarkers Prev*, 1994 **3** 413–421.

79. YOKOI T, SAWADA M, KAMATAKI T, 'Polymorphic drug metabolism: studies with recombinant Chinese hamster cells and analyses in human populations,' *Pharmacogenetics*, 1995 **5** S65–S69.
80. MACLEOD S L, TANG Y, YOKOI T, 'The role of recently discovered genetic polymorphism in the regulation of the human CYP1A2 gene [abstract],' *Proc Am Assoc Cancer Res*, 1998 **39** 396.
81. NAKAJIMA M, YOKOI T, MIZUTANI M, KINOSHITA M, FUNAYAMA M, KAMATAKI T, 'Genetic polymorphism in the 5′-flanking region of human CYP1A2 gene: effect on the CYP1A2 inducibility in humans,' *J Biochem*, 1999 **125** 803–808.
82. INGELMAN-SUNDBERG M, DALY A K, NEBERT D W, 'Home Page of the Human Cytochrome P450 (CYP) Allele Nomenclature Committee,' http://www.imm.ki.se/CYPalleles/, 2003.
83. GAGO-DOMINGUEZ M, BELL D A, WATSON M A, YUAN J M, CASTELAO J E, HEIN D W, CHAN K K, COETZEE G A, ROSS R K, YU M C, 'Permanent hair dyes and bladder cancer: risk modification by cytochrome P4501A2 and N-acetyltransferases 1 and 2,' *Carcinogenesis*, 2003 **24** 483–489.
84. LANG N P, BUTLER M A, MASSENGILL J, LAWSON M, STOTTS R C, HAUER-JENSEN M, KADLUBAR F F, 'Rapid metabolic phenotypes for acetyltransferase and cytochrome P4501A2 and putative exposure to food-borne heterocyclic amines increase the risk for colorectal cancer or polyps,' *Cancer Epidemiol Biomarkers Prev*, 1994 **3** 675–682.
85. SACHSE C, BHAMBRA U, SMITH G, LIGHTFOOT T J, BARRETT J H, SCOLLAY J, GARNER R C, BOOBIS A R, WOLF C R, GOODERHAM N J, COLORECTAL CANCER STUDY GROUP, 'Polymorphisms in the cytochrome P450 CYP1A2 gene (CYP1A2) in colorectal cancer patients and controls: allele frequencies, linkage disequilibrium and influence on caffeine metabolism,' *Br J Clin Pharmacol*, 2003 **55** 68–76.
86. ISHIBE N, SINHA R, HEIN D W, KULLDORFF M, STRICKLAND P, FRETLAND A J, CHOW W H, KADLUBAR F F, LANG N P, ROTHMAN N, 'Genetic polymorphisms in heterocyclic amine metabolism and risk of colorectal adenomas,' *Pharmacogenetics*, 2002 **12** 145–150.
87. ZHOU W, LIU G, THURSTON S W, XU L L, MILLER D P, WAIN J C, LYNCH T J, SU L, CHRISTIANI D C, 'Genetic polymorphisms in N-acetyltransferase-2 and microsomal epoxide hydrolase, cumulative cigarette smoking, and lung cancer,' *Cancer Epidemiol Biomarkers Prev*, 2002 **11** 15–21.
88. MCGLYNN K A, ROSVOLD E A, LUSTBADER E D, HU Y, CLAPPER M L, ZHOU T, WILD C P, XIA X L, BAFFOE-BONNIE A, OFORI-ADJEI D, CHEN G C, LONDON W T, SHEN F M, BUETOW KH, 'Susceptibility to hepatocellular carcinoma is associated with genetic variation in the enzymatic detoxification of aflatoxin B1,' *Proc Natl Acad Sci*, 1995 **92** 2384–2387.
89. CHEN S Y, CHEN C J, TSAI W Y, AHSAN H, LIU T Y, LIN J T, SANTELLA R M, 'Associations of plasma aflatoxin B1–albumin adduct level with plasma selenium level and genetic polymorphisms of glutathione S-transferase M1 and T1,' *Nutr Cancer*, 2000 **38**(2) 179–185.
90. SUN C A, WANG L Y, CHEN C J, LU S N, YOU S L, WANG L W, WANG Q, WU D M, SANTELLA R M, 'Genetic polymorphisms of glutathione S-transferases M1 and T1 associated with susceptibility to aflatoxin-related hepatocarcinogenesis among chronic hepatitis B carriers: a nested case-control study in Taiwan,' *Carcinogenesis*,

2001 **22**(8) 1289–1294.

91. OMER R E, VERHOEF L, VEER P V, IDRIS M O, KADARU A M Y, KAMPMAN E, BUNSCHOTEN A, KOK F J, 'Peanut butter intake, GSTM1 genotype and hepatocellular carcinoma: a case-control study in Sudan,' *Cancer Causes and Control*, 2001 **12** 23–32.
92. CHEN J, STAMPFER M J, HOUGH H L, GARCIA-CLOSAS M, WILLETT W C, HENNEKENS C H, KELSEY K T, HUNTER D J, 'A prospective study of N-acetyltransferase genotype, red meat intake, and risk of colorectal cancer,' *Cancer Res*, 1998 **58** 3307–3311.
93. LIN H J, PROBST-HENSCH N M, LOUIE A D, KAU I H, WITTE J S, INGLES S A, FRANKL H D, LEE E R, HAILE R W, 'Glutathione transferase null genotype, broccoli, and lower prevalence of colorectal adenomas,' *Cancer Epidemiology, Biomarkers and Prevention*, 1998 **7** 647–652.
94. SLATTERY M L, KAMPMAN E, SAMOWITZ W, CAAN B J, POTTER J D, 'Interplay between dietary inducers of GST and the GSTM1-genotype in colon cancer,' *Int J Cancer*, 2000 **87** 728–733.
95. SPITZ M R, DUPHORNE C M, DETRY M A, PILLOW P C, AMOS C I, LEI L, DE ADRADE M, GU X, HONG W K, WU X, 'Dietary intake of isothiocyanates: evidence of a joint effect with glutathione S-transferase polymorphisms in lung cancer risk,' *Cancer Epidemiol Biomarkers Prev*, 2000 **9** 1017–1020.
96. LONDON S J, YUAN J M, CHUNG F L, GAO Y T, COETZEE G A, ROSS R K, YU M C, 'Isothiocyanates, glutathione S-transferase M1 and T1 polymorphisms, and lung-cancer risk: a prospective study of men in Shanghai, China,' *Lancet*, 2000 **356** 724–729.
97. ZHAO B, SEOW A, LEE E J, POH W T, THE M, ENG P, WANG Y T, TAN W C, YU M C, LEE H P, 'Dietary isothiocyanates, glutathione S-transferase -M1, T1 polymorphisms and lung cancer risk among Chinese women in Singapore,' *Cancer Epidemiol Biomarkers Prev*, 2001 **10** 1063–1067.
98. MACLEOD S, SINHA R, KADLUBAR F F, LANG N P, 'Polymorphisms of CYP1A1 and GSTM1 influence the in vivo function of CYP1A2,' *Mol Pharmacol*, 1997 **376** 135–142.
99. PROBST-HENSCH N M, TANNENBAUM S R, CHAN K K, COETZEE G A, ROSS R K, YU M C, 'Absence of the glutathione S-transferase M1 gene increases cytochrome P450 1A2 activity among frequent consumers of cruciferous vegetables in a Caucasian population,' *Cancer Epidemiol Biomarkers Prev*, 1998 **7** 635–638.
100. SINHA R, ROTHMAN N, MARK S D, MURRAY S, BROWN E D, LEVANDER O A, DAVIES D S, LANG N P, KADLUBAR F F, HOOVER R N, 'Lower levels of urinary 2-amino-3,8-dimethylimidazo[4,5-f]-quinoxaline (MeIQx) in humans with higher CYP1A2 activity,' *Carcinogenesis*, 1995 **16** 2859–2861.
101. LAMPE J W, CHEN C, LI S, PRUNTY J, GRATE M T, MEEHAN D E, BARALE K V, DIGHTMAN D A, FENG Z, POTTER J D, 'Modulation of human glutathione S-transferases by botanically defined vegetable diets,' *Cancer Epidemiol Biomarkers Prev*, 2000 **9** 787–793.
102. INGELMAN-SUNDBERG M, 'Polymorphism of cytochrome P450 and xenobiotic toxicity,' *Toxicology*, 2002 **181–182** 447–452.
103. EATON D L, BAMMLER T K, 'Concise review of the glutathione S-transferases and their significance to toxicology,' *Toxicol Sci*, 1999 **49** 156–164.
104. GLATT H, BOEING H, ENGELKE C E, MA L, KUHLOW A, PABEL U, POMPLUN D, TEUBNER W, MEINL W, 'Human cytosolic sulphotransferases: genetics, characteristics, toxicological aspects,' *Mutat Res*, 2001 **482** 27–40.
105. TUKEY R H, STRASSBURG C P, 'Human UDP-glucuronosyltransferases: metabolism,

expression, and disease,' *Annu Rev Pharmacol Toxicol*, 2000 **40** 581–616.
106. OMIECINSKI C J, HASSETT C, HOSAGRAHARA V, 'Epoxide hydrolase–polymorphism and role in toxicology,' *Toxicol Lett*, 2000 **112–113** 365–370.

3

Assessing the mutagenicity of chemicals in food: the case of pesticides

J. M. Parry, University of Wales–Swansea, UK

3.1 Introduction: mutagenicity test programmes

The interaction of chemical or physical agents with the genetic material (i.e. the DNA of the nucleus or mitochondria) and/or components of cell division cycle can result in the production of modifications of individual genes or the structure and number of chromosomes of an exposed organism. Modifications of genes and/or chromosomes have been implicated in the development of cancer and the production of aberrant gametes and thus to inherited disease (for review see COM 2000). The aims of mutagenicity test programmes are to detect any potential hazard at an early stage in compound development, and to evaluate whether this hazard represents an actual risk to exposed individuals and populations.

Test system development can be considered to have involved the design and application of experimental models which

- have a high sensitivity and are capable of detecting potential mutagenic hazards (such test systems primarily involve the use of *in vitro* models),
- evaluate whether the hazard is reproduced under relevant exposure conditions and provide measures of risk under various exposure scenarios (such test systems primarily involve the use of *in vivo* models).

In the case of chemical residues that may be present in foods, the critical question is whether such residues represent a quantifiable risk to exposed populations. Routine analysis of foods performed by regulatory bodies indicates the presence of pesticides in various foods (FDA 2003) and thus, the need to ensure that exposure to such residues does not represent a significant risk to the human population.

Concern over the potential mutagenicity of chemicals such as pesticides and their potential effect on human health has resulted in the development of more than 90 test systems. Many of the test systems are better described as 'genotoxicity test systems' because they evaluate the induction of endpoints broader than those which directly lead to the production of inherited changes in the genetic material of a cell. The methods developed range from the use of viruses to those involving intact rodents and cover both the measurement of mutagenic activity itself and a range of indirect endpoints such as DNA adduct formation, DNA repair activity and the production of chromosomally aberrant rodent embryos. Table 3.1 illustrates the variety of test methods which have been approved by the European Union for the assessment of the mutagenicity of chemicals including pesticides. Many of these assays currently have only a limited usage and/or may only be available in a few laboratories.

A consequence of the proliferation of test systems was their application (with varying levels of quality control) to investigate the potential mutagenicity of various types of pesticides including both the individual active ingredients and various commercial preparations. For example, the fungicide carbendazim has been evaluated for mutagenic potential in more than 30 assay systems and the herbicide chlorpropham in more than 50 assay systems. A consequence of these studies has been the development of compound data sets which show confusing patterns of positive and negative results. In such cases, the regulator is faced with drawing conclusions based upon conflicting data and in doing so assessing the relative importance of results derived from different assay systems. It has thus become important to provide guidance on an effective strategy for the mutagenicity testing of chemicals such as pesticides which recommends the most relevant assays and where they should be utilized in chemical assessment programmes.

Table 3.1 The genotoxicity tests listed in EU Directive 6/548 Annex V

B.10	Mutagenicity – *in vitro* mammalian chromosome aberration test
B.11	Mutagenicity – *in vitro* mammalian bone marrow chromosome aberration test
B.12	Mutagenicity mammalian erythrocyte micronucleus test
B.13/14	Mutagenicity – reverse mutation test using bacteria
B.15	Gene mutation – *Saccharomyces cerevisae*
B.16	Mitotic recombination – *Saccharomyces cerevisae*
B.17	Mutagenicity – *in vitro* mammalian cell gene mutation test
B.18	DNA damage and repair – unscheduled DNA synthesis – mammalian cells *in vitro*
B.19	Sister chromatid exchange assay *in vitro*
B.20	Sex-linked recessive lethal test in *Drosophila melanogaster*
B.21	*In vitro* mammalian cell transformation test
B.22	Rodent dominant lethal test
B.23	Mammalian spermatogonial chromosome aberration test
B.24	Mouse spot test
B.25	Mouse heritable translocation
B.39	Unscheduled DNA synthesis (UDS) test with mammalian liver cells *in vivo*

3.2 Criteria for the testing of pesticides

When evaluating the potential mutagenic activity of a pesticide there are two prime considerations:

1. Which assay systems should be selected for use?
2. How can the selected test systems be used to develop an effective, efficient and cost-effective testing strategy which is capable of detecting most if not all potential mutagens and indicate whether any activity detected is biologically relevant to non-target (in the case of pesticides) species including humans?

The aims of mutagenicity testing programmes can be varied but I have focused here upon the development and application of a testing strategy which is

- capable of detecting intrinsic mutagenic hazard, an exercise which can primarily be based upon the use of *in vitro* test systems,
- capable of determining whether mutagenic hazard detected *in vitro* is also reproduced *in vivo* and
- if mutagenic potential is detected *in vivo* whether the activity represents a potential quantifiable risk to somatic cells such as the development of cancer and/or to germ cells such as an elevation in inherited defects.

The development of effective testing programmes requires a strategy which primarily utilizes assay systems which have a number of key properties.

- They are well validated, preferably at the international level.
- The methods are widely used and have a large database for comparative purposes.
- The methods are well characterized in terms of their sensitivity and reliability.
- The methods have a high sensitivity and thus they detect most if not all of the potential mutagenic hazards.
- The methods have a high level of specificity and thus avoid the generation of false positive results.

When deciding upon the most appropriate test system, an ideal balance between specificity and sensitivity can be difficult to achieve. In general, it is most convenient to use assay systems of high sensitivity at an early stage of testing. However, it is important to appreciate that not all mutagenic activity detectable in the high sensitivity *in vitro* systems represents a hazard and risk to intact animals including humans.

3.3 Selecting appropriate tests

In 2000 the UK Advisory Committee on the Mutagenicity of Chemicals in Food, Consumer Products and the Environment (COM) initiated an exercise to develop a strategy for mutagenicity testing which involved a review of the application of the currently available test systems which could be considered suitable for the assessment of a wide range of chemicals (including pesticides). The conclusions of this evaluation exercise were published in December 2000 (COM 2000). As indicated earlier, potentially more than 90 assay methods can be used to identify the genotoxic hazard of chemicals. However, the COM decided that it should develop a strategy of mutagenicity testing based upon the use of a limited number of well validated and informative test systems.

A key feature in the selection and application of mutagenicity test systems is that they should be capable of providing information on the three basic levels of mutation which are of relevance to both the induction of cancer and birth defects:

1. gene or point mutations
2. clastogenicity, the induction of structural chromosome aberrations
3. aneugenicity, the induction of numerical chromosome aberrations.

This selection of mutagenicity endpoints is more focused and biologically relevant than those covered by the term genotoxicity, which has generally been used to cover any effect which has the potential to modify the integrity of the genome.

The mutagenicity testing strategy developed by the COM is based upon three basic stages.

1. *Stage 1* – The *in vitro* evaluation of the potential of a chemical to induce point or gene mutations and the induction of chromosome aberrations of structure and number.
2. *Stage 2* – The *in vivo* testing of the chemical in somatic cells with two aims, namely to determine whether *in vitro* activity is reproduced *in vivo*, and to determine whether a chemical has *in vivo* mutagenic activity which was not detected under *in vitro* test conditions.
3. *Stage 3* – *In vivo* testing of the chemical in germ cells to determine whether *in vivo* somatic cell activity is reproduced in germ cells and thus represents a potential to induce inherited defects.

Stage 1 tests can in many cases be used to determine the mechanism of mutagenic activity of a test chemical but are not appropriate for the quantification of risk. The assessment of risk is dependent upon the application using appropriate numbers of animals in the Stage 2 and 3 test systems.

The separation of the stages of mutagenicity testing is important as the European Union Directive 93/21/EEC classifies mutagenic hazard into three basic categories:

- **Category 1: 90**. These are substances known to be mutagenic to man. There is sufficient evidence to establish a causal association between human exposure to a substance and heritable genetic damage.
- **Category 2: 91**. These are substances which should be regarded as if they are mutagenic to man. There is sufficient evidence to provide a strong

presumption that human exposure to the substance may result in the development of heritable genetic damage, generally on the basis of:
  - appropriate animal studies
  - other relevant information.
- **Category 3: 93**. These are substances which cause concern for man owing to possible mutagenic effects. There is evidence of activity from appropriate mutagenicity studies but it is insufficient to place the substance in Category 2.

The mutagenicity testing strategy developed by the COM will provide information relating to the European Union classification categories in a step-wise manner by following the three stages of testing.

3.3.1 Stage 1: The *in vitro* methodologies recommended by the COM

(1) Bacterial tests for the measurement of induced gene mutation

The use of bacterial assays for gene mutations (point, insertions, deletions) using specialised strains of *Salmonella typhimurium* and/or *Escherichia coli*. The tests should be performed in the presence and absence of an exogenous source of mammalian metabolic activity (generally liver S9 mix from a rat treated with an enzyme inducing preparation).

(2) Tests for the measurement of clastogenicity and aneugenicity

The current methodology recommended by the Organisation for Economic Cooperation and Development (OECD) involves the analysis of metaphase cells generated from cell cultures derived from permanent cell lines (generally from Chinese hamster cultures) or from human lymphocytes from an 'appropriate' (e.g. no previous mutagen exposure) donor (OECD 1997). These assays provide information on changes in the structure and number of chromosomes.

(3) Mammalian cell mutation assay

Although a range of point or gene mutations assays are available, the COM expressed its preference for the mouse lymphoma L5178Y assay which measures the induction of drug resistance due to homozygosity of defective alleles of the thymidine kinase gene. This assay has been validated extensively and has adequate 'statistical power' to allow the detection of weak mutagenic activity.

In the case of the selection of an *in vitro* assay for the detection of the potential clastogenicity and aneugenicity of chemicals, the COM expressed a preference for the use of the *in vitro* binucleate cell micronucleus assay originally developed by Fenech and colleagues (Fenech *et al.* 1999). In this assay, cultures treated with a test pesticide undergo nuclear division in the presence of the actin inhibitor cytochalasin B which prevents the completion of cytokinesis and thus produce binucleate cells. Micronuclei are produced by chromosome breakage (clastogenicity) or the failure of individual chromosomes to segregate to either of the two nuclei of the binucleate cells (chromosome loss as an indicator of induced aneuploidy). Micronuclei containing acentric chromosome fragments (produced by breakage) can be distinguished from those containing whole chromosomes (produced by chromosome loss) by the use of an antibody to the kinetochore protein present at the centromere of the segregating chromosome or by using molecular probes for the centromere region itself. The *in vitro* binucleate cell assay can also be used to measure the induction of the malsegregation of chromosomes leading to non-disjunction which produces nuclei which contain either a missing or an extra chromosome by the use of centromere probes for specific chromosomes. The combination of the various developments of the *in vitro* binucleate cell assay provides a powerful tool for the identification of clastogenic and aneugenic (both chromosome loss and non-disjunction) activity *in vitro*.

Not all positive responses detected in the *in vitro* test systems can be considered biologically relevant to intact animals. For example, positive results in cytogenetic assays in cultured mammalian cells may have been detected only at high toxic doses which could not be achieved in any tissue of an intact animal. The significance of positive responses under such test conditions should be evaluated using appropriate expertise. For each test system for which an OECD guideline is available recommendations for maximum test concentrations have been made. Following such guidance can substantially reduce the generation of 'false positive' results.

3.3.2 Stage 2: Strategy for the *in vivo* testing of pesticides in somatic cells

Following *in vitro* Stage 1 testing of a pesticide, the assessor can be presented with three potential outcomes in any of the test systems used:

1. a positive response
2. a negative response
3. an equivocal response.

Stage 2 of testing involves the evaluation of the three responses in the somatic tissue of an intact rodent.

In the case of a positive response the question is 'whether the *in vitro* activity is also produced *in vivo*'. There are a number of reasons why *in vitro* positives may not be reproducible *in vivo* such as effective detoxification in an intact animal and the inability to reproduce conditions such as high dose toxicity at target sites. Detailed consideration including expert advice of the *in vitro* data at this stage can result in a considerable saving in animal usage and clarification as to whether the *in vitro* response observed is relevant to the overall toxicological profile of a compound.

In the case of a negative response *in vitro*, the primary consideration is whether there is some deficiency in the *in vitro* assay such as a lack of appropriate activating enzymes which could lead to a failure to detect potential *in vivo* activity. In the case of a pesticide for which there may be human exposure via operator use or via residues in the diet then confirmation of negative mutagenic activity will require *in vivo* studies to confirm the lack of *in vitro* activity.

In the case of an equivocal response *in vitro,* it is generally unproductive to undertake further *in vitro* studies if the data from the recommended package of *in vitro* tests is available and consideration has been made of factors such as high dose toxicity. In such a case, *in vivo* testing is most likely to produce clarifying data. However, the selection of an appropriate *in vivo* strategy should be based upon expert judgement of the nature of the equivocal response. For example, if only equivocal results have been obtained in a bacterial gene mutation tester strain, then clarification of the response would not be helped by studying clastogenic activity in an intact rodent by, for example, using the rodent bone marrow micronucleus assay (see later).

When the decision is made to test a pesticide for potential mutagenic activity *in vivo* this should be influenced by the available *in vitro* database. In most cases the *in vivo* test of first choice will be the rodent bone marrow micronucleus assay. This test measures the induction of micronuclei (see earlier in the discussion of the *in vitro* assay) in the newly formed erythrocytes of the bone marrow, a tissue which is accessible to a wide range of chemicals. The induction of micronuclei in the rodent bone marrow indicates that a test chemical has aneugenic and/or clastogenic activity. These two activities can be identified by the use of kinetochore or centromere staining (see earlier) to distinguish between micronuclei containing whole chromosomes and/or fragments.

In the case of a pesticide that was either negative or equivocal *in vitro* then a negative result in a rodent bone marrow micronucleus assay which is supported by data confirming that the substance had reached the tissue would provide reassurance of a lack of mutagenic activity. However, in the case of a pesticide with mutagenic activity *in vitro* a negative result in a bone marrow micronucleus might not provide sufficient reassurance of a lack of activity *in vivo* and information will be required from another test system which measures genotoxic potential using a different endpoint or target tissue.

The selection of a second *in vivo* test system should be based upon expert consideration of a range of factors such as the profile of the *in vitro* response(s), known or postulated metabolism and potential target tissues (for example site-of-contact activity only).

Of the available second *in vivo* somatic assays the choice of a method capable of detecting mutagenic endpoints covers cytogenetic (including micronucleus assays) in proliferating tissues, gene mutation assays using transgenic rodents such as Big Blue™ and Muta™ mouse (reviewed by Schmezer and Eckert 1999) and the analysis of mutation frequencies at specific sites within genes such as restriction enzyme recognition sites (Jenkins *et al.* 1999). In the case of the second *in vivo* assay the choice can be extended to include indirect genotoxicity assays. These include methods which measure:

- an indication of DNA damage directly – such as the Comet assay and DNA unwinding
- DNA adduct formation – such as P^{32} post-labelling, covalent binding and mass spectrometer analysis for the quantification of modified nucleotides
- DNA repair activity such as the induction of unscheduled DNA synthesis (UDS) assay in the liver of rats.

The rat liver UDS assay has been widely used as an indirect measure of potential mutagenic activity in an organ responsible for the metabolism of an extensive range of pesticides and is described in OECD Guideline 486.

If a pesticide has been shown to be mutagenic *in vivo* then it is reasonable to assume that it will also be capable of inducing mutations in germ cells and that there is little to be gained from performing germ cell studies. In those cases where negative results have been obtained in both a comprehensive range of *in vitro* test systems and in a recommended *in vivo* assay, it has generally been considered that there is no need to extend testing to germ cells, i.e. Stage 3 of the COM strategy. However, this situation may not continue as on theoretical grounds one might predict the existence of substances which interact with cell targets unique to germ cell production such as the pairing of chromosomes during the first division of germ cells meiosis. It can be expected that the development of techniques such as gene expression analysis (see later) may result in the detection of interactions with specific genes whose activities are involved in potential cellular targets, for example gene products active in mitosis and meiosis which may indicate a requirement for the analysis of germ cell effects.

It has generally been assumed that those chemicals which produce negative results in somatic *in vivo* micronucleus assays will not be capable of inducing a positive response in rodent germ cells (Adler and Ashby 1989, Waters *et al.* 1994, Shelby 1996, Tinwell *et al.* 2001, Ashby and Tinwell 2001). Thus, even when positive results have been produced *in vitro*, a negative *in vivo* result in somatic tissue would indicate that there is no need to undertake germ cell studies. This assumption requires reconsideration following the demonstration by Chaplin *et al.* (1995) that *N*-hydroxymethylacrylamide produced a positive response in the dominant lethal gene cell assay. This positive response was produced in spite of negative results of *N*-hydroxymethylacrylamide in comprehensive mouse bone marrow micronucleus studies (Witt *et al.* 2003). A similar profile of negative bone marrow results but positive female germ cell results also appears to be true for the plastics component bisphenol A (Hunt *et al.* 2003).

3.3.3 Stage 3: Strategy for the *in vivo* testing of pesticides in germ cells

A decision to undertake germ cell testing will in most cases be based on the results obtained in the various assays recommended for Stage 1 and 2 testing. However, there are situations where data derived from other forms of toxicological testing (e.g. reproductive toxicity testing) indicates that germ cell effect may be predicted. Currently, the assays routinely available for the analysis of germ cell effects are limited to male rodents. However, developments are taking place which enable the analysis of female specific effects by the analysis of effects upon rodent oocytes chemically treated either *in vitro* or *in vivo* (Yin *et al.* 1998, Hunt *et al.* 2003).

The available test systems for the measurement of germ cell effects include assays which measure the induction of a range of genotoxic endpoints. If germ cell studies are performed because of positive results observed in somatic cells, then it is important that the correct test system is selected which measures a genetic endpoint which corresponds to that observed in somatic cells. For example, there is no value in following up the observation of the unique induction of gene mutations in somatic cells with the measurement of chromosome aberrations in germ cells.

The currently available methods for the analysis of mutagenic effects in germ cells include the measurement of the following endpoints:

1. Clastogenic effects in spermatogonial cells described in OECD Guideline 483.
2. Micronuclei in spermatocytes.
3. Aneuploidy in sperm using chromosome specific molecular probes.
4. Dominant lethal effects in rodents following the mating of treated males mated with untreated females, described in OECD Guideline 478 (OECD 1984).
5. Gene mutations in transgenic rodents.

Assays 1 to 5 provide evidence of mutagenic hazard in male germ cells. Indirect evidence of DNA interaction can be obtained using methods such as the P^{32} post-labelling assay for the quantification of DNA adduct formation. However, the demonstration of DNA adduct formation in male germ cells does not provide unambiguous evidence that the adducts detected will produce mutations in germ cells. Such adduct formation requires confirmation in an assay system which measures a mutagenic response.

In those cases where human exposure has been shown to have occurred to a pesticide which is a germ cell mutagen there may be a case for providing an estimate of the risks of such exposure. The risk assessment of germ cell mutations can currently be obtained by the application of two methodologies:

1. The specific locus assay which involves the exposure of male mice to a test substance, mating to untreated females over the period of spermatogenesis and the quantification of mutations present in offspring. The assay provides a measure of the production of gene mutations for characters such as coat and eye colour.
2. The heritable translocation assay, which measures the production of clastogenic effects by the detection and quantification of broken and rearranged chromosomes which are transmitted to embryos.

Both assays involve the use of large numbers of animals and their usage can only be justified in special circumstances. In the future the application of transgenic animal models (see later) should provide estimates of risks of germ cell mutagenicity.

3.4 Assessing dose-response relationships

Following the identification of a potential hazard, the estimation of risk requires the generation of detailed dose response. In most areas of toxicology experience has demonstrated that exposure doses can be determined below which no toxicological effects can be detected and no observable effect levels (NOEL) can be determined and thresholds of activity estimated. However, when mutagenic activity has been detected it has generally been assumed that mutagenic response is directly related to exposure dose and that it is precautionary to assume a linear dose relationship for the production of mutations, i.e. no threshold of activity can be assumed. However, as our understanding increases concerning the mechanisms of mutagenesis of an increasing range of chemicals, it has become clear that there are a range of interactions which may modify the dose-response relationships.

In the case of DNA reactive chemicals, the activity of a test chemical may be modified by the cellular metabolic events of the intact animal such as phase II conjugations leading to deactivation and potentially to excretion before the chemical can interact with target cells and produce DNA reactions which may lead to mutagenic changes. Even when DNA adducts are produced they may be repaired before they are processed into mutations. The potential interactions which may modify the dose-response relationships of DNA reactive chemicals are illustrated in Fig. 3.1. If the mechanisms of compound deactivation and DNA adduct repair can be demonstrated, then it would be reasonable to assume that thresholds of mutagenic activity exist and NOELs may be determined experimentally.

There are also mutagenic chemicals which produce their effects by interacting with cellular targets other than DNA. Examples of such chemicals include chemicals which modify the cell division spindle apparatus (e.g. the fungicide carbendazim) and induce aneuploidy, and inhibitors of the topoisomerase enzymes involved in the winding and unwinding of DNA which can produce both numerical and structural chromosome changes. In both cases the presence of multiple cellular targets which require inactivation to produce genetic changes also suggests that threshold dose-response relationships can be determined (Parry *et al.* 1994). In the case of a pesticide which induces aneuploidy by interactions with the spindle apparatus, a strategy can be developed which would allow the experimental demonstration of thresholds of activity. Such a strategy of testing is illustrated in Fig. 3.2.

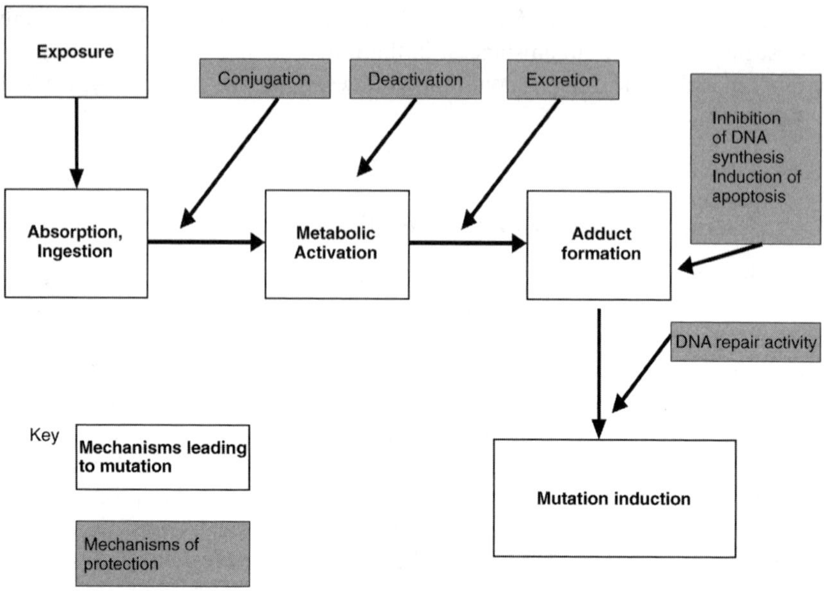

Fig. 3.1 Potential reasons which may lead to thresholds of activity for DNA reactive pesticides.

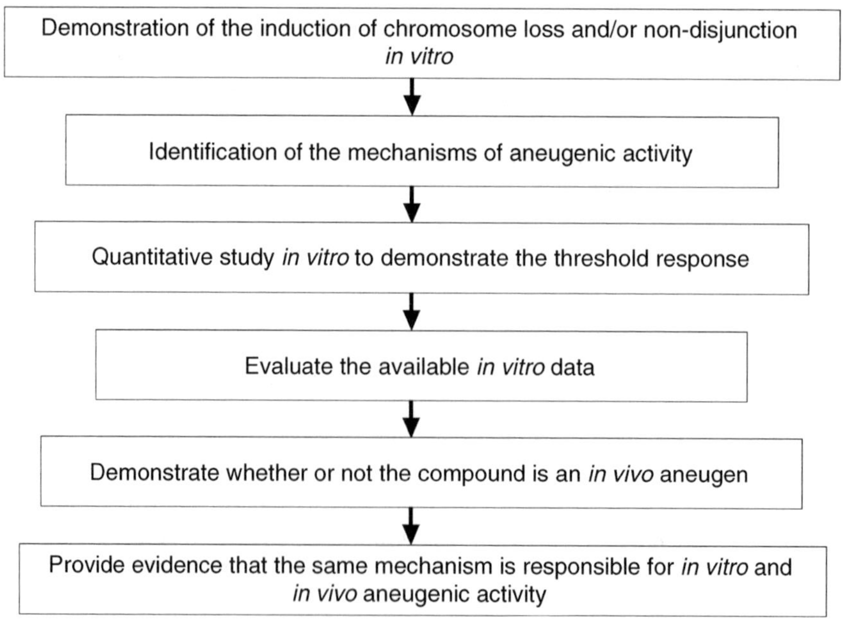

Fig. 3.2 Demonstrating a threshold response for an aneugenic pesticide.

3.5 Developing test methodologies

3.5.1 The application of toxicogenomics

The increasing availability of information concerning the role of specific genes and their protein products on the activity of cells and intact organisms has led to the development of a series of related methodologies grouped under the term 'omic' technologies. These include the measurement of gene expression (or transcriptomics), the analysis of specific proteins in cells (or proteomics), and the analysis of the metabolism of cellular molecules such as lipid and carbohydrates (or metabolomics).

In gene expression studies, messenger RNAs derived from organisms are reverse transcribed into c-DNAs which are then analysed by their binding to so-called 'gene expression chips and microarrays' which can contain DNA copies of many thousands of genes (Rockett and Dix 1999, Celias *et al.* 2000).

The relative binding of the prepared c-DNA to the chip can provide indications of modifications of the expression of genes, for example under conditions of exposure to chemicals. Such data can be used to produce gene expression 'fingerprints' which many authors have suggested may have considerable value in the assessment of the toxicological activity of individual chemicals i.e. toxicogenomics (e.g. Corton *et al.* 1999, Farr and Dunn 1999, Nuwaysir *et al.* 1999). Advances in the analysis of specific proteins provides the ability to identify specific proteins associated with toxicological responses (Anderson *et al.* 1996, MacBeath and Schreiber 2000).

The currently available technologies are unlikely to provide any significant changes to the strategy of mutagenicity screening programmes. However, the combination of these techniques has the potential to provide a considerable advance in our understanding of the mechanisms of action of specific mutagenic chemicals. In particular, the methods may be of value in identifying those chemicals which interact with cellular targets other than DNA such as carbendazim which induce aneuploidy by modification of the synthesis of the mitotic division spindle. With appropriate modifications, the gene expression chips probably represent the only available technologies suitable for identifying potential additive and/or synergetic interactions between combinations of pesticides.

3.5.2 The application of molecular cytogenetics

The current methods for the detection of chromosome damaging (clastogenic) activity of chemicals (see Stage 1 testing) are based upon the microscopic observation and quantification of chromosome changes such as fragments and micronuclei which are generally lethal to the cell. Such methods do not provide information about the inheritance of chromosome rearrangements but rather indicate the potential for the formation of chromosome rearrangements.

The development of molecular probes capable of interacting with and identifying specific chromosomes and chromosome regions provides the potential to characterize chromosome rearrangements induced by chemical treatments. The use of these methods, grouped under the general term *in situ* hybridization, will be reflected increasingly in chemical screening programmes (for review see Parry 1996), particularly when assessments are made of the consequences of induced chromosome rearrangements upon target cells.

3.5.3 Transgenic rodent gene mutation assay

To detect and quantify the ability of a chemical to induce gene mutations *in vivo*, a range of transgenic rodent models has been developed. These models involve the incorporation of bacterial or bacteriophage genes into the genomes of mice and rats. Examples of these models include the insertion of Lac I (Tas *et al.* 1993), Lac Z (Cosentino and Heddle 1996), cII (Swinger *et al.* 2001), gpt-delta (Swinger *et al.* 1999) and phi x174 (Cosentino and Heddle 2000) into the rodent genome. The basic principles of these models involve the exposure of animals to the test agents, the extraction of transgenic DNA from a range of target tissues and the recovery and expression of mutated genes in bacteria or bacteriophages. Key to the use of the systems is the use of experimental designs which involve sampling times which allow the estimation of maximum and/or plateau levels of mutations from the tissues sampled (see Heddle *et al.* 2003).

In the case of the current transgenic animals the inserted transgenes are not transcriptionally active and are assumed to be selectively neutral. Thus, the current transgenic test systems can provide valuable information concerning the mutagenic effects of chemicals upon the inserted transgene, but they cannot reproduce the selective effects (generally negative) of mutations induced in transcriptionally active genes.

3.6 Conclusions

By the nature of their intended use (i.e. to kill or inhibit the growth of specific species), pesticides can be predicted to produce at least some toxicological effects. The critical question is whether toxicity is produced in non-target species including humans. Mutagenicity testing identifies pesticide activity which may potentially lead to the induction of mutations which can lead to elevations in birth defects, reductions in fertility and in somatic cells to some of the stages involved in the initiation and progression of cancer.

Mutagenic changes are the produce of interactions with cellular targets that are common to all species (i.e. the information store DNA or RNA and the components of the mammalian cell division cycle). Thus, if mutagenic activity of a pesticide is detected then it is highly unlikely that the mutagenic hazard will be limited to the target species. Rather, data is required to determine the potential risks of exposure to non-target species.

The mutagenicity testing strategy described here is based upon an extensive database of chemical testing and can be predicted to be capable of detecting most if not all mutagenic hazard and provide estimates of risk. The assays were selected for their sensitivity, specificity and cost effective application. The application of the strategy will allow the identification of mutagenic hazard at an early stage of pesticide development and when necessary provide clarification as to whether the identified hazard represents an actual mutagenic risk to operators and to consumers of pesticide-containing food stuffs.

Thus far, the methods developed for mutagenicity testing have provided little information concerning the detection and quantification of potential additive and/or synergistic interactions of pesticide mixtures, particularly at the levels that have been detected in food stuffs. The developing technologies of gene and protein microassays have the potential to identify quantitative and qualitative changes in targets of pesticide interactions. However, the detection of mutated genes and their products will require further development to enable the quantification of rare mutant genes.

3.7 Acknowledgements

The studies of the author were supported in part by funding from the European Union Funded Project, Protection of the European Population from Aneugenic Chemicals (PEPFAC) and the UK Food Standards Agency.

3.8 References and further reading

ADLER, I-D. and J. ASHBY (1989). The present lack of evidence for unique rodent germ cell mutagens. *Mutat. Res.*, **213**, 55–66.

ANDERSON, N.L., J. TAYLOR, J.P. HOFMANN, R. ESQUER-BALSEO, S. SWIFT and N.G. ANDERSON (1996). Simultaneous measurement of hundreds of liver proteins: application in assessment of liver function. *Toxicol. Pathol.*, **24**, 72–76.

ASHBY, J. and H. TINWELL (2001). Continuing ability of the rodent bone marrow micronucleus assay to act as a predictor of the possible germ cell mutagenicity of chemicals. *Mutat. Res.*, **478**, 211–213.

CELIAS, J.E., M. KRUHFFER, I. GROMOVA, C. FREDRIKSON, M. OSTERGAARD, T. THYKJAAR, J. GROMOV, J. YU, H. PALSDOTTIR, N. MAGNUSSON and T.F. ORNTOFT (2000). Gene expression profiling: monitoring transcription and translation products and proteomics. *FEBS Lett*, **480**, 2–16.

CHAPLIN, R.E., P.A. FAIL, J.D. GEORGE, T.B. GRIZZLE, J.J. HEINDEL, G.J. HARRY, B.J. COLINS and J. TEAGUE (1995). The reproductive and neural toxicities of acrylamide and three analogues in Swiss mice, evaluated using the continuous breeding protocol. *Fundam. Appl. Toxicol.*, **27**, 9–24.

COM (2000). Committee on the Mutagenicity of Chemicals. Guidance on a Strategy for Testing Chemicals for Mutagenicity. Department of Health, London, UK.

CORTON, J.C., S.P. ANDERSON, A.J. STAUBER, D.B. JANSZEN, J.S. KIMBELL and R.B. CONOLLY (1999). Entering the era of toxicogenomics with DNA microarrays. *CIIT Activities*, **19**, 1–9.

COSENTINO, L. and J.A. HEDDLE (1996). A test for neutrality of mutations of the Lac Z transgene. *Environ. Mol. Mutagen.*, **28**, 313–316.

COSENTINO, L. and J.A. HEDDLE (2000). Differential gene expression of transgenic and endogenous loci *in vivo*. *Mutat. Res.*, **454**, 1–10.

FARR, S. and R.T. DUNN (1999). Concise review: gene expression applied to toxicology. *Toxicol. Sci.*, **50**, 1–9.

FDA (2003). FDA Pesticide Program Residue Monitoring 1993–2001 http:/ www.cfsan.fda.gov./~dms/pesrpts.html

FENECH, M., J. GOTT, J. TURNER and S. BROWN (1999). Necrosis, apoptosis, cytokinesis and DNA damage in human lymphocytes measured simultaneously with the cytokinesis-block micronucleus assay. *Mutagenesis* **14**, 605–612.

HEDDLE, J.A., H-J. MARTUS and G.R. DOUGLAS (2003). Treatment and sampling protocols for transgenic mutations assays. *Environ. Mol. Mutagen.*, **41**, 1–6.

HUNT, P.A., K.E. KOEHLER, M. SUSIARGO, C.A. HODGES, A. IIAGEN, R.C. VOIGT, S. THOMAS. B.F. THOMAS and T.J. HASSOLD (2003). Bisphenol A exposure causes meiotic aneuploidy in the female mouse. *Current Biology*, **13**, 546–553.

JENKINS, G.J.S., H.S. SUZEN, R. A. SUEIRO and J. M. PARRY (1999). The restriction site mutation assay: a review of methodology development and the current status of the techniques. *Mutagenesis* **14**, 439–448.

MACBEATH, G. and S.L. SCHREIBER (2000). Printing proteins as microarrays for high throughput function determination. *Science*, **289**, 1760–1763.

NUWAYSIR, E.F., M. BITTNER, J. TRENT, J.C. BARRETT and C.A. AFSHAR (1999). Microarrays and toxicology: the advent of toxicogenomics. *Mol. Carcinogen.*, **24**, 153–59.

OECD (1984). Organisation for Economic Co-operation and Development. Guidelines for Testing Chemicals No. 478. The Dominant Lethal Assay, OECD, Paris.

OECD (1997). Organisation for Economic Co-operation and Development. Ninth addendum to the OECD Guidelines for the Testing of Chemicals. Update of Section 4, Health Effects, Revised Guidelines, 471, 473, 474, 475, 476, 483, 486, OECD, Paris.

PARRY, J.M. (1996). Molecular Cytogenetics. *Mutat. Res.* Special Issue, **372**, 151–294.

PARRY, J.M., P.J. FIELDER and A. MCDONALD (1994). Thresholds for aneuploidy-inducing chemicals. *Mutagenesis* **9**, 503–504.

ROCKETT, J.C. and D.J. DIX (1999). Application of DNA arrays to toxicology. *Environ. Health Perspect.*, **107**, 681–685.

SCHMEZER, P. and C. ECKERT (1999). Induction of mutations in transgenic animal models. Big Blue^{JM} and MutaTH Mouse. In: *The use of short and medium term tests for carcinogens and data on genetic effects in carcinogen hazard evaluation*. IARC Publication No. 146, Lyon, pp. 367–394.

SHELBY, M.A. (1996). Selecting chemicals and assays for assessing mammalian germ cell mutagenicity. *Mutat. Res.*, **352**, 159–167.

SWINGER, R.R., L. COSENTINO, K.I. MASUMURA, T. NOHMI and J.A. HEDDLE (2001). Further characterisation and validation of gpt deltra transgenic mice for quantifying somatic mutations *in vivo*. *Environ. Mol. Mutgen.*, **37**, 297–303.

SWINGER, R.R., L. COSENTINO, N. SHIMA, J.H. BIELAS, W. CRUZ-MUNOZ and J.A. HEDDLE (1999). The CII locus in the Muta Mouse System. *Environ. Mol. Mutagen.*, **34**, 201–207.

TAS, K.S., C. URLANDO and J.A. HEDDLE (1993). Comparison of somatic mutations in a transgenic versus host locus. *Proc. Natl. Acad. Sci. USA*, **90**, 10681–10685.

TINWELL, H., M.H. BRINKWORTH and J. ASHBY (2001). Further evidence for the rodent bone marrow micronucleus assay acting as a sensitive predictor of the possible germ cells mutagenicity of chemicals. *Mutat. Res.*, **473**, 259–261.

WATERS, M., H.F. STACK, M.A. JACKSON, B.A. BRIDGES and I-D. ADLER (1994). The performance of short-term tests in identifying potential germ cell mutagens: a qualitative and quantitative analysis. *Mutat. Res.*, **341**, 109–131.

WITT, K.L., L.A. HUGHES, L.T. BURBA, A-F. MCFEE, J.M. MATTHEW, S.L. BLACK and J.B. BISHOP (2003). Mouse bone marrow micronucleus test results do not predict the germ cells mutagenicity of N-hydroxymethylacrylamide in the mouse dominant lethal assay. *Environ. Mol. Mutagen.*, **41**, 111–120.

YIN, H., E. BAART, I. BETZENDAHL and U. EICHENLAUB-RITTER (1998). Diazepam induces meiotic delay, aneuploidy and predivision of homologues and chromatids in mammalian oocytes. *Mutagenesis*, **13**, 567–580.

4

The impact of chemical residues: the case of polychlorinated biphenyls (PCBs)

H. C. Gallagher, I. E. J. De Souza and C. M. Regan, University College Dublin, Ireland

4.1 Introduction: risks posed by organohalogen compounds

Organohalogen compounds are persistent and ubiquitous environmental pollutants. These compounds include fabricated chemicals, such as polychlorinated biphenyls (PCBs), as well as dioxins and dibenzofurans, which are not intentionally produced but are by-products of various industrial processes such as bleaching, herbicide production and incineration of chlorinated products. For many years there has been considerable concern that organohalogens, in particular the PCBs, may pose a neurotoxic threat to human health by adversely affecting cognitive performance and/or motor skills in populations exposed to environmental levels of these compounds.

PCBs were widely synthesised in the USA, Germany, Japan, France, Spain and Italy until increasing safety concerns led to their production being banned by many individual countries in the 1970s. They are, however, still being produced in North Korea and Russia. Manufactured by reacting gaseous chlorine with molten biphenyl, the resultant PCB products are complex mixtures of over 200 distinct chlorobiphenyl congeners with different chlorine substitution patterns, although the numbers of congeners actually detected in biological samples is much lower (Brouwer *et al.*, 1998). Different manufacturing methods have resulted in the production of PCB mixtures with different degrees of chlorination and, thus, different physical and chemical properties. For example, in the United States, Monsanto produced Aroclor mixtures that ranged from 21–68% chlorine by weight (Aroclors 1221–1268). The lightly chlorinated PCB mixtures (e.g. Aroclors 1221–1248) are clear oils, whereas the more highly chlorinated mixtures are viscous resins (Safe, 1983). PCB compounds are efficient energy conductors and as a consequence were widely used in industrial products such as capacitors, plastics, fire retardants and carbonless copy paper (World Health Organization, 1993).

The environmental levels of PCBs peaked (in the USA) in the 1970s and the World Health Organization (WHO) estimated that, by 1980, over 1 million tonnes of these chemicals had been produced worldwide. Their high stability and propensity to bioaccumulate means that despite not being widely manufactured currently, PCBs persist in significant quantities in the environment. The WHO has reported that PCBs are contaminants of almost every component of the global ecosystem including air, soil, water and sediments (Tanabe, 1988). The major form of human exposure to PCBs is the food chain, particularly fish, beef and dairy products that are relatively high in fat. When ingested, these compounds are readily absorbed, reflecting their lipophilicity. Moreover, they are present in breast milk and readily cross the placenta. PCB concentrations in different tissues largely reflect the tissue lipid content, yet their levels are relatively low in brain tissue despite its high lipid content (Dewailly *et al.*, 1999). This is assumed to reflect differences in the polarity of lipids that predominate in different tissues. The lipid content of the brain is composed of membranes and, therefore, mainly comprises phospholipids and cholesterol, which have lower affinity for PCBs than triglycerides and cholesterol esters that are prevalent in adipose tissue.

Worldwide, there have been several accidental incidences of major PCB contamination that have resulted in huge public health interest about the potential impact of environmental exposure to organohalogens on neurodevelopment and behavioural outcome. These include pesticide spills into Lakes Michigan and Ontario (Jacobson *et al.*, 1985; Lonky *et al.*, 1996) and contamination of cooking oil in Japan and Taiwan (Kuratsune *et al.*, 1971; Hsu *et al.*, 1984). Several human epidemiological studies have been conducted on population cohorts that have been exposed to high levels of PCBs through these incidences of environmental pollution, and other studies have attempted to correlate background levels of PCB exposure with adverse neurodevelopmental sequelae (Huisman *et al.*, 1995; Rogan *et al.*, 1986a, b). These include longitudinal studies of the offspring of mothers exposed to high and background levels of PCBs. In this chapter, we will focus on the potential cognitive implications of exposure to organohalogen compounds both in humans and in animal models. Emphasis will be placed on perinatal exposure as this has been identified as a sensitive epoch during development for the potential detrimental effects of organohalogens.

4.2 Organohalogens as neurotoxins

Similar to other neurotoxicants like mercury and lead, the adverse effects of PCBs on neurodevelopmental outcome were first recognised following calamitous exposures to high doses in accidental poisoning episodes. Children who had been exposed to high levels of PCBs *in utero* and through later consumption of contaminated breast milk were much more sensitive to PCB-induced toxicity than their mothers indicating that, like other toxicants, the perinatal period of brain development is a sensitive epoch for PCB action. As newborn infants, these children had various developmental deficits including reduced birth weight, altered reflexes, and in later childhood they also exhibited behavioural abnormalities and IQ deficits. However, subsequent prospective studies on populations exposed to lower and/or background levels of PCBs increased the relevance of PCB-induced neurotoxicity, as these provided evidence of adverse effects for these chemicals at exposure levels that are commonly experienced by the general population. Some controlled animal studies further supported the premise that PCB exposure, particularly in the prenatal period, results in some neurodevelopmental perturbations but with very limited evidence to implicate these chemicals in persistent or profound deficits on cognition or behaviour.

4.2.1 Measuring exposure levels

Although the most common route of human exposure to organohalogens is the ingestion of contaminated foodstuffs, *in utero* placental and breast milk transfer together constitute the most important routes of exposure during the sensitive perinatal period. Overall, levels of organohalogen exposure in humans have been difficult to estimate. While some epidemiological studies have directly measured PCB levels in biological samples (cord blood, colostrum, milk and maternal or offspring serum), others have simply relied on questionnaires that estimated exposure levels on the basis of location and diet. It should also be noted that the accidental PCB exposure of the Japanese and Taiwanese cohorts produced serum and/or cord blood levels that are orders of magnitude higher than those observed in general populations, with the Japanese children exhibiting the highest levels of all (Harada, 1976). Information on the specific PCB congeners present in biological samples has only been collected in three human studies. Thus, one of the obvious strengths of animal studies lies in their ability to control organohalogen exposure levels, routes and congener specificity.

4.2.2 Neurodevelopmental outcome measures and confounders

Confounding variables complicate human studies in particular and it can be difficult to define ‘normal’ neurodevelopment outcomes given the heterogeneity of the general population. Neonatal tests of neurodevelopment generally involve assessing muscle tonicity, reflexes, responsiveness and alertness. Childhood tests are broadly divided into behavioural assessment (including activity scaling), motor skills (fine and coarse motor function) and mental tests, which monitor linguistic ability, memory, cognition and social skills. For both neonates and children, several of these outcome measures have been standardised, and the employment of such tests facilitates the validation and comparison of exposure outcome between different studies. These standardised testing methodologies include the Prechtl, Kaufman, Fagan and Neonatal Behavioural Assessment Scale (NBAS) scoring systems for neonates and infants, as well as the McCarthy Scales of Children's Abilities, Peabody Vocabulary and IQ tests for older children (Table 4.1). However, given that the effects of organohalogens on neurodevelopment sequelae are generally subtle, they tend to be smaller than those effects that are attributable to other significant variables such as socioeconomic status, smoking, breastfeeding and Home Observation for Measurement of the Environment (HOME) scores. Thus, as highlighted below, the consideration of confounders is of prime importance in the interpretation of human epidemiological data on organohalogen exposure.

4.3 Neurobehavioural consequences of PCB exposure

Human epidemiological studies on the neurobehavioural sequelae that follow PCB exposure have been conducted in eight separate population cohorts. There is considerable heterogeneity between these studies, however, in terms of outcome measures, control of confounding variables and the use of exposure markers. This variance in approach means that comparisons between studies can be difficult and as a consequence there is considerable controversy and disagreement regarding the actual effects (if any) that PCBs have on neurodevelopment. All studies conducted to date have been prospective rather than retrospective and several have now been continued as longitudinal studies.

4.3.1 Exposed populations

The Japanese and Taiwanese population cohorts consisted of children that had been exposed in the perinatal period to high levels of PCBs via their mothers' consumption of contaminated cooking oils in 1968 and 1979, respectively. The Michigan and Oswego studies were conducted on children born to mothers who had consumed large quantities of contaminated fish from Lakes Michigan and Ontario, respectively. In the Faroe Islands cohort, the children studied had been exposed prenatally to elevated levels of PCBs and methylmercury, through their mothers' consumption of whale meat. The three remaining population cohorts that have been investigated include children from the general populations in the Netherlands, North Carolina and Germany exposed to 'background' levels of PCBs.

4.3.2 Influence of PCB exposure on neonate neurodevelopmental endpoints

Of the cohorts mentioned above, the effects of PCB exposure on neonatal measures of neurodevelopment were only specifically assessed in four of these

Table 4.1 Standardised neurodevelopmental, motor and cognitive scoring systems referred to throughout this review

	Assessment age; Details	Employed within
Neonates		
Neonatal Behavioural Assessment Scale (NBAS)	<3 days; Reflexes, responsiveness	Rogan and Gladen, 1991; Rogan *et al*., 1986b; Jacobson *et al*., 1985
Newborn Neurological Exam (Prechtl)	10–21 says; Age-appropriate neurodelvelopment	Huisman *et al*., 1995
Children		
Bayley Scalers of Infant Development	<2.5 years; Age-appropriate cognitive and motor ability	Rogan *et al*., 1988; Yu *et al*., 1994; Lai *et al*., 1994; Rogan and Gladen, 1991; Koopman-Esseboom *et al*., 1996
Kaufman Assessment Battery for Children (K-ABC)	2.5–12.5 years; Age-appropriate cognitive ability	Walkowiak *et al*., 2001; Winneke *et al*., 1998; Patandin *et al*., 1999
McCarthy Scales of Children's Ability	>3 years; Age-appropriate cognitive ability	Jacobson and Jacobson, 1996; Jacobson *et al*., 1990
Weshler Intelligence Scale for Children (WISC-R)	>6 years; General intelligence	Lai *et al*., 1994
The Neurological Exam for Toddler Age (Hempel)	1–3 years; Age-appropriate motor ability	Huisman *et al*., 1995
Fagan Test of Infant Intelligence	3–12 months; Short-term memory, novelty reactions	Jacobson *et al*., 1985; Darvill *et al*., 2000

populations – those in the Netherlands, North Carolina, Lake Michigan and Oswego (Lake Ontario). In all four studies some adverse effects on neonatal neurodevelopment were reported. In the Dutch study, postnatal exposure to PCBs, PCDDs and PCDFs was associated with reduced neonatal optimality as assessed by the Prechtl test, although this was not directly correlated with PCB levels in the cord blood (Huisman *et al.*, 1995). In North Carolina, higher levels of PCBs in maternal milk were linked to hypotonicity and reduced reflexes (Rogan *et al.*, 1986a,b). In the Michigan study, the level of fish consumption by mothers was correlated with motor immaturity, emotional lability, exaggerated startle responses and reduced reflexes in the Neonatal Behavioural Assessment Scale (NBAS; Jacobson *et al.*, 1984). Although the two Great Lake studies were initiated ten years apart, similar effects were observed in the Oswego study, with newborns exposed to high levels of chlorinated PCBs scoring poorly on autonomic and habituation elements of the NBAS (Lonky *et al.*, 1996).

4.3.3 Influence of PCB exposure on childhood neurodevelopmental endpoints

Mental, motor and behavioural consequences of prenatal PCB exposure have been quantified in children ranging from 6 months to 12 years in several original and follow-up publications. The most profound cognitive deficits were observed in the Taiwanese group with an inverse association between PCB exposure and mental development being recorded at several ages up to and including 12 years (Rogan *et al.*, 1988; Yu *et al.*, 1994; Lai *et al.*, 1994, 2002). In various studies of this population, the average test scoring difference between exposed and non-exposed control children using the Bayley Scales was in the region of −4 to −6 percentage points. Studies on the Michigan and Oswego cohorts also revealed deficits in cognitive skills during the first few months of life as measured by the Fagan Test of Infant Intelligence (Jacobson *et al.*, 1985; Lonky *et al.*, 1996) despite the exposure levels being significantly less than that of the Taiwanese population. Moreover, in the Michigan cohort, the children exhibited deficits in tasks requiring short-term memory such as visual recognition tests (Jacobson *et al.*, 1985). Longitudinal studies have been performed on both of these populations, mainly by employing the McCarthy Scales of Children's Abilities. These indicated deleterious cognitive effects persisting to 11 years of age in the Michigan cohort. In the Oswego studies only small, but measurable, deficits were evident at 38 months, with full recovery observed at 54 months (Jacobson and Jacobson, 1996; Stewart *et al.*, 2003). Importantly, the PCB exposure levels were higher in the Michigan group, suggesting that functional recovery may be possible following lower exposures.

In the Netherlands, a significant association between PCB cord blood levels and psychomotor deficits was recorded particularly at 3 months, while mental impairment was observed at 42 months using the Kaufman Assessment Battery for Children. However, the Dutch authors reported that PCB cord blood levels were not predictive for motor development deficits at 7 or 42 months (Patandin *et al.*, 1999; Huisman *et al.*, 1995). Similar negative associations between cognitive performance and PCB exposure have also been reported in the German group (Walkowiak *et al.*, 2001; Winneke *et al.*, 1998). Although similar to the Dutch and German studies in measuring consequences of background exposure, studies on the North Carolinian population did not find any association between cognitive deficits and PCB exposure at 3–5 years of age, although some psychomotor disturbances were recorded in children up to 2 years (Rogan *et al.*, 1986a,b; Rogan and Gladen, 1991; Gladen and Rogan, 1991).

The Japanese children, despite being exposed to the highest levels of PCBs, have not been subjected to standardised quantitative longitudinal testing. However, in a group of 127 exposed children, a mean IQ level of 70 was recorded and the children were described as being 'sullen, expressionless and hypoactive' (Harada, 1976). This suggests that severe cognitive and behavioural deficits may persist in this group.

4.3.4 Consensus view

There are a number of factors that hamper forming conclusions from human PCB studies. Following the original reports of Jacobson *et al.* (1984, 1985, 1990) detailing a relationship between reduced performance on the McCarthy scales and prenatal PCB exposure in Michigan, other authors failed to replicate this data in the North Carolinian population cohort (Gladen and Rogan, 1991; Rogan *et al.*, 1986a,b). This apparent discrepancy led to the demand for longer-term analysis of multiple independent studies as the only means by which a robust effect of PCBs could be identified (Darvill *et al.*, 1996; Rice *et al.*, 1996). In recent years, this has been achieved to some degree with several independent authors extending and confirming the findings of Jacobson and colleagues by reporting deleterious effects of PCBs in populations exposed to relatively high concentrations of PCBs (Patandin *et al.*, 1999, Walkowiak *et al.*, 2001; Stewart *et al.*, 2003). Moreover, when considered in parallel with the extensive animal data from prenatal and perinatal PCB exposure studies discussed below (Rice, 1995, 1998, 1999; Schantz and Bowman, 1989; Schantz *et al.*, 1995) the overall evidence appears to support the premise that PCBs are predictors of small, albeit significant, cognitive deficits in pre-school children. However, the persistence of these cognitive deficits is still debatable. Although Jacobson *et al.*, reported PCB-related deficits at 11 years of age (Jacobson and Jacobson, 1996), Gray and colleagues (2000) failed to detect any association between PCB exposure and cognitive performance at age 7. A recent longitudinal report of the Oswego cohort also indicated that children who had exhibited PCB-related deficits in McCarthy scores at 38 months, were normal at 54 months suggesting that functional recovery may occur (Stewart *et al.*, 2003).

Clearly, unless and until several independent population cohorts have been methodically assessed in the longer term, up to and including adulthood, firm conclusions on the relevance of PCB exposure for mature brain function cannot be drawn. However, it is notable that it is the more significantly exposed cohorts which to date have shown some persisting PCB-related cognitive deficits in the pre-teen years. Of the Great Lake studies, levels of PCB contamination were significantly higher in the Michigan population than the Oswego population. Furthermore, the Japanese group, who were exposed to the highest levels of PCBs also appeared to exhibit persisting deficits, but unfortunately these have not been systematically analysed. The potential for functional recovery or 'catch-up' following toxicant exposure is not without precedent. Bellinger *et al.* (1990) reported similar effects in lead-exposed children who exhibited deficits in cognitive function at 2 years of age but did not differ from control populations at 5 years.

4.3.5 Confounding factors

As mentioned above, there are other important considerations in analysing studies of organohalogen exposure. These effects include concomitant exposure to other toxicants, notably methylmercury, as well as breast-feeding status, socioeconomic factors and smoking. In general, practices involved in controlling for such confounders varied widely between studies and this has made meta-analysis and comparisons between studies difficult to perform accurately. In several studies, however, adequate statistical analyses of multifactorial parameters were performed that concluded PCB-induced effects on human neurobehavioural endpoints to remain significant after adjustment for many common confounders. Methylmercury is of particular relevance since co-exposure with PCBs is common and it is one of the few chemicals that has been unequivocally reported to act synergistically with PCBs, as evidenced by modulation of dopamine levels *in vitro* (Bemis and Seegal, 1999). Moreover, methylmercury alone has been linked to deficits in linguistic ability, memory and attention in children (Grandjean *et al.*, 1997, 1999). In a study of Faroe Islanders with elevated levels of both PCB and methylmercury, the deleterious effects of PCBs on cognitive performance disappeared after adjustment for methylmercury (Grandjean *et al.*, 1998). In the Seychelles, however, children that had high levels of methylmercury, but low levels of PCBs, did not exhibit neurobehavioural deficits (Davidson *et al.*, 1995, 1998, 1999) suggesting that in the Faroe study PCBs may have potentiated the deleterious effects of methylmercury on these endpoints (Grandjean *et al.*, 2001).

Breast-feeding patterns are also of relevance to PCB studies since breast milk contains relatively high levels of these compounds and breast-fed infants, therefore, consume a significant proportion of their total lifetime dose of PCBs in the first few months of life. However, even in breast-fed children born to mothers with a high PCB burden, the beneficial effects of breast-feeding seem to outweigh the risks of PCB exposure (Koopman-Esseboom *et al.*, 1996; Weisglas-Kuperus *et al.*, 2000). Although transplacental PCB exposure levels are much lower than those attained through breast milk, the former seem to exert a more harmful outcome. This presumably reflects temporal differences in sensitivity to neurodevelopmental insult.

4.3.6 Neurodevelopmental endpoints in animal models of PCB exposure

In view of the inherent complexities associated with measuring neuro-behavioural consequences of PCB exposure in humans, animal models have been particularly useful in providing more controlled experimental conditions with primate and, more commonly, rodent models being employed (Table 4.2). Accumulating evidence now supports the conclusion that developmental exposure to organohalogens can produce subtle cognitive deficits in animals. However, diverse behavioural effects are observed following developmental organohalogen exposure and the nature of these effects seems to be exquisitely sensitive to both the behavioural paradigm and exposure protocol employed (Table 4.3). It is also noteworthy that the exposure doses utilised in studies examining neurobehavioural effects are lower than doses that cause overt reproductive or developmental toxicity in the offspring.

In primates, prolonged exposure to commercial PCB mixtures, e.g Aroclor 1248 by placental transfer during gestation and lactation, produced deficits in delayed spatial alternation learning and spatial discrimination reversal learning tasks (Bowman *et al.*, 1978; Levin *et al.*, 1988; Schantz *et al.*, 1989, 1991). By contrast, in studies where monkeys were postnatally exposed to PCBs, no impairments in spatial reversal learning were observed (Rice, 1998, 1999). This suggests that perinatal exposure to organohalogens may have more profound

Table 4.2 Animal behavioural paradigms referred to throughout this review

Paradigm	Details
Water maze	Test developed to map spatial orientation in rats. Consists of a pool of water in which a rat swims and searches for a hidden platform. The time taken for the animal to find the platform is measured, along with other parameters such as swim angle and speed.
Radial arm maze	Test used to measure reference or working memory. Consists of a central area with arms emanating radially outwards. Food-deprived rats enter the arms in search of food. Working memory is tested when all arms are baited with food, whereas reference memory is tested when baited arms are interspersed with non-baited arms.
Passive avoidance	An avoidance task is usually based on an electric shock as an adverse stimulus. The animal must refrain from performing some act by remaining passive and its latency to do so reflects its ability to avoid.
Spontaneous alternation	Spatial alternation which represents a tendency to avoid stimulus re-exposure during exploratory behaviour, usually in a T-maze task.
Object recognition task	Based on the spontaneous exploration of novel and familiar objects. Normal animals will spend more time exploring a novel object than a familiar one.

Table 4.3 Summary of PCB-induced animal behavioural changes

Species	Altered behaviour	PCB(s) employed	Reference
Rat	Impaired T-maze ability	PCB118; PCB153	Schantz *et al.*, 1995
Rat	Impaired water maze	Aroclor 1254	Provost *et al.*, 1999
Rat	Impaired/facilitated radial arm maze	Aroclor 1254; PCB77; PCB95	Roegge *et al.*, 2000; Schantz *et al.*, 1996, 1997; Corey *et al.*, 1996
Rat	Hypoactivity	PCB95	Schantz *et al.*, 1997; Nishida *et al.*, 1997
Rat	Impaired active avoidance	Fenclor 42	Pantaleoni *et al.*, 1988
Rat	Hyperactivity	Clophen A30; PCB153; PCB126; Aroclor 1248	Agrawal *et al.*, 1981; Lilienthal *et al.*, 1990; Holene *et al.*, 1998; Berger *et al.*, 2001
Rat	Changes in operant behaviour	Clophen A30	Lilienthal *et al.*, 1990
Rat	Altered visual discrimination	PCB118; PCB126	Holene *et al.*, 1998
Mouse	Hyperactivity	PCB77	Tilson *et al.*, 1979
Mouse	Circling	3,4,3′,4′-tetrachlorobiphenyl	Chou *et al.*, 1979
Mouse	Hypoactivity	Fenclor 54	Fanini *et al.*, 1990
Mouse	Impaired active avoidance	PCB77	Tilson *et al.*, 1979
Monkey	Impaired delayed spatial alternation	Aroclor 1248; Aroclor 1016; PCB mixture	Levin *et al.*, 1988; Rice 1998, 1999; Schantz *et al.*, 1989
Monkey	Altered operant behaviour	PCB mixture	Rice 1998, 1999
Monkey	Altered discrimination	Aroclor 1248	Bowman *et al.*, 1978, 1981; Mele *et al.*, 1986
Monkey	Hyperactivity	Aroclor 1248	Bowman *et al.*, 1981

effects as compared to postnatal exposure. In addition, deficits in visual discrimination, delayed spatial alternation and reversal learning and fixed interval response tasks have been observed in rodents following gestational and lactational exposure to commercial PCBs (Lilienthal *et al.*, 1990; Lilienthal and Winneke, 1991; Schantz *et al.*, 1995, 1996; Widholm *et al.*, 2001). In the radial maze task, however, Aroclor 1254, but not ortho-substituted PCB congeners, produce learning deficits (Schantz *et al.*, 1995; Roegge *et al.*, 2000). Exposure to Aroclor 1254 has also been found to impair performance of rodents in the water maze (Provost *et al.*, 1999), as has exposure to the organohalogen 2,3,7,8-tetrachlorodibenzo-para-dioxin (TCDD) (Mundy *et al.*, 1998). Paradoxically, however, Seo *et al.* (1999) have demonstrated TCDD exposure impairs visual reversal learning but facilitates radial arm maze learning. It should also be noted that evidence exists for sex-selective effects of these compounds in both delayed spatial alternation and radial maze tasks, the deficits being observed in both females and males respectively (Schantz *et al.*, 1995; Roegge *et al.*, 2000; Widholm *et al.*, 2003). Overall, the effects of organohalogen exposure on neurobehavioural tasks are quite variable with impairment most often seen in working memory paradigms. In addition, some organohalogen compounds can have effects that are sex-selective.

It is not surprising then, given the ability of specific organohalogens to influence behaviour, that some authors have investigated whether perinatal organohalogen exposure to these compounds influences synaptic plasticity. Long-term potentiation (LTP) is a long-lasting increase in synaptic response following electrical stimulation and has been purported as a model for learning-induced synaptic plasticity. Thus, it can be utilised as a measure of synaptic efficacy following exposure to environmental chemicals. Gilbert and Crofton (1999) demonstrated *in vivo* impairment of LTP in the rat dentate gyrus following perinatal exposure to Aroclor 1254. In this study, the authors reported a reduction in the magnitude of LTP in both population spike intensity and excitatory postsynaptic potential slope. In addition, Hong *et al.* (1998) and Niemi *et al.* (1998) have demonstrated a reduction in the magnitude of LTP in the CA1 region of the hippocampus following PCB exposure. Significantly, however, the organohalogen-induced deficits in *in vivo* LTP do not correlate with impaired spatial learning ability in the water maze (Gilbert *et al.*, 2000). This indicates that, at least in some behavioural paradigms, LTP impairment following organohalogen exposure does not necessarily reflect alterations to behaviour.

4.4 Molecular mechanisms of organohalogen-induced toxicity

It is well established that PCBs and dioxins produce many of their biological effects by binding to the aryl hydrocarbon (Ah) receptor and inducing gene expression (Safe, 1994; Okey *et al.*, 1994). The aryl hydrocarbon (Ah) receptor is a member of the basic helix-loop-helix family of receptor-type transcription factors. Binding of a ligand such as TCDD activates the receptor causing it to disassociate from a heat shock protein complex and bind to the aryl hydrocarbon receptor nuclear translocator. This complex translocates to the nucleus where it binds to a response element and influences gene transcription, in particular the induction of cytochome P-450 subtypes 1A1 and 1A2 . The Ah receptor has been detected in the brain albeit at lower levels than in other organs (Gasiewicz and Rucci, 1984) and activation of these receptors in the brain results in expression of metabolizing enzymes such as cytochrome P450 1A1 isoform or aldehyde dehydrogenase isozme 3 (Unkila *et al.* 1995). TCDD and some so-called dioxin-like PCBs, which can assume a coplanar configuration and include PCB congeners with no ortho-chlorines, two para-chlorines, and at least two meta-chlorines, bind to the Ah receptor (Safe, 1994). However, PCBs with two or more ortho-chlorines are very weak Ah-receptor agonists and there is some evidence that these PCB congeners may be the main PCB compounds responsible for producing the neurobehavioural effects observed as a result of PCB exposure (Levin *et al.*, 1988; Lilienthal and Winneke, 1991; Schantz *et al.*, 1989; Seegal and Schantz, 1994).

There have been several studies aimed at elucidating the molecular basis of PCB effects in the CNS and many of these studies suggest mechanisms of action of PCBs that are independent of the Ah receptor. Organohalogens with weak Ah affinity have been shown to perturb normal calcium homeostasis (Kodavanti *et al.*, 1995, 1998; Kodavanti and Tilson, 2000; Seegal, 1996). The mechanism by which this increase in calcium occurs was shown to be through inhibition of calcium uptake into mitochondria and microsomes by an ortho-substituted PCB congener (Voie *et al.*, 1998). Moreover, in rats exposed to Aroclor 1254, microsomal calcium uptake is also impaired (Sharma *et al.*, 2000). Perinatal exposure to PCBs also leads to protein kinase C translocation to the membrane. Specifically, ortho-substituted PCBs increase PKC translocation (Kodavanti and Tilson, 2000) while Aroclor 1254 decreases PKC activity and calcium buffering in the brain (Yang *et al.*, 2003).

In addition, both *in vivo* and *in vitro* studies have demonstrated that PCBs can perturb neurotransmitter function (Bemis and Seegal, 1999; Mariussen and Fonnum, 2001; Seegal *et al.*, 2002), although there is scant evidence to relate these effects to memory deficits. Brain dopamine concentration and receptor binding is decreased in mice following perinatal exposure to 3,4,3′,4′-tetrachlorobiphenyl (Tilson *et al.*, 1979; Agrawal *et al.*, 1981). However, effects on dopamine following exposure to PCB mixtures are variable. For example, developmental and adult exposure to Aroclor 1016 and Aroclor 1260 was shown to decrease brain dopamine levels in earlier studies (Seegal *et al.*, 1991a,b; 1994). Interestingly, Seegal *et al.* (1994) demonstrated that the reduced dopamine concentrations inhibited by early PCB exposure were not reinstated by stopping PCB exposure even though brain PCB levels themselves were reduced. This suggests that prolonged suppression of brain dopamine concentrations may reflect enduring biochemical alterations induced by the early exposure to PCB and as a consequence may account for persisting behavioural changes.

The structure of the PCB compound may also play an important role in its effects on dopamine. This was aptly demonstrated by Seegal and colleagues where exposure to coplanar PCB congeners led to elevations in dopamine concentrations whereas exposure to ortho-substituted PCB congeners had the opposite effect (for review see Brouwer *et al.*, 1995). Although Zahalka *et al.* (2001) reported perinatal exposure to Aroclors 1016 and 1254 to have no effect on dopamine or noradrenaline, and similar results have been obtained by Morse *et al.* (1996a), with the exception that the latter authors reported an increased serotonin turnover rate, markers of structural and functional brain development such as synaptophysin have been shown to decrease following perinatal exposure to Aroclor 1254 (Morse *et al.*, 1996b). These latter findings suggest that brain plasticity may be altered by exposure to organohalogens.

A morphological basis for the cognitive impairments mediated by Aroclor 1254 has been proposed by Pruitt *et al.* (1999). These authors found that continuous organohalogen exposure reduced the relative size of rat hippocampal intra- and infra-pyramidal mossy fibres without influencing fibres in other hippocampal regions. As reduced thyroid levels are known to reduce the thickness of the intra- and infra-pyramidal mossy fibre bands, suggesting loss of synapse density between hippocampal granule and pyramidal neurons, it has been suggested that this structural abnormality may underpin long-term behavioural deficits produced by organohalogens. This is consistent with the steady-state in thyroid levels that accompanies PCB exposure (Byrne *et al.*, 1987; Juarez de Ku *et al.*, 1994; Morse *et al.*, 1993). Moreover, thyroxin supplementation is known to enhance maze learning (Schwegler and Crusio, 1995) as well as increasing intra- and infra-pyramidal mossy fibre growth. Thus, it is possible that these PCB-induced morphological effects, mediated through

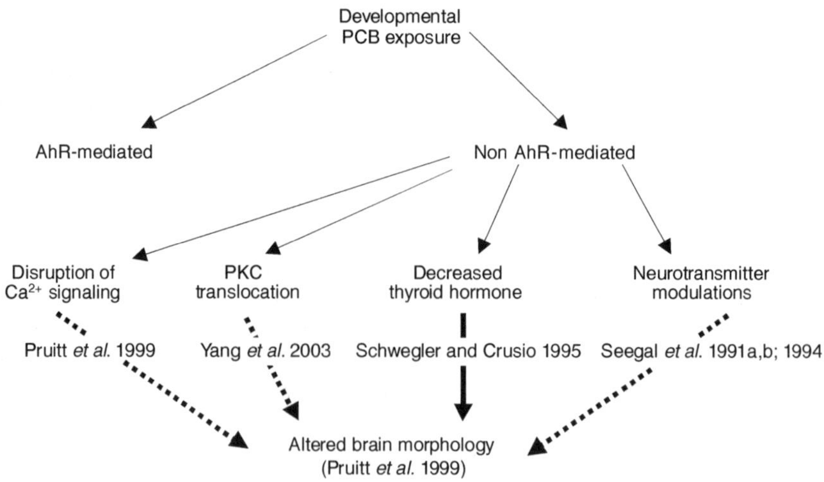

Fig. 4.1 Potential mechanisms for behavioural changes following developmental PCB exposure in experimental animals.

altered thyroid hormone levels, explain the associated cognitive deficits (Fig. 4.1).

4.5 Conclusion

There are interesting parallels between the human cognitive studies and controlled laboratory-based animal studies reviewed here. In essence the Jacobson studies on the Michigan cohort revealed that *in utero* exposure to PCBs is associated with poorer short-term memory functioning, as evidenced by spatial tasks such as visual recognition memory. However, there was no evidence of perceptual motor impairment in these children, and their uncompromised performances in the vocabulary testing also suggested long-term memory to be unaffected. Similarly, both primates and rodents exposed to PCBs *in utero* and during lactation are later impaired in their ability to learn tasks (particularly spatial tasks) requiring the use of short-term memory (Schantz *et al.*, 1991, 1995, 1996). An obvious drawback of the animal-based studies is that they generally underestimate toxic threats by evaluating only one chemical or commercial mix in any given study, whereas in reality children are exposed to complex mixes of other toxicants. It is now accepted that complexes comprising multiple chemicals can be much more potent and that synergism can occur between chemicals such that single exposure protocols in animals are of limited value (Bemis and Seegal, 1999; Jett *et al.*, 1999). Furthermore, animal studies tend to underestimate higher order dysfunction reflecting obvious difficulties in monitoring uniquely human aspects of cognition, language and behaviour. It has been suggested that for PCBs, lead and mercury, the underestimation of toxic effects may be as high as 100- to 100,000-fold (Rice *et al.*, 1996).

Despite these drawbacks, animal studies do present the opportunity to dissect structure activity relationships and determine the influence of individual organohalogen congeners on neurobehavioural outcome. This is of particular relevance given that the neurobehavioural effects of PCBs appear to be quite distinct from the other toxic effects of these compounds in that they exhibit different structure activity relationships, with non-coplanar ortho-substituted compounds more likely to be neuroactive. This has been demonstrated in both rats and monkeys where exposure to commercial mixtures of PCB shows deficits in delayed spatial alternation whereas much more subtle effects were seen following exposure to TCDD. In addition, one effect observed in both rats and monkeys – deficits in delayed spatial alternation – is induced by exposure to ortho-substituted PCBs, defined experimental mixtures, and commercial Aroclors (Faroon *et al.*, 2001). Studies from both human and experimental data suggest that early developmental exposures to PCBs are far more likely to result in adverse neurobehavioural effects than exposure during adulthood. Moreover, few effects on neurodevelopment can be ascribed to lactational or postnatal exposure. Since there is evidence that the ortho-substituted compounds are the most prevalent form of PCB in the environment (Porte and Albaiges, 1994), the elucidation of potential neurotoxic or other toxic effects associated with these chemicals is of utmost importance.

Improved monitoring of the potential deleterious neurobehavioural effects of chemicals generally cannot realistically rely on *in vivo* testing, given the large number of animals that would be required. There is, therefore, an urgent need to develop and validate *in vitro* alternatives that may serve as initial indicators of neurobehavioural toxicity. With regard to organohalogens, it is clear that further efforts towards elucidating the molecular mechanisms that contribute to their neurobehavioural toxicity are imperative. Both neurochemical and signalling studies performed to date indicate that *in vitro/ex vivo* systems may indeed be useful in predicting the *in vivo* effects of these compounds. Elucidating signalling mechanisms other than dioxin-like effects and/or those mediated by the aryl hydrocarbon receptor must also be prioritised since these appear to be of particular importance in distinguishing neurobehavioural from other forms of organohalogen-induced toxicity. If this mechanistic approach can yield validated screens for the prediction of deleterious neurobehavioural effects induced by organohalogens, then this may serve to reduce the numbers of compounds proceeding to animal studies. Ultimately, *in vivo* analysis of neurobehaviour will always be of particular importance in comparing the effects of individual congeners and complex mixtures of organohalogens and in investigating synergistic effects.

Neurodevelopmental abnormalities arise from complex interactions between environmental and genetic factors. Although human studies reveal that overall neurobehavioural effects of organohalogens are relatively subtle and may not be detectable at the level of the individual, they may have implications at the level of the population. Most chemicals in current use have only been produced within the last 50 years and their effects on humans are still largely unknown from an evolutionary perspective (Stein *et al.*, 2002). In this regard, exposure to environmental factors such as toxicants is of particular concern, not least because this is arguably the most preventable source of neurodevelopmental insult.

4.6 Acknowledgements

The authors work on this subject is currently supported by an EU 5th Framework Program Grant (QLK4-CT-2000-00261). CMR is a Science Foundation Ireland Investigator.

4.7 References

AGRAWAL AK, TILSON HA, BONDY SC (1981) 3,4,3',4'-Tetrachlorobiphenyl given to mice prenatally produces long-term decreases in striatal dopamine and receptor binding sites in the caudate nucleus. *Toxicol Lett.* 7, 417–424.

BELLINGER D, LEVITON A, SLOMAN J (1990) Antecedents and correlates of improved cognitive performance in children exposed in utero to low levels of lead. *Environ Health Perspect*. 89, 5–11.

BEMIS JC, SEEGAL R (1999) Polychlorinated biphenyls and methylmercury act synergistically to reduce rat brain dopamine content in vitro. *Environ Health Perspect*. 107, 879–885.

BERGER DF, LOMBARDO JP, JEFFERS PM, HUNT AE, BUSH B, CASEY A, QUIMBY F (2001) Hyperactivity and impulsiveness in rats fed diets supplemented with either Aroclor 1248 or PCB-contaminated St. Lawrence river fish. *Behav Brain Res*. 126, 1–11.

BOWMAN RE, HEIRONIMUS MP, ALLEN JR (1978) Correlation of PCB body burden with behavioral toxicology in monkeys. *Pharmacol Biochem Behav*. 9, 49–56.

BOWMAN RE, HEIRONIMUS MP, BARSOTTI DA (1981) Locomotor hyperactivity in PCB-exposed rhesus monkeys. *Neurotoxicology* 2, 251–268.

BROUWER A, AHLBORG UG, VAN DEN BERG M, BIRNBAUM LS, BOERSMA ER, BOSVELD B, DENISON MS, GRAY LE, HAGMAR L, HOLENE E, HUISMAN M, JACOBSON SW, JACOBSON JL, KOOPMAN-ESSEBOOM C, KOPPE JG, KULIG BM, MORSE DC, MUCKLE G, PETERSON RE, SAUER PJJ, SEEGAL RF, SMITS-VAN PROOIJE AE, TOUWEN BCL, WEISGLAS-KUPERUS N, WINNEKE G. (1995) Functional aspects of developmental toxicity of polyhalogenated aromatic hydrocarbons in experimental animals and human infants. *Eur J Pharmacol*. 293, 1–40.

BROUWER A, AHLBORG UG, VAN LEEUWEN FX, FEELEY MM (1998) Report of the WHO working group on the assessment of health risks for human infants from exposure to PCDDs, PCDFs and PCBs. *Chemosphere* 37, 1627–1643.

BYRNE JJ, CARBONE JP, HANSON EA (1987) Hypothyroidism and abnormalities in the kinetics of thyroid hormone metabolism in rats treated chronically with polychlorinated biphenyl and polybrominated biphenyl. *Endocrinology* 121, 520–527.

CHOU SM, MIIKE T, PAYNE WM, DAVIS GJ (1979) Neuropathology of 'spinning syndrome' induced by prenatal intoxication with a PCB in mice. *Ann NY Acad Sci*. 320, 373–395.

COREY DA, JUAREZ DE KU LM, BINGMAN VP, MESERVE LA (1996) Effects of exposure to polychlorinated biphenyl (PCB) from conception on growth, and development of endocrine, neurochemical, and cognitive measures in 60 day old rats. *Growth Dev Aging* 60, 131–143.

DARVILL T, LONKY E, REIHMAN J, DALY H (1996) Critical issues for research on the neurobehavioral effects of PCBs in humans. *Neurotoxicol Teratol*. 18, 265–270.

DARVILL T, LONKY E, REIHMAN J, STEWART P, PAGANO J (2000) Prenatal exposure to PCBs and infant performance on the Fagan test of infant intelligence. *Neurotoxicology* 21, 1029–1038.

DAVIDSON PW, MYERS GJ, COX C, SHAMLAYE CF, MARSH DO, TANNER MA, BERLIN M, SLOANE-REEVES J, CERNICHIARI E, CHOISY O, CHOI A, CLARKSON T (1995) Longitudinal neurodevelopmental study of Seychellois children following in utero exposure to methylmercury from maternal fish ingestion: outcomes at 19 and 29 months. *Neurotoxicology* 16, 677-688.

DAVIDSON PW, MYERS GJ, COX C, AXTELL C, SHAMLAYE C, SLOANE-REEVES J, CERNICHIARI E, NEEDHAM L, CHOI A, WANG Y, BERLIN M, CLARKSON TW (1998) Effects of prenatal and postnatal methylmercury exposure from fish consumption on neurodevelopment: outcomes at 66 months of age in the Seychelles Child Development Study. *JAMA* 280, 701–707.

DAVIDSON PW, MYER GJ, SHAMLAYE C, COX C, GAO P, AXTELL C, MORRIS D, SLOANE-REEVES J, CERNICHIARI E, CHOI A, PALUMBO D, CLARKSON TW (1999) Association between prenatal exposure to methylmercury and developmental outcomes in Seychellois children: effect modification by social and environmental factors. *Neurotoxicology* 20, 833–841.

DEWAILLY E, MULVAD G, PEDERSEN HS, AYOTTE P, DEMERS A, WEBER JP, HANSEN JC (1999) Concentration of organochlorines in human brain, liver, and adipose tissue autopsy samples from Greenland. *Environ Health Perspect.* 107, 823–828.

FANINI D, PALUMBO G, GIORGI R, PANTALEONI G (1990) Behavioral effects of PCBs in mice. *Behav Pharmacol.* 1, 505–510.

FAROON O, JONES D, DE ROSA C (2001) Effects of polychlorinated biphenyls on the nervous system. *Toxicol Ind Health* 16, 305–333.

GASIEWICZ TA RUCCI G (1984) Cytosolic receptor for 2,3,7,8-tetrachlorodibenzo-p-dioxin. Evidence for a homologous nature among various mammalian species. *Mol Pharmacol.* 26, 90–98.

GILBERT ME, CROFTON KM (1999) Developmental exposure to a commercial PCB mixture (Aroclor 1254) produces a persistent impairment in long-term potentiation in the rat dentate gyrus *in vivo*. *Brain Res.* 850, 87–95.

GILBERT ME, MUNDY WR, CROFTON KM (2000) Spatial learning and long-term potentiation in the dentate gyrus of the hippocampus in animals developmentally exposed to Aroclor 1254. *Toxicol Sci.* 57, 102–111.

GLADEN BC, ROGAN WJ (1991) Effects of perinatal polychlorinated biphenyls and dichlorodiphenyl dichloroethene on later development. *J Pediatr.* 119, 58–63.

GRANDJEAN P, BUDTZ-JORGENSEN E, WHITE RF, JORGENSEN PJ, WEIHE P, DEBES F, KEIDING N (1999) Methylmercury exposure biomarkers as indicators of neurotoxicity in children aged 7 years. *Am J Epidemiol.* 150, 301–305.

GRANDJEAN P, WEIHE P, BURSE VW, NEEDHAM LL, STORR-HANSEN E, HEINZOW B, DEBES F, MURATA K, SIMONSEN H, ELLEFSEN P, BUDTZ-JORGENSEN E, KEIDING N, WHITE RF (2001) Neurobehavioral deficits associated with PCB in 7-year-old children prenatally exposed to seafood neurotoxicants. *Neurotoxicol Teratol.* 23, 305–317.

GRANDJEAN P, WEIHE P, WHITE RF, DEBES F (1998) Cognitive performance of children prenatally exposed to 'safe' levels of methylmercury. *Environ Res.* 77, 165–172.

GRANDJEAN P, WEIHE P, WHITE RF, DEBES F, ARAKI S, YOKOYAMA K, MURATA K, SØRENSEN N, DAHL R, JØRGENSEN PJ (1997) Cognitive deficit in 7-Year-old children with prenatal exposure to methylmercury. *Neurotoxicol Teratol.* 19, 417–428.

GRAY K, LONGNECKER N, KLEBANOFF M, BROCK J, ZHOU H, NEEDHAM L (2000) In utero exposure to background levels of polychlorinated biphenyls and cognitive functioning among school-aged children. *Am J Epidemiol.* 151, S24.

HARADA M (1976) Intrauterine poisoning: clinical and epidemiological studies and significance on the problem. *Bull Inst Const Med Kumamoto Univ.* 25, 169.

HOLENE E, NAFSTAD I, SKAARE JU, SAGVOLDEN T (1998) Behavioural hyperactivity in rats following postnatal exposure to sub-toxic doses of polychlorinated biphenyl congeners 153 and 126. *Behav Brain Res.* 94, 213–224.

HONG SJ, GROVER CA, SAFE SH, TIFFANY-CASTIGLIONI E, FRYE GD (1998) Halogenated aromatic hydrocarbons suppress CA1 field excitatory postsynaptic potentials in rat hippocampal slices. *Toxicol Appl Pharmacol.* 148, 7–13.

HSU ST, MA CI, HSU SK, WU SS, HSU NH, YEH CC (1984) Discovery and epidemiology of PCB poisoning in Taiwan. *Am J Ind Med.* 5, 71–79.

HUISMAN M, KOOPMAN-ESSEBOOM C, FIDLER V, HADDERS-ALGRA M, VAN DER PAAUW CG,

TUINSTRA LG, WEISGLAS-KUPERUS N, SAUER PJ, TOUWEN BC, BOERSMA ER (1995) Perinatal exposure to polychlorinated biphenyls and dioxins and its effect on neonatal neurological development. *Early Hum Dev.* 41, 111–127.

JACOBSON JL, JACOBSON SW (1996) Intellectual impairment in children exposed to polychlorinated biphenyls *in utero*. *N Engl J Med.* 335, 783–789.

JACOBSON JL, FEIN GG, JACOBSON SW, SCHWARTZ PM, DOWLER JK (1985) The effect of intrauterine PCB exposure on visual recognition memory. *Child Dev.* 56, 853–860.

JACOBSON JL, JACOBSON SW, HUMPHREY HE (1990) Effects of *in utero* exposure to polychlorinated biphenyls and related contaminants on cognitive functioning in young children. *J Pediatr.* 116, 38–45.

JACOBSON JL, JACOBSON SW, SCHWARTZ P, FEIN G, DOWLER J (1984) Prenatal exposure to an environmental toxin: a test of the multiple effects model. *Dev Psychol.* 20, 523–532.

JETT DA, NAVOA RV, LYONS MA JR. (1999) Additive inhibitory action of chlorpyrifos and polycyclic aromatic hydrocarbons on acetylcholinesterase activity in vitro. *Toxicol Lett.* 105, 223–229.

JUAREZ DE KU LM, SHARMA-STOKKERMANS M, MESERVE LA (1994) Thyroxine normalizes polychlorinated biphenyl (PCB) dose-related depression of choline acetyltransferase (ChAT) activity in hippocampus and basal forebrain of 15-day-old rats. *Toxicology* 94, 19–30.

KODAVANTI PR, TILSON HA (2000) Neurochemical effects of environmental chemicals: in vitro and in vivo correlations on second messenger pathways. *Ann NY Acad Sci.* 919, 97–105.

KODAVANTI PR, WARD TR, MCKINNEY JD, TILSON HA (1995) Increased [^{3}H]phorbol ester binding in rat cerebellar granule cells by polychlorinated biphenyl mixtures and congeners: structure-activity relationships. *Toxicol Appl Pharmacol.* 130, 140–148.

KODAVANTI PR, DERR-YELLIN EC, MUNDY WR, SHAFER TJ, HERR DW, BARONE S, CHOKSI NY, MACPHAIL RC, TILSON HA. (1998) Repeated exposure of adult rats to Aroclor 1254 causes brain region-specific changes in intracellular Ca2+ buffering and protein kinase C activity in the absence of changes in tyrosine hydroxylase. *Toxicol Appl Pharmacol.* 153,186–198.

KOOPMAN-ESSEBOOM C, WEISGLAS-KUPERUS N, DE RIDDER MA, VAN DER PAAUW CG, TUINSTRA LG, SAUER PJ (1996) Effects of polychlorinated biphenyl/dioxin exposure and feeding type on infants' mental and psychomotor development. *Pediatrics.* 97, 700–706.

KURATSUNE M, YOSHIMURA T, MATSUZAKA J, YAMAGUCHI A (1971) Yusho, a poisoning caused by rice oil contaminated with polychlorinated biphenyls. *HSMHA Health Rep.* 86, 1083–1091.

LAI TJ, GUO YL, YU ML, KO HC, HSU CC (1994) Cognitive development in Yucheng children. *Chemosphere* 29, 2405–2411.

LAI TJ, LIU X, GUO YL, GUO NW, YU ML, HSU CC, ROGAN WJ (2002) A cohort study of behavioral problems and intelligence in children with high prenatal polychlorinated biphenyl exposure. *Arch Gen Psychiatry.* 59, 1061–1066.

LEVIN ED, SCHANTZ SL, BOWMAN RE (1988) Delayed spatial alternation deficits resulting from perinatal PCB exposure in monkeys. Arch Toxicol. 62, 267–273.

LILIENTHAL H, WINNEKE G (1991) Sensitive periods for behavioral toxicity of polychlorinated biphenyls: determination by cross-fostering in rats. *Fundam Appl Toxicol.* 17, 368–375.

LILIENTHAL H, NEUF M, MUNOZ C, WINNEKE G (1990) Behavioral effects of pre- and postnatal exposure to a mixture of low chlorinated PCBs in rats. *Fundam Appl Toxicol.* 15, 457–467.

LONKY E, REIHMAN J, DARVILL T, MATHER J, DALY H (1996) Neonatal Behavioural Assessment Scale performance in humans influenced by maternal consumption of environmentally contaminated Lake Ontario fish. *J. Great Lakes Res.* 22, 198–212.

MARIUSSEN E, FONNUM F. (2001) The effect of polychlorinated biphenyls on the high affinity uptake of the neurotransmitters, dopamine, serotonin, glutamate and GABA, into rat brain synaptosomes. *Toxicology* 159, 11–21.

MELE PC, BOWMAN RE, LEVIN ED (1986) Behavioral evaluation of perinatal PCB exposure in rhesus monkeys: fixed-interval performance and reinforcement-omission. *Neurobehav Toxicol Teratol.* 8, 131–138.

MORSE DC, GROEN D, VEERMAN M, VAN AMERONGEN CJ, KOETER HB, SMITS VAN PROOIJE AE, VISSER TJ, KOEMAN JH, BROUWER A (1993) Interference of polychlorinated biphenyls in hepatic and brain thyroid hormone metabolism in fetal and neonatal rats. *Toxicol Appl Pharmacol.* 122, 27–33.

MORSE DC, SEEGAL RF, BORSCH KO, BROUWER A (1996a) Long-term alterations in regional brain serotonin metabolism following maternal polychlorinated biphenyl exposure in the rat. *Neurotoxicol.* 17, 631–638.

MORSE DC, PLUG A, WESSELING W, VAN DEN BERG KJ, BROUWER A (1996b) Persistent alterations in regional brain glial fibrillary acidic protein and synaptophysin levels following pre- and postnatal polychlorinated biphenyl exposure. *Toxicol Appl Pharmacol.* 139, 252–61.

MUNDY WR, BUSHNELL PJ, CROFTON KM, HERR DW, MOSER, VC, KODAVANTI, PRS (1998) Neurobehavioral effects of developmental Aroclor 1254 exposure. *The Toxicologist* 42, 34.

NIEMI WD, AUDI J, BUSH B, CARPENTER DO (1998) PCBs reduce long-term potentiation in the CA1 region of rat hippocampus. *Exp Neurol.* 151, 26–34.

NISHIDA N, FARMER JD, KODAVANTI PR, TILSON HA, MACPHAIL RC. (1997) Effects of acute and repeated exposures to Aroclor 1254 in adult rats: motor activity and flavor aversion conditioning. *Fundam Appl Toxicol.* 40, 68–74.

OKEY AB, RIDDICK DS, HARPER PA (1994) The Ah receptor: mediator of the toxicity of 2,3,7,8-tetrachlorodibenzo-p-dioxin (TCDD) and related compounds. *Toxicol Lett.* 70, 1–22.

PANTALEONI GC, FANINI D, SPONTA AM, PALUMBO G, GIORGI R, ADAMS PM (1988) Effects of maternal exposure to polychlorobiphenyls (PCBs) on F1 generation behavior in the rat. *Fundam Appl Toxicol.* 11, 440–449.

PATANDIN S, LANTING CI, MULDER PG, BOERSMA ER, SAUER PJ, WEISGLAS-KUPERUS N (1999) Effects of environmental exposure to polychlorinated biphenyls and dioxins on cognitive abilities in Dutch children at 42 months of age. *J Pediatr.* 134, 33–41.

PORTE C, ALBAIGES J (1994) Bioaccumulation patterns of hydrocarbons and polychlorinated biphenyls in bivalves, crustaceans, and fishes. *Arch Environ Contam Toxicol.* 26, 273–281.

PROVOST TL, JUAREZ DE KU LM, ZENDER C, MESERVE LA (1999) Dose- and age-dependent alterations in choline acetyltransferase (ChAT) activity, learning and memory, and thyroid hormones in 15- and 30-day old rats exposed to 1.25 or 12.5 PPM polychlorinated biphenyl (PCB) beginning at conception. *Prog Neuropsychopharmacol Biol Psychiatry.* 23, 915–928.

PRUITT DL, MESERVE LA, BINGMAN VP (1999) Reduced growth of intra- and infra-pyramidal mossy fibers is produced by continuous exposure to polychlorinated biphenyl.

Toxicology 138, 11–17.

RICE DC (1995) Neurotoxicity of lead, methylmercury, and PCBs in relation to the Great Lakes. *Environ Health Perspect.* 103 (Suppl 9), 71–87.

RICE DC (1998) Effects of postnatal exposure of monkeys to a PCB mixture on spatial discrimination reversal and DRL performance. *Neurotoxicol Teratol.* 20, 391–400.

RICE DC (1999) Behavioral impairment produced by low-level postnatal PCB exposure in monkeys. *Environ Res.* 80, S113–S121.

RICE DC, EVANGELISTA DE DUFFARD AM, DUFFARD R, IREGREN A, SATOH H, WATANABE C (1996) Lessons for neurotoxicology from selected model compounds: SGOMSEC joint report. *Environ Health Perspect.* 104 (Suppl 2), 205–215.

ROEGGE CS, SEO BW, CROFTON KM, SCHANTZ SL (2000) Gestational-lactational exposure to Aroclor 1254 impairs radial-arm maze performance in male rats. *Toxicol Sci.* 57, 121–130.

ROGAN WJ, GLADEN BC. (1991) PCBs, DDE, and child development at 18 and 24 months. *Ann Epidemiol.* 1, 407–413.

ROGAN WJ, GLADEN BC, MCKINNEY JD, CARRERAS N, HARDY P, THULLEN J TINGELSTAD J, TULLY M (1986a) Polychlorinated biphenyls (PCBs) and dichlorodiphenyl dichloroethene (DDE) in human milk: effects of maternal factors and previous lactation. *Am J Public Health.* 76, 172–177.

ROGAN WJ, GLADEN BC, MCKINNEY JD, CARRERAS N, HARDY P, THULLEN J TINGELSTAD J, TULLY M (1986b) Neonatal effects of transplacental exposure to PCBs and DDE. *J Pediatr.* 109, 335–341.

ROGAN WJ, GLADEN BC, HUNG KL, KOONG SL, SHIH LY, TAYLOR JS, WU YC, YANG D, RAGAN NB, HSU CC (1988) Congenital poisoning by polychlorinated biphenyls and their contaminants in Taiwan. *Science* 241, 334–336.

SAFE S (1983) Polychlorinated biphenyls (PCBs) and polybrominated biphenyls (PBBs): Biochemistry, toxicology and mechanism of action. *CRC Crit. Rev. Toxicol.* 13, 319–395.

SAFE SH (1994) Polychlorinated biphenyls (PCBs): environmental impact, biochemical and toxic responses, and implications for risk assessment. *Crit Rev. Toxicol.* 24, 87–149.

SCHANTZ SL, BOWMAN RE. (1989) Learning in monkeys exposed perinatally to 2,3,7,8-tetrachlorodibenzo-p-dioxin (TCDD). *Neurotoxicol Teratol.* 11, 13–19.

SCHANTZ SL, LEVIN E, BOWMAN R (1991) Long-term neurobehavioural effects of perinatal PCB exposure in monkeys. *J Environ Toxicol Chem.* 10, 747–756.

SCHANTZ SL, LEVIN ED, BOWMAN RE, HEIRONIMUS MP, LAUGHLIN NK (1989) Effects of perinatal PCB exposure on discrimination-reversal learning in monkeys. *Neurotoxicol Teratol.* 11, 243–250.

SCHANTZ SL, MOSHTAGHIAN J, NESS DK (1995) Spatial learning deficits in adult rats exposed to ortho-substituted PCB congeners during gestation and lactation. *Fundam Appl Toxicol.* 26, 117–126.

SCHANTZ SL, SEO BW, MOSHTAGHIAN J, PETERSON RE, MOORE RW (1996) Effects of gestational and lactational exposure to TCDD or coplanar PCBs on spatial learning. *Neurotoxicol Teratol.* 18, 305–313.

SCHANTZ SL, SEO BW, WONG PW, PESSAH IN (1997) Long-term effects of developmental exposure to 2,2',3,5',6-pentachlorobiphenyl (PCB 95) on locomotor activity, spatial learning and memory and brain ryanodine binding. *Neurotoxicology* 18, 457–467.

SCHWEGLER H, CRUSIO WE (1995) Correlations between radial-maze learning and structural variations of septum and hippocampus in rodents. *Behav Brain Res.* 67, 29–41.

SEEGAL RF (1996) Epidemiological and laboratory evidence of PCB-induced neurotoxicity. *Crit. Rev. Toxicol.* 26, 709–737.

SEEGAL RF, SCHANTZ SL (1994) Neurochemical and behavioural sequelae of exposure to dioxins and PCBs. In: *Dioxins and Health* (Schector A, ed.). New York: Plenum Press, pp. 409–447.

SEEGAL RF, BUSH B, BROSCH KO (1991a) Sub-chronic exposure of the adult rat to Aroclor 1254 yields regionally-specific changes in central dopaminergic function. *Neurotoxicology* 12, 55–65.

SEEGAL RF, BUSH B, BROSCH KO (1991b) Comparison of effects of Aroclors 1016 and 1260 on non-human primate catecholamine function. *Toxicology* 66, 145–163.

SEEGAL RF, BUSH B, BROSCH KO. (1994) Decreases in dopamine concentrations in adult, non-human primate brain persist following removal from polychlorinated biphenyls. *Toxicology* 86, 71–87.

SEEGAL RF, OKONIEWSKI RJ, BROSCH KO, BEMIS JC (2002) Polychlorinated biphenyls alter extraneuronal but not tissue dopamine concentrations in adult rat striatum: an in vivo microdialysis study. *Environ Health Perspect.* 110, 1113–1117.

SEO BW, SPARKS AJ, MEDORA K, AMIN S, SCHANTZ SL (1999) Learning and memory in rats gestationally and lactationally exposed to 2,3,7,8-tetrachlorodibenzo-p-dioxin (TCDD). *Neurotoxicol Teratol.* 21, 231–239.

SHARMA R, DERR-YELLIN EC, HOUSE DE, KODAVANTI PR (2000) Age-dependent effects of Aroclor 1254R on calcium uptake by subcellular organelles in selected brain regions of rats. *Toxicology* 156, 13–25.

STEIN J, SCHETTLER T, WALLINGA D, VALENTI M (2002) In harm's way: Toxic threats to child development. *J. Devel. Behav. Pediat.* 23, S13–22.

STEWART PW, REIHMAN J, LONKY EI, DARVILL TJ, PAGANO J (2003) Cognitive development in preschool children prenatally exposed to PCBs and MeHg. *Neurotoxicol Teratol.* 25, 11–22.

TANABE S (1988) PCB problems in the future: Foresight from current knowledge. *Environ. Poll.* 50, 5–28.

TILSON HA, DAVIS GJ, MCLACHLAN JA, LUCIER GW (1979) The effects of polychlorinated biphenyls given prenatally on the neurobehavioral development of mice. *Environ Res.* 18, 466–474.

UNKILA M, POHJANVIRTA R, TUOMISTO JT, TUOMISTO J (1995) Alterations in plasma tryptophan binding to albumin in 2,3,7,8-tetrachlorodibenzo-p-dioxin-treated Long-Evans rats. *Eur J Pharmacol.* 293, 115–121.

VOIE OA, FONNUM F (1998) Ortho-substituted polychlorinated biphenyls elevate intracellular [Ca^{2+}] in human granulocytes. *Environ. Toxicol. Pharmacol.* 5, 105–112.

WALKOWIAK J, WIENER JA, FASTABEND A, HEINZOW B, KRAMER U, SCHMIDT E, STEINGRUBER HJ, WUNDRAM S, WINNEKE G (2001) Environmental exposure to polychlorinated biphenyls and quality of the home environment: effects on psychodevelopment in early childhood. *Lancet.* 358, 1602–1607.

WEISGLAS-KUPERUS N, PATANDIN S, BERBERS GA, SAS TC, MULDER PG, SAUER PJ, HOOIJKAAS H (2000) Immunologic effects of background exposure to polychlorinated biphenyls and dioxins in Dutch preschool children. *Environ Health Perspect.* 108, 1203–1207.

WIDHOLM JJ, CLARKSON GB, STRUPP BJ, CROFTON KM, SEEGAL RF, SCHANTZ SL (2001) Spatial reversal learning in Aroclor 1254-exposed rats: sex-specific deficits in associative ability and inhibitory control. *Toxicol Appl Pharmacol.* 174, 188–198.

WIDHOLM JJ, SEO BW, STRUPP BJ, SEEGAL RF, SCHANTZ SL (2003) Effects of perinatal exposure to 2,3,7,8-tetrachlorodibenzo-p-dioxin on spatial and visual reversal learning in rats. *Neurotoxicol Teratol.* 25, 459–471.

WINNEKE G, BUCHOLSKI A, HEINZOW B, KRAMER U, SCHMIDT E, WALKOWIAK J, WIENER JA, STEINGRUBER HJ (1998) Developmental neurotoxicity of polychlorinated biphenyls (PCBS): cognitive and psychomotor functions in 7-month old children. *Toxicol Lett.* 28, 423–428.

WORLD HEALTH ORGANIZATION (1993) International Programme on Chemical Safety. *Polychlorinated Biphenyls and Terphenyls.* 2nd edn. Geneva.

YANG JH, DERR-YELLIN EC, KODAVANTI PR. (2003) Alterations in brain protein kinase C isoforms following developmental exposure to a polychlorinated biphenyl mixture. *Brain Res Mol Brain Res.* 111, 123–135.

YU ML, HSU CC, GUO YL, LAI TJ, CHEN SJ, LUO JM (1994) Disordered behavior in the early-born Taiwan Yucheng children. *Chemosphere* 29, 2413–2422.

ZAHALKA EA, ELLIS DH, GOLDEY ES, STANTON ME, LAU C (2001) Perinatal exposure to polychlorinated biphenyls Aroclor 1016 or 1254 did not alter brain catecholamines nor delayed alternation performance in Long-Evans rats. *Brain Res Bull.* 55, 487–500.

5

Targeted and rapid methods in analysing residues in food

E. P. Meulenberg, ELTI Support, The Netherlands, M. M. Rhemrev-Boom, ResQ Lab, The Netherlands and C. G. J. Koopal, TNO Nutrition and Food Research, The Netherlands

5.1 Introduction

Since ancient times man has been fascinated by the phenomenon that people surviving serious infectious diseases were not susceptible to subsequent infections. Long before Christ, it was found in China, Western Asia and Greece that applying wound excretion onto healthy persons made them 'immune' against the same disease. This may be considered as the most primitive form of vaccination. At the end of the eighteenth century, Jenner discovered that humans living through cowpox were subsequently protected against smallpox. He concluded that similar forms of infections led to different symptoms in different hosts. About the same time, Pasteur made the first vaccine consisting of attenuated bacterial strains by sub-culturing virulent bacteria.

The theoretical aspects of immune systems were elaborated by Ehrlich (1900). He suggested that the body contained specialized cells that synthesized protecting substances, antibodies, which were secreted into the blood and functioned to rapidly eliminate intruding microorganisms. In addition, his hypothesis was that this immunological reaction had a chemical basis. Kraus, at the end of the nineteenth century, was the first to perform an *in vitro* immunochemical reaction. He observed that when serum containing antibodies against typhus bacilli was combined with cell free extract of this bacillus, a visible precipitate was formed. It appeared that the same reaction in the body could be reproduced in a test tube leading to visible antigen-antibody complexes. Based on this finding, in the following years a whole range of immunochemical assays was developed, both in solution and in gel format.

Due to the work of Felton, Heidelberger, and Kendall in the early twentieth century (Heidelberger, 1939), it was established that antiserum contained certain proteins belonging to the family of the gamma-globulins. These soluble proteins were called antibodies and they appeared to be divalent proteins that were able to form networks with antigens (target substance), an agglutination reaction leading to immune complexes or precipitates. It was also demonstrated that these networks were only formed at optimal ratios of antigen and antibody. An example of the agglutination reaction is the titration of antigen by adding serial dilutions of the corresponding antibody. The difference in diffusion behavior between antigen, antibody and complexes between them, was used to develop several techniques, e.g. the Ouchterlony test, radial immunodiffusion, immuno-electrophoresis and nowadays immunoblots (Western blots) (Benjamini and Leskowitz, 1991). However, concentrations of antigen are sometimes too small to allow precipitates to be formed. Berson and Yalow (1959) solved this problem by labelling the antigen, insuline, using ^{125}I. In this case, immune complexes can be measured by radioactivity counting. Their technique provided the breakthrough to the modern application of immunoassay for clinical diagnostics and later onto other fields of investigation.

5.2 The principles of the immunoassays

The basis of the immunoassay is the reversible high-affinity binding between a target compound, antigen, and the corresponding antibody as depicted in the following equation:

$$Ab + Ag \leftrightarrow Ab{-}Ag \qquad [5.1]$$

where Ab = antibody, Ag = antigen (analyte), Ab–Ag = immune complex. To be able to detect and/or quantify the immune complex, Ab–Ag, in most present immunoassays one of the components is labelled, giving:

$$Ab + Ab^* + Ag \leftrightarrow Ab^*{-}Ag + Ab{-}Ag \qquad [5.2]$$

or

$$Ab + Ag^* + Ag \leftrightarrow Ab{-}Ag^* + Ab{-}Ag \qquad [5.3]$$

where Ab* = labelled antibody, Ag* = labelled antigen, Ag = sample antigen (unknown concentration) and Ab, Ab* or Ag* is added in a defined amount to the reaction system. This can be shown as a standard curve constructed using equation (5.3) as depicted in Fig. 5.1. As can be seen, the higher the concentration of antigen (analyte), the lower the concentration of complex detected.

The first immunoassays were developed in solution using radioisotopes, e.g. ^{125}I, ^{131}I, ^{3}H, Cr, ^{32}P, etc. as a label, the so-called radioimmunoassay (RIA). Such formats required separation of the free and bound phase. Several means are used for such separation. By adding activated charcoal, followed by

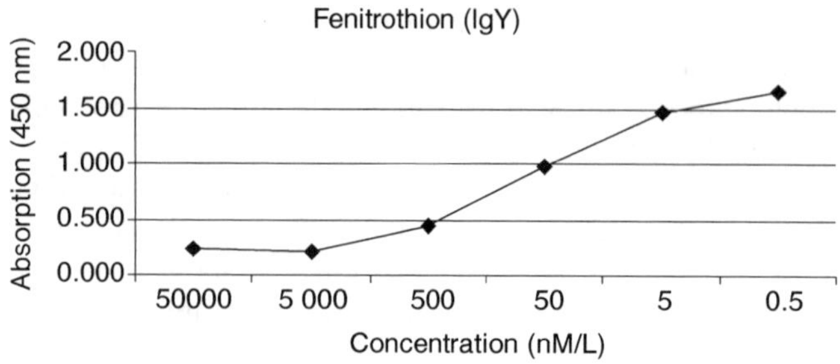

Fig. 5.1 Standard curve for fenitrothrion.
Note: Chicken antibody (IgY) against fenitrothion was used to make a standard curve.

centrifugation, the free fraction is precipitated and the supernatant, bound fraction is measured. In the case of small antigens, ethanol can be used to precipitate the protein (bound) fraction leaving the supernatant for analysis. In contrast, PEG, ammonium sulfate, sodium sulfate are used to precipitate and determine the bound fraction, especially in combination with gamma-counting. Further, gel chromatography may be used as an alternative means.

Two main modifications marked the development of the modern immunoassay, the ELISA (Enzyme Linked Immuno Sorbent Assay):

- the use of a solid support, whereon either Ab or Ag is coated
- the use of enzyme labels.

Solid supports made of plastic, glass or paramagnetic particles, may be used in various shapes and forms, such as tubes, rods, beads, plates, etc. Among these the micro-titre plate is used most commonly. In addition, radioisotopes posing health and waste disposal problems have been replaced by enzyme labelling in combination with a chromogenic or other detectectable substrate. Figure 5.2 illustrates the simplest format of an ELISA, the direct immunoassay. A defined amount of antibody is coated onto the wells of a micro-titre plate. A labelled antigen in a defined amount and a sample are added. After incubation, the wells are decanted and enzyme substrate plus chromogen is added. The enzymatic reaction is stopped using a strong acid or base and the colour developed is measured spectrophotometrically.

It will be appreciated that fluorogenic substrates can similarly be used and be measured using a fluorometer (Franek *et al.*, 2000). Further, phosphorescent, bioluminescent or chemiluminescent and electrochemical formats may be designed (Rongen *et al.*, 1994; Schobel *et al.*, 2000; Warsinke *et al.*, 2000). A review of the technique of chemiluminescence flow-injection immunoassays has been given by Gübitz *et al.* (2001).

Although the direct ELISA as described above is widely used for analysis at the field of clinical chemistry, veterinary, environmental and food control (Nilsson, 1990; Rosner *et al.*, 1991; Samarajeewa *et al.*, 1991; Dankwardt *et al.*, 1998), various alternative formats are envisaged. Among these are:

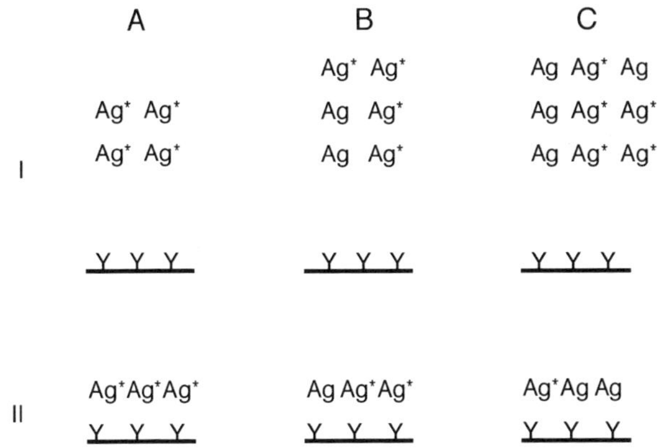

Fig. 5.2 Principle of the direct immunoassay.
Note: Ag = Antigen; Ag* = labelled antigen; Y = antibody; A = no antigen in sample; B = low amount of antigen in sample; C = high amount of antigen in sample; I = plate coated with antibody; II = antigen and labelled antigen bound to antibody on plate after the immunochemical competition reaction.

- the indirect immunoassay
- the sandwich assay
- assays using secondary or even tertiary antibody
- homogeneous assays requiring no separation step, among which the polarized fluorescent assay is well known (Önnerfjord *et al.*, 1998; Eremin and Smith, 2003).

In the indirect immunoassay the antigen is coated onto micro-titre plates; this is incubated with a sample and antibody. In this case the antibody is labelled, generally with an enzyme, and after washing, the bound fraction is measured by adding chromogen and substrate in the same way as above. Optionally, a second antibody directed against the primary antibody and labelled with an enzyme is used as a tracer as secondary antibodies are readily available both as such and labelled. Such antibodies may be used for several different immunoassays including primary antibodies from the same species, whereas in the former format for each assay the corresponding primary antibody must be labelled. Indirect immunoassays may pose problems in coating low molecular weight antigens due to failing adsorption or the fact that after adsorption they are no longer recognized by the antibody. In this case the antigens are coupled to a carrier protein such as BSA, HSA or a polymer such as polylysine. Coupling procedures will be discussed later.

Sandwich assays use two antibodies raised against different epitopes on the antigen. It will be clear that only larger antigens may contain more than one epitope. In this format, one of the antibodies is coated onto micro-titre plates and the second one is labelled and used as a tracer. The coated plate is incubated with a sample, washed and incubated with the second antibody. The more antigen is present, the more second antibody is bound to the plate leading to higher colour development in the enzyme reaction. A modification of this format is the use of a tertiary antibody raised against the second antibody and labelled instead of the second antibody. Sandwich immunoassays are generally used for proteins, peptides and microorganisms.

The above formats are all heterogeneous assays wherein bound and unbound phases are separated. In contrast, in homogeneous assay no separation is required due to a difference in signal between antigen-bound and free antibody. Generally, in such formats the tracer is fluorescently labelled. One specific embodiment is FPIA, fluorescence polarization immunoassay, wherein the binding of a fluorescently labelled antigen results in a change of the polarization of fluorescence. FPIA requires special instrumentation and also the detection limit is not as high as in common ELISA. FPIA has been described in several reviews both from a theoretical point of view and with regard to various applications (Eremin and Smith, 2003; Franek *et al.*, 2000). The applicability of a homogeneous fluoroimmunoassay was demonstrated for the detection of a pyrethroid metabolite in urine (Matveeva *et al.*, 2001). Another example of homogeneous immunoassay involves an apoenzyme covalently bound to glucose oxidase in combination with a tracer consisting of antigen-FAD conjugate. Displacement of tracer from antibody by sample antigen results in activation of the enzyme which then is able to participate in the colour development reaction.

5.3 The use of immuno-affinity chromatography

Analytical techniques used to measure the concentration of target compounds in a mixture usually involve a separation step followed by detection. For instance, high performance liquid chromatography (HPLC) is a frequently used technique in which the separation is accomplished by the differential migration of species through a packed column of particles, followed by detection of the separated compounds. Using this technique, fully automated analyses are performed quickly and with high precision. To improve chromatographic assays, however, considerable effort has been undertaken to develop sensitive and selective detection techniques (Krull *et al*, 1997). Conventional detectors include those based on the analyte's optical (ultraviolet absorption and fluorescence detection), chemical (electrochemical detection) or physical (mass spectrometry) properties. Contrary to HPLC, when an immunoassay is used for analysis, the target compound is separated from other components in the sample by binding specifically to an antibody or other binding molecule. Immunoassays combine the selectivity of antibody binding with the sensitivity of a particular label (enzyme, radioactivity, fluorophore or chemiluminescent tag). Because many immunoassay formats have been developed on a static reaction vessel (tube, well or membrane surface) to which reagents are added concurrently or sequentially, due to long incubation times (several hours), these assays are usually slow and relatively labour intensive (Fulton *et al.*, 1991).

Immuno-affinity chromatography combines the advantages of both LC and immunoassay (Afeyan *et al.*, 1992). Basically, an immuno-affinity column, which consists of an immobilized ligand (in this case the antibody), a solid phase support and a flow-through guard column, selectively isolates and/or concentrates target compounds from a complex mixture and, therefore, reduces detection limits. Because its selectivity is derived from the immobilized antibody, immuno-affinity chromatography is undoubtedly one of the most powerful techniques, when the objectives are (Hermanson, 1992):

1. *Isolation and purification* of target compounds. The inherent selectivity of immuno-affinity techniques offers and delivers high purities at high yields under the mildest of conditions.
2. *Concentrate, capture and detect* target compounds for analytical purposes. Immuno-affinity binding of low-concentration analyte to a high selective solid phase support will lead to a selective concentration and significant enhancement of analytical sensitivity.
3. *Selective removal* of undesirable contaminants from process streams, buffer or media. The selective nature of immuno-affinity techniques allows the removal of trace amounts of contaminants.

Species which are immunogenic are candidates for immuno-affinity chromatography, provided the complementary antibodies can be raised and isolated in the quantities required. The potential advantages of using HPLC to perform an immunoassay are automated capabilities, greater precision as a result of performing replicate measurements with the same equipment and readily available detection schemes. Although, compared to conventional HPLC, very fast analysis (within several minutes) can be performed this way, a realistic drawback is that sample throughput with serial processing HPLC systems is not as great as using parallel processing plate immunoassays. However, fully automated HPLC systems have been described that can reduce this limitation (Krull *et al.*, 1997).

When applying immuno-affinity chromatography, ideally, a sample passed through an immuno-affinity column separates into two bands (Walters, 1985, Leonard, 1997). The first band elutes with a capacity ratio $k' = 0$ and contains all the compounds which are not recognized by the immobilized antibody. The target compound should be strongly adsorbed to the immobilized antibody and should not elute. By adjusting the mobile phase, elution of the captured target compound is performed in a second band (see Fig. 5.3).

The correct choice of binding conditions can have a dramatic effect on the performance of the immuno-affinity column. The binding buffer establishes a favourable affinity environment and should be used to initially wash and equilibrate the immobilized antibody in preparation for binding the target molecule (Hermanson, 1992). For most antibodies, affinity interaction is optimal at about pH 7–8. For this reason, 0.01–0.1 M sodium phosphate, pH 7.0–7.4 (PBS) is frequently used as binding buffer. Sodium chloride is usually included at physiological concentration (0.15 M) for stabilization and/or to prevent nonspecific interactions. Selection of elution strategies, in general, has largely

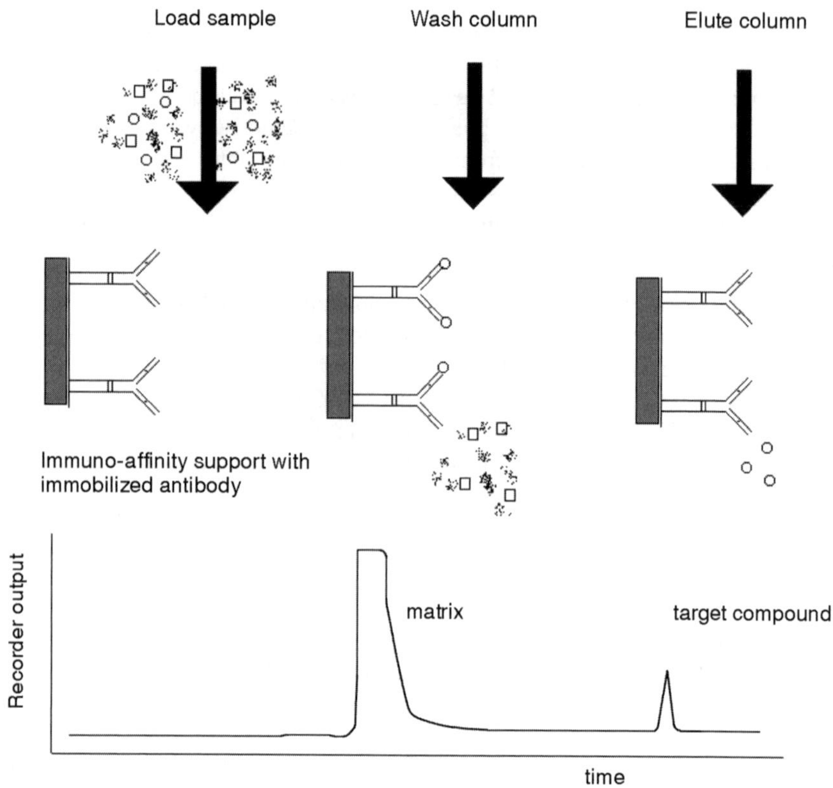

Fig. 5.3 Schematic demonstration of immuno-affinity chromatography.

been an empirical art, balancing stability of the immuno-affinity column and the eluted product and efficiency (Yarmush *et al.*, 1992). An optimal elution buffer will elute the target compound instantly without altering the target compound immobilized antibody and/or solid phase support. Deactivation of the immuno-affinity support is caused by a number of factors, including loss of antibody, structural change of the support matrix, and nonspecific adsorption of contaminating compounds, incomplete antigen elution and loss of antibody function. In most cases, this degradation is associated with repeated exposure to harsh elution conditions.

Although the choice of the elution buffer is a matter of trial-and-error, at first the properties of the antigen itself (isoelectric point, solubility, etc.) should be taken into account. Most antibody-antigen interactions are dissociated at low or high pH, and elution in immuno-affinity chromatography is mostly performed using a buffer at pH 2–3 (0.1 M glycine) or at pH 10–11 (0.1 M glycine/sodium hydroxide). Changing the pH is not always effective, as some antibodies lose their function and other methods of elution must be found. For instance, chaotropic agents may be used to effect elution by changing the structure of water in and around the site of the affinity interaction. These elution conditions work well when the bond between the ligand and target molecule is primarily formed from hydrophobic interactions. Thiocyanate (as the ammonium, sodium or potassium salt) is among the more powerful agents; at high concentration (3 M) it is capable of dissociating antigen-antibody bonds and partly unfolding protein structures. From that standpoint, it is not desirable to choose a chaotropic agent for antigen elution when either antigen or antibody is sensitive to this. Raising the ionic strength of the solvent, for instance, is an extremely mild elution technique, although it might be too mild to be effective. Concentrations of sodium chloride have been used in the range 0.75–1.2 M for that purpose. Presumably, sodium chloride is effective in those cases where charge-charge interactions play a particularly important role.

When antibodies with extremely high affinity are used, and antigen has to be recovered in the denatured form, denaturants, such as urea and guanidine hydrochloride, are sometimes chosen. Denaturants are particularly harsh eluents, and if possible, it is recommended to select another antibody. Over the years, various water miscible organic solvents have been used as elution buffer. Of all organic solvents, ethylene glycol seems to be the best choice because it denatures proteins only at very high concentrations (> 60%). In our laboratory good results have been obtained with elution buffers containing 10–35% acetonitrile (see Fig. 5.4).

Besides loading and elution conditions, the flow rate through the immuno-affinity column is another important parameter to be considered. Normally, porous beaded supports contain internal volume that is accessible to the mobile phase. Compounds are convected in the flowing stream into these pores minimizing the diffusion path length between the antigen and antibody (Afeyan *et al.*, 1992). Consequently, target compounds are rapidly brought into intimate contact with the immobilized antibody, thereby eliminating long incubation steps. However, the rate at which the mobile phase moves through the solid phase support governs the efficiency of this process. Too fast a flow will cause the mobile phase to move past the beads faster than the required diffusion time; too slow a flow will create secondary diffusion effects, a decrease in resolution and an unnecessarily long chromatographic separation.

To summarize, defining the appropriate loading and elution conditions is not only desirable for the optimum working conditions, in relation to the high costs of most antibodies, immuno-affinity columns should be reused at least hundreds of times. In most cases, the successful development of an assay based on immuno-affinity chromatography is primarily determined by the stability of the antibody under the elution conditions with respect to the affinity of antibody for the antigen. A good example of a successful application based on immuno-affinity chromatography is given in Fig. 5.5. This immuno-affinity column, an anti-testosterone column, could be used for more than 5,000 injections for the fully automatic determination of, respectively, testosterone in urine or, due to the cross-reactivity of the antibody, cholesterol in high density lipoprotein and low density lipoprotein fractions after on-line fractionation of serum by means of ion exchange chromatography.

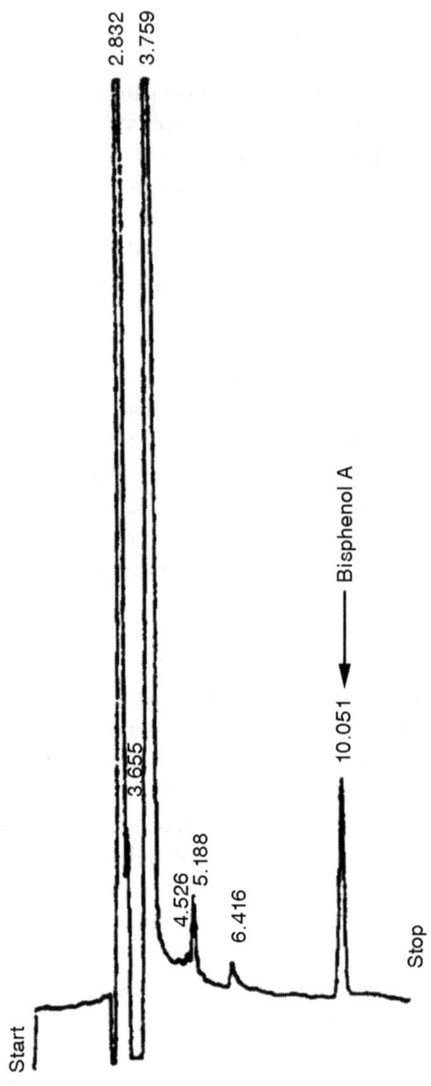

Fig. 5.4 Determination of Bisphenol A in surface waters and effluents by means of immuno-affinity chromatography with anti-bisphenol A (Elti Support, Nijmegen, the Netherlands) covalently coupled to RiFlex-HY (ResQ lab, Nijeveen, the Netherlands). Note: Immuno-affinity conditions: injection volume: 30 ml; loading buffer: PBS buffer pH 7.0, elution buffer: 35%v/v acetonitrile in water; RP-HPLC conditions: analytical column: Zorbax SB-C8, 5 μm, 250 × 4.6 mm; flow: 0.8 $ml.min^{-1}$; mobile phase: 45%v/v acetonitrile in water; detection: UV-VIS 230 nm. Performance: reproducibility: 2% RSD; Dynamic range: 3–100 ng; LOD: 100 $ng.l^{-1}$.

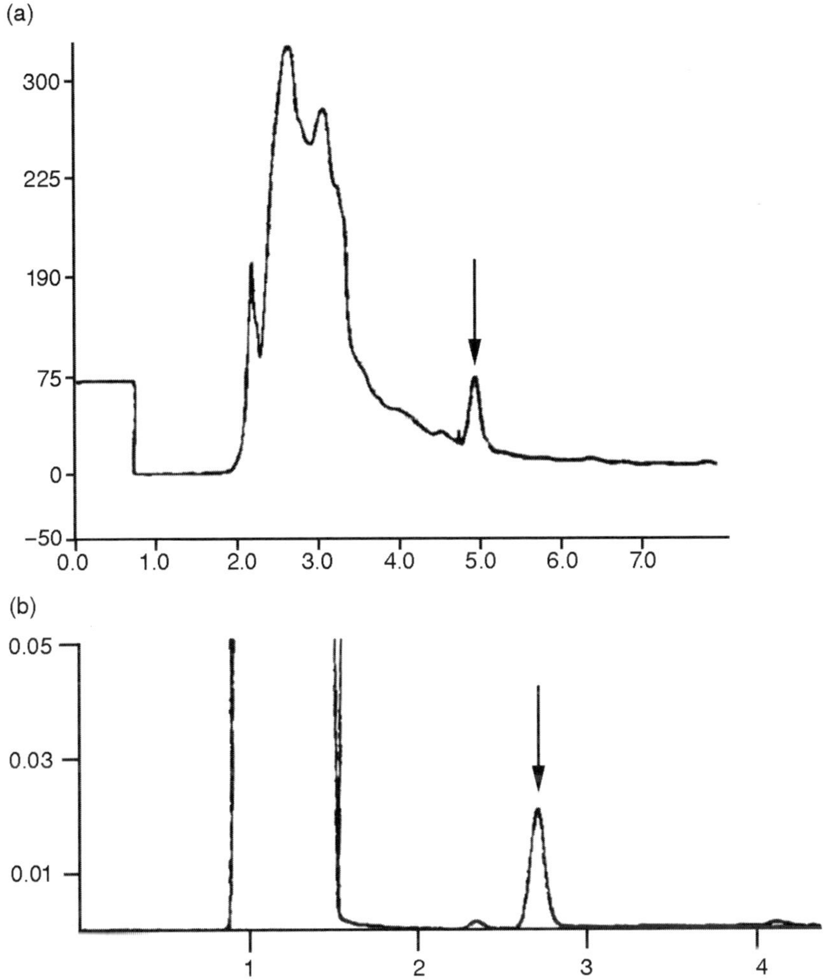

Fig. 5.5 Determination of testosterone in urine (a) respectively total cholesterol in HDL and LDL fractions (b) by means of immuno-affinity chromatography with anti-testosterone (Pierce, Illinois, USA) covalently coupled to POROS XL (PerSeptive Biosystems, Cambridge, USA).

Note: (a) Immuno-affinity conditions: injection volume: 200 ml; loading buffer: PBS buffer pH 7.0, elution buffer: methanol. RP-HPLC conditions: analytical column: Inertsil ODS-2, 5 μm, 250 × 4.6 mm; flow: 1.2 ml.min^{-1}; mobile phase: 81%v/v methanol in water; detection: UV-VIS 240 nm. Performance: reproducibility: 1% RSD; Dynamic range: 10–200 ng.

(b) Immuno-affinity conditions: injection volume: 100 μl; loading buffer: PBS buffer pH 7.0, elution buffer: methanol. RP-HPLC conditions: analytical column: Inertsil ODS-2, 5 m, 250 × 4.6 mm; flow: 1.2 ml.min^{-1}; mobile phase: 81%v/v methanol in water; detection: UV-VIS 240 nm.

Prior to determination, cholesterol is enzymatically converted by means of a cholesterol esterase/cholesterol oxidase solution.

Performance: reproducibility: 2% RSD; Dynamic range: 0.5–4.0 g.l^{-1}.

5.4 Developing immunoassays to detect residues in food and water

Each immunoassay is basically designed and/or applied in order to detect compounds or microorganisms that may be harmful for humans or animals. It can be envisaged that, consequently, target compounds vary from high molecular weight to very small molecular weight entities. Furthermore, these targets may be present in various matrices such as water, soil, food, air, rain, snow, plants, meat, bodily fluids, tissues, etc. The list of target compounds is extremely long and includes proteins, peptides, carbohydrates, growth factors, hormones, etc., in the field of clinical chemistry; pesticides, metabolites, toxins and industrial pollutants in the field of environmental analysis; drugs and growth factors in the field of pharmacology and veterinary control; microorganisms such as bacteria, viruses, fungi, and GMO, allergens, vitamins in the field of clinical chemistry, food, environmental and veterinary analysis; industrial compounds or by-products for environmental analysis or process control and many others. Development of immunoassays for such target compounds has been logarithmically increasing and several review articles have been published (Ferguson, 1984; Kaufman and Clower, 1991; Sherry, 1992; Colbert, 1994; Deshpande, 1994; Meulenberg *et al.*, 1995; Meulenberg, 1997; Gamble and Murrell, 1998; Meulenberg, 1998; Pimbley and Patel, 1998; Chapman *et al.*, 2000; Stead, 2000; Lac, 2001).

Due to the properties of speed, low sample volume, no need for pretreatment, specificity, and sensitivity, immunoassays are very useful in early warning programmes for water quality control. In our laboratory we performed several projects aimed at the detection and quantification of chlorophenoxy herbicides, phenylurea herbicides and microcystines (Meulenberg, 2000; Meulenberg and Peelen, 2002a; Meulenberg and Peelen, 2002b). Herbicides are predominantly used in spring time depending on weather conditions. Their presence in surface water is therefore unpredictable, but may reach peak concentrations above maximal admissible levels for surface water used for the production of drinking water. To avoid high costs in conventional analytical methods, where more than 90% of the samples are negative, we used commercial kits to analyze daily samples once a week. Such a protocol allows for a sufficient period of time to take measurements at the intake point of the drinking water production plant.

Microcystines present a completely different class of compounds. They are produced by blue algae (*Microcystis sp.*) especially during the summer when the temperature is high and there is little or no wind. These microcystines are excreted by the algae and pose a serious health problem in water recreation areas. They may affect the skin and lead to pulmonary problems and, in the long term, hepatic even cancer. In view of the rapid bloom of these blue algae it is important to monitor the concentration of microcystines and give a warning to people when the levels become too high (ELTI Report, 2000–2002). Figure 5.6 presents the results of a monitoring project performed in 2002 for microcystines.

For the development of an immunoassay several factors should be taken into account. First,

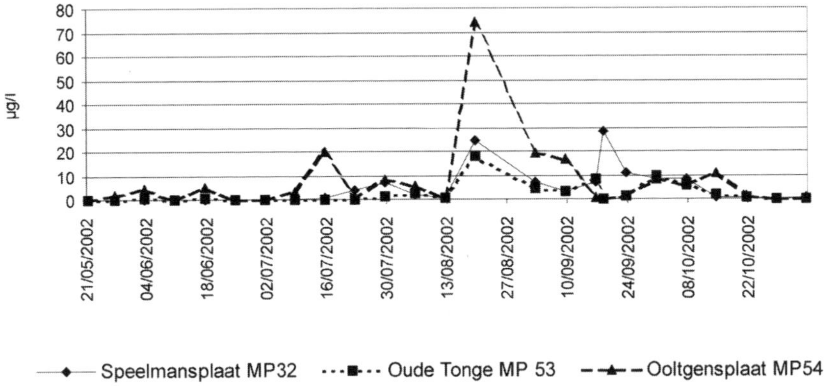

Fig. 5.6 Overview of the concentration of microcystines in surface water.
Note: Surface water was sampled at three different points in Zeeland (The Netherlands) from May–October, 2002. The samples were filtered through 0.45 μm filters and analyzed using an immunoassay kit from SDI (G.B.)

- the target compound and its physico-chemical properties
- the matrix to be analyzed for presence of the compound and whether an isolation method should be included
- the required working range of detection in association with relevant regulations.

5.4.1 Antibody production

The development of an immunoassay starts with the production of antibodies. Various animals may be chosen to raise antibodies, e.g. rabbit, rats, mice, sheep, goat, horses, chickens, even camels and llamas, depending on the use of the antibody, the amount needed, the ease of handling, costs, available facilities, etc. Immunization is performed according to standard protocols that generally involve an initial injection of immunogen in, for example, Freunds complete adjuvant, followed by several booster injections in Freunds incomplete adjuvant. Other adjuvants include mineral oils, bacterial cell wall component, alumina, etc. It should be taken into account that small compounds (< 5000 Dalton), i.e. haptens, are not immunogenic as such. In this case, conjugates with carrier proteins are used to render them immunogenic. It can be envisaged that conjugates may also lead to antibodies to the carrier protein, which may interfere in the immunoassay. Inherently, antibodies produced in animals are polyclonal, i.e. a heterogeneous population of various antibodies showing differences in affinity for the target compound. To circumvent the limited availability of polyclonal antibodies and the heterogeneity of polyclonal antiserum, an alternative *in vitro* hybridoma technique for the production of antibodies has been developed by Kohler and Milstein (1975). In principle, the properties of the antibody-producing cell are combined with the property of unlimited propagation of a myeloma cell from the same species by fusion of both. The myeloma cell is selected based on a high fusion frequency and selectability due to the lack of one or more enzymes. Further, it should be a non-secreting non-antibody producing cell line. As the antibody-producing cell usually spleen cells of an immunized mouse are isolated. Protocols for fusion of such cells have been described. As an example, suspensions of myeloma cells and spleen cells are mixed with 50% PEG (MW 1000–6000) and incubated for 1 minute at 37°C. Then the mixture is diluted with medium, centrifuged and re-suspended into selective medium, e.g. HAT medium. Unfused myeloma and spleen cells will not grow in this selection medium, only fused cells. The resultant cells are termed hybridoma cells. These are cultured further and those showing sufficient growth are used for selection of desired antibody. Most commonly, the limited dilution method is adopted, which means that the suspension of hybridoma cells is diluted such that each well in a culture plate contains only one such cell. After culturing, the supernatants of the wells are analyzed for binding to the target molecule, antigen, in an indirect immunoassay using antigen coated onto micro-titre plates and species specific labelled second antibody for detection. Those wells that contain specific antibody are used for *in vitro* antibody production. An alternative procedure for selection of useful hybridoma cells involves the isolation of the appropriate cells from the suspension on micro-titre plates, on solid support or magnetic particles coupled with the corresponding antigen. After selection the bound cells are then detached and sub-cultured in diluted form. The resulting antibodies are termed monoclonal antibodies, because they essentially originate from one single hybridoma cell.

5.4.2 Titration of antibody

During immunization, the concentration of the antibody, i.e. the titre, should be monitored to determine at what point antibodies can be collected from the blood for development of the immunoassay. Generally it takes more than two months until a sufficiently high titre is obtained. Titration of antibody involves the determination of binding to the antigen. For this, micro-titre plates are coated with the antigen, serum is added in several dilutions and binding is detected using labelled second antibody. Small molecules, haptens, cannot be coated directly onto plates and require a conjugate consisting of the hapten coupled to a carrier protein. Such conjugates are called selection conjugates.

5.4.3 Isolation of antibody

Subsequently, the antibody has to be characterized for several parameters that define a useful assay as discussed below. Isolation and optionally purification of antibody may be performed in several ways. Although crude immune serum may be used, better results are often achieved when the IgG fraction is isolated from the serum. Various protocols are available such as differential precipitation using ammonium sulfate, sodium sulfate, PEG, gel permeation chromatography, electrophoresis, and affinity chromatography on protein A, protein G, or antigen-coupled solid phase columns. In the latter case, the specific antigen is coupled onto a solid phase, immune serum is passed through the column and the antibody is then eluted (see also section 5.3).

5.4.4 Synthesis of conjugates

Depending on the format to be used, either the antibody is labelled or the antigen/hapten is labelled with a selected signal-producing tag. Covalent coupling of, for example, an enzyme or fluorophore to a protein or peptide is easy to perform according to standard protocols (Haugland, 2002; Perbio Catalog 2001–2002). However, small molecules may pose several problems. A prerequisite for coupling is the presence of one or more functional groups in the molecule. If an antigen/hapten lacks such functional groups, a derivative containing it may be used. The use of a derivative or labelled conjugate as such should not affect recognition by or affinity for the antibody. Coupling protocols have been reviewed by several authors (Szurdoki *et al.*, 1995; Szekacs *et al.*, 1995; Brandon *et al.*, 1995; Skerritt and Lee, 1996). In principle, the same chemistry is used for the synthesis of hapten-based immunogens or selection conjugates.

5.4.5 Standard curve

The first step in designing a direct immunoassay is to determine optimal concentrations of antibody and tracer in a so-called checkerboard analysis. Then displacement of the tracer is checked by adding increasing concentrations of analyte to the binding reaction mixture for the construction of a standard curve. From this standard curve the detection limit and working range may be determined. Both of these parameters should cover regulatory levels. It will be appreciated that such levels vary for most target compounds as well as possible matrices. The lowest range may be taken as the main goal, because samples with levels exceeding the highest detectable concentration may be diluted. When the detection level and working range do not meet the definitions set, the conditions of the immunochemical reaction may be modified, for example, by changing the buffer used, pH, reaction temperature and period, and concentrations of the components in the reaction mixture. For instance, by lowering the amount of antibody coated, the sensitivity of the assay may be lowered.

5.4.6 Specificity

Subsequently, the specificity of the antibody should be determined by measuring cross-reactivities of related and unrelated compounds. As mentioned above, the molecular size of a target compound will determine whether it fits into the binding site of an antibody as a whole or that more than one epitope for antibody binding is present. For example, certain groups of pesticides contain common chemical functionalities, for example, the organophosphate insecticides chlorpyrifos, fenitrothion and pirimifos. By selecting this common part for coupling of carrier protein, the opposite site containing the compound-specific part will be available for exposure to the immune system and resulting antibodies. Following such an approach will yield compound-specific assays. On the other hand, coupling carrier proteins to the compound-specific site will yield group-specific antibodies and corresponding assays. Larger molecules such as proteins, peptides or even whole microorganisms sometimes contain a large number of epitopes and hence related compounds or microorganisms may show cross-reactivity with the antibody produced. Cross-reactivities are determined by comparing the standard curve (analyte) with those of the compounds to be tested and calculating the ratio of the concentrations at the 50% binding point (IC_{50}) times 100%.

5.4.7 Matrix effects

Next, matrix effects, i.e. interferences derived from the particular matrix containing the analyte to be measured, are determined by measuring the analyte in several different matrices. For example, analytes present in surface water are added in various concentrations including zero concentration and compared to analyte in assay buffer. Although aqueous samples may in principle be measured directly without any pretreatment, care should be taken with samples at high or low pH, e.g. fruit juices, because this may interfere with the binding reaction. Difficulties are to be expected when analytes are to be measured in solid and liquid matrices that have to be extracted, such as food, crops, plants, soil, sediments, serum, urine, tissues, etc. Depending on the physico-chemical properties of the analyte and the occurrence at the surface or dispersed in a particular matrix, a suitable solvent should be selected, optionally in combination with a suitable extraction technique. As a result the analyte will be contained in the selected solvent. Aqueous buffers may be applied in the immunoassay as such, but organic solvents generally have an adverse effect. The effect of such solvents in various concentrations may be determined and subsequently the extract has either to be diluted in buffer, the solvent exchanged or the extract further cleaned up. An overview of current generic extraction and clean up procedures is given in several reports (Jourdan *et al.*, 1996; Skerrit and Rani, 1996; Scippo and Maghuin-Rogsister, 2000; Barker, 2000; Stolker *et al.*, 2000).

5.4.8 Linearity

The linearity in an assay is determined by diluting a high concentration sample several times in either assay buffer or sample matrix. In comparing expected and found levels, at best a 45 degree regression line is found.

5.4.9 Precision and accuracy

Furthermore, for each immunoassay the precision and accuracy have to be determined. Precision involves the calculation of intra- and inter-assay variation at three different levels and variation preferably is below 10%. Accuracy is an important parameter in validation of immunoassays. It means that amounts present in a sample are measured accurately comparable with or better than conventional methods, if available. Recoveries should preferably and reproducibly be in the range of 80 to 100%. Both spiked and real samples are analyzed and compared with the corresponding conventional method such as HPLC, GC, MS.

5.4.10 Evaluation and validation

Protocols and ISO norms for the immunoassay method are established and available at the US EPA, FDA and the NEN Institute (The Hague, The Netherlands). By following these protocols and meeting the norms, any immunoassay may be evaluated and used as a validated analytical method to detect and quantify target compounds. Further regulatory aspects and requirements have been reviewed by MacNeil and Kay (2000). Guidelines for the validation of genetically engineered and transgenic crops are given by Lipton *et al.* (2000).

5.4.11 Alternative formats

In addition to the conventional immunoassays (ELISA, CIA, FIA, etc.) on micro-titre plate or in flow systems, two alternative useful formats have been developed, the immunofiltration assay and the dipstick (comparable to the pregnancy test). In immunofiltration the antibody is coated onto a membrane in a container. The sample is passed, followed by tracer and then chromogen/substrate in order to arrive at the colour reaction. The advantage of such a system is that a high sample volume may be used, leading to a kind of concentration factor for the analyte. If performed in micro-titre plates, this assay is suitable for automation (Morais *et al.*, 1999). Dipstick assays are predominantly for qualitative or semi-quantitative detection of analytes. For example, the peanut protein conarachin, an allergen, has been detected in all kinds of food samples at a contamination level of 0.1% after simple buffer extraction using a dipstick consisting of an immunostick coated with polyclonal antibodies. This stick is successively immersed in extract, a solution of biotine-labelled antibody, avidine-HRP, TMB substrate, and sulfuric acid. Aliquots of the resulting coloured solution are added to a micro-titre plate and analyzed in a reader (Mills *et al.*, 1997). Another dipstick comparable to the pregnancy test was designed to dectect the antibiotic sulfadimidine. Onto a flow membrane a sulfadimidine-OVA conjugate as well as total sheep IgG was immobilized at two membrane sites. Specific antibody coupled to gold particles and samples are added and allowed to migrate through the membrane. If no analyte is present in the sample, the antibody will bind to the OVA-conjugate which is visible as a red line; in contrast, analyte in the sample will prevent this binding and the antibody will migrate to the sheep IgG giving a red line at the second spot

(Verheijen *et al.*, 1998). Even a homogeneous dipstick has been developed for the detection of TNT in drinking water at a detection level of 0.7 μg/l using a combination of a FAD-TNT-conjugate, specific antibody, glucose oxidase (GOD) and apo-GOD. The presence of TNT in a sample will prevent the binding of apo-GOD to GOD and consequently an enzyme reaction does not occur (Heiss *et al.*, 1999).

5.5 Recent developments in immunoassays

Regarding the enormous list of immunoassays described up to now, it appears that most of the polyclonal and monoclonal antibodies developed satisfy the needs of most researchers and other users. However, there always remain situations where conventional antibodies and/or immunoassays are not suitable because of a lack of specificity and/or affinity. Advances in molecular biology and genetic engineering have allowed the isolation of the genes coding for antibodies. An IgG antibody presents the well known Y-shape consisting of two identical large or heavy peptide chains and two identical short or light peptide chains linked together by S-bridges. The portion formed by the stem of the antibody comprises predominantly highly conserved amino acids and defines the species specificity of the antibody for binding to receptors on cells and organs. The two arms of the Y-shaped protein are formed by the light chains linked to the corresponding part of the long chains. These portions of the antibody consist of the variable parts and the antigen specific binding sites.

At DNA level there exist three clusters of gene segments distributed over three different chromosomes coding for regions of the heavy chains and, for the mouse, only one segment for the variable domain. Triggering of a lymphocyte results in differentiation of the cell and rearrangement or translocation of the DNA segments. Splicing of the transcribed RNA yields mRNA which can now be used for the synthesis of heavy and light chains. Regarding the infinite combinations possible, this explains the capability of the body to produce millions of different antibodies. The gene segments may be isolated from the DNA and are then available for either direct introduction into microorganisms through the use of plasmids or vectors leading to recombinant antibodies. Pesticide analysis using recombinant antibodies has been described in general by Ward *et al.* (1995).

Genetic engineering is more directed to the variable part of antibodies, the binding sites, and optionally modification of the nucleotides in order to vary the properties of the resulting antibodies or fragments thereof. A very useful technique was developed using bacteriophages as recipients of antibody DNA fragments. It has been demonstrated that for some bacteriophages, i.e. the filamentous phages such as lambda, Fd, etc., genes may be inserted such that the corresponding antibody fragments are expressed at the tip of the phage. By infecting appropriate bacteria the 'phage antibodies' may be produced *in vitro* in large amounts. Selection of desired phage antibodies is performed in a similar way as for polyclonal or monoclonal antibodies by coupling the target antigen onto a solid phase, incubating with phage suspension and isolating antigen-bound phages for further characterization. Production and use of such recombinant and phage antibodies has been described by several authors (Choudray *et al.*, 1995; Alcocer *et al.*, 2000; Benhar 2001; Daly *et al.*, 2001; Lange *et al.*, 2001). For example, an assay for atrazine was developed using recombinant FAB fragments produced in the yeast Pichia (Lange *et al.*, 2001). Production of phage antibody fragments has been especially successful in clinical medicine (Prof. van Venrooij, personal communication).

Immunoassays have proven to be comparable to conventional analytical methods with regard to sensitivity, specificity/selectivity, and other analytical parameters. The advantage of the immunoassays relative to methods such as HPLC, LC or MS, is the capability to measure large amounts of sample sometimes without any pretreatment from a very small sample volume within a very short time (about 2–3 hours for most assays). The disadvantage is that for each target compound a different assay has to be developed and used for measurement. For example, when it is desired to control surface water for the presence of both herbicides such as triazine and phenylurea compounds, and insecticides such as organophosphates, for each target compound or group of compounds, assay kits are commercially available, but have to be used separately with the same sample.

A solution to this drawback is the development of multi-analyte immunoassays. One multi-analyte immunoassay for drugs in urine, based on the agglutination reaction was developed by Parsons *et al.* (1993) using the Advisor reaction disc system. In a multi-channel system coated with different selection-conjugates of hapten and fluorescein, a mixture of sample, primary antibodies and anti-fluorescein second antibodies coupled to micro-particles is added to a central sample reservoir. If one or more of the target compounds is present in the sample the agglutination reaction between both antibodies and fluorescein-drug conjugate is unable to occur, because the primary antibodies are occupied by the corresponding analyte.

The group of Dr A. Montoya has designed an indirect multi-analyte immunoassay for N-methylcarbamates (Montoya *et al.*, 2001). Herein selection conjugates of several haptens coupled to OVA were coated on micro-titre plates divided into four parts. The plates are incubated with sample or standard and the corresponding antibodies for each target compound. After washing, secondary antibodies labelled with HRP are added and the colour reaction allowed to take place. Each part of the micro-titre plate thus yields results for the particular analyte. This type of assay for N-methylcarbamates was validated for use in fruits (Montoya, 2002). A direct multi-analyte immunoassay for the organophosphate insecticides fenitrothion, chlorpyrifos and pirimiphos was developed in our own laboratory. Here highly specific antibodies against these compounds were coated onto the wells of a micro-titre plate, for each target compound two rows of the plate and the last two rows for a combination of the three antibodies. Then the plate was incubated with a mixture of the corresponding tracers and standards. Due to the high specificity and very low cross-reactivity of the antibodies, this type of assay allows for the simultaneous determination of several different insecticides in a group-specific and a compound-specific fashion (Meulenberg *et al.*, 2001). Essentially an unlimited combination of antibodies may be used in such format and applied for environmental, food and veterinary uses by combining antibodies, various tracers, etc. (Bilitewski, 1998). All the multi-analyte assays described above are based on enzyme reactions in discrete wells for each target compound or group of compounds. However, the use of tracers with different fluorescent tags, i.e. showing different excitation/emission spectra, may enable the simultaneous detection of several analytes. Such fluorophores are commercially available, including coupling protocols (Haugland, 2002).

Micro-array immunoassay is a recently developed format and involves the spotting of various antibodies on a biochip. In a flow cell system sample or standard, followed by tracer and chemiluminescent substrate are allowed to react. Signal detection is made using a CCD camera. This system has been used for the identification and quantification of cross-reacting triazines and metabolites (Winklmair *et al.*, 1999). Immunoarray assays based on the calculation of cross-reactivities of triazine herbicides using complex mathematics have also been described (Wortberg *et al.*, 1995). Further research is needed for optimization of micro-array immunoassay systems.

It will be appreciated that the above description of the immunoassay is by no means exhaustive. Many more examples can be found in the literature as well as alternative forms of embodiments. Reference is made particularly to the review articles cited.

5.6 Recent developments in immuno-affinity chromatography

Undoubtedly, immuno-affinity chromatography is one of the most powerful techniques to selectively isolate and/or concentrate minor target compounds from complex mixtures. If used in combination with other modes of chromatography, for instance HPLC, the immuno-affinity column can serve as a selective (on-line) clean-up step. Antibodies for this purpose may be selected that are specific for a single analyte or cross-react with a set of related analytes sharing a common epitope. After elution of the captured analytes by means of the immuno-affinity column, quantitative analysis can be performed by HPLC (Rhemrev-Boom *et al.*, 2001). Today, a variety of antibodies with the required characteristics can be produced even at large scale, making this technique more and more accessible in a large field of applications. Due to this, many researchers put a lot of effort in the development of reliable solid-phase supports (Hermanson *et al.*, 1992). The term 'support' or 'media' is usually understood to refer to a combination of a ligand (in this case an antibody) that is firmly attached or immobilized, mostly covalently, to a matrix (an insoluble substance, with a defined particle diameter). When designing an immuno-affinity support, perhaps the most important question is whether a reliable commercial source exists for the desired solid-phase support in the quantities required. Despite a significant improvement in the characteristics of commercially available supports over the years, no 'perfect' support for every application is available. In general, these supports should be chemically stable to withstand regeneration and cleaning procedures and have low non-specific adsorption or interaction. High ligand accessibility in order to obtain high capacity immuno-affinity supports as well as particle size, pore-size distribution and low costs are also important parameters. Furthermore, these supports should be mechanically stable to allow high flow rates and withstand the high pressures normally used in HPLC.

To be more specific, a solid-phase support contains two aspects, the core particle and the stationary phase, which determines the functionality of the support and is immobilized onto the core. Over time, a wide variety of materials, each with its own advantages and disadvantages, have been proposed for the design of these solid-phase supports (Hermanson *et al.*, 1992; Phillips, 2000; Scouten, 1981). Among the first materials introduced were natural polysaccharides, such as agarose, cellulose and cross-linked dextran (Cuatrecasas *et al.*, 1968). These materials have an abundance of primary hydroxyl groups, which are easily activated to a wide range of activation procedures, and do not contribute to non-specific binding of non-target molecules. Agarose for instance has a large population of both primary and secondary hydroxyls. Due to these secondary hydroxyls, which are not consumed during or after activation and cross-linking reactions, the hydrophilic nature of the matrix is preserved. Although stable over a wide pH-range, their major drawback is their poor mechanical strength related to their swelling ability, and they are therefore not suitable as solid phase support for immuno-affinity chromatography when combined with HPLC. Synthetic organic polymers, such as polyacrylamide, polyacrylate, polystyrene/divinylbenzene and combinations thereof, exhibit, in most cases, a better pressure tolerance compared to natural polymers (Hermanson *et al.*, 1992). Many of those supports are also more tolerant towards changes in buffer composition, withstand organic solvents and tolerate extremes in pH. In addition, because of their synthetic nature, these materials are, unlike natural polymers, usually microbe resistant. Although surface derivatization of these particles provides enough ligand density for many immuno-affinity-based separations, their capacity is generally less when compared to natural polymers. In addition, due to the hydrophobic character of some synthetic polymers, for certain applications non-selective adsorption can be a problem. The inorganic silica is, undoubtedly, the most widely used chromatographic material. These materials, including alumina and certain zeolites have the inherent advantage of rigidity over soft gels of agarose or beaded cellulose. Although functional groups can be easily introduced and a variety of protocols have been proposed throughout the years to modify the surface of silica, its main disadvantage is the instability at mild alkaline pH (Hofstee, 1975).

Although the core plays a dominant role in the mechanical, chemical and thermal stability of the solid-phase support, the functionality of the solid-phase support should be such that relatively unstable biomolecules, such as antibodies, can be covalently coupled preferably under physiological conditions (Hermanson *et al.*, 1992; Phillips, 2000).

For immuno-affinity based separations, protocols for the activation of the solid-phase support have been developed for the so-called site-directed coupling of antibodies. When coupled at random, even stable antibody preparations can lose effective activity if their antigen-binding sites are blocked. Preferably, the immobilized antibody should be oriented such that its bivalent binding potential for antigen can be fully realized (O'Shannessy and Wilchek, 1990). For instance immobilized protein A can be used to orient the antibody with its antigen-binding sites pointing away from the matrix. The Fc binding properties of protein A leave the antigen-specific sites of the antibody free to interact with antigen. Cross-linking of this complex with a bifunctional cross-linker, such as dimethyl pimelimidate, creates a stable immuno-affinity support with good antigen-binding activity. However, this method of antibody immobilization works well if there are no other immuno-globulins present in the matrix from which the antigen should be isolated. If so, unexpected non-specific interactions may occur, and for this reason it is recommended to use another method of antibody immobilization.

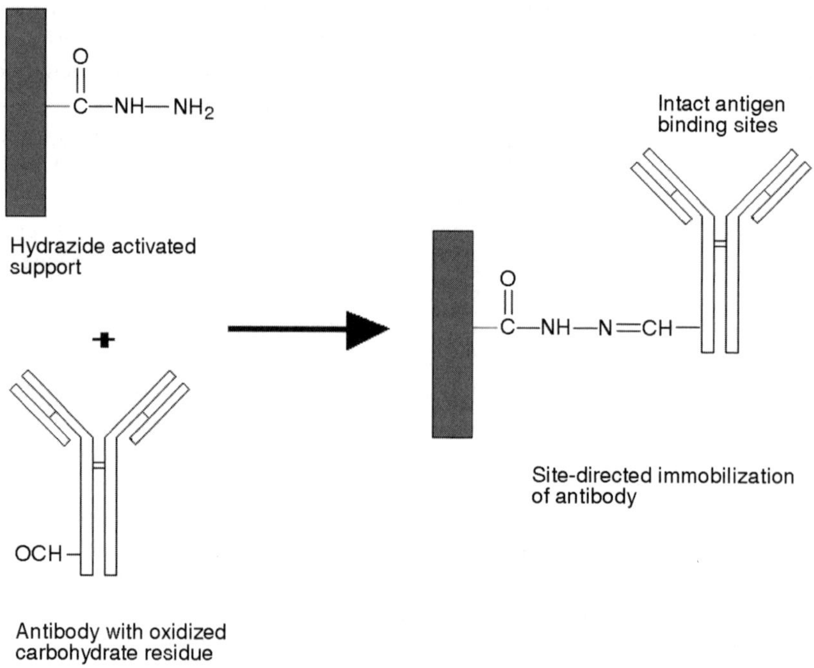

Fig. 5.7 Site-directed coupling of antibodies to a hydrazide-activated solid-phase support.

A frequently used procedure is coupling of the antibody to a hydrazide activated support (see Fig. 5.7). These supports permit the coupling of aldehyde or ketone-containing ligand through the formation of stable hydrazone linkages. By mildly oxidizing the sugar residues from the heavy chains in the CH_2 domain of the antibody, formyl groups will be generated, which can be used for site-directed immobilization of the antibody. In general, this method results in the coupling of intact antibody molecules and usually gives a high yield of antigen-binding site activity. In fact, only the site-directed method of coupling to the oxidized carbohydrate residues using hydrazide chemistry resulted in theoretical maximum antigen binding activity.

Recently, our laboratory developed a new solid-phase support, based on a rigid inorganic polymer (Rhemrev-Boom, 2001). By shielding the surface of the core with a hydrophilic polymer, the chemical stability is improved and non-selective adsorption of, in particular, lipophilic target compounds is minimized. By cross-linking the polymer around the surface of the core, the coating is stabilized and functional groups are introduced for activation of the solid-phase support. Based on this material, several activated supports have been made: an aldehyde activated support for the covalent coupling of proteins, receptors, enzymes, etc., through the primary amine of the ligand via reductive amination and a Protein A and hydrazide activated support for the covalent coupling of antibodies. In this way, materials have been obtained with good mechanical, physical and chemical stability. The solid-phase support demonstrated a low non-selective interaction and adequate capacity for separations on analytical scale. An example of a successful application developed with this material based on immuno-affinity chromatography is given in Fig. 5.8.

5.7 The use of immunosensors in residue analysis

Immunosensors are a subgroup of the larger class of biosensors. By definition, a biosensor utilizes a biological compound, e.g. an enzyme, immunoglobulin, receptor or even a whole cell, to detect specific substances in the measurement environment (Turner *et al.*, 1989). Consequently, immunosensors are biosensors that utilize immunochemical moieties for detection. The fundamental principles of biosensors in general and more specifically the immunosensors as described here, can be found elsewhere (Wise, 1989; Cahn, 1993; Scott, 1998).

In principle, any immunoassay can be translated into an immunosensor format and the usefulness of the result is merely dependent on the quality of the antibodies that are applied. Furthermore, the detection limit and the dynamic range is only marginally determined by the sensor platform utilized; the properties of the antibodies and the antigens used in conjunction with these antibodies are largely responsible for the end results of the immunosensor. Naturally, the quality of the physical principle behind the sensor needs to be sufficient in order to sustain the statement above.

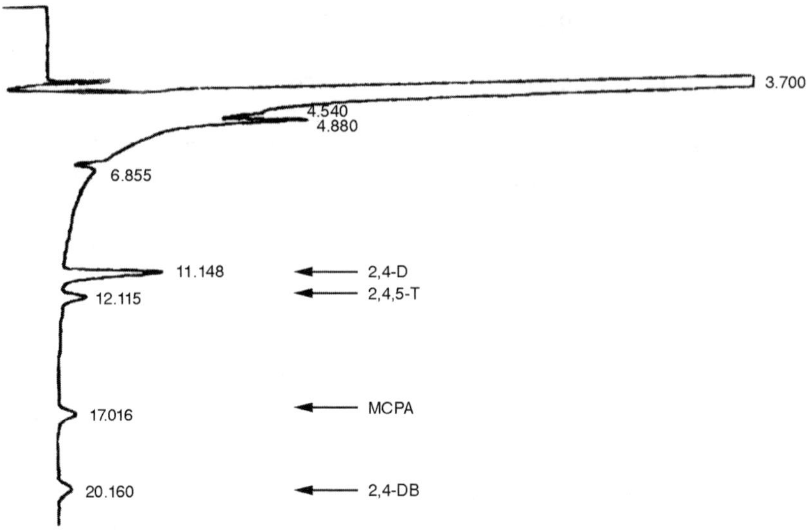

Fig. 5.8 Determination of chlorophenoxyacetic acid herbicides in surface waters and effluents by means immuno-affinity chromatography with antibody (Elti Support, Nijmegen, the Netherlands) covalently coupled to RiFlex-HY (ResQ lab, Nijeveen, the Netherlands).

Note: Immuno-affinity conditions: injection volume: 30 ml; loading buffer: PBS buffer pH 7.0, elution buffer: 10%v/v acetonitrile in water; RP-HPLC conditions: analytical column: Zorbax SB-C8, 5 μm, 250 $\times$ 4.6 mm; flow: 0.8 ml.min^{-1}; mobile phase: 60%v/v methanol in 0.1 N HCl; detection: UV-VIS 230 nm.

Performance: reproducibility: 4–6% RSD; Dynamic range: 5–1000 ng; LOD: 1–5 ng.

Only a small number of biosensor principles, suitable for the difficult task to tackle the small concentrations in the complex matrix in residue analysis, is available commercially at present. Principles like fluorescence and surface plasmon resonance (SPR) are the most popular techniques for these applications, while techniques based on electrochemical, acoustic and optical wave-guide sensors can also be found in the literature. However, reliable applications for the latter alternatives are rare at the present time.

5.7.1 Formats for immunosensors

The format for an immunosensor assay is normally the same as can be found in the plate immunoassays as described previously in this chapter, i.e. there are direct and indirect immunosensor assays, while in the latter case the assay can be further defined as either an inhibition assay or a competition assay.

Direct assay

The direct immunosensor is based on the principle of the straightforward capture and measurement of an analyte by an immobilized antibody on the surface of the biosensor. The direct immunosensor for trace analysis is not very popular, as it normally lacks the necessary sensitivity. This is rather obvious if one considers that most transducers in biosensor technology are essentially based on some change in the surface properties of the sensor during the binding event of the immunochemical partners involved (e.g. mass increase, refractive index change, change of viscosity). The small analytes present only very small changes in this respect. An exception would be an analyte displaying fluorescent properties (see below; example fluorescent sensor). Therefore, direct immunosensor assays are normally not applied to residue analysis. Instead, several forms of indirect formats are utilized, as discussed below.

Indirect inhibition assay

While immunoassays always need labelled antibodies in indirect formats, immunosensors can be designed in such a way that label-free detection is possible. This is a great advantage of the immunosensor approach. The large mass of antibodies makes this label-free detection possible. However, labelled antibodies may also be used, as for example in fluorescence-based immunosensors. In this case, the antibodies are modified with a fluorescent label. The antigen (analyte) is immobilized on the sensor surface, similar to in micro-titre plate coating. Often some kind of covalent chemistry for surface immobilization is applied to the antigen or the protein conjugate with the antigen. This is done in order to obtain a more stable sensor surface, as a biosensor is supposed to have a longer life span than the (disposable) micro-titre plate. Simple surface adsorption would lack the desired stability for a sensor application. Furthermore, the regeneration of the sensor surface for repeated use (see below) is performed under conditions which will certainly destroy the weak physical bonds involved in simple surface adsorption.

The antibody in solution, labelled or not, is then passed over the sensor surface, which is modified with the antigen. Consequently, when the antibody is captured by the antigens on the surface, the concomitant sensor response can be measured.

In order to measure the analyte concentration in solution, an inhibition immunosensor assay is performed. In this inhibition format, the analyte of interest (which is also bound on the sensor surface) is incubated in solution with the antibodies. The antibodies are present in a known concentration. The sensor response of this antibody concentration, i.e. without any analyte present, is known to the user. This is the maximum sensor response that can be expected. If one is able to construct a biosensor, which provides a significant signal due to the binding of a highly diluted antibody solution, very sensitive measurements can be performed with this indirect sensor assay. This is due to the fact that the highly diluted antibody solution becomes easily saturated with the analyte antigen present at low concentrations. The antibodies which are saturated with the analyte are no longer capable of binding to the sensor surface, leading to a decreased signal (inhibited response). The high molecular mass of antibodies makes the inhibition approach very feasible in combination with mass or refractive index sensitive sensors.

Competition assay

If the inhibition approach cannot be used for some reason, e.g. if a fluorescent sensor principle is utilized, the competition sensor assay may be used in order to improve the sensitivity with respect to the direct sensor assay. As with the other alternatives, the competition immunosensor assay is designed in a similar manner as the corresponding plate immunoassay (see equation 5.2). The sensor surface may be coated with the antibody, as in the direct assay, while the measurement is performed by mixing the analyte with a known amount of a labelled antigen, e.g. carrying a fluorescent label. The mixed sample solution is then passed over the sensor surface, where the free analyte and the labelled antigen compete for the binding sites on the sensor surface. As in the competition sensor assay, a decrease in signal is observed with increasing concentration of analyte, leading to a highly sensitive measurement format. For this competition format, one needs to work with labelled substances, which is a drawback with respect to the label-free mass sensitive sensor alternatives.

5.7.2 Example: SPR sensor

Numerous examples of immunosensors can be found in the literature. The sensor formats deal with, e.g. HCG (human chorionic gonadotropin), vitamin H (biotin), cardiolipin (see Cahn, 1993; Scott, 1998); many more examples can be found on the websites of Biacore AB (Biacore.com) and IASys (Affinity-

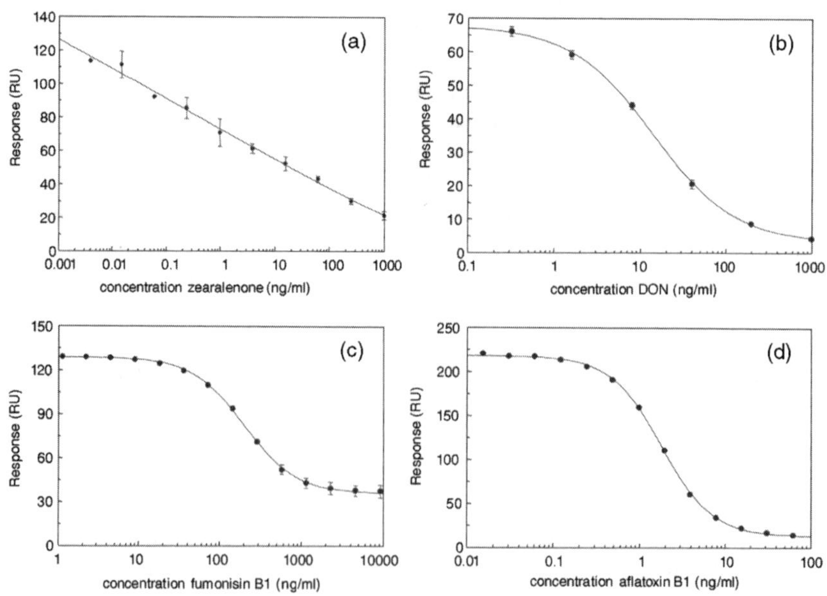

Fig. 5.9 Calibration curves for mycotoxins (a) zearalenone, (b) DON, (c) fumonisin B1 and (d) aflatoxin B1.

Table 5.1 Legal and/or advisory levels, detection limits and reproducibility of multi-analyte immunosensors.

Mycotoxin	Level (ng/g)	Detection limit (ng/g)	RSD (%)
Aflatoxin B1	2	0.2	2–10
Zearalenone	200	0.01	16–19
Ochratoxin A	3	50	4–9
Fumonisin B1	1000	0.5	2–8
DON	500		2–5

sensors.co.uk), two commercial system manufacturers for imunosensor technology. As a primary example of the immunosensor for residue analysis, an application of an SPR immunosensor is described below (Van der Gaag *et al.*, 2003). The example deals with the detection of various mycotoxins, utilizing an inhibition immunosensor assay. The sensor system used is a Biacore 2000 in combination with Biacore CM5 sensor surfaces (Biacore AB, Sweden).

In order to perform an inhibition immunosensor format, the mycotoxins were modified in order to enable the immobilization onto the CM5 sensor surface (Thouvenot, 1983). This immobilization was then performed using standard procedures, as recommended by Biacore (Jönsson *et al.*, 1991). A total of five mycotoxins were immobilized – aflatoxin B1, zearalenone, ochratoxin A, fumonisin B1 and deoxynivalenol (DON). The sensors were then calibrated using diluted antibody solutions for the various mycotoxin antigens on the sensor surface, in combination with the appropriate mycotoxin standard solutions. Calibration curves for four standards are shown in Fig. 5.9.

In order to express the practical potential of this example, the performance of the mycotoxin sensors is summarized in Table 5.1, where the results are compared to the legal and/or advisory levels for these mycotoxins in raw food materials (e.g. cereals). It can be seen from the table that the immunosensor consequently has detection limits for the tested mycotoxins that are well below the legal limits. Furthermore, these detection limits can compete very well with plate immunoassays. The sensor may be even more quantitative than a plate immunoassay, provides faster results and is reusable.

5.7.3 Future potential of immunosensors

The example above deals with an expensive and large laboratory version of SPR technology. However, to find practical application in industry or in the field, e.g. at collection and/or import facilities and environmental screening, miniaturized sensor systems would be very desirable. A promising development is the chip version of SPR as provided by Texas Instruments; the SPREETA device (Nomadics, Inc, Stillwater, OK, USA). This chip houses the full optics and electronics for SPR measurement in a housing which is smaller than a two Euro coin (see Fig. 5.10 for recent version of this device). With this kind of

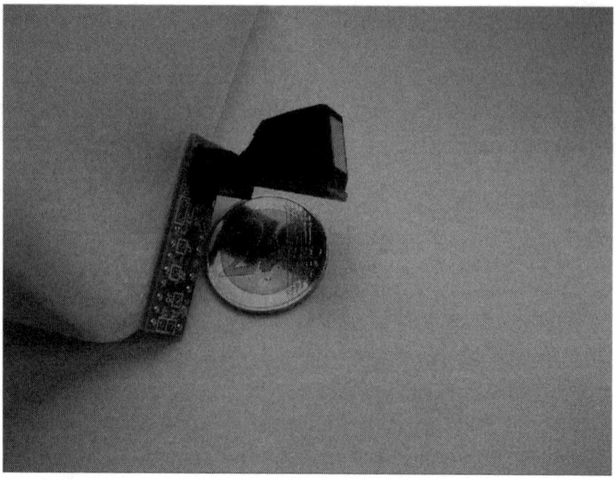

Fig. 5.10 SPREETA TSPR2K11 miniature SPR sensor from Texas Instruments.

development, a miniaturized version of the technology described in the example, becomes feasible.

It is likely that the development of a sophisticated laboratory instrument like the Biacore 2000 towards a miniaturized device like the SPREETA will give some trade off in performance of the technology. This need not be a problem, as the laboratory version proved to be very sensitive. Furthermore, reflecting the various technologies described in this chapter, appropriate combinations can be made between sensor systems and immuno-affinity chromatography. The advantages of IAC (e.g. sample pre-concentration and cleaning) can be merged with those of the immunosensor (fast and quantitative measurement results, calibration and regeneration capability). Smart combinations of the various possibilities for immunochemical technology may lead to sophisticated and still low cost instruments for residue analysis, applicable in any environment imaginable.

5.8 References

AFEYAN NB, GORDON NF, REGNIER FE (1992), 'Automated real-time immunoassay of biomolecules', *Nature* 358 603–604.

ALCOCER MJC, DOYEN C, LEE HA, MORGAN MRA (2000), 'Functional scFv antibody sequences against the organophosphorus pesticide chlorpyrifos', *J. Agric. Food Chem.*, 48, 335–337.

BARKER SA (2000), 'Sorbent technologies: Principles and applications', in O'Keeffe M, *Residue analysis in food: Principles and applications*, Australia, Harwood Academic Publishers, 37–71.

BENHAR I (2001), 'Biotechnological applications of phage and cell display', *Biotechnol. Adv.*, 19, 1–33.

BENJAMINI E, LESKOWITZ S (1991), 'Immunology: A short course', New York, Wiley-Liss, 106–117.

BERSON SA, YALOW RS (1959), 'Recent studies on insulin-binding antibodies', *Ann. N.Y.*

Acad. Sci., 82, 338–344.

BILITEWSKI U (1998), 'Simultaneous determination of several analytes using immunochemical techniques An overview', *Food Technol Biotechnol.*, 36(2), 135–144.

BRANDON DL, BINDER RG, BATES, AH, MONTAGUE WC (1995), *New Frontiers in Agrochemical Immunoassay*, Arlington, AOAC Int., 77–89.

CAHN TM, (ed). (1993), *Biosensors*, Chapman & Hall, London.

CHAPMAN MD, VAILES LD, ICHIKAWA K (2000), 'Immunoassays for indoor allergens', *Clin. Rev. Allergy Immunol.*, 18, 285–300.

CHOUDRAY PV, LEE HA, HAMMOCK BD, MORGAN MRA (1995), ' Recombinant antibodies: New tools for immunoassays', in Kurtz DA, Skerritt JH and Stanker L, *New Frontiers in Agrochemical Immunoassay*, Arlington, AOAC Int., 171–185.

COLBERT DL (1994), 'Drug abuse screening with immunoassay: unexpected cross-reactivities and other pitfalls', *Br. J. Biomed. Sci.*, 51, 136–146.

CUATRECASAS P, WILCHEK M, ANFINSEN CB (1968), 'Selective enzyme purification by affinity chromatography', *Proc. Nat. Acad. Sci. USA* 61 636.

DALY SJ, DILLON PP, BRENNAN J, DUNNE L, FITZPATRICK J, O'KENNEDY R (2001), 'Production and analytical applications of scFv antibody fragments', *Anal. Lett.*, 34(11), 1799–1827.

DANKWARDT A, PULLEN S, HOCK B (1998), 'Immunoassays: Applications for the aquatic environment', in Wells PG, Lee K and Blaise C, *Microscale testing in aquatic toxicology*, Boca Rota, CRC Press, 13–29.

DESHPANDE SS (1994), 'Immunodiagnostics in agricultural, food, and environmental quality control', *Food Technol.*, June, 136–141.

EHRLICH P (1900), 'On immunity, with special reference to cell life', *Proc. Roy. Soc.*, 424, 1366.

EREMIN S, SMITH DS (2003), 'Fluorescence polarization immunoassays for pesticides', *Combinatorial Chemistry, High Troughput Screening*, 6, 79–99.

FERGUSON DB (1984), 'Physiological considerations in the use of salivary steroid estimation for clinical investigations', in Kawamura Y and Ferguson DB, *Steroid hormones in saliva*, Basel, Karger, 1–20.

FRANEK M, DENG A, KOLAR V (2000), 'Performance characteristics for flow injection immunoassay using monoclonal antibodies against s-triazine and 2,4–D herbicides', *Anal. Chim. Acta* 412, 19–27.

FULTON SP, MEYS M, VARADAY L, JANSEN R, AFEYAN NB (1991), 'Antibody quantification in seconds using affinity perfusion chromatography', *BioChromatography* 11(2), 226–231.

GAMBLE HR, MURRELL KD (1998), 'Detection of parasites in food', *Parasitology*, 117, S97–S111.

GÜBITZ G, SCHMID MG, SILVIAEH H, HASSAN Y (2001), 'Chemiluminescence flow-injection immunoassays', *Crit. Rev. Anal. Chem.*, 31(3), 167–174.

HAUGLAND RP (2002), 'Handbook of fluorescent probes and research products', Gregory J and Spence MTZ, Leiden, Molecular Probes Inc.

HEIDELBERGER M (1939), 'Quantitative absolute methods in the study of antigen-antibody reactions', *Bact. Rev.*, 3, 39.

HEISS C, WELLER MG, NIESSNER R (1999), 'Dip-and-read test strips for the determination of trinitrotoluene (TNT) in drinking water', *Anal. Chim. Acta*, 396, 309–316.

HERMANSON GT, MALLIA AK, SMITH PK (1992), *Immobilized Affinity Ligand Techniques*, Academic Press, San Diego.

HOFSTEE BHJ (1975), 'Accesible hydrophobic groups of native proteins', *Biochem.*

Biophys. Res. Commun. 63, 618.
JÖNSSON B, LÖFÅS S,. LINDQUIST G (1991) Immobilization of proteins to a carboxymethyldextran-modified gold surface for biospecific interaction analysis in surface plasmon resonance sensors, *Anal. Biochem.*, 198, 268–277.
JOURDAN SW, SCUTELLARO AM, HAYES MC, HERZOG DP (1996), 'Adapting immunoassays to the analysis of food samples', in Beier RC and Stanker LH, *Immunoassays for residue analysis: Food safety*, Washington, ACS Series 621, 17–28.
KAUFMAN BM, CLOWER M (1991), 'Immunoassay of pesticides', *J. Assoc. Off. Anal. Chem.*, 74(2), 239–247.
KÖHLER G, MILSTEIN C (1975), 'Continuous cultures of fused cells secreting antibody of predefined specificity', *Nature*, 256, 495.
KRULL IS, CHO B-Y, STRONG R, VANDERLAAN M (1997), 'Principles and practice of immunodetection in FIA and HPLC', *LC-GC International* 10, 178–292;
LAC G (2001), 'Saliva assays in clinical and research biology', *Pathol. Biol.*, 49, 660–667.
LANGE S, SCHMITT J. SCHMID RD (2001), 'High-yield expression of the recombinant, atrazine-specific Fab fragment K411B by the methylotrophic yeast *Pichia pastoris*', *J. Immunol. Methods*, 255, 103–114.
LEONARD M (1997), 'New packing materials for protein chromatography', *J. Chromatogr.* B699, 3–27.
LIPTON CR, DAUTLICK JX, GROTHAUS GD, HUNST PL, MAGIN KM, MIHALIAK CA, RUBIO FM, STAVE JW (2000), 'Guidelines for the validation and use of immunoassays for determination of introduced proteins in biotechnology enhanced crops and derived food ingredients', *Food Agric. Immunol.*, 12, 153–164
MACNEIL JD, KAY JF (2000), 'Regulatory aspects of residue analysis', O'Keeffe M, *Residue analysis in food: Principles and applications*, Australia, Harwood Academic Publishers, 277–299.
MATVEEVA EG, SHAN G, KENNEDY IM, GEE SJ, STOUTAMIRE DW, HAMMOCK BD (2001), 'Homogeneous fluorimmunoassay of a pyrethroid metabolite in urine', *Anal. Chim. Acta*, 444, 103–117.
MEULENBERG EP (1997), 'Immunochemical detection of environmental and food contaminants: Development, validation and Appliaction', *Food Technol. Biotechnol.*, 35(3), 153–163.
MEULENBERG EP (1998), 'Pesticides, immunoassays', in Meyers RA, *Encyclopedia of Environmental Analysis and Remediation*, John Wiley & Sons.
MEULENBERG EP (2000), 'Determination of microcystines in surface water and floating layers using an immunoassay', ELTI-Report, Nijmegen, The Netherlands.
MEULENBERG EP, PEELEN G (2002a), 'Phenylurea herbicides: monitoring in the river Meuse using Elisa kits', ELTI-Report, Nijmegen, The Netherlands.
MEULENBERG EP, PEELEN G (2002b), 'Determination of microcystines in surface water and floating layers using an immunoassay', ELTI-Report, Nijmegen, The Netherlands.
MEULENBERG EP, MULDER WH, STOKS PG (1995), 'Immunoassays for pesticides', *Environ. Sci. Technol.*, 29(3), 553–561.
MEULENBERG EP, CLARK S, PEELEN G (2001), Abstr. L-18, VIth International Conference on Agri-Food Antibodies, Prague, Czech Republic.
MILLS ENC, POTTS A, PLUMB GW, LAMBERT N, MORGAN MRA (1997), 'Development of a rapid dipstick immunoassay for the detection of peanut contamination of food', *Food Agric. Immunol.*, 9, 37–50.
MONTOYA A (2002), 4th European Pesticide Residue Workshop, EPRW, Rome.
MONTOYA A, ABAD A, MORENO MJ, MANCLUS JJ, MERCADER JV (2001), Abstr. L-19, VIth

International Conference on Agri-Food Antibodies, Prague, Czech Republic.

MORAIS S, MAQUIEIRA A, PUCHADES R (1999), 'Immunofiltration: A methodology for preconcentration and determination of organic pollutants', *Anal. Chem.*, 71, 1905–1909.

NILSSON B (1990), 'Enzyme-linked immunosorbent assays', *Current Opinion in Immunology*, 2, 898–904.

ÖNNERFJORD P, EREMIN S, EMNEUS J, MARKO-VARGA G (1998), 'A flow immunoassay for studies of human exposure and toxicity in biological samples', *J. Mol. Recog.*, 11, 182–184.

O'SHANNESSY DJ, WILCHEK M (1990), 'Immobilization of glycoconjugates by their oligosaccharides: use of Hydrazido-derivatized matrices', *Anal. Biochem.* 191, 1.

PARSONS RG, KOWAL R, LEBLOND D, YUE VT, NEARGARDER L, BOND L, GARCIA D, SLATER D, ROGERS P (1993), 'Multianalyte assay system developed for drugs of abuse', *Clin. Chem.*, 39(9), 1899–1903.

PERBIO CATALOG (2001–2002), Pierce, Brunschwig Chemie, Amsterdam, The Netherlands.

PHILLIPS TM, DICKENS BF (2000), *Affinity and Immunoaffinity Purification techniques*, Eaton Publishing, Natick, USA.

PIMBLEY DW, PATEL PD (1998), 'A review of analytical methods for the detection of bacterial toxins', *J. Appl. Microbiol. Symp. Suppl.*, 84, 98S–109S.

RHEMREV-BOOM MM, YATES M, RUDOLPH M, RAEDTS M (2001), '(Immuno) affinity chromatography: a versatile tool for fast and selective purification, concentration, isolation and analysis', *J. Pharm. Biomed. Analysis* 24, 825–833.

RONGEN HAH, HOETELMANS RMW, BULT A, VAN BENNEKOM WP (1994), 'Chemiluminescence and immunoassays', *J. Pharmac. Biomed. Anal.* 12(4), 433–462.

ROSNER MH, GRASSMAN JA, HAAS RA (1991), 'Immunochemical techniques in biological monitoring', *Environ. Health Persp.*, 94, 131–134.

SAMARAJEEWA U, WEI CI, HUANG TS, MARSHALL MR (1991), 'Application of immunoassay in the food industry', *Crit. Rev. Food Sci. Nutr.*, 29(6), 403–434.

SCHOBEL U, BARZEN C, GAUGLITZ G (2000) 'Immunoanalytical techniques for pesticide monitoring based on fluorescence detection', *Fres. J. Anal. Chem.* 366, 646–658.

SCIPPO M-L, MAGHUIN-ROGISTER G (2000), 'Primary extraction technologies', in O'Keeffe M, *Residue analysis in food: Principles and applications*, Australia, Harwood Academic Publishers, 17–36.

SCOTT AO, (ed.) (1998), *Biosensors for Food Analysis*, Athenaeum Press, Gateshead, UK.

SCOUTEN WH (1981), *Affinity Chromatography Bioselective Adsorption on Inert Matrices*, John Wiley & Sons, Inc., Canada.

SHERRY JP (1992), 'Environmental chemistry: The immunoassay option', *Crit. Rev. Anal. Chem.*, 23, 217–300.

SKERRITT JH, LEE N (1996), 'Approaches to the synthesis of haptens for immunoassay of organophosphate and synthetic pyrethroid insecticides', in Beier RC and Stanker LH, *Immunoassays for residue analysis: Food safety*, Washington, ACS Series 621, 124–149.

SKERRITT JH, RANI BEA (1996), 'Detection and removal of sample matrix effects in agrochemical immunoassays', in Beier RC and Stanker LH, *Immunoassays for residue analysis: Food safety*, Washington, ACS Series 621, 29–43.

STEAD DA (2000), 'Current methodologies for the analysis of aminoglycosides', *J. Chromat. B* 747, 69–93.

STOLKER AAM, STERK S, VAN GINKEL LA (2000), 'Automated extraction/clean-up technologies', O'Keeffe M, *Residue analysis in food: Principles and applications*, Australia, Harwood Academic Publishers, 73–105.

SZEKACS A, JUNG F, HAMMOCK BD (1995), Chemical modification of haptens: Selective amino group protection by chromophores for an immunoassay for aminotriazoles', in Kurtz DA, Skerritt JH and Stanker L, *New Frontiers in Agrochemical Immunoassay*, Arlington, AOAC Int., 65–75.

SZURDOKI F, BEKHEIT HKM, MACRO M-P, GOODROW MH, HAMMOCK BD (1995), 'Important factors in hapten design and enzyme-linked immunosorbent assay development', in Kurtz DA, Skerritt JH and Stanker L, *New Frontiers in Agrochemical Immunoassay*, Arlington, AOAC Int., 39–63.

THOUVENOT D, MORFIN RF (1983) Radioimmunoassay for zearalenon and zearalanol in human serum: production, properties and use in porcine antibodies. *Applied and Environmental Microbiology*, 45, 16–23.

TURNER APF, KARUBE I, WILSON GS, Eds., (1989), *Biosensors. Fundamentals and Applications*, Oxford University Press, Oxford.

VAN DER GAAG B, SPATH S, DIETRICH H, STIGTER 2 E, BOONZAIJER G, VAN OSENBRUGGEN T, KOOPAL K (2003) Biosensors and Multiple Mycotoxin Analysis, *Food Control*, 14(4), 251–254.

VERHEIJEN R, STOUTEN P, CAZEMIER G, HAASNOOT W (1998), 'Development of a one step strip test for the detection of sulfadimidine residues', *Analyst*, 123, 2437–2441.

WALTERS RR (1985), 'Affinity chromatography', *Anal. Chem.*, 57(11), 1099A–1106A.

WARD VK, HAMMOCK BD, MAEDA S, CHOUDRAY PV (1995), 'Development and application of recombinant antibodies to pesticide residue analysis', in Kurtz DA, Skerritt JH and Stanker L, *New Frontiers in Agrochemical Immunoassay*, Arlington, AOAC Int., 197–216.

WARSINKE A, BENKERT A, SCHELLER FW (2000), 'Electrochemical immunoassays', *Fres. J. Anal. Chem.* 366, 622–634.

WINKLMAIR M, SCHUETZ AJ, WELLER MG, NIESSNER R (1999), 'Immunochemical array for the identification of cross-reacting analytes', *Fres. J. Anal. Chem.*, 363: 731–737.

WISE DL, (ed.) (1989), *Applied Biosensors*, Butterworths, Boston.

WORTBERG M, KREISSIG SB, JONES G, ROCKE DM, HAMMOCK BD (1995), 'An immunoassay for the simultaneous determination of multiple triazine herbicides', *Anal. Chim. Acta*, 304, 339–352.

YARMUSH ML, ANTONSEN KP, SUNDARAM S, YARMUSH DM (1992), 'Immunoadsorption: strategies for antigen elution and production of reusable adsorbents', *Biotechnol. Progr.* 8, 168–178.

6

Good agricultural practice and HACCP systems in the management of pesticides and veterinary residues on the farm

R. Early, Harper Adams University College, UK

6.1 Introduction

The term 'food safety' is defined as the 'Assurance that food will not cause harm to the consumer when it is prepared and/or eaten according to its intended use' (CCFH, 1997). The production of food that is safe to eat is predicated on the concept that hazards that might be present in foodstuffs, or which might arise as a result of the processing of foodstuffs, will either be prevented, eliminated, or reduced to acceptable levels. The word 'hazard' is defined as 'A biological, chemical or physical agent in, or condition of, food with the potential to cause an adverse health effect' (CCFH, 1997). In food processing and manufacturing, strategies for the production of safe food concern the selection of raw materials that are free from hazards, the use of processing technologies intended specifically to control hazards, and the management of processes in ways that prevent the occurrence of hazards and the production of unsafe foods.

The use of pesticides and veterinary substances (medicines and zootechnical additives, etc.) in agricultural food production brings an interesting dimension to the concept of food safety and practical requirements for the production of safe food. Whereas most activities in the production of food involve the removal of hazards from food, the use of pesticides and veterinary substances involves the application of toxic substances (chemical hazards) to foodstuffs or, more accurately, plants and animals destined to become foodstuffs. Food is necessary for the growth and survival of human beings. The right to food is recognised in The United Nations Declaration of Human Rights (UN, 1948) which states, in Article 25, that 'Everyone has the right to a standard of living adequate for the health and well-being of himself and his family, including food, clothing, housing and medical care and necessary social services . . .'. Food that is capable of contributing to the health and well-being of people must be of the right quality (including safety), contain the right nutrients in the right amounts, and it must be provided in the right quantities. Food is consumed and becomes part of people. Though food-borne hazards may affect people as the consumers of food, most, such as bacterial pathogens and physical hazards, will not become part of people and the consequences of their action will be seen relatively quickly. The potential exists for the residues of pesticides and veterinary substances contained within foodstuffs to become part of people and to adversely affect health and well-being, often in ways that do not become immediately apparent and then maybe only over a long period of time.

It is critical that the use of pesticides and veterinary drugs is done in such ways, and under such methods of control, that the safety of consumers is assured. During the last 20 years or so, the Hazard Analysis Critical Control Point (HACCP) system for food safety management has been widely adopted by the food manufacturing industry. The occurrence throughout the world of various food safety scares originating at farm level has focussed attention on the need to manage food safety at all levels of the food chain, and, as appropriate, to adopt systematic methods of food safety management at farm level. Consequently, many public health and food safety authorities now recommend the use of HACCP in the agricultural production of food. In some instances HACCP can be relatively easily applied in agriculture. In others caution must be taken regarding the interpretation of HACCP in relation to products which, in truth, are not yet food. In all cases HACCP ought to be carried out in conjunction with Good Agricultural Practice (GAP) which provides a foundation for HACCP in the same way that Good Manufacturing Practice (GMP) is used to support HACCP in the food processing and manufacturing industries.

This chapter concerns the use of HACCP to manage food safety in relation to the use of pesticides and veterinary substances in farming and growing. There is no intention to give detailed accounts of the ways to control the use of specific pesticides or veterinary substances in agriculture. The purpose of the chapter is to explain what GAP and HACCP are, and to outline the rationales and methodologies for their use in controlling activities at farm level that have the potential to damage the health of consumers.

6.2 Safety issues in the food supply chain

Food safety is an issue of significant concern for governments and public health authorities throughout the world. In many developing countries food poisoning is a major cause of infant mortality and poor health in people. The root cause is often contaminated water used for drinking and food preparation, as well as generally unsanitary living conditions. In the developed, industrialised societies of the world food safety takes on a different complexion. Illness and disease caused by food in western societies are frequently traced back to bad practices in the way foodstuffs are handled, prepared and stored, in both commercial and domestic settings. During the last 20 years, however, the agricultural production of food has received increasing scrutiny for the part it plays in the creation and propagation of food safety problems. The majority of food poisoning incidents can be traced to failures in food safety management in food processing and manufacturing, and in food service (restaurants, cafes and fast-food establishments) as well as the home. Recognition of the part that agriculture plays in the generation of food safety problems has come from the nature of food poisoning incidents and specifically the causes. Perhaps the best way to make safe food is to grow foodstuffs locally and prepare meals in the home for immediate consumption. This traditional model of food production and supply has served society well for many generations, but it is not without the potential to cause harm. Historically people suffered from naturally occurring food-borne hazards such as ergot toxin caused by the fungus *Claviceps purpurea* associated with cereals and particularly rye, or botulism caused by the growth of *Clostridium botulinum* in badly preserved meats and vegetables. Even so people generally learned how to handle food and prepare meals, and how to keep themselves and their families safe.

During the last quarter of the twentieth century the expansion and globalisation of the food industry has brought increasing complexity to the food supply system and lengthened the food supply chain. At the same time, in many countries, the growth of supermarkets and fast-food establishments has distanced most consumers from the sources of food and raw food materials; and the opportunity to learn in the home how to handle food safely has been diminished. Significantly, the growth of supermarkets and fast-food establishments has shifted the power in the food supply system from farmers and growers to the supermarkets and fast-food corporations themselves. Increased competition in the food marketplace resulting from globalisation and the growing dominance of the supermarkets and fast-food retailers, and pressure brought to bear on suppliers by supermarkets and fast-food corporations demanding cost reductions for the benefit of competitive advantage, has forced many farmers and growers to adopt new, industrialised approaches to the agricultural production of food. Indeed, many traditional, small farmers and growers have gone out of business to be replaced by large, intensive agricultural enterprises operating on the basis of a belief system that regards the land, crops and food animals as assets to be 'sweated'.

The changes that have occurred in agriculture during the last quarter of a century or more have brought increased productivity, but at the cost of degradation of the environment, biodiversity and the quality of the soil. Significantly, these changes have brought many new and problematical issues of food safety. In the late 1980s it became apparent that the intensive production of broiler chickens brought with it the problem of *Salmonella enteritidis* PT4 infection and an increased risk of food poisoning for consumers. Indeed, in the UK food poisoning notifications rose from 14,253 cases in 1982 to 85,464 cases almost two decades later (PHLS, 2003). The increase was mainly caused by *Salmonella enteritidis* PT4 associated with eggs and poultry meat. The problem of salmonella infection in intensively reared poultry has been controlled to a great extent in recent years by the use of vaccines. But it has now been replaced by *Campylobacter* spp. and these organisms account for most food poisoning in the UK today.

Another food safety issue arising from the intensification of food animal production and, to a great extent, the concentration of meat processing in the hands of a small number of large meat businesses, is that of *E. coli* O157: H7. This organism has been responsible for many deaths and much illness in consumers in Europe, Japan and notably the USA. While *E. coli* O157: H7 was unheard of 20 years ago, today it is a common cause of food poisoning mainly associated with improperly cooked hamburgers. In the USA the organism is responsible for around 60 deaths a year and some 70,000 cases of food poisoning. In the UK a major incident in 1996/97 resulted in 496 cases and 21 deaths (The Pennington Group, 1997). It would seem that the intensification of beef production, and particularly the use of beef-lot systems in the USA, has created the problem of *E. coli* O157: H7. In 2001 ConAgra, an American agri-business super-corporation, was forced to recall 19 million pounds of ground beef after 19 people became ill from *E. coli* O157: H7 (Nestle, 2003) in hamburgers made from beef produced in feed-lot systems and processed in high-speed meat processing plants (Schlosser, 2001). Intensively reared cattle fed on corn, soy and by-products from the meat processing industry are more likely to carry and shed *E. coli* O157: H7 than are grass-fed animals.

Another food safety issue linked with the intensification of agricultural production is found in the bovine spongiform encephalopathy (BSE) disaster of the 1990s in the UK. Part of the belief system on which intensive agriculture is founded concerns minimising costs to maximise profits. The concept of utilising the remains of cattle and sheep in the production of feedstuffs for herbivores, i.e., cattle, was consistent with the consequentialist, and probably egoistic, thinking in existence in the rendering and animal feed industries during the 1980s and early 1990s. Tragically, the practice of recycling animal remains through cattle appears to have given rise to BSE and its occurrence may have caused the deaths of people from variant Creutzfeldt-Jacobs Disease (vCJD). The occurrence of BSE has brought the UK's agricultural practices under scrutiny and many significant changes have been made in the hope that food safety problems can be eliminated. The recycling of animal remains through food animals is still practised in some countries.

Much of the focus on food safety concerns microbial food poisoning because this is the greatest food safety problem world-wide. The reduction of microbial food poisoning is considered by most governments and public health authorities to be a key priority. This is reflected in the objectives of the UK's Food Standards Agency (established in 2000) which aims to reduce food poisoning by 20% in the first five years' operation (FSA, 2003a). Even the achievement of this objective will not bring food poisoning cases in the UK back to 1980s levels and it is sobering to reflect that while the attention of government agencies and public health authorities is focused on microbial food poisoning, many more people in many western societies suffer and die from disease associated with the over-consumption of food and poor diet, another topic being addressed by the Food Standards Agency.

Alongside microbial issues of food safety, the food industry and consumers must be concerned with issues of the chemical contamination of food and, probably to a lesser extent, physical contamination, because this form of contamination tends to be dealt with more easily. There are many sources of chemical contamination that can affect the safety of food. Given the nature of the global food production system today and the dependence of the food supply and consumers on intensive methods of agriculture, pesticides and veterinary substances are a cause for concern in matters of chemical hazard and food safety. Warnings about the dangers of pesticides for human health and biodiversity have been well reported over the years. As far back as the 1960s Carson (2000) was writing in *Silent Spring* of the harms that pesticides bring. There can be no doubt that dangers are inherent in the use of pesticides and in the consumption of foodstuffs containing unacceptable levels of pesticide residues. Since the publication of *Silent Spring* much has been learned about the safe handling and use of pesticides, and many improvements have been made in the formulation of biodegradable pesticides with reduced levels of residual toxicity. Even so, the World Health Organisation estimates that there are 25 million cases of pesticide poisoning globally each year with some 20,000 deaths, mainly in developing countries (Anon, 2002). Illness and death from pesticides result mainly from mistakes and poor education in pesticide handling, environmental contamination, and illegal use or illegal levels of residues in food.

Harm resulting from the legal use of pesticides is unlikely and Grierson (1997) says there have been no such cases in the USA. If pesticides are used properly and, for instance, the correct pre-harvest intervals are observed, the risk of harm to consumers ought to be negligible. In principle, in most countries the use of pesticides is regulated by law. In the UK the Control of Pesticides Regulations 1986 and the associated Plant Protection Products Regulations 1995 govern their sale, supply, storage, advertisement and use. Of specific importance to human health and food safety is the use of pesticides in developing countries where regulation and control may be flawed relative to that in developed countries. Globalisation and the movement of food throughout the world makes pesticide control a critical issue for all consumers. The use of pesticides in food production is of specific concern to food safety because of the actual or potential dangers that pesticides pose to the immediate and long-term health of consumers. Pesticides are generally toxic to humans (as well as other biological organisms) and some have been shown to be carcinogenic, mutagenic and teratogenic. Concern is also raised over the ability of some pesticides to act as endocrine-disruptors, causing, for instance, the impairment of brain and other bodily functions, disruption in the development of the brain and reproductive system, weakening of the immune system and the development of behavioural disorders. Also of concern is the degree to which pesticides are absorbed by the body and deposited in fatty tissues and the liver, as demonstrated by the organochlorine compound, DDT, amongst others.

While concerns may be raised about the toxicity of the active agents in pesticides other components may be worrying. Some pesticides contain polyacrylamide to aid the adhesion of the active agents to plant leaves. Polyacrylamide is converted to acrylamide at high temperatures such as those used in food processing and cooking. Recently the presence of acrylamide in fried and baked foods has caused concern (FSA, 2003b) because of its carcinogenic potential. In contrast to food poisoning bacteria which are generally fast acting causes of illness, the action of pesticides in causing illness and death may be very slow and may be dependent on long-term accumulation within the tissues and the presence of different compounds acting in synergy.

An understanding of the potential hazards that pesticides represent to human health is essential to those who aim to control their use and minimise the risks they represent to human health. It is likely, however, that even though much is known about pesticides and their effects on human health, some relevant questions will be impossible to answer. For such reasons the adoption of Integrated Pest Management in many parts of the world is seen as a way to minimise and, possibly, almost eliminate the use of pesticides.

Veterinary substances sit alongside pesticides as a source of concern for the health of consumers. Like pesticides, if they are used properly and according to the regulations that govern them they should, in principle, represent no more than an acceptable level of risk. In the UK The Medicines (Restrictions on the Administration of Veterinary Medicinal Products) Regulations 1994 allow only the administration to animals of products which have been given marketing authorisation for the treatment of specific conditions in specific species. It is usual practice in the UK for veterinarians to prescribe and dispense veterinary medicines, though persons acting under the supervision of veterinarians may administer licensed products to food animals provided proper procedures are adhered to and records of treatments are kept. Many kinds of veterinary substances are used in food animal production for the treatment of infection and disease, and to increase productivity and yield. Provided veterinary medicines are used under the right conditions, at the right rates and provided appropriate withdrawal periods are observed, little risk should exist for the consumers of meat derived from treated animals.

Concern is associated with the use of zootechnical substances, for instance, prophylactics and hormones used to promote growth and increase yield. The use of antibiotics as growth promoters in agriculture far exceeds their use in medicine to treat human disease. This contributes to the worrying levels of antibiotic resistant bacteria now seen throughout the world and brings many of the values on which intensive agriculture is predicated into question. Another source of concern for the health of consumers is the use of hormones to increase productivity. Though the practice is permitted in some countries, e.g. the USA, in others it is illegal, e.g. the EU. Consequently, US beef produced with the use of hormone growth promoters cannot be imported into EU countries. Also permitted in the US is bovine growth hormone (BGH), known as bovine somatotrophin (BST) in the EU, which is used to increase milk yield in dairy cows. Though the presence of the hormone as a residue in milk raises no safety concerns as it is also naturally present, the use of BST causes increased levels of IGF-1 (insulin-like growth factor 1) which some suggest may be associated with breast cancer in women. Milk produced with the use of BST cannot be imported into the EU and the use of BST is banned within the EU. Though hormones and antibiotics may be used as growth promoters in some instances, their use should be carefully regulated by law. Unfortunately, at times they are used illegally and such practice raises concerns for public health (Meikle, 2003). Those who use these substances illegally are unlikely to manage their use under GAP or HACCP. It is realistic to believe, therefore, that farmers who use GAP and/or HACCP will tend to compliance with the law and their produce will, consequently, be free from residues of illegal hormones or antibiotics.

Conceptually, food safety is a sub-set of food quality. A food that is poor quality and unappetising can still be safe to eat, but a food that is not safe to eat will not be of the right quality. Rancid butter is not quality butter but should do no harm if eaten. A slice of ham contaminated with *Staphylococcus aureus* may look, smell and taste right, but cause food poisoning because of the presence of toxin, and it cannot be regarded as a quality product. The term 'quality' is defined as 'The degree to which a set of inherent characteristics fulfils requirements' (ISO, 2000a). Agricultural produce destined for the food chain should comply with the quality requirements of customers and consumers, and requirements ought to be defined in documented product specifications. Food safety requirements will normally be reflected in product specifications. However, food businesses have moral and legal duties to protect consumers from food-borne harms irrespective of what is written into specifications. When consumers buy food they expect it to be safe and not to cause them harm either immediately or in the long term, for example, through gradual and progressive poisoning by toxic substances contained in foods at low levels.

In practice absolute food safety is impossible to commit to in the case of all food products, so food businesses have to work with the concept of 'commercial food safety'. The canning industry cannot guarantee that every one of billions of cans sterilised will be free from *Clostridium botulinum*, so the industry works with the concept of 'commercial sterility' (Hersom and Hulland, 1980). Within western societies the requirement for food producers to protect consumers is embodied in law and in the UK the principal food legislation is the Food Safety Act 1990. Section 8 of the Food Safety Act 1990 states that

> Any person who (a) sells for human consumption, or offers, exposes or advertises for sale for such consumption, or has in his possession for the purpose of such sale or of preparation for such sale; or (b) deposits with, or consigns to, any other person for the purpose of such sale or of preparation for such sale, any food which fails to comply with food safety requirements shall be guilty of an offence.

Food producers must be sure that the foodstuffs they make available for sale, use and consumption will cause no harm to consumers or risk prosecution. Section 14 of the Food Safety Act 1990 states that 'Any person who sells to the purchaser's prejudice any food which is not of the nature or substance or quality demanded by the purchaser shall be guilty of an offence'. This section confirms food safety as a sub-set of quality. Within the context of pesticides and veterinary substances it makes it clear that if a foodstuff contains substances that consumers might reasonably expect not to be present then an offence may have been committed. However, the Food and Environment Protection Act 1985, part III section 16(k), not the Food Safety Act, provides statutory powers to control pesticide residues in food. Also, the substances present in a foodstuff need not necessarily be harmful for a prosecution to ensue. For instance, cigarette ash in a food product may cause no harm, but the product will not be of the 'nature, substance and quality' demanded and its presence constitutes an offence.

To be sure that safe foods are produced, food businesses ought to operate systematic methods of quality management and quality assurance incorporating food safety systems. Though food businesses may take whatever measures are deemed necessary to ensure food safety and protect consumers, the Food Safety Act offers the 'due diligence' defence as a way to avoid prosecution. Section 21 of the Act states that 'it shall be a defence for the person charged to prove that he took all reasonable precautions and exercised all due diligence to avoid the commission of the offence by himself or by a person under his control'. Taking 'all reasonable precautions' is interpreted as having in place, within the resources that might be expected to be available to a particular type of business, the systems required to prevent the occurrence of circumstances that could constitute an offence, i.e., the production of unsafe food. Exercising 'due diligence' is taken to mean operating the (food safety) systems effectively. The scope of the Food Safety Act does not apply to agricultural produce while it is being grown, i.e., crops in the field and animals on the hoof. However, at the point of harvesting or slaughter, crops and animals become food and are encompassed by the Act. If what happened prior to harvesting or slaughter influences the safety of food products post-harvest or -slaughter then care must be taken to comply with the requirements of the Act, and subordinate legislation. With regard to the control of pesticides and veterinary substances in foodstuffs, compliance with the terms of the Food Safety Act is best done through the use of Good Agricultural Practice and the Hazard Analysis Critical Control Point system.

6.3 Good agricultural practice

The principles upon which GAP is based reflect those of Good Manufacturing Practice used in the food processing and manufacturing industry. The Institute of Food Science and Technology (IFST, 1998) says that GMP consists of 'effective manufacturing operations' and 'effective food control'. In use, GMP constitutes a systematic approach to the control of food production operations and food products such that the requirements stated in product specifications are met consistently. Effectively GMP correlates with the development of quality control procedures and a quality assurance system to ensure that product specifications are adequately defined and documented, and that manufacturing operations and food control are carried out according to the documented requirements which, essentially, form a quality plan. GAP is essentially the application of quality management and quality assurance theory at farm level. Quality management is defined as the 'Coordinated activities [used] to direct and control an organisation with regard to quality' (ISO, 2000a). Quality management should be thought of as the systematic control of quality planning and operational activities required to meet the objectives of the business. Quality management encompasses quality assurance which is defined as that 'Part of quality management focussed on providing confidence that quality requirements will be fulfilled' (ISO, 2000a) and which exists to ensure customer requirements are met. Quality control is 'Part of quality management focussed on fulfilling quality requirements' (ISO, 2000a). It concerns, for example, inspections and measurements undertaken to ensure processes are operating correctly and products meet specifications. In recent years we have seen the development of approaches to Integrated Farm Management (IFM), usually incorporating, as relevant, Integrated Pest Management (IPM) and Integrated Crop Management (ICM), such as that advocated by LEAF [Linking Environment And Farming] (2000). IFM and GAP are effectively the same thing. They represent an intelligent approach to moderating conventional, intensive agricultural methodologies which have been based on the use of high levels of off-farm inputs and the transfer of control from the farmer to agricultural corporation farm advisers. The principal objective of GAP is the management of agricultural resources to fulfil the human needs of agriculture while, at the same time:

- protecting the environment and preventing pollution
- maintaining and enhancing the quality of the soil such that food production remains sustainable
- maximising the welfare of animals in food production systems
- maintaining and enhancing the amenity value of the land and landscape
- promoting conditions that restore and enhance biodiversity.

The concept of reducing off-farm inputs is central to the developing belief system that provides the foundation and justification for GAP. Reducing dependence on fossil fuels, artificial fertilisers and pesticides is considered crucial to maintaining sustainability and promoting biodiversity. In some ways elements of the belief system on which organic farming is based are being incorporated into the GAP philosophy. Clearly, in matters of food safety the reduction or avoidance of pesticides eliminates the need to manage this source of potential food-borne harm. Economics decisions will undoubtedly influence the commitment to a particular agricultural belief system, but with increasing awareness of the environmental impacts of agriculture, and the need to preserve the land for future generations, many farmers are committing to more environmentally sensitive methods of agricultural food production.

GAP has a starting point. It is the recognition that farmers and growers, as well as the businesses that interact with them, such as agricultural inputs businesses, food manufacturers and supermarkets, have moral, social and legal responsibilities for developing sustainable methods of food production that are socially and economically viable, protective of human health and well-being and animal health and welfare, and sustain biodiversity and the environment. GAP is a strategic approach to farm management which equates to quality management in other industries. It is achieved through a structured and systematic approach to managing and controlling agricultural activities and it comprises the following elements, each with specific objectives:

1. *Planning and management*: establishing plans for the overall operation of the farm and implementing management techniques and procedures for farming activities that aim to enhance the farm's value and productivity as a source of food, and sustain or increase its contribution to society and the economy, without damaging the land and landscape or eliminating wildlife.
2. *Staff training and development*: the identification of staff training and development requirements; providing and updating staff training and development; ensuring that staff are adequately trained for the work they do and in compliance with legal requirements concerning health and safety or specialist operations and activities.
3. *Soil preservation*: maintaining soil fertility; preventing soil erosion; preventing runoff, leaching and the production of effluents that contaminate watercourses and harm wildlife and the environment.
4. *Water protection*: preserving and re-cycling water; using water efficiently and in ways that prevent soil erosion, runoff and leaching; protecting water supplies from contaminants that might harm human and animal health.
5. *Crop and fodder production*: the selection of crops, cultivars and varieties according to constraints of specific locations, e.g. nutrient requirements and natural availability, and their effect on wildlife and biodiversity; selection according to requirements for soil protection, and potential to replenish soil nutrients and build soil quality as well as taking into account factors concerning proximity to processors and the consumer marketplace.
6. *Crop protection*: the selection of crops for pest and disease resistance and tolerance of climatic conditions; rotation to provide disease breaks; tactical use of pesticides, e.g. to control pests, diseases and weeds; evaluative use of agro-chemicals based on recognised need and weighing of advantages versus disadvantages, benefits versus harms; legal and safe storage and use of chemicals; record keeping; protection of humans and the environment from chemicals.
7. *Animal production*: the provision of space, feed, water and appropriate protection from the climate to ensure animal welfare and productivity; use of stocking rates appropriate to maintenance of health and welfare, and to

the prevention of environmental contamination from waste; planning and managing methods of waste disposal; protecting the environment and food chain from waste; providing nutritionally balanced feeds and supplements appropriate to circumstances in which animals are kept; avoiding chemical and biological contaminants in feedstuffs; planning and recording breeding activities; maintaining traceability in all aspects of animal production; protecting the human food chain from zoonoses and chemical contamination.

8. *Animal health and welfare*: preventing disease through use of appropriate stocking rates; proper pasture management; providing hygienic and adequately maintained housing; providing clean and sufficient bedding; maintaining social groupings; use of the Farm Animal Welfare Council's '5 Freedoms'[1] to sustain animal health and welfare, and corresponding additional good practices (see Spedding, 2000); appropriate veterinary supervision of livestock; preventing disease through the purchase of healthy stock; inspection, treatment, vaccination and segregation; recording injury, sickness, treatments and mortality; using veterinary medicines and zootechnical substances in legal and safe ways.
9. *Harvesting and on-farm processing and storage*: harvesting in compliance with pre-harvest requirements; maintaining pesticide use intervals; maintaining veterinary substance intervals; providing clean and hygienic harvesting equipment and facilities; providing adequate, clean and hygienic storage facilities; storing harvested products under conditions that prevent damage, deterioration and contamination; preventing pest damage and contamination of harvested products; handling and holding animals appropriately pre-slaughter; maintaining welfare standards in animal slaughter and shearing operations; transporting harvested products under clean, hygienic conditions; maintaining harvest and slaughter records; maintaining routes of produce traceability.
10. *Energy conservation and waste management*: designing buildings and facilities to conserve energy; selecting machinery that is energy efficient; using energy saving methods of cultivation; adopting alternative technologies based on sustainable energy sources; planning for minimal waste production and handling; using safe and efficient methods of waste disposal; recycling organic wastes; minimising use of non-recyclable materials; minimising off-farm inputs; planning corrective action for pollution incidents, e.g. pesticide or fertiliser spillage, leakage from silage; buying farm inputs locally and regionally; exploiting local and regional markets to reduce transport energy consumption.
11. *Human welfare, health and safety*: training staff in safe working practices; implementing procedures for safe working; maintaining equipment in a

---

[1] The Farm Animal Welfare Council's 5 Freedoms are: freedom from hunger and thirst; freedom from discomfort; freedom from pain, injury and disease; freedom to express normal behaviour; and freedom from fear and distress.

condition suitable for safe use; restricting work time to safe working periods; allowing rest breaks; providing (as appropriate) adequate housing, security of housing and food security for employees; preventing the exploitation of workers, women and children; supporting local businesses to keep money within the local economy; recognising a duty of care for staff; planning farm activities to achieve farm objectives and to provide social, economic and environmental benefits.

12. *Landscape amenity and protection of biodiversity*: planning farm activities to prevent or minimise damage to the landscape and biodiversity; enhancing the aesthetics of the landscape and success and security of flora and fauna; selecting and organising agricultural operations to minimise adverse effects on the land and biodiversity; managing field margins to encourage wildlife; creating and maintaining areas of wild habitat to support biodiversity; managing wetlands to support wildlife; minimising or eliminating the use of artificial fertilisers and pesticides; preventing the pollution of watercourses.

The concept of 'externalities' is now coming to the fore in considerations of agriculture, food production, sustainability and the environment. Mautner (1997) defines 'externality' as 'A consequence considered irrelevant in deliberation or evaluation; especially, a cost or benefit not included in the accounts. Things that have value but no price, e.g. environmental beauty, are, from the standpoint of accountancy, externalities'. Pretty (2002) explains that externalities are the side effects of economic activity and are, therefore, external to markets so their costs are not included in the prices paid by producers and consumers. He also says that externalities often damage the interests of those without representation and the identity of the source, or producer of the externality is not always known. As so-called conventional, or intensive, agriculture has developed during the twentieth century, within the framework of neo-classical economics, many of the externalities associated with this approach to food production have not been incorporated into the economic models of farm operation and the calculation of food production costs. For instance, as agricultural inputs businesses have encouraged the use of fertilisers or pesticides with claims of direct economic benefit for farmers, so they have excluded from the calculation the true costs of using such inputs for society, the environment and biodiversity. Though a grower may gain direct benefit in terms of yield from the use of pesticides, the social costs associated with the need to remove pesticide residues from drinking water and the environmental costs due to loss of biodiversity are not usually reflected in the cost-benefit analysis that justifies pesticide use in the first place.

Other food-related externalities include the cost to people, the health services, the economy and society of poisoning and disease caused by the use of pesticides and veterinary substances in food production. Much work is now being done to calculate the external costs of agricultural food production. Pretty *et al.* (2000) estimate the external costs of UK agriculture in 1996 to have been £2,343 million. Of this £120 million is the cost of removing pesticides from drinking water and £71 million the cost of removing nitrates, phosphates and soil. The use of GAP offers many benefits to farmers and growers. Significantly it can offer social and environmental benefits through helping to reduce negative externalities.

In relation to the control of pesticides and veterinary substances GAP should be managed to meet specific objectives. Considering the control of pesticides first, it should be realised that control through HACCP is not possible unless certain requirements are in place under GAP. For example, food safety cannot be controlled if illegal pesticides or the wrong pesticides are purchased and used. As part of GAP only approved suppliers of off-farm inputs should be used, and only approved products should be purchased for specific duties. The secure storage and safe handling of pesticides should also be encompassed by GAP as should the maintenance and cleaning of spraying and other pesticide application equipment. The planned maintenance of equipment is essential to its correct performance. Equipment that has begun to wear, or that may fail, can lead to both food safety and environmental problems as well as extra cost through the overuse of pesticide, or even the under-use which leads to repeat applications. In this respect the calibration of spraying equipment is an important activity within GAP. It might be argued that calibration is a critical control point within HACCP. Logic dictates that it falls within GAP. There is little point in attempting to control pesticide by any means if the equipment used to apply it cannot perform to required targets and tolerances. The application of HACCP to food safety control is predicated on the existence of processes that work properly according to pre-determined requirements. The control of pesticides using HACCP presumes the use of properly maintained and calibrated equipment. The training of staff in the safe handling of pesticides and in maintaining, cleaning and calibrating equipment also falls within GAP, as does keeping records associated with activities concerning the use of pesticides. The management of veterinary substances through GAP has parallels with the management of pesticides. The legitimate sourcing, secure storage and safe handling of veterinary substances for use in specific and legitimate applications should be specified and managed as part of GAP. So should the training of staff to handle and administer veterinary substances. Records of the activities associated with use of veterinary substances should be kept within the GAP system. As required, audits of GAP should be able to reconcile the purchase of both pesticides and veterinary substances to materials stored and materials used.

6.4 The Hazard Analysis Critical Control Point (HACCP) system

The HACCP concept was originally developed for the US space programme as a method of making safe foods for astronauts. It is now recommended by the Codex Alimentarius Commission of the Food and Agriculture Organization and the World Health Organisation of the United Nations (UN), many governments, and many food industry organisations as the best way to manage food safety.

HACCP is entirely compatible with (and ought to be part of) quality management systems developed to ISO 9001: 2000 (ISO 2000b) though it is not itself a quality management system, or quality assurance system, in the proper sense of these terms. HACCP is used expressly to manage food safety. The concept of HACCP can be translated to other issues of quality and QA systems and, based on these concepts, can be implemented to control factors affecting aspects of food quality not related to food safety. HACCP itself should be used specifically for the management of food safety. Any liberal reinterpretation as a dual method of food safety management and quality assurance can lead to confusion. At times businesses are tempted, or advised, to use HACCP principles for both food safety and quality purposes leading to the combination of requirements critical to food safety with those important to the control of quality factors unrelated to food safety. This can create confusion and problems. Even though food safety is logically an element of quality, clarity of purpose in food safety management comes through discrete food safety systems operating in parallel to those used for controlling other aspects of food quality.

6.4.1 Applying the HACCP concept

The Hazard Analysis Critical Control Point concept provides a methodology for the systematic management of food safety. It is based on the seven principles of HACCP (CCFH, 1997):

Principle 1: Conduct a hazard analysis.
Principle 2: Determine the Critical Control Points (CCPs).
Principle 3: Establish critical limit(s).
Principle 4: Establish a system to monitor control of the CCP(s).
Principle 5: Establish the corrective action to be taken when monitoring indicates that a particular CCP is not under control.
Principle 6: Establish procedures for verification to confirm the HACCP system is working effectively.
Principle 7: Establish documentation concerning all procedures and records appropriate to these principles and their application.

The HACCP concept is implemented through a logical sequence of activities. A HACCP study is undertaken which yields a HACCP plan that is implemented as a HACCP system. A HACCP plan is defined as 'A document prepared in accordance with the principles of HACCP to ensure control of hazards which are significant for food safety in the segment of the food chain under consideration' (CCFH, 1997). A HACCP system is 'A system which identifies, evaluates and controls hazards which are significant for food safety' (CCFH, 1997). The term 'hazard analysis' refers to the development of an understanding of the hazards associated with a food product and its associated production process. A hazard is 'A biological, chemical or physical agent in, or condition of, food with the potential to cause an adverse health effect' (CCFH, 1997). Biological hazards include:

- food-borne disease causing bacteria, e.g., *Vibrio cholerae*, *Mycobacterium tuberculosis*, and viruses
- infective food poisoning bacteria, e.g., *E. coli* O157: H7, *Listeria monocytogenes*, *Salmonella* spp., *Shigella* spp., *Yersinia enterocolitica*
- intoxicating food poisoning bacteria, e.g., *Staphylococcus aureus*, *Clostridium botulinum*
- toxigenic fungi, e.g., *Aspergillus flavus*, *Aspergillus clavatus, Fusarium* spp.
- food poisoning viruses, e.g., Norwalk virus, hepatitis A
- protozoan parasites, e.g., *Cryptosporidium parvum*, *Toxoplasma gondii*
- poisonous plants and plant materials, e.g., deadly nightshade berries
- poisonous fungi, e.g. *Amanita phalloides, Amanita virosa, Amanita mascaria*
- allergenic materials, e.g., nuts and wheat gluten.

Many microbial pathogens are responsible for a variety of food-borne illnesses. While some pathogens cause short-term inconvenience with symptoms such as vomiting and diarrhoea, others may cause serious and immediate effects or long-lasting illness or death. *E. coli* O157: H7 is linked with haemolytic uraemic syndrome (HUS) causing kidney failure and death, often in children. *Campylobacter* spp. have been associated with Guillain-Barré syndrome (a cause of paralysis in adults and children). *Listeria monocytogenes* can cause abortion as well as meningitis. Consumers who are allergic to nuts can rapidly suffer anaphylactic shock and die. Chemical hazards can cause short-term illness from which a full recovery is usual, or long-term illness and death. While the health effects of some chemical contaminants are well documented, the effects (or freedom from effects) of some pesticides and veterinary residues may be a matter of conjecture rather than proven science. This may be so particularly where freedom from effects over many years of exposure is concerned, or where the understanding of toxicity is based on research concerning a single substance but little is known of the so-called 'cocktail effect', when residues of the substance exist in combination with others. Those who use pesticides and veterinary substances should ensure that records are kept of their correct use, as advised by manufacturers and in compliance with legal requirements. Records allow traceability to manufacturers in the event that questions are asked about product safety or issues of legal liability arise. A benefit of HACCP is that sources of food-borne hazard within the food chain are known and accountability for food safety problems can be identified. Chemical hazards include:

- naturally occurring environmental contaminants, e.g., some heavy metals
- industrial contaminants, e.g., dioxins, PCBs
- pesticide (insecticide, herbicide and fungicide) residues in cereals, fruit and vegetables, etc.
- nitrates (mainly leafy crops) and other fertiliser residues
- pesticides and nitrates in drinking water
- residues of veterinary medicines and other zootechnical substances in animal products, e.g., meat, milk, eggs

- contaminants arising from the handling, storage and processing of foodstuffs, e.g., grain treatment compounds, machine lubricants, cleaning agents, rodenticides and other pest control poisons
- contaminants arising from food packaging, e.g., plasticisers and other packaging material additives, adhesives, inks, metals leached from cans.

Physical hazards can be problematic to food processors, but may be less so to farmers and growers. They can represent a source of harm to consumers in that they may damage tissue (externally and internally) through laceration, damage teeth and block airways. Physical hazards include:

- slicing hazards – sharp glass fragments, sharp plastic fragments, wood splinters, sharp metal filings and swarf
- dental hazards – glass particles, pieces of wood, pieces of hard plastic, stones, metal fragments and parts, e.g., nuts, washers
- choking hazards – wood, stones, metal fragments, string, nuts, e.g., peanuts.

6.5 The HACCP study

The HACCP study provides the information used to develop the HACCP plan which is implemented as the HACCP system. The HACCP study is a twelve-stage process (though variation on the number of stages is possible).

6.5.1 Stage 1: Assemble the HACCP team (and define the scope and terms of reference of the study)

Conventionally, a HACCP study is carried out by a HACCP team. In the case of agricultural enterprises there may not be enough people available to constitute a team. This does not mean that HACCP systems cannot be developed and used. Ideally, a HACCP team will be multidisciplinary, consisting of members with the expertise required to deal with the range of issues that can arise during the study. In food manufacturing a HACCP team will usually contain representatives from the technical, production and engineering areas of the business and often someone with knowledge of food microbiology. At farm level it may be that only one person is available to undertake the HACCP study. Clearly that person should be conversant with the theory and practice of HACCP and, ideally, will have completed an appropriate unit of training in HACCP. While a single person (or a team) may undertake the development of HACCP systems, there may be times when questions arise that cannot be answered easily. External sources of information may then be needed. Specialist consultants can be used to carry out, or supplement HACCP studies, at a cost. Other sources of advice may be experts within farm inputs businesses, e.g., pesticide and veterinary substance manufacturers, university academics and government advisers.

The scope and terms of reference of the HACCP study must be set before any work commences. HACCP studies are conventionally product-based studies, carried out in relation to a specific food product and its associated production process. However, in food manufacturing it may be that a single process is used to make many different products so, for reasons of convenience and time saving, a process-based study may be undertaken. When HACCP is applied at farm level it is likely that most studies will be carried out as product-based studies, i.e., studies concerning a named crop and its associated production process, or breed of animal and its associated breeding and/or production process.

The scope of the HACCP study confines the HACCP system and dictates its start and end point. It can be important to break HACCP studies into 'bite-sized chunks', especially where complex production processes are concerned. This can make the study simpler and allow less opportunity for something critical to be missed. On completion of a series of studies the HACCP systems covering an entire production process can be linked together to form the overall HACCP system. For instance, seed preparation and propagation may form one HACCP study, with crop production, harvesting and post-harvest pre-treatments forming others. Alternatively, the breeding of animals might be covered in one HACCP study, while another encompasses the keeping of animals to meet customer and market requirements.

The terms of reference of the study dictate which hazards are to be analysed. It may be more convenient to select only biological, or chemical or physical hazards, or a specific form of hazard from one of the categories. When the specific hazards of pesticides and veterinary substances are under consideration effectively the terms of reference are already set. The use of generic HACCP plans is sometimes advocated as a short-cut to the development of HACCP systems. Generic HACCP plans can be useful as sources of ideas and information, but they can lead to difficulties as local factors and hazards may be overlooked. It is generally accepted that HACCP plans developed in relation to existing products and processes provide greater security than plans based on theory, as generic plans often are. However, in the context of using HACCP for the control of pesticides and veterinary substances generic plans may have some benefits. Compared with the complexities of many food manufacturing processes the application of pesticides or use of veterinary substances may be relatively simple. The principles used to define food safety control may readily apply to most agricultural enterprises irrespective of their differences. For instance, even though two pesticides are different, and are applied to different crops using different equipment, the principles upon which control is based may be the same. The principles might then be embodied in generic HACCP plans for pesticide use that compensate for the lack of expertise in HACCP application at farm level. The same logic applies to HACCP and veterinary substances.

6.5.2 Stage 2: Describe the product

At this stage it is usual to develop a complete description of the food product to provide information that enables the identification of hazards associated with intrinsic characteristics of the product itself, or hazards arising from conditions concerning, for example, its packaging, storage, transport, distribution and use. Foods possess intrinsic preservation factors such as pH, salt-in-moisture content and low water activity (a_w) that affect the survival and growth of bacterial pathogens. They are also influenced by extrinsic preservation factors such as heat treatments and hygienic or aseptic packaging that affect food safety. These factors along with factors such as the presence of allergens, for example, peanuts, in the food, or the need to store the food under refrigeration to keep it safe, are encompassed by the product description stage.

With the terms of reference of the HACCP study confined to pesticides or veterinary substances, the product description stage should consider the application of named pesticides to a given crop, or the use of named veterinary substances in relation to a given breed of animal. Essentially, the crop or the animal are the product (or food product to be) and, in effect, HACCP Principle 1 (Stage 6) has been pre-empted as the hazards are already identified because they are applied to the product by choice. In this interpretation of HACCP for use at farm level it is important at this stage to gather information about the pesticides or veterinary substances to be used, the rates at which they will be used (e.g. pesticide concentrations or strength of veterinary substance), the frequency of use, advised intervals between use and harvest or slaughter, withdrawal periods (e.g. in relation to dairy cattle, etc.). Such information will enable the degree of risk to consumers to be assessed and points of control to be identified. During the preparation of a HACCP plan a variety of sources may be consulted to understand the nature of pesticides and veterinary substances as hazards associated with crops and animals. These include text books, scientific journals, food research organisations, consultants and academics, national and local government organisations with responsibility for food safety, and sources on the Internet. Perhaps the best sources of information concerning pesticides and veterinary substances are the manufacturers who, effectively, bear some accountability for the safety of the products they supply.

6.5.3 Stage 3: Identify the intended use of the product

At this stage the intended use of the product should be defined to identify whether the way(s) in which the product is used (by a processor or consumer) could give rise to a hazard, or whether the product itself might be intrinsically harmful to any sensitive consumer groups (children, the elderly, people with depressed immune systems, etc.). It is also important to identify whether specific market requirements need to be observed. For example, organic markets will not take crop products containing pesticides and some markets will not accept animal products containing some types of veterinary residues (e.g., growth promoters). In the context of pesticides and veterinary substances it is important to consider whether food safety issues could arise even though residues might be within legal limits. Consideration should also be given to the nature of food safety issues if control fails. For instance, if fruit sold without previously being washed is not washed by the consumer before being eaten could permitted levels, or accidentally high levels of pesticide cause illness? If peaches and nectarines, for example, are consumed whole, without removal of the skin, might there be the potential to poison consumers if the skins are contaminated with pesticides? Could potatoes intended for mashing be harmful if they are baked as jacket potatoes and the skins contain pesticide residues? If animals are treated with certain veterinary substances might residues present in the meat affect all consumers, or just sensitive consumers, e.g. babies? Asking such questions is an important part of the HACCP study and allows the possibility of hazards to be properly evaluated. When fruit and vegetables are sold for processing or use by consumers the responsibility lies with the producer (and also retailers) to ensure that the products are free from hazards. Crop production methods should therefore ensure that pesticide residues do not exceed the permitted maximum residue levels (MRLs). The same principles apply to the use of veterinary substances.

6.5.4 Stage 4: Construct a flow diagram

Stage 3 of the HACCP study generates information that helps in the identification of hazards associated with the product and with characteristics of the product. In food production and processing the potential exists for hazards to arise directly as a result of the process itself. In Stage 4 a flow diagram of the production process (Figs 6.1 and 6.2) should be prepared that identifies the inputs to, and the outputs from, the process, as well as the operating conditions and parameters required to make the product. In the case of crop production, inputs include seed, seed treatment agents, irrigation water, manure, fertilisers and pesticides, as well as, for example, water used in post-harvest operations such as hydro-cooling to remove field heat and washing to remove soil and contaminants, etc. The product itself is the principal output. Others may be product rejected in grading due to damage or deterioration, waste botanical material, for example, from trimming and other preparation processes, soil from washing operations, etc., all of which, given the right circumstances, could give rise to hazards.

The crop production process will consist of various operations including seed treatment and propagation, field or site preparation, fertiliser applications, planting, growing, irrigation, pesticide applications, harvesting, post-harvest handling and post-harvest pre-treatments (e.g., cleaning, trimming), as well as storage and transport, etc. In a HACCP study confined to the consideration of pesticides, focus will be drawn to pesticides as inputs to the process, the application of pesticides as operations and crops carrying pesticide residues as outputs. Similar concepts apply to the development of process flow diagrams concerning animal production and the use of veterinary substances as inputs affecting the safety of the animal products that constitute outputs. The scope of the flow diagram should be constrained by the scope of the HACCP study. It

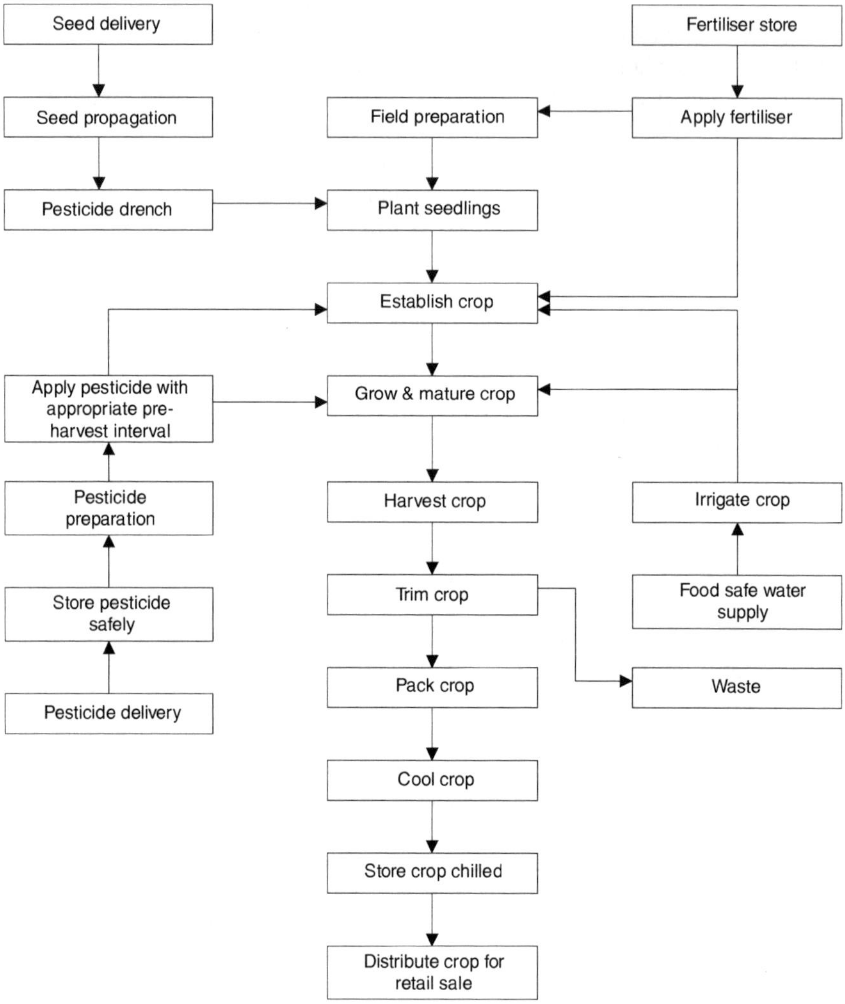

Fig. 6.1 Flow diagram for field crop production.

should be structured logically and systematically, and provide a level of detail that allows evaluation and the identification of hazards without constant reference to additional information.

A flow diagram may be drawn by referring to information and data concerning the production process and any operations carried out as part of the process. Sources of information will include specifications or data sheets for pesticides and veterinary substances, other information provided by manufacturers, government agencies, and legal requirements concerning use, etc. Procedures and information concerning crop or animal production processes, harvesting and post-harvest management of crops, the transport and

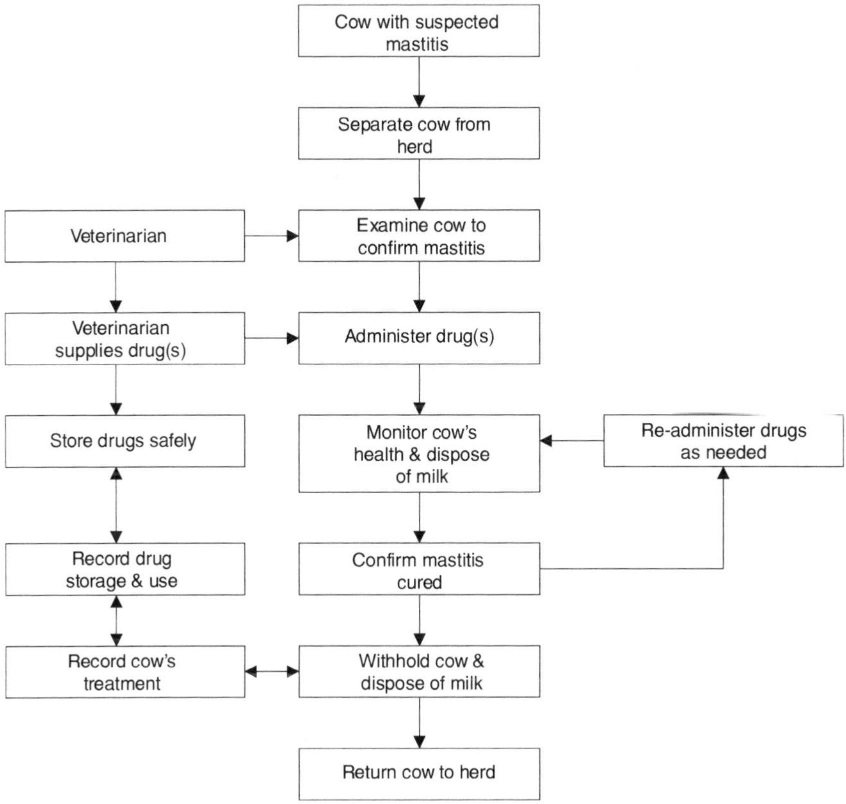

Fig. 6.2 Flow diagram for the treatment of a cow suffering from mastitis.

slaughtering of animals, etc., may all inform the development of a process flow diagram.

6.5.5 Stage 5: Confirm the flow diagram

The completed flow diagram should be confirmed as a true representation of the production process and not a reflection of a theoretical process differing from the true process because things have been overlooked or unauthorised changes have been made. The process flow diagram should be confirmed by comparing it with what actually happens, as it happens. Given the nature of agricultural food production it may not be practical to observe the complete growing cycle of a crop or animal in the first instance. So, reference may need to be made to procedures, records and the experience of personnel to confirm as best as possible the accuracy and veracity of the diagram, at least until a cycle has been completed.

6.5.6 Stage 6: Identify and analyse all potential hazards, assess the risks and identify the preventive measures (HACCP Principle 1)

The hazards associated with a product and its intended use, and the hazards occurring in, or associated with the production processes, are now identified and analysed. Identification means recognising every hazard that might arise as a result of factors associated with the product, what it is and the way it is used, or the way the product is made. Analysis concerns understanding the nature of the hazards, assessing their risk in terms of their likely occurrence and severity of effects for consumers, and identifying the means of control or preventive measures. Each hazard should be analysed in turn.

When a HACCP study focuses on pesticides and veterinary substances the hazards should be identified automatically. The analysis should aim to assess the risks associated with the pesticides and veterinary substances of concern, especially with regard to the presence of residues in products and the effects on consumers. Risk assessment will be concerned with, for example, recognising when and how frequently pesticides and veterinary substances are used, and the nature of consequences for consumers (a) if they are used correctly according to recommended and legal requirements, and (b) if they are inadvertently used at levels exceeding recommended and legal requirements. Risk analysis is not easy and risk can be difficult to quantify, but it is a necessary part of HACCP and has the benefit of allowing hazards that prove to be of negligible risk to be dispensed with. There is no point in spending time and effort controlling hazards that are unlikely to arise. When the nature of each hazard has been evaluated control methods can then be determined to either prevent or eliminate them, or to reduce them to acceptable levels. Preventive measures for pesticides and veterinary substances are likely to involve establishing concentrations and/or use rates to prevent use at levels that might represent harm to consumers, and setting post-treatment intervals or withdrawal periods to prevent crop or animal products that contain unsafe residues from reaching consumers.

6.5.7 Stage 7: Determine the Critical Control Points (CCPs) (HACCP Principle 2)

A Critical Control Point (CCP) is 'A step at which control can be applied and is essential to prevent or eliminate a food safety hazard or reduce it to an acceptable level' (CCFH, 1997). Preventive measures are applied at CCPs. Each hazard identified in Stage 6 must be assessed in relation to each step in the process, as recorded on the process flow diagram, to decide whether a particular step in the process constitutes a CCP for a given hazard. Experience and judgement are used to decide whether a process step is a CCP. The CCP decision tree (Fig. 6.3) can be used as an aid to the identification and clarification of CCPs. Effectively, a CCP can be thought of as the last line of defence and a point beyond which control of a specific hazard is not possible. Thus, if control is not exercised at the CCP then safe food will not be produced. CCPs for pesticides and veterinary substances are likely to concern checking the

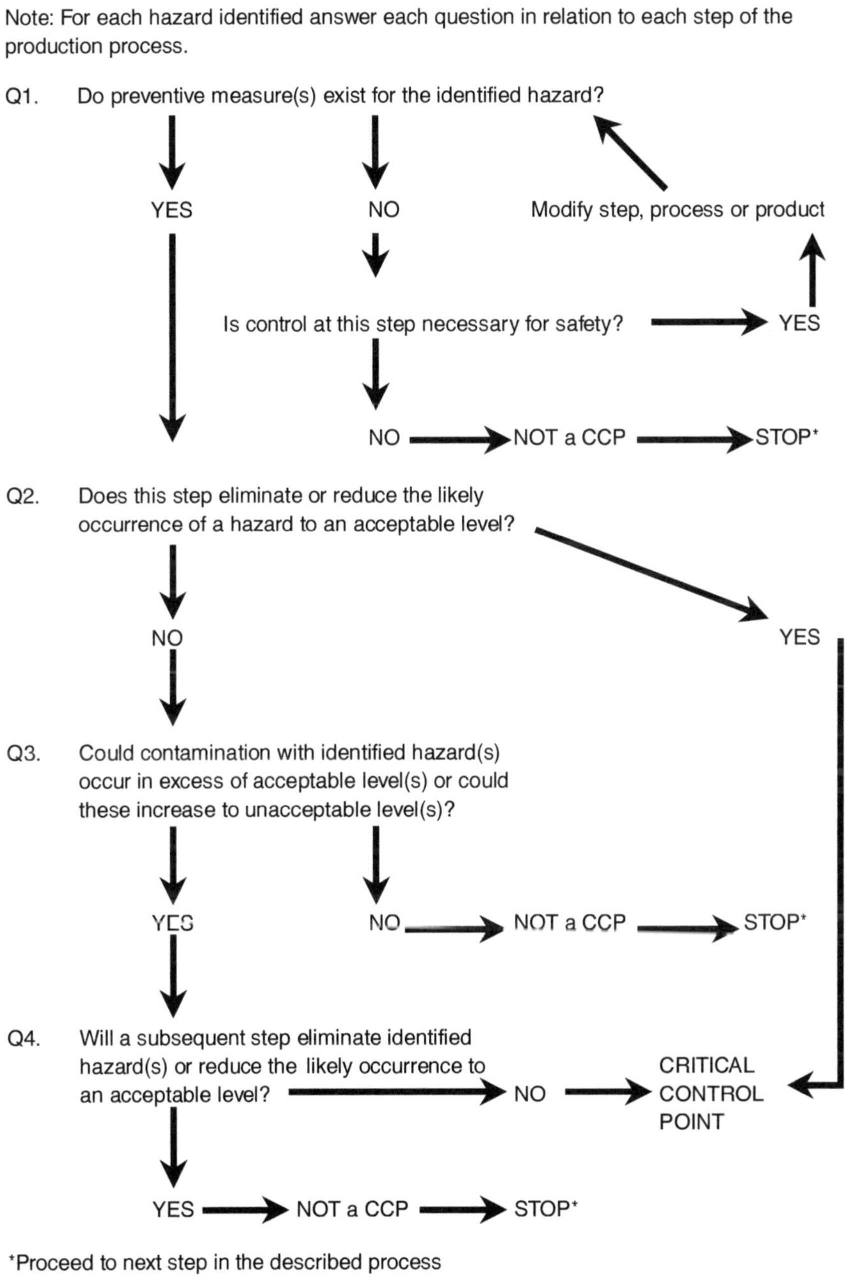

Fig. 6.3 CCP decision tree.
Source: FLAIR. Undated. HACCP User Guide. Concerted Action No. 7. Food Linked Agro Industrial Research, 191, rue de Vaugirard – 75015, Paris.

concentration or dosage of substances, confirming and controlling usage rates and maintaining harvest intervals or withdrawal periods.

Care must be taken not to create more CCPs than are needed to ensure food safety as the complexity and costs of maintaining the HACCP system will increase unnecessarily. Also, an intelligent interpretation of HACCP is required if the creation of false CCPs is to be avoided. Take abattoirs and meat packing, for example. A number of microbial hazards might be thought of as hazards that require control in the production of raw meat for the retail food market. Significant amongst them is *E. coli* O157: H7 and many abattoirs and meat packing plants implement preventive measures and CCPs in relation to this organism. For instance, it is not uncommon to see visual inspection of the coat of cattle designated as a preventive measure for *E. coli* O157: H7, with a point before slaughter designated as a CCP. If animals are considered to be visually unacceptable they are rejected on the grounds that they might risk bringing the organism into the processing plant and contaminating meat. Clipping or tying back animal hides to prevent the contamination of meat may also be designated a preventive measure applied as a CCP during the early stages of processing. Similarly, the prevention of cross-contamination between gut contents and meat may also be seen as a preventive measure with evisceration processes constituting the CCP. The measures taken to reduce *E. coli* O157: H7 contamination in meat processing amount to good hygiene practices. They are an important part of GMP. However, their designation as preventive measures and corresponding CCPs defies a logical understanding of HACCP.

Hazards are either prevented, or eliminated, or reduced to acceptable levels by preventive measures applied at CCPs. It is difficult, therefore, to justify the interpretation of HACCP used in some abattoirs and meat packing plants because none of the actions described will prevent or eliminate *E. coli* O157: H7, or reduce it to acceptable levels. Indeed, as an organism with a very low infective dose level of 10–100 cells, there can be no acceptable level. There will always be a chance that *E. coli* O157: H7 will be present on some meat, irrespective of the measures taken in processing, and given that few meat packing plants actually test for the organism how can they know their CCPs are working effectively? The way to ensure meat is safe from *E. coli* O157: H7 is to cook it properly and prevent post cooking re-contamination. In my opinion abattoirs and meat packing plants misinterpret HACCP and create work that offers no food safety or business benefit. Hygiene in abattoirs and meat packing would be better controlled through aspects of GMP. This example, though not directly related to crops and animal production, can be of value to those using HACCP in agriculture and who will have to decide whether preventive measures and CCPs are valid or whether to use GAP instead.

6.5.8 Stage 8: Establish critical limits for each CCP (HACCP Principle 3)

A critical limit is 'A criterion which separates acceptability from unacceptability' (CCFH, 1997). Critical limits establish parameters for the operation of preventive measures at CCPs. They may concern quantitative values such as time, temperature, pH, a_w, concentration, application rates, etc., or qualitative values proven to indicate food safety. In the use of pesticides, values for concentration and application rates may be set as quantitative critical limits, as may intervals between application and harvesting. Legally defined maximum residue limits (MRLs) may also serve as critical limits. Similarly, in the use of veterinary substances the potency, usage and withdrawal periods may be designated as critical limits. Critical limits are set in relation to specific hazards, so provided they are adhered to a product can be regarded as safe. Records of control activities at CCPs and adherence to critical limits should be kept for HACCP system verification and maintenance, and to provide evidence of due diligence and the production of safe food.

6.5.9 Stage 9: Establish a monitoring system for each CCP (HACCP Principle 4)

Monitoring activities or procedures are carried out to confirm that the controls exercised at CCPs remain effective to ensure food safety or to detect that control has been lost. Monitoring usually consists of a planned sequence of observations or measurements used to show the HACCP system is operating effectively. Monitoring methods should be kept as simple as possible. They may be quantitative or qualitative and will often be linked to the nature of preventive measures. In crop and animal production monitoring activities will be designed to ensure that controls over the use of pesticides and veterinary substances are effective and that critical limits are being complied with. The measurement of substance residues in crops and animal products, for example through government surveillance programmes to ensure MRLs are not exceeded, is an approach to monitoring, but its value to issues of immediate control at farm level is limited.

The HACCP plan should identify how each CCP is to be monitored, the frequency of monitoring and who is responsible for ensuring that monitoring is carried out. Records of monitoring activities should be maintained for HACCP system verification and maintenance, as well as for due diligence purposes. Conventionally, monitoring activities show that control has been lost at CCPs. It is beneficial to use monitoring to indicate that a CCP is going out of control. Rather than allow control to be lost and then have to take corrective action, it makes sense to use preventive action to ensure control is maintained at all times.

6.5.10 Stage 10: Establish corrective action procedures (HACCP Principle 5)

If monitoring shows that control at a CCP has been lost, corrective action must be taken. Corrective action has a dual purpose: to return the CCP to a state of control, and to identify and manage any potentially non-conforming (unsafe) product. A corrective action procedure should be written for each CCP stating the actions required to restore control. The procedures should also state requirements for identifying, segregating and testing implicated product to prevent it being inadvertently used or despatched to customers. The personnel responsible for taking action and controlling product should be identified, as should those responsible for confirming control has been restored. Government surveillance may initiate corrective action, but often notifications of non-compliance with critical limits will be after the event and corrective action then means improvement in the future.

6.5.11 Stage 11: Establish verification procedures (HACCP Principle 6)

When the HACCP plan is complete it can be implemented as the HACCP system. Prior to implementation the plan should be validated. This means answering the question: Will the system work when we put it into practice? (ILSI, 1999). Validation is defined as 'Obtaining evidence that the HACCP plan is [likely to be] effective' (CCFH, 1997). Validation amounts to an assessment of the scientific and technical content of the HACCP plan, checking that the elements of the plan are complete, that decisions and assumptions made during the study are sound, and that the plan is adequate to create a workable and effective food safety management system. ILSI (1999) recommends a series of validation activities intended to collect objective evidence that confirms the adequacy of the plan in relation to the seven principles of HACCP:

- Principle 1 (Hazard analysis): Confirm (a) that the skills of those undertaking the HACCP study were adequate for the task, (b) that the flow diagram was suitable for the purposes of the study, and (c) that all significant hazards and appropriate preventive measures have been identified.
- Principle 2 (Identify CCPs): Confirm (a) that CCPs have been identified for the application of preventive measures for each significant hazard and (b) that the CCPs are at appropriate stages of the process.
- Principle 3 (Critical limits): Confirm (a) that critical limits are established for each hazard and (b) that the limits are appropriate to the preventive measures applied at the relevant CCPs.
- Principle 4 (Monitoring): Confirm (a) that monitoring methods and systems can demonstrate the effectiveness of preventive measures, and (b) that procedures exist for the calibration of monitoring methods and systems, as appropriate.
- Principle 5 (Corrective action): Confirm (a) that corrective action procedures exist for each preventive measure and CCP, (b) that procedures exist to prevent non-conforming product reaching customers, and (c) that responsibility for taking and verifying corrective action is identified, as well as that for approving the disposition of non-conforming product.
- Principle 6 (Verification): Confirm that procedures and a plan for the verification of the HACCP system have been established.
- Principle 7 (Documentation): Confirm that documentation describing the entire HACCP system and records required to support the system have been established.

Validation should seek to confirm that the HACCP plan is comprehensive and will be effective as a means of protecting consumers when implemented as the HACCP system. Auditing techniques, such as those employed in quality systems auditing, should be used for validation.

Verification is carried out on the operational HACCP system. It means answering the question: Are we doing what we planned to do? (ILSI, 1999). Verification is defined as 'The application of methods, procedures, tests and other evaluations, in addition to monitoring, to determine compliance with the HACCP plan' (CCFH, 1997). Verification is a check that what the HACCP plan says will be done, is done. Verification activities should confirm that the HACCP system has been implemented in compliance with the plan. Procedures (and any other methods or tests thought necessary) should be established for this purpose. Verification should confirm that:

- hazard analysis and the identification of preventive measures was carried out properly (also a check on validation)
- the identification of CCPs and setting of critical limits was carried out properly (also a check on validation)
- the control of hazards at CCPs is effective and records of CCP control are kept
- monitoring methods are effective and monitoring records are kept
- corrective action procedures work effectively, that customers are protected from receiving non-conforming product and records of corrective action are kept
- verification procedures themselves are carried out properly
- documentation covering the entire HACCP system has been established and records to support the system are completed properly and retained for an appropriate period of time.

The length of crop and animal production cycles may make it necessary to extend verification activities throughout the year. So that modifications and improvements can be made to the HACCP plan, as required, it can be important to take into account deviations from intended production processes, such as those caused by the weather, pests, disease, etc., when analysing verification results.

6.5.12 Stage 12: Establish documentation and record keeping requirements (HACCP Principle 7)

Various documents and records constitute the HACCP plan and support the HACCP system. Most will result from the HACCP study. A key output of the study should be the HACCP control chart (Tables 6.1 and 6.2). This is central to the plan and defines the operation and control of the system. Other documents that may be part of, or referenced in the plan include pesticide and veterinary substance specifications, the process flow diagram, crop and animal production procedures, CCP control and monitoring procedures, preventive and corrective

Table 6.1 Example of a HACCP control chart for field crop production

Process step	Step no.	CCP no.	Hazard	Control measure	Critical limit(s)	Monitoring*		Corrective action**
						Procedure	Frequency	Procedure
Seed delivery.	1	1	Unacceptable pesticide residues in seed.	Seed meets spec.	As stated in spec.	Check certificate of analysis on delivery.	Each delivery.	Reject delivery. Review supplier.
Seed propagation	2							
Pesticide drench.	3	2	Microbial pathogens in drench water.	Use potable water.	Absence of pathogens.	Confirm water quality with supplier.	Annually.	Agree measures for improvement with supplier.
Field preparation.	4	3	Contamination with pathogens from un-rotted manure.	Check history of manure use on site.	No un-rotted manure used in past two years.	Confirm site history.	Prior to site preparation.	Use site only if free from manure deposits or choose another site.
Fertiliser application (P & K) during field preparation	5							
Planting of seedlings	6							
Irrigation during crop establishment and growth	7	4	Microbial pathogens in water.	Use clean water.	Absence of pathogens.	Confirm water quality with supplier.	Prior to use.	Agree measures for improvement with supplier or use another source.
Fertiliser (N) application during growth	8							
Pesticide preparation	9	5	Pesticide(s) prepared at excessive concentration giving unacceptable residue levels.	Use calibrated equipment for preparation.	As defined by manufacturer for named pesticide(s).	Observe preparation procedures complied with and check usage of pesticides against stocks.	Periodically when pesticide(s) used.	Calibrate equipment, revise procedures, or test crop for excess residue, according to nature of failure.
		6	Microbial pathogens in water.	Use clean water.	Absence of pathogens.	Confirm water quality with supplier.	Prior to use.	Agree measures for improvement with supplier or use another source.

Pesticide application	10	7	Pesticide(s) applied at excessive concentration giving unacceptable residue levels.	Apply with appropriate and calibrated equipment. Use trained staff for job.	As defined by manufacturer for named pesticide(s) and/or legally defined limits.	Check pesticide usage and observe application procedure.	Periodically when pesticide(s) used.	Calibrate equipment, revise procedures, or test crop for excess residue, according to nature of failure.
Pesticide post-application period	11	8	Pesticide(s) remain in crop at unacceptable residue levels.	Observe pre-harvest interval. Do not harvest until interval elapses.	Pre-harvest interval as advised by manufacturer for named pesticide(s).	Record dates of pesticide applications and observe interval to harvest.	Each crop.	Test crop for excess residue and reject if levels exceed requirements.
Harvesting (Glass control)	12	9	Contamination with glass from machinery.	Glass policy – only use glass when needed and care taken when glass involved.	No glass contamination of product.	Check all glass for damage.	Daily.	Segregate and check implicated product before approving for use.
Harvesting (Wood control)	13	10	Contamination with wood from packaging.	Care taken when wood is involved.	No wood contamination of product.	Check packaging materials for damage.	Daily.	Segregate and check implicated product before approving for use.
Harvesting (Staff control)	14	11	Contamination with microbial pathogens from staff.	Good personal hygiene practised by staff.	Staff adhering to personal hygiene policy.	Observation and supervision of staff.	Continuous.	Appropriate management of staff breaking the rules.
Storage	15	12	Growth of microbial pathogens on produce.	Select temperature and humidity suitable to prevent growth.	Adequate temperature and humidity to maintain product quality, but unsuitable for microbial growth.	Check storage temperature and humidity.	Daily.	Segregate and check implicated product before approving for use. Rectify temperature and humidity.
Transport	16	13	Contamination with microbial pathogens from transport vehicles.	Use only approved vehicles and hauliers. Check vehicles before use.	Vehicles clean, hygienic and fit for use.	Check records of vehicle inspection.	Daily.	Agree measures for improvement with haulier or use another approved haulier.
		14	Growth of microbial pathogens.	Check temperature and humidity suitable to prevent growth prior to despatch.	Temperature/humidity suitable to maintain product quality, but unsuitable for microbial growth.	Check records of vehicle temperature and humidity assessment.	Daily.	Review control procedures. Agree measures for improvement with haulier or use another approved haulier.

Note: This table is not as detailed as should be possible, because specific crops and pesticides are not identified. Some other hazards are identified for illustrative purposes.

* The responsibility for monitoring and corrective action would normally be given.

Table 6.2 Example of HACCP control chart for treating cows suffering from mastitis

Process step	Step no.	CCP no.	Hazard	Control measure	Critical limit(s)	Monitoring*		Corrective action**
						Procedure	Frequency	Procedure
Suspect cow with mastitis.	1	1	Milk with mastitis causing micro organisms (some bacterial pathogens) entering bulk milk and placing consumers at risk.	Remove cow from herd.	Cow physically separated from herd until infection is cured.	Observe separation is effective.	Daily checks.	Review procedure for managing cows with mastitis.
Separate cow from herd	2		Cow is source of infection for other cows which places milk and consumers at risk.					
Veterinarian examines cow.	3							
Veterinarian confirms mastitis.	4							
Veterinarian administers drug treatment.	5	2	Drug(s) residues due to excessive usage rates entering milk supply after cow cured.	Check usage rate for drug(s).	Use at rate(s) defined by manufacturer.	Observe drug(s) being administered and compliance with usage rate(s).	Each time drug(s) used.	Review procedure for drug(s) administration.
Cow milked during segregation period.	6	3	Milk with mastitis causing micro organisms (some bacterial pathogens) entering bulk milk.	Dispose of milk.	No milk from infected cow enters bulk milk.	Observe milking and correct disposal.	Each time cow milked.	Review procedure for managing cows with mastitis.
Monitor cow's health during segregation period.	7							
Drugs re-administered according to need.	8	4	Drug(s) residues due to excessive usage rates entering milk supply after cow cured.	Check usage rate for drug(s).	Use at rate(s) defined by manufacturer.	Observe drug(s) being administered and compliance with usage rate(s).	Each time drug(s) used.	Review procedure for drug(s) administration.
Confirm that infection is cured but withhold cow from herd for post-treatment period.	9	5	Drug(s) residues entering milk supply.	Keep cow separate from herd for withdrawal period. Continue to dispose of milk.	Withdrawal period advised by drug(s) manufacturer or veterinarian. No milk from infected cow enters bulk milk.	Observe separation is effective and lasts required time. Observe milking and correct disposal.	Daily checks. Each time cow milked.	Review procedure for managing cows with mastitis.
Return cow to herd.	10							

* Those responsible for monitoring and corrective action would normally be identified.

action procedures, and verification procedures. The records kept within the system will be those relating to CCP control and monitoring, preventive and corrective action, HACCP system validation and verification, and HACCP plan and system modification.

6.6 Implementing and maintaining HACCP systems

The HACCP plan must be properly implemented and the HACCP system maintained if food safety is to be ensured. Mortimore and Wallace (2001) define an eight-step approach to implementation. Adaptation of this approach (Early, 2002) to emphasise the implementation of preventive measures, or confirmation of their adequacy if they already exist, leads to a ten-step process, as follows:

1. *Determine the approach to implementation* – the HACCP system may be implemented as a complete system or broken down into more manageable units.
2. *Agree the activities to be undertaken and the timetable* – this requires the identification of implementation activities, those responsible for them and a timetable for completion. Project management techniques, e.g. Gantt charts, can be useful.
3. *Confirm the existence of adequate preventive measures, or implement preventive measures, as necessary* – preventive measures may exist as part of an operational process or may have been identified in the HACCP study and require implementation. Either way they must be confirmed to exist.
4. *Conduct training in the operation of preventive measures or confirm adequate operation exists* – preventive measures must be shown to be effective. Staff training may be needed for the operation of new preventive measures.
5. *Set up CCP monitoring methods* – methods for monitoring the control of CCPs must be established.
6. *Conduct training in CCP monitoring* – staff must be adequately trained and competent in CCP monitoring activities.
7. *Complete 'once-only' activities* – activities required to put everything in place to finish the HACCP system, e.g., procedure writing, creating records, establishing document and record control systems, process engineering and modification, and staff training, must be completed.
8. *Confirm the monitoring systems are in place* – confirmation must be made that monitoring systems are in place and operating adequately, through the use of adequate procedures by trained staff.
9. *Confirm implementation is complete and operate the HACCP system* – when confirmation is made that implementation activities have been completed the HACCP system can become fully operational.
10. *Audit to confirm adequate implementation* – correct implementation of the HACCP system should be confirmed by audit using standard quality

assurance auditing techniques. The system will need running for an agreed time to generate records that allow the state of implementation and operational effectiveness to be confirmed. One (or more) complete production cycle may be needed to have complete confidence in the system.

Although the HACCP plan may be operational in the form of the HACCP system, both the plan and the system will need to be maintained. Ideally, the HACCP plan will be reviewed annually to confirm that it still addresses all food safety requirements. When changes to crop or animal production procedures are made, and specifically in the use of pesticides and veterinary substances, the plan should be revised and the system modified. HACCP system audits should be carried out periodically to confirm that it complies with the plan and corrective action should be taken to rectify non-compliances.

6.7 Future trends

Although HACCP was developed for use in food processing and manufacturing its application throughout the food chain is now being advocated by many authorities as a key element of the 'field to fork' approach to food safety control. Though food safety authorities may encourage its use in agriculture, practical problems concerning the interpretation of HACCP and the development of HACCP systems will be encountered at farm level. An area of development that we might hope to see is in ways to use HACCP for food safety management in crop and animal production that are consistent with the need to manage food safety at farm level, and commensurate with the nature and operational restrictions of farming and growing. It is naive to believe that farms can be operated to the same hygiene standards as food manufacturing businesses, yet there are those who take such a view.

There is possibly no better demonstration than the BSE crisis that what happens at one end of the food chain can have disastrous consequences at the other. Yet BSE was not caused by farmers. It was caused by the animal feed industry, a food manufacturing industry. Even if all farmers involved in animal production in the 1980s had used HACCP it is unlikely that the hazards associated with the practices that led to BSE would have been spotted. The official advice at the time was that feeding meat and bone meal to cattle was an acceptable, safe practice.

If HACCP is to be used beneficially at farm level it should only be used where:

- a proven need for food safety management exists
- HACCP is shown to be the only practical way to ensure food safety
- the use of HACCP does not become detrimental to the ability of farmers and growers to remain in business.

The risk exists that HACCP could be used as a technical barrier to trade and a means of eliminating small agricultural enterprises that do not have the resources to maintain HACCP systems to the standards advocated at government levels by large agricultural and food businesses. We can hope that developments will be made in the interpretation and simplification of HACCP at farm level.

The possibility of HACCP functioning as a technical barrier to trade also exists where the food safety authorities in one country act with greater zeal to ensure its application than do the authorities in another country. Such a possibility exists within, for instance, the European Union, where the authorities in different member states may not act equally in interpreting food safety regulations. We can hope to see developments in the consistent interpretation of food safety regulations and the application of HACCP throughout all trading nations. We might also hope to see developments in the international standardisation of training for the use of HACCP in different business sectors, as well as in the maintenance and improvement of HACCP systems. Problems of inequality in the interpretation of food safety regulations by national food safety authorities might be overcome by the implementation and use of internationally accepted training standards. Such standards could also aid the integration of HACCP with quality management and quality assurance systems, and with GAP.

Mayes (2001) sees the globalisation of the world's food industry as a driving force for the use of HACCP throughout the food supply chain and suggests that HACCP will become the benchmark method for food safety management, as advocated by Codex Alimentarius. He suggests that World Trade Organisation (WTO) member countries that adopt Codex standards will not have to justify their sanitary measures under the WTO's Sanitary and Phytosanitary (SPS) agreement. Although working to Codex standards may offer advantages, Mayes suggests that the global acceptance of HACCP as the standard for food safety management raises issues about standardised methods of application, and assessment of the effectiveness of implementation and the ability to control food-borne hazards.

The development of global food supply chains increases the potential for the movement of food-borne pathogens from one country to another. This potential has been demonstrated by the occurrence of SARS (Sudden Acute Respiratory Syndrome) in China, which rapidly affected other parts of the world through the movement of people by air travel. Due to the speed at which the globalisation of food supply is being encouraged by western governments, major food manufacturers and major supermarket companies, some urgency would seem to be justified in establishing a standardised, water-tight, approach to food safety management at all levels of the international food supply system. HACCP may provide the necessary approach, but it should be remembered that the effectiveness of HACCP is contingent on the identification of known hazards. By definition, the unpredicted hazard is the hazard that we do not expect and will not plan for. A body of scientific knowledge and experience is needed if food-borne hazards are to be controlled. Yet the continually increasing global movement of foodstuffs, particularly unprocessed and minimally processed foods, such as fresh vegetables and meat sold through supermarkets, seems only to increase the potential to expose consumers to new food-borne hazards. Whether the world's public health experts will stay ahead of the threats that globalisation brings remains to be seen.

6.8 Conclusion

This chapter has described the use of GAP and HACCP with particular emphasis on the control of pesticides and veterinary substances. Though HACCP can be used to good effect by some farmers and growers, it should be remembered that not all will need to use HACCP. Indeed, caution should be taken in any decision to use HACCP at farm level. It should only be used where there is a genuine need to manage food safety with HACCP methodology, and where clear benefits can be seen. In many cases HACCP will not be needed and will not be practical as, for instance, the circumstances will be such that hazards cannot be prevented, eliminated or reduced to acceptable levels. Its use will only bring unnecessary complications and in such instances GAP is probably the better solution. This said, there is not the intention here to diminish the value of HACCP, just to urge that reason, judgement and proportionality are used in its recommendation as a tool for food safety management in areas of the food chain beyond food manufacturing for which it was originally designed.

6.9 Acknowledgements

I would like to thank my colleagues, Steve Baugh (veterinarian), Martin Hare (crop scientist) and Lorna White (animal scientist) for their advice and comments on this chapter.

6.10 Sources of further information and advice

Campden and Chorleywood Food Research Association (CCFRA), Chipping Campden, Gloucestershire, GL55 6LD, United Kingdom. http://www.campden.co.uk (Information and training).

The European Commission Food Safety website. Food Safety: From the Farm to the Fork. http://www.europa.eu.int/comm/food/index_en.html

the Food Business Initiative, Harper Adams University College, Newport, Shropshire, TF10 8NB, United Kingdom. http://www.foodbusinessinitiative.com (Information and training on HACCP, ICM, AMTRA & BASIS).

ILSI (International Life Sciences Institute) USA. One Thomas Circle, 9th Floor, Washington DC, 20005, USA. http://www.ilsi.org/

ILSI (International Life Sciences Institute) Europe. Avenue E. Mounier 83, Box 6, B-1200 Brussels, Belgium. http://europe.ilsi.org/

UK Pesticide Safety Directorate. PSD, Mallard House, Kings Pool, York YO1 7PX, United Kingdom. http://www.pesticides.gov.uk/

UK Veterinary Medicines Directorate. Veterinary Medicines Directorate, Woodham Lane, New Haw, Addlestone, Surrey, KT15 3LS, United Kingdom. http://www.vmd.gov.uk/

US Government Centres for Disease Control. Centres for Disease Control and Prevention, 1600 Clifton Road, Atlanta, GA., 30333, U.S.A. http://www.cdc.gov/

US Food & Drug Administration, 5600 Fishers Lane, Rockville, MD 20857-0001, USA. http://www.fda.gov/default.htm. See also: the USFDA Foodborne Pathogenic Microorganisms and Natural Toxins Handbook (Bad Bug Book) at, http://vm.cfsan.fda.gov/~mow/intro.html

6.11 References and bibliography

ANON. 2002. U.N. Food agency adopts updated pesticide standards. Press release of the United States Embassy, Tokyo, Japan. http://usembassy.state.gov/tokyo/wwwhenv20021107a2.html. Accessed: 30/04.02.

CCFH. 1997. Hazard Analysis Critical Control Point (HACCP) System and Guidelines for its Application. Annex to CAC/RCP-1 (1969), Rev. 3 (1997). Codex Committee on Food Hygiene. In: *Codex Alimentarius Commission Food Hygiene Basic Texts, Food and Agriculture Organization of the United Nations*, World Health Organization, Rome.

CARSON, R. 2000. *Silent Spring*. London, Penguin Books. First published 1964.

DILLON, M. and GRIFFITH, C. (eds.) 2001. *Auditing in the Food Industry*. Cambridge, Woodhead Publishing Limited.

EARLY, R. 2002. Use of HACCP systems in fruit and vegetable production and post-harvest pre-treatment. In: Jongen, W. (ed.). *Fruit and Vegetable Processing*. Cambridge, Woodhead Publishing Limited. pp. 91–118.

FSA. 2003a. *About Us*. Food Standards Agency. http://www.foodstandards.gov.uk/aboutus/ Accessed: 06/06/03.

FSA. 2003b. *Acrylamide*. Food Standards Agency. http://www.foodstandards.gov.uk/safereating/acrylamide branch/. Accessed: 02/04/03.

GRIERSON, B. 1997. Food safety through the ages. American Council on Science and Health. http://www.acsh.org/publications/priorities/0903/foodsafety.html. Accessed: 07/05/03.

HERSOM, A.C. and HULLAND, E.D. 1980. *Canned Foods: Thermal Processing and Microbiology*. 7th edn. Edinburgh, Churchill Livingstone.

IFST. 1998. *Food and Drink: Good Manufacturing Practice*. 4th edn. London, Institute of Food Science and Technology (UK).

ILSI. 1999. *Validation and Verification of HACCP*. Brussels, International Life Sciences Institute.

ISO. 2000a. ISO 9000: 2000 *Quality management system – Fundamentals and vocabulary*. Geneva, International Organization for Standardization.

ISO 2000b. ISO 9001: 2000 *Quality management system – Requirements*. Geneva, International Organization for Standardization.

LEAF. 2000. *The LEAF handbook for integrated farm management*. Stoneleigh, Linking Environment and Farming.

MAUTNER, T. (ed.) 1997. *Penguin dictionary of philosophy*. London, Penguin Books.

MAYES, T. 2001. The Future of HACCP. In: T. Mayes and S. Mortimore (eds), *Making the*

Most of HACCP. Cambridge, Woodhead Publishing Limited.

MEIKLE, J. 2003. Chicken farmers reintroduce growth drugs despite public fear. *Guardian Unlimited*. http://politics.guardian.co.uk/green/story/0,9061,964007,00.html. Accessed: 06/06/03.

MORTIMORE, S. and WALLACE, C. 1998. *HACCP: a practical approach*, 2nd edn. Gaithersburg, Aspen Publishers.

MORTIMORE, S. and WALLACE, C. 2001. *HACCP*. Oxford, Blackwell Science.

NESTLE, M. 2003. *Safe Food: Bacteria, Biotechnology and Bioterrorism*. Berkeley, University of California Press.

PRETTY, J. 2002. *Agri-culture: Reconnecting People, Land and Nature*. London, Earthscan Publications.

PRETTY, J.N., BRETT, C., GEE, D., HINE, R., MASON, C.F., MORISON, J.I.L., RAVEN, H., RAYMENT, M. and VAN DER BIJL, G. 2000. An assessment of the total external costs of UK agriculture. *Agricultural Systems*, 65, 113–136.

PHLS. 2003. *Food poisoning notifications: annual totals for England and Wales, 1982–2001*. Public Health Laboratory Service. http://www.phls.co.uk/topics_az/noids/foodAnnNots.htm. Accessed: 06/06/03.

SCHLOSSER, E. 2001. *Fast Food Nation*. London, Allen Lane, The Penguin Press.

SHAPTON, D.A. and SHAPTON, N.F. (eds) 1993. *Principles and Practices for the Safe Processing of Food*. Cambridge, Woodhead Publishing Limited.

SPEDDING, C. 2000. *Animal Welfare*. London, Earthscan.

THE PENNINGTON GROUP. 1997. *Report on the circumstances leading to the 1996 outbreak of infection with E. coli O157 in Central Scotland*. Edinburgh, The Stationery Office.

UN. 1948. Universal Declaration of Human Rights. Adopted and proclaimed by General Assembly resolution 217A (III) of 10 December 1948. United Nations, New York. http://www.un.org/Overview/rights.html. Accessed: 24/03/03.

Part II

Veterinary residues

7

Assessing the safety of veterinary drug residues

K. N. Woodward, International Federation for Animal Health, Belgium

7.1 Introduction

Most developed and many developing countries have in place schemes for the pre-marketing authorisation of veterinary medicines. Veterinary medicinal products generally have to satisfy three major criteria before they are authorised, licensed or approved (depending on the terminology in place in the country or region concerned). These criteria are quality, efficacy and safety (Beechinor, 1993a,b; Kloos, 1993; Woodward, 1999) and it is largely the latter which concerns this chapter. Safety is a broad term which covers a number of areas including microbiological safety and environmental safety. From a classical toxicological aspect, safety relates to three main areas: consumer safety, operator safety and, to a lesser extent, target animal (the animal to be treated) safety.

The tissues of food animals, and their other produce such as milk and honey, are destined for consumption by humans. Regulatory authorities need to be convinced that residues of veterinary drugs which may persist in edible tissues after slaughter, or that are excreted in milk or find their way into honey, are not going to elicit toxic responses in consumers who have eaten such produce. Over the last 30 years or so, authorities regulating a wide variety of chemical substances, from pesticides to human medicines, and industrial chemicals to biocides, have recognised a series of toxicological studies, or more accurately toxicity tests, that enable them to characterise the toxic properties of the substances which they aim to regulate, and often, but not always, to identify concentrations or doses which serve as safety limits (Diggle, 1999a,b,c). These might include occupational exposure limits or safe concentrations for drinking water. Veterinary drugs are no exception to this, and toxicologists have devised testing strategies to investigate the potential toxic properties of substances used in veterinary medicine, particularly from the viewpoint of consumer safety (Farber, 1985; Woodward, 1999). Quantitative indices have also been identified to allow safe concentrations of these materials to be identified in food of animal origin.

7.2 Types of toxicity study

The toxicity studies demanded by regulatory authorities for a range of chemical types, including human medicines, veterinary medicines, pesticides, biocides and industrial chemicals have a degree of similarity. They include studies designed to examine acute effects (single dose) and repeated exposure as well as those designed to examine specific effects such as adverse effects on pregnancy, fertility and reproductive performance, neurotoxicity and the ability or otherwise of the substance to induce cancer, and these are combined with careful clinical observations of the animals involved as well as rigorous investigations on organ systems (Dayan, 1986).

Acute toxicity is generally not an important issue in the assessment of the safety of veterinary drug residues. This is because concentrations of residues of veterinary medicines are unlikely to be sufficiently high to pose an acute toxic hazard and these studies serve greater purpose in attempting to predict what might occur following accidental contamination with a veterinary medicine, for example in the occupational setting (Woodward and Atkinson, 1992; Woodward, 1996, 1999). However, there are some exceptions. For example, concentrations of potent pharmacologically active drugs in animal tissues could conceivably elicit adverse reactions in human consumers. Indeed, this has occurred following the ingestion of meat containing residues of the β-agonist drug clenbuterol. Clenbuterol is a drug which is authorised in a number of countries for a variety of uses in food animals, including relaxation of the uterus in cattle prior to parturition. However, it has also been used illegally as a growth promoter. The drug acts as a repartitioning agent, lowering the amount of adipose tissue while increasing the muscle mass (Brambilla, 1992). In 1990, a total of 22 patients from 8 families suffered toxic effects, including headaches, tremors, dizziness and tachycardia after consuming veal liver later shown to contain relatively high concentrations of clenbuterol (Pulce *et al.*, 1991). Similar episodes have occurred in Spain and Italy (Brambilla *et al.,* 1997; Maistro *et al.*, 1995; Martinez-Navarro, 1990; Salleras *et al.,* 1995).

Properly conducted acute toxicity studies, with rigorous observation of the experimental animals, can provide indications of potential for toxicity in longer-term studies, for example, evidence of liver or kidney damage, and signs of neurotoxicity and other effects on physiological systems (Rhodes, 1999). Longer-term studies are designed to investigate the effects of repeat dosing. Such studies are generally of 28 (short-term repeat dose studies) or 90 days (subchronic studies) duration, and occasionally they may be of life-time duration, namely 24 months in the rat and 18 months in the mouse as part of chronic toxicity tests (Ballantyne, 1999). It is in these studies that target organ toxicity is observed, either directly by histological examination of tissues or indirectly through clinical biochemistry and examination and analysis of urine and faeces, for example.

More specialised studies are employed to investigate a drug's potential to induce malformations in the offspring of animals exposed to the material during pregnancy. These are usually referred to as teratology studies and animals are given the drug at sensitive periods of organogenesis in the developing foetus to determine if a potential to produce birth defects exists or to examine whether the drug is generally toxic to the embryo or foetus. Similarly, some chemicals are known to affect sperm cells or otherwise have deleterious effects on reproductive performance, and these aspects too form part of toxicological screening.

A drug's potential to cause cancer is of major concern and drugs may be tested in long-term carcinogenicity studies in rodents. However, the results of such studies are notoriously difficult to interpret because of species-specific tumours, non-specific effects, and the generation of tumours which may have no relevance to human risk assessment. The causes of cancer are manifold, but underlying the majority are genetic events involving damage to DNA, mutations, and disruption of chromosomes. Chemicals which cause such genotoxic effects are immediately suspect from the point of view of their carcinogenic potential and a number of screening tests have been developed to determine the genotoxic effects, if any, of substances. These involve studies using bacteria or mammalian cells, studies in experimental animals and other techniques to investigate effects on DNA and genetic material. If positive results are obtained in such studies, there arises a suspicion that the material tested is a genotoxic carcinogen and this then leaves the investigator with two main choices: to abandon the substance on the grounds that further development of a potentially carcinogenic material is likely to be a costly waste of time and money, as it is unlikely to gain regulatory approval; or to conduct animal carcinogenicity studies which may only serve to prove that the material is indeed a genotoxic carcinogen. Even if the substance gives negative results in a carcinogenicity bioassay, the investigator, and therefore the company developing the product, has to attempt to explain why the material produced evidence of genotoxicity as this may still suggest a potential to affect germ-line cells and create hereditary mutations, or to otherwise have a deleterious effect on offspring.

Nevertheless, it has been argued that on pharmacological grounds testing of veterinary drugs for carcinogenicity is unnecessary, first, because many veterinary drugs are similar to human drugs, and many of these have been shown to be carcinogenic in rodents but on mechanistic grounds are considered not to pose a human health risk, and second, because the concentrations of veterinary drugs in animal tissues means that human exposure is likely to be very low (Galer and Monro, 1998). While these assertions might be true, it seems likely that on precautionary grounds, veterinary drugs will have to demonstrate a lack of genotoxic, and possible carcinogenic potential, before regulatory authorities will authorise their use in food animals. Furthermore, it seems likely that in an increasingly open regulatory climate, with the decisions of regulators open to increasing public scrutiny, and with the concerns of society reflected in decision making (Illing 1991, 1999, 2001), that testing of substances for genotoxic, and where appropriate for carcinogenic potential will persist for the foreseeable future, while the presence of residues of carcinogenic drugs, unless they can be shown to be irrelevant to human risk assessment, will not be tolerated, contrary to earlier views that zero tolerance might not be a pragmatic solution (Somogyi, 1979).

The need to conduct other studies is usually dependent on either the results from longer-term investigations such as the 90-day study, or structural alerts in the molecule. Thus, if signs of adverse effects on the immune system are noted in the 90-day study, then investigations of the substance's immunotoxic potential may be considered necessary. If the drug is structurally related to substances known to be neurotoxic, then specific investigations into its neurotoxicity may be deemed necessary.

The studies described above allow toxicologists to characterise the toxicological properties of substances, to build up an overall picture of their toxicity profiles and to identify quantitative parameters based on the dosages used in the tests. As toxicological data for older drugs may be available from a number of sources, including the open literature, the final toxicological profile constructed may well depend on a weight of evidence approach (Doull *et al.*, 1996). Of the latter, the most important from a regulatory perspective is the no observed effect level, or NOEL. The NOEL is identified for each study where toxic effects have been observed; for each study, it is the lowest dose at which toxic effects seen at higher doses did not occur, or more precisely, where they were not seen as it can never be excluded that subtle effects *did* occur but that they were beyond the observational capabilities of the test system. In fact the NOEL, or no effect level (NEL) as it was once called, has been criticised because toxicity standardised tests do not investigate the full biological profile of a substance and specialised tests are rarely conducted; hence specific adverse effects may be missed (Zbinden, 1979). It can be argued that the use of the term NOEL avoids this pitfall as it is clearly aimed at toxic effects noted in those studies that have been conducted, rather than toxic effects too subtle to observe, or those that might have been seen had other studies been employed. As mentioned earlier, it is now common practice to conduct specialised tests on the basis of either structure activity alerts or because of effects seen in the standard tests, so perhaps the criticism is partly assuaged, if not entirely removed. A suggestion that the NOEL could be refined by defining it as the dose which is statistically different from both the control group and the lowest observable (adverse) effect level (Calabrese and Baldwin, 1994) appears to have met with universal indifference, possibly because toxicity studies in general do not provide sufficient data to draw these distinctions with any confidence.

When it is not possible to identify an NOEL for a particular study, it is often necessary to repeat it using more carefully chosen doses so that an NOEL can be identified. The NOEL plays a crucial role in the safety assessment of substances to which consumers are likely to be exposed including food additives such as colorants and antioxidants, residues of pesticides, and of course residues of veterinary drugs. To see how this works in practice, it is useful at this point to consider an example. A convenient example lies in the establishment of maximum residue limits (MRLs) for residues of veterinary drugs in the European Union.

7.3 Elaboration of maximum residue limits (MRLs) for veterinary drugs in the EU

In the EU, veterinary medicinal products are subjected to a system of rigorous legislative requirements in order to demonstrate safety, quality and efficacy. The operation of this legislation is beyond the scope of this chapter and the interested reader is referred elsewhere (Woodward, 1997, 1999). However, before any veterinary medicinal product intended for use in food animals can be authorised it must first be entered into one of the Annexes of Council Regulation No. (EEC) 2377/90, the so-called MRL Regulation. The prime purpose of this legislation is to ensure that pharmacologically active substances, a definition which includes other constituents of the medicine in addition to the active ingredient or ingredients, are adequately assessed for their toxic potential, and that consumers of food of animal origin are adequately protected. In fact, as we shall see, these assessments take into account factors other than toxicity. As noted with the example of clenbuterol, pharmacologic properties which may be desirable for the treated animal, may not be at all desirable if they occur in the consumer who has eaten animal products. This sentiment applies not only to pharmacodynamic effects of drugs expressed in the animal (e.g. β-adrenergic effects, various hormonal effects, anaesthesia, analgesia), but it is also true of more indirect effects. For example, it is evidently desirable that the antimicrobial effects of antibiotics are seen in the treated animal, i.e. that the drug exerts its bacteriostatic or bactericidal effects on the pathogenic bacteria causing the disease, while it is not desirable that active residues of such drugs adversely affect the normal gastrointestinal flora of consumers eating meat containing antimicrobially active residues. This issue, although not essentially a problem of toxicity (although it is related to the toxicity of the drug to bacteria), will be discussed later as it is relevant to safety assessment and needs to be considered along with pharmacological and toxic properties of the drug in question. Finally, the presence of a particular drug in an edible product is not in itself problematic. What is critical is how much of the drug (and its metabolites) is present, and how long it persists. Veterinary drug residues may be composed of the original substance, the parent drug and various metabolites. These are subject to various metabolic processes such as eventual conversion to non-toxic metabolic products including eventually water and carbon dioxide, and excretion in the urine, expired air or bile. In other words, they will eventually decrease in concentration as time passes, as a result of the animal's metabolism. This is known as residue depletion or depuration. So, the risks posed by residues of a veterinary drug depend not only on its toxic, pharmacological and microbiological activities, and those of its metabolites, but also on its rate of disappearance from the animal. It is obvious from this that another factor therefore is the ability to measure the concentration of the drug and its metabolites, which in turn is dependent on having an adequate analytical method. All of these factors are important in the elaboration of MRLs.

In the EU, MRLs are established by the Committee for Medicinal Products for Veterinary Use (CVMP), a part of the structure of the European Medicines Agency (EMEA). In fact, the CVMP issues an opinion after consideration of the toxicological and residues depletion data. This opinion is for entry into one of the four Annexes of Regulation (EEC) No. 2377/90. The actual decision, in legal terms, is taken by the European Commission, and the Annex entries are published in the *Official Journal of the European Union*. The nature of the Annexes is shown below:

- Annex I: Full MRLs; the data supplied are adequate to address safety and residues concerns.
- Annex II: On public health grounds, MRLs are not necessary. These entries include those for simple salts, innocuous substances and compounds which are rapidly converted in the animal to non-toxic metabolites.
- Annex III. Provisional MRLs. The majority of data in the supporting dossiers is satisfactory but some relatively minor points need addressing. Satisfactory resolution leads to Annex I (or possibly Annex II) entry.
- Annex IV: Substances are not considered safe on public health grounds. Annex IV entries include nitrofurans, nitroimidazoles, chloramphenicol and dapsone.

Companies wishing to market a veterinary medicinal product for use in food producing animals must therefore supply sufficient data to satisfy the CVMP that the drug is safe for consumers and that MRLs can therefore be established. It will come as no surprise therefore from what has been said above to find that the main components of these data are toxicological, pharmacological and microbiological, along with data on residues depletion and analytical methodologies. In fact, the two major components of an MRL application are termed the safety file and the residues file, and the outline contents of these are shown in Tables 7.1 and 7.2.

From the studies outlined in the safety file, the critical areas of toxicology, microbiology and pharmacology can be identified and a toxicological profile, or perhaps more appropriately, a biological profile, can be constructed. Equally importantly, NOELs can be identified and from the point of view of hazard assessment, the lowest NOEL is usually chosen unless there is good reason to discount it (e.g. because the toxicity noted is irrelevant to human risk assessment, usually because it is species-specific to the animal used in the test system).

Table 7.1 Major contents of the safety file

- Safety Expert Report
- Characterisation (e.g. name, structure, impurities, molecular weight)
- Physico-chemical properties (e.g. melting and boiling points, vapour pressure, solubility in water and organic solvents, pH, density)
- Pharmacology
  - Pharmacodynamics
  - Pharmacokinetics
- Toxicological studies
  - Single dose (acute toxicity)
  - Repeat dose (at least 90 days' duration)
  - Reproductive toxicity
    - Study of effects on reproduction
    - Embryotoxicity/teratology
  - Genotoxicity
  - Carcinogenicity
- Microbiological effects on human gut flora
- Pharmacological, microbiological and toxicological observations in humans (where available)

The NOEL forms the basis of the MRL because it forms the basis of the calculation of the acceptable daily intake or ADI. The ADI concept was developed in 1957 by the Joint FAO/WHO Expert Committee on Food Additives (JECFA) of which more will be said later (JECFA, 1957) and its use described by the World Health Organisation's *Environmental Health Criteria 70* (WHO, 1987). This concept was largely based on the ideas of René Truhaut (Poulsen, 1995). In the ADI calculation, the NOEL is divided by a suitable safety factor, usually 100 to give the ADI value. The 100-fold safety factor concept is empirical and arises from the contention that there is a ten-fold intra-species variability in toxicity, and a ten-fold animal-human variability, giving the overall safety factor of 100. It follows from this that in those (few) examples where the ADI is based on human-derived

Table 7.2 Major contents of the residues file

- Residue Expert Report
- Characterisation (e.g. name, structure, impurities, molecular weight)
- Physico-chemical properties (e.g. melting and boiling points, vapour pressure, solubility in water and organic solvents, pH, density)
- Pharmacokinetics in target animals (sheep, pigs, cattle, fish, etc.)
- Residues studies
  - Residues depletion studies in each target species
    - Radiolabelled studies
    - Studies with unlabelled drug
- Elaboration of MRLs
- Routine analytical methods
  - Description of the method
  - Validation of the method (e.g. precision, accuracy, limit of detection, limit of quantification, susceptibility and interference, practicability and applicability)

data, the safety factor is usually 10. However, higher safety factors may also be used, for instance where there are minor flaws in the data package or because of the nature of the toxicity observed. As an example, irreversible effects such as teratogenicity may sometimes attract a higher safety factor. As the NOEL is usually expressed as mg of substance per kg body weight, mg/kg body weight/day, the ADI is based on the same units:

$$\text{ADI} = \frac{\text{NOEL}}{100}\ \text{mg/kg body weight}$$

Note that as the term 'daily' is built into the ADI, the value is not expressed in terms of 'per day'. It is often considered useful to factor in the average human body weight, taken by most regulatory authorities including the EU as 60 kg, to give the ADI in terms of mg per person:

$$\text{ADI} = \frac{\text{NOEL} \times 60}{100}\ \text{mg per person}$$

The ADI has received critical attention over the years, not least because of the arbitrary nature of the safety factor and the lack of scientific justification for its ten by ten-fold nature. It has been suggested that increased scientific knowledge of pharmacokinetics and pharmacodynamics for specific molecules could be used to determine safety factors that are more scientifically sound than the 100 factor usually employed. Thus, rather than a factor of ten for species differences, and a further factor of ten for human differences, there would be subfactors for species differences in kinetics and dynamics, and human differences in kinetics and dynamics for specific substances (Renwick, 1991) and so differences in absorption, first pass metabolism, renal plasma flow and plasma half-life could be taken into account (Renwick, 1993).

However, the major drawback to such an approach is the lack of relevant data, particularly from human exposure that would leave part of the safety factor incomplete, and would require more animal data to contribute to other aspects of the calculation. There are few examples where all the necessary data are available (Kroes *et al.*, 1993). Other approaches, including graphical representation of data (Dourson *et al.*, 1985) and the fitting of dose-response models to toxicological data (Crump, 1984) suffer from other drawbacks, but as with the pharmacokinetic and pharmacodynamic approach, require more data than is currently provided by routine toxicity testing.

The ADI is defined as the quantity of a substance, in the context of this chapter, residues of a veterinary drug, that can be ingested by humans over the course of a life-time without causing adverse effects. Clearly this definition too presents some problems although these could be considered semantic in most cases. Consider a drug which is otherwise non-toxic, but causes some degree of foetotoxicity. The NOEL is established on the basis of foetotoxicity, and the ADI calculated accordingly. It is likely that this ADI is applicable to only a small part of the population, pregnant women, and probably for only a limited period of gestation. As it is the lowest NOEL that has been employed, then it can be argued that the entire population is protected. However, it does call into question the ADI definition and its concept of life-time exposure. Similar criticisms could be made when the ADI concept is applied to substances where the major effects are acute rather than subchronic or chronic. Of particular importance is the question: does the current ADI concept protect groups who might be more sensitive to the toxic effects of a substance such as the elderly, pregnant women and the very young? (Somogyi, 1992.) While this is probably addressed by the current very large safety factors used in the ADI calculation, it cannot be answered with certainty.

Microbiological safety of residues, although not a toxicological issue, must also be considered. The concerns here arise from several areas (Boisseau, 1993; Corpet, 1987, 1993; Gorbach, 1993; Kidd, 1994) as residues of microbiologically active drugs such as antibiotics could conceivably:

- perturb the bacterial ecology of the gastrointestinal tract, particularly that of the colon
- weaken the barrier effect of the gastrointestinal flora allowing the ingress and growth of pathogens
- as a result, thus increase the susceptibility and vulnerability of the consumer to pathogenic bacteria, and significantly, to bacteria pathogenic to the gastrointestinal tract
- provide conditions that could lead to the colonisation of the gastrointestinal tract by other organisms, not necessarily pathogens, including bacteria and fungi
- provide conditions that could be conducive to the development of antimicrobial resistance.

Many of these concerns arise from the use of antimicrobial drugs in humans as therapeutic doses may lead to some of these effects. Indeed, sometimes the perturbations in colonic flora can be dramatic following the therapeutic use of antibiotics in humans. However, there is no firm evidence that residues present in food of animal origin can have such effects in humans and as the concentrations of residues in food to which humans are exposed are extremely low, it seems highly unlikely that major adverse effects would occur. Nevertheless, it is considered prudent to investigate the potential of residues of antimicrobial drugs to adversely affect the human gastrointestinal flora.

Unfortunately, there are no validated or even widely accepted experimental models for this, but several approaches are available:

Studies in humans
These involve human volunteers given doses of the test compound. The faeces are then examined for population changes in species of bacteria.

Studies in gnotobiotic animals
Gnotobiotic animals are animals whose own gut flora is absent. They are then given human gut flora and treated with antibiotic drugs to determine whether

there are any adverse effects on the adopted bacteria. These studies are notoriously difficult to interpret, not least because the effects of the host animal on the gut flora may be greater than that of the administered drug.

In vitro *studies*
These *in vitro* studies may examine a number of end-points, including the development of resistance (Cerniglia and Kotarski, 1999; Rumney and Rowland, 1992; Woodward, 1998). They generally involve determination of the so-called minimum inhibitory concentrations (MIC_{50} values) or some similar measurement, either through serial dilution or using continuous culture methodologies that aim to model microflora interactions, the ecology of the human colon and the effects of pH and anaerobiosis. It seems likely that a more systematic approach, using both *in vitro* and *in vivo* models, is likely to be employed in the future (Cerniglia and Kotarski, 1999).

Occasionally, the main effects may be pharmacological rather than toxicological, and again may be noted in animal studies or in investigations in humans. Such effects may be more significant with some substances such as anaesthetics, analgesics and β-agonists, as noted earlier with clenbuterol, than classical toxicological effects, and in those circumstances the NOEL, and the subsequent ADI, may be based on the pharmacological properties (van Leeuwen, 1990).

7.4 Elaboration of MRLs for particular foods in the EU

Elaboration of MRLs is far more problematic in many ways than the calculation of MRLs. There is no simple equation which can be applied and the approach is much more iterative. This is because a number of factors have to be taken into account. Fundamentally, the magnitude of the MRLs has to be such that the ADI is not exceeded. In addition to this, the MRL values established for different tissues has to be practicable; there is little point in setting the MRL for muscle at an order of magnitude higher than that for liver for a particular species if pharmacokinetics and residues depletion data show that in reality the values are likely to be the other way around. Consequently, patterns of tissues depletion must also be considered.

Some information on the distribution and metabolism of a specific drug in a particular animal species is provided by pharmacokinetic studies in that animal. However, the main information is provided by residues depletion profiles. Groups of the intended target species, cattle, sheep, pigs or fish, for example, are given the drug at the therapeutic dose, in the intended market formulation, and groups of animals are then serially slaughtered (or milk collected at sequential time points) and tissues (or milk) collected for chemical analysis. In practice, the major tissues collected for analysis are muscle, liver, kidney and fat except for pigs, fish and poultry where skin, which is also eaten, is additionally analysed.

The amount of residue consumed by humans depends not only on how much is present in tissues and organs, but also on how much food containing the residue is eaten. Consequently, a 'market basket' approach to food intake has been adopted as the pragmatic solution. This makes use of food intakes that are certainly in excess of what might be considered normal but in doing so, it does take into account individuals who might be considered to be extreme consumers. The values used in the EU are given in Table 7.3.

Thus, MRLs are elaborated (rather than calculated) by considering the practical aspects of pharmacokinetic factors and residues time-depletion profiles, while bearing in mind the ADI, and ensuring that in considering the magnitude of the MRLs, the ADI values will not be exceeded. Under the requirements of Regulation No. (EEC) 2377/90, MRLs must be practicable, and that is taken to mean that there is an adequate analytical method with which to determine the drug or its metabolites. Indeed, there is a direct requirement for the provision of an analytical method (Table 7.2).

Similar requirements for toxicity and residues depletion data exist under legislation in the United States (Frank and Schafer, 2001; Guest, 1990; Guest and Fitzpatrick, 1990; Miller and Flynn, 2000; Sundlof, 2001; Teske, 1992; Woodward, 1999). Not surprisingly, many of the issues surrounding the calculations of ADI values, the types of toxicity and residues studies to be conducted, the use of microbiological safety studies, to name but a few, apply here also (Friedlander *et al.*, 1999; Paige *et al.*, 1999a; Perez, 1977). In the US, there is no separate MRL legislation as such, and in fact the approach to determining safety limits is subtly different from that of the EU. Having calculated an ADI, the next step is to calculate a safe concentration for a particular tissue. For example, for liver and using an ADI value of 0.1 μg per kg per day, the safe concentration calculation (SC) is:

$$SC = \frac{\text{ADI} \times \text{human weight}}{\text{daily tissue intake}}$$

$$= \frac{0.1\mu\text{g/kg per day} \times 60\text{ kg}}{0.1\text{ kg/day}} = 60\mu\text{g/kg} = 60\text{ ppb}$$

Using this figure, and data from total residues depletion studies, a tolerance for liver can be established for the drug. The same process can then be

Table 7.3 Daily food intake factors (grams) used in the EU in the elaboration of MRLs

Large animals		Poultry		Fish/bees	
Muscle	300	Muscle	300	Muscle + skin	300
Liver	100	Liver	100	Honey	20
Kidney	50	Kidney	10		
Fat	50	Fat + skin	90		
Milk	1500	Eggs	100		

conducted for other tissues and for milk (Frank and Schafer, 2001; Friedlander *et al.*, 1999). Food consumption values used in the United States are essentially similar to those used in the EU and shown in Table 7.3. The tolerance is essentially equivalent to the MRL although the use of simple arithmetic to derive it makes it somewhat easier to understand.

The MRL and tolerance values are used to derive withdrawal periods for marketed veterinary medicines. The withdrawal period is the time from administration of the medicine, or last administration in a multi-dose regime, to the point where residues have depleted to below the MRL or tolerance. This is done by conducting studies where animals are treated with the medicine in question, as the formulation to be marketed, and then slaughtering the animals at intervals and analysing the key tissues of muscle, fat, liver and kidney. Similar studies are conducted with dairy cattle for milk. A withdrawal period is then derived by examining the time dependent tissue depletion (or depletion in milk), against the MRL or tolerance values. In practice, use is made of various statistical models in calculating the withdrawal period. The withdrawal period, or milk withhold time then becomes part of the terms of the marketing authorisation, and appears as such in the product literature and on the product label (Friedlander *et al.*, 1999; Woodward, 1999). Farmers are then required to observe these withdrawal times after their animals have been treated with veterinary medicines to ensure that any residues present are below the relevant MRL or tolerance values.

The EU and the United States have in place extensive systems for residues surveillance so that residues can be monitored and violations of statutory limits such as MRLs can be detected (Paige *et al.*, 1997, 1999b; Sundlof *et al.*, 2000; Van Dresser and Wilcke, 1989; Woodward, 1997, 1999). This not only provides significant confidence for consumers but also allows offenders who have allowed violations to occur, to be prosecuted. The results of residues monitoring are published in many countries including the US and the UK. These results demonstrate that residues of veterinary medicines are indeed very low in food of animal origin, and that MRL and tolerance violations are extremely rare (Paige *et al.*, 1999b; Pullen, 1990; Sundlof *et al.*, 2000; Veterinary Residues Committee, 2002).

7.5 International regulation: the role of the Joint Expert Committee on Food Additives (JECFA)

JECFA began evaluating the toxicity and residues data on veterinary drugs in the mid-1980s, with a view to establishing MRL values. The MRLs developed are taken into the Codex Alimentarius system, which like JECFA is a joint FAO and WHO body, as part of its food standards programme, through the Codex Committee on Residues of Veterinary Drugs in Food (Herrman, 1993; Luetzow, 2003). In practice, this means that veterinary drug assessments and MRL values are available to developing countries that might not have the means to do this for themselves, and that scientific monographs on toxicity and residues characteristics are readily available in the public domain. It also means that the deliberations and decisions of the JECFA are transparent as these are published in a separate report series.

Occasionally, the MRLs set by JECFA are different from those set by the EU or from US tolerances. Or JECFA might set an MRL whereas other bodies felt unable to do so. For example, the EU has not published an MRL for the anabolic steroid trenbolone acetate, whereas JECFA has established an MRL (Van Leeuwen, 1991). This raises the spectre of trade disputes between the EU and countries which adopt the JECFA MRL, or at least its scientific approach. There are differences in scientific opinion for a number of reasons including variations in scientific approaches, attitudes to risk assessment and risk-benefit conclusions (Illing, 1991, 1999, 2001; Nilsson *et al.*, 1993). However, some of the variations in MRLs which arise from various national, multinational (e.g. the EU) and international bodies (e.g. JECFA and Codex) arise not because of differences in the interpretation of toxicity data, but because different food intake values are used in their elaboration. Approaches to resolve this problem, which could lead to disputes between various trading blocks, would either be to harmonise food intake values across regulatory authorities and international bodies, or to determine the equivalence of MRLs to reveal whether or not the ADI values in each country are being exceeded (Fitzpatrick *et al.*, 1995, 1996).

On this final point, because of the definition of the ADI, and because of the magnitude of the safety factors involved, it has to be appreciated that occasional intakes of a specific residue in excess of the ADI does not necessarily mean that human health is compromised. Similarly, although MRL violations are undesirable from a legal viewpoint, because of the uncertainty factor built into these, and the safety factors built into the ADI which underpins them, residues concentrations above the MRL values do not in themselves constitute a threat to public health (McEvoy, 2001).

7.6 Conclusions

Veterinary medicines are subject to considerable assessment prior to marketing and nowhere is this truer than in the assessment of consumer safety. At the national, multistate and global levels, toxicity and residues data on veterinary medicines are examined in minute detail to determine whether or not they pose a risk to the consumer. The safety assessment is largely based on toxicity data but other aspects are also considered, for example pharmacological activity and, for antimicrobial drugs, potential effects on the gastrointestinal flora. Studies are designed so that appropriate NOELs can be determined and toxicological, pharmacological and microbiological ADIs calculated and MRLs elaborated using these ADI values as a basis. An exceptional amount of financial, intellectual, scientific and regulatory resource is employed so that consumers can be assured that the food which they eat is free from potentially harmful

Table 7.4 Substances in Annex IV of Regulation (EEC) No. 2377/90, substances withdrawn from the EU MRL procedure or substances for which the CVMP could not make a recommendation

Annex IV	
Aristolochia spp. and preparations	Dapsone
Chloramphenicol	Dimetridazole
Chloroform	Metronidazole
Chlorpromazine	Nitrofurans (including furazolidone)
Colchicine	Ronidazole
No recommendation	
2-ethyl-1,3-hexanediol	Populeum ointment
Phenylbutazone	*Chelidonii herba*
Suxibutazone	Benzylidenacetone
Ramifenazone	Metesculetol sodium
	Phenazone
Withdrawn	
Decoquinate	Testosterone
Niclosamide	Fenprostalene
Bromopropylate	methylprednisolone
Heptenophos	Benzonaphthol
Camylofine	Clanobutin
Narcobarbital	Haloquinol
Thiopental sodium	Benzonicotinate
Propionylpromazine	Copper naphthenate
Dextrometorphan hydrobromide	Cuproxoline
Ammonium phthalamate	Glycofurol
Pentetrazol	Polyethylene terephthalates

residues. The MRL, while not in itself a safety limit, has become the measure in many countries of whether the ADI, the true yardstick of human safety, is likely to be exceeded. Numerous substances used in veterinary medicinal products have now been assessed for their safety. For example, by mid-2004, there were 110 Annex I and 5 Annex III entries – i.e. 115 susbtances – with full or provisional MRLs. Approximately 300 substances had been entered into Annex II after scientific evaluation and in addition, there were over 160 Annex II entries on the basis that the substances were 'generally recognised as safe' or of 'vegetable' origin. Some 40 susbtances were entered as ingredients in homeopathic remedies, largely because of the huge dilutions at which they are employed.

There are ten substances in Annex IV (Table 7.4) and, as explained earlier, these are prohibited from use in food animals. However, further to these, there are a further 22 substances whose applications were later withdrawn, presumably in the face of questions raised by the CVMP and a further nine substances for which the CVMP was unable to make a recommendation because of lack of data or in the absence of satisfactory responses to its questions by the applicant (Table 7.4). Around 65 substances fall into the non-defended category

– they were known to be used in food animals in the EU, but no MRL application was made. These include nalidixic acid, ipronidazole, codeine phosphate, halothane, diazepam and ranitidine. None of the drugs which have been withdrawn, which have received no recommendation or for which no applications were made, may be used in food animals in the EU.

Calculating ADI values and elaborating MRLs alone is not sufficient to guarantee consumer safety. These are the limits but are they adhered to in practice by the observation of withdrawal periods by farmers and others producing food of animal origin for human consumption? This question can only be answered in detail by the results of residues monitoring programmes such as the one used in the European Union. Unfortunately, only the UK routinely published the results of its residues monitoring in the European Union. This gives considerable reassurance; the numbers of MRL violations are very low and the detection of illegal drugs is very rare (Veterinary Residues Committee, 2002). Similar findings are made by other surveillance schemes such as the one operating in the United States (Paige *et al.*, 1999b; Van Dresser and Wilke, 1989). Overall, the regulatory schemes in operation provide the consumer with considerable reassurance about the safety of food of animal origin. It should also be remembered that food from healthy animals, which may have been treated with medicines at some point in their lives, is almost certainly likely to be more wholesome than food derived from sick animals.

7.7 References

BALLANTYNE B. (1999). Repeat exposure toxicity. In: Ballantyne B, Marrs TC and Syversen T. (eds), *General and Applied Toxicology*, Macmillan, London, 55–66.

BEECHINOR JG. (1993a). Quality, safety and efficacy criteria for product licensing. Part I. *Ir Vet J*, **46**, 116–118.

BEECHINOR JG. (1993b). Quality, safety and efficacy criteria for product licensing. Part III. *Ir Vet J*, **46**, 122–124.

BOISSEAU J. (1993). Basis for the evaluation of microbiological risks due to veterinary drug residues in food. *Vet Microbiol,* **35**, 187–192.

BRAMBILLA G. (1992). Health aspects of the use of beta-2 adrenergic drugs in animal production. *Ann 1st Super Sanita,* **28**, 437–439.

BRAMBILLA G, LOIZZO A, FONTANA L, STROZZI M, GUARINO A and SOPRANO V. (1997). Food poisoning following consumption of clenbuterol treated veal in Italy. *JAMA,* **276**, 635.

CALABRESE EJ and BALDWIN L. (1994). Improved method for the selection of the NOAEL. *Regul Toxicol Pharmacol,* **19**, 48–50.

CERNIGLIA CE and KOTARSKI S. (1999). Evaluation of veterinary drug residues in food for their potential to affect human intestinal microflora. *Regul Toxicol Pharmacol.,* **29**, 238–261.

CORPET, E. (1987). Antibiotic residues and drug resistance in human intestinal flora. *Antimicrob Agents Chemother,* **31**, 587–593.

CORPET DE. (1993). An evaluation of the methods to assess the effects of antimicrobial residues on the human gut flora. *Vet Microbiol,* **35**, 199–212.

CRUMP KS (1984). A new method for determining allowable daily intakes. *Fundam Appl Toxicol*, **4**, 854–871.

DAYAN AD (1986). Interpretation of data. In: Richardson ML (ed.), *Toxic Hazard Assessment of Chemicals*, Royal Society of Chemistry, London, 87–97.

DIGGLE G. (1999a). Overview of regulatory affairs. Regulation of veterinary drugs. In:. Ballantyne B, Marrs TC and Syversen T. (eds), *General and Applied Toxicology*, Macmillan, London, 1543–1580.

DIGGLE G. (1999b). Regulatory affairs and the role of toxicology – Part 1. *Regulatory Review*, **2** (Issue 6), 3–9.

DIGGLE G. (1999c). Regulatory affairs and the role of toxicology – Part 2. *Regulatory Review*, **2** (Issue 7), 3–7.

DOULL J, ROZMAN KK and LOWE MC. (1996) Hazard evaluation in risk assessment: Whatever happened to sound scientific judgment and weight of evidence? *Drug Metab Rev,* **28**, 285–299.

DOURSON ML, HERTZBERG RC, HARTUNG R and BLACKBURN K. (1985). Novel methods for the estimation of acceptable daily intake. *Toxicol Ind Health,* **1**, 23–33.

FARBER T. (1985). Regulatory requirements for the approval of drugs used in food animals. In: Homburger F and Marquis JK. (eds), *Chemical Safety Evaluation, Regulation and Compliance,* Karger, London, 11–23.

FITZPATRICK SC, BRYNES SD and GUEST GB. (1995). Dietary intake values as a means to harmonization of maximum residue levels for veterinary drugs. I. Concept. *J Vet Pharmacol Ther,* **18**, 325–327.

FITZPATRICK SC, VILIM A, LAMBERT G, YONG MS and BRYNES SD. (1996). Dietary intake estimates as a means to harmonization of maximum residue levels for veterinary drugs. II. Proposed application to the Free Trade Agreement between the United States and Canada. *Regul Toxicol Pharmacol,* **24**, 177–183.

FRANK P and SCHAFER JH. (2001). Animal health products. In: Gad SC (ed.). *Regulatory Toxicology,* Taylor and Francis, London, 70–84.

FRIEDLANDER LG, BRYNES SD and FERNANDEZ AH. (1999). The human food safety evaluation of veterinary drugs. *Vet Clin North Am,* **15**, 1–11.

GALER DM and MONRO AM. (1998). Veterinary drugs no longer need testing for carcinogenicity in rodent bioassays. *Regul Toxicol Pharmacol,* **28**, 115–123.

GORBACH SL. (1993). Perturbation of intestinal microflora. *Vet Hum Toxicol,* **35** (Supplement 1), 15–23.

GUEST GB. (1990). Veterinary drug registration in the United States. In: Simon F, Lees P and Semjen G (eds), *Veterinary Pharmacology. Toxicology and Therapy in Food Producing Animals,* University of Veterinary Science, Budapest, 269–272.

GUEST GB and FITZPATRICK SC. (1990). Overview on bound residue issue – regulatory aspects. *Drug Metab Rev,* **22**, 595–599.

HERRMAN J. (1993). The role of the World Health Organisation in the evaluation of pesticides. *Regul Toxicol Pharmacol,* **17**, 282–286.

ILLING HPA. (1991). Possible risk considerations for toxic risk assessment. *Hum Exp Toxicol,* **10**, 215–219.

ILLING HPA. (1999). Are societal judgments being incorporated into the uncertainty factors used in toxicological risk assessment? *Regul Toxicol Pharmacol*, **29**, 300–308.

ILLING HPA. (2001). The importance of risk perception and risk communication for toxicological risk assessment. In *Toxicity and Risk. Context, Principles and Practice.* Taylor and Francis, London, 43–56.

JECFA. (1957). *Procedures for the testing of intentional food additives to establish their safety for use.* Second Report of the Joint FAO/WHO Expert Committee on Food Additives, WHO Technical report Series 144, WHO, Geneva.

KIDD ARM. (1994). *The Potential Risk of Effects of Antimicrobial Residues on Human Gastro-Intestinal Microflora.* Report prepared at the invitation of Fédération Européen de la Santé Animal (FEDESA), FEDESA, Brussels, Belgium.

KLOOS CM. (1993). Quality, safety and efficacy criteria for product licensing. Part II. *Ir Vet J*, **46**, 119–121.

KROES R, MUNRO I and POULSEN E. (1993). Workshop on the scientific evaluation of the safety factor for the acceptable daily intake (ADI): editorial summary. *Food Add Contam,* **10**, 269–273.

LUETZOW M. (2003). Harmonisation of exposure assessment for food chemicals; the international perspective. *Toxicol Letters,* **140–141**, 419–425.

MAISTRO S, CHIESA E, ANGELETTI R and BRAMBILLA G. (1995). Beta blockers to prevent clenbuterol poisoning. *Lancet,* **346**, 180.

MARTINEZ-NAVARRO JF. (1990). Food poisoning related to consumption of illicit β-agonist in liver. *Lancet,* **336**, 1311.

MCEVOY J. (2001). Safe limits for veterinary drug residues: what do they mean? *Northern Ireland Veterinary Today,* Spring Edition, 37–40.

MILLER MA and FLYNN WT. (2000). Regulation of antibiotic use in animals. In: Prescott J, Baggott JD and Walker RD. (eds) *Antimicrobial Therapy in Veterinary Medicine.* Iowa State University Press, Ames, 760–771.

NILSSON R, TASHEVA M and JAEGER B. (1993). Why different regulatory decisions when the scientific information base is similar? – Human risk assessment. *Regul Toxicol Pharmacol,* **17**, 292–332.

PAIGE JC, TOLLEFSON L and MILLER M. (1997). Public health impact on drug residues in animal tissues. *Vet Hum Toxicol,* **39**, 162–169.

PAIGE JC, TOLLEFSON L and MILLER MA. (1999a). Health implications of residues of veterinary drugs and chemicals in animal tissues. *Vet Clin North Am,* **15**, 31–43.

PAIGE JC, CHAUDRY MH and PELL FM. (1999b). Federal surveillance of veterinary drugs and chemical residues (with recent data). *Vet Clin North Am,* **15**, 45–61.

PEREZ MK. (1977). Human safety data collection and evaluation for the approval of new animal drugs. *J Toxicol Environ Health*, **3**, 837–857.

POULSEN E. (1995). René Truhaut and the acceptable daily intake: A personal note. *Teratog Carcinog Mutagen,* **15**, 273–275.

PULCE C, LAMAISON D, KECK G, BOSTVIRONNOIS C, NICOLAS J and DESCOTES J. (1991). Collective human poisonings by clenbuterol residues in veal liver. *Vet Hum Toxicol,* **33**, 480–481.

PULLEN MM. (1990). Residues. In: Pearson AM and Dutson TR. (eds), *Meat and Health. Advances in Meat Research.* Elsevier, London, 135–156.

RENWICK AG. (1991). Safety factors and establishment of acceptable daily intakes. *Food Add Contam,* **8**, 135–150.

RENWICK AG. (1993). Data-derived safety factors for the evaluation of food additives and environmental contaminants. *Food Add Contam,* **10**, 275–305.

RHODES C. (1999). Principles of testing for acute toxic effects. In: Ballantyne B, Marrs TC and Syversen T. (eds), *General and Applied Toxicology*, Macmillan, London, 33–54.

RUMNEY CJ and ROWLAND IR. (1992). *In vivo* and *in vitro* models of the human colonic flora. *Crit Rev Food Sci Nutr,* **31**, 299–331.

SALLERAS L, DOMINGUEZ A, MATA E, TABERNER JL, MORO I and SALVA P. (1995). Epidemiologic study of an outbreak of clenbuterol poisoning in Catalonia, Spain. *Public Health Rep*, **110**, 338–342.

SOMOGYI A. (1979). Residues of carcinogenic animal drugs in food: difficulties in evaluation of human safety. In *Carcinogenic Risks. Strategies for Intervention*, International Agency for Research on Cancer (IARC) Scientific Publication No. 25, IARC, Lyon, France.

SOMOGYI A. (1992). The objective of the legislator. Safety evaluation of veterinary drug residues. *Adv Vet Med,* **42**, 10–17.

SUNDLOF SF. (2001). Legal controls of veterinary drugs. In Adams HR (ed.), *Veterinary Pharmacology and Therapeutics.* 8th edn, Iowa State Press, Ames, 1149–1156.

SUNDLOF SF, FERNANDEZ AH and PAIGE JC. (2000). Antimicrobial drug residues in food-producing animals. In: Prescott J, Baggott JD and Walker RD. (eds), *Antimicrobial Therapy in Veterinary Medicine*. Iowa State University Press, Ames, 744–759.

TESKE RH. (1992). Chemical residues in food. *J Am Vet Med Assoc,* **201**, 253–256.

VAN DRESSER WR and WILCKE JR. (1989). Drug residues in food animals. *J Am Vet Med Assoc,* **194**, 1700–1710.

VAN LEEUWEN FXR. (1990). The use of pharmacological data in the evaluation of veterinary drugs. *Tijdschr Diergeneeskd,* **115**, 774–779.

VAN LEEUWEN FX. (1991). The approach taken and conclusions reached by the Joint FAO-WHO Expert Committee on Food Additives. *Ann Rech Vet,* **22**, 253–256.

VETERINARY RESIDUES COMMITTEE. (2002). Annual Report on Surveillance for Veterinary Residues in 2001. Available from: Veterinary Medicines Directorate, Addlestone, Surrey, UK.

WOODWARD KN. (1996). The regulation of fish medicines – UK and European Union aspects. *Aquaculture Res,* **27**, 725–734.

WOODWARD KN. (1997). Progress with the establishment of maximum residue limits for veterinary drug in the European Union. *Toxicol Ecotoxicol News/Reviews,* **4**, 46–54.

WOODWARD KN. (1998). The use of microbiological end-points in the safety evaluation and elaboration of maximum residue limits for veterinary drugs intended for use in food producing animals. *J Vet Pharmacol Ther,* **21**, 47–53.

WOODWARD, KN. (1999). Regulation of veterinary drugs. In: Ballantyne B, Marrs TC and Syversen T. (eds), *General and Applied Toxicology*, Macmillan, London, 1633–1652.

WOODWARD KN and ATKINSON K. (1992). The Control of Substances Hazardous to Health (COSHH) Regulations and their application to veterinary medicines. *British Institute of Regulatory Affairs Journal,* **10**, 22–24.

WORLD HEALTH ORGANISATION. (1987). *Principles for the Safety Evaluation of Food Additives and Contaminants in Food. Environmental Health Criteria 70.* World Health Organisation, Geneva.

ZBINDEN G. (1979). The no-effect level, an old bone of contention in toxicology. *Arch Toxicol,* **43**, 3–7.

8

The toxicity of particular veterinary drug residues

K. N. Woodward, International Federation for Animal Health, Belgium

8.1 Introduction

It is a useful and interesting exercise to look at some of the substances reviewed by both the Committee for Medicinal Products for Veterinary Use (CVMP) in the calculation of ADI values, and where possible, compare these with the acceptable daily intake (ADI) values calculated by the Joint FAO/WHO Expert Committee on Food Additives (JECFA). Unfortunately, not all of the toxicity data are readily available but the JECFA monographs mentioned in this chapter summarise the information in some detail, while other data are available in the published literature. Some examples which illustrate the principles involved in assessing toxicity data and the difficulties in identifying no-observed effect levels (NOELs) and calculating ADI values are given below. These examples also show, to some extent, how different expert bodies can arrive at different conclusions.

By far the largest group of drugs used in veterinary medicine is the antimicrobial substances (Black, 1984; MacNeil and Ellis, 1995; Wingfield and Appelbe, 1984; Woodward and Shearer, 1995; Ziv, 1986). So, most of the examples discussed below are chosen from that category. However, a number of other drugs has also been selected as these illustrate some particularly useful points.

8.2 Griseofulvin

Griseofulvin is a fungal metabolite produced by *Penicillium griseofulvum* and *Penicillium patulum* strains. It is used in human medicine for the treatment of dermatomycoses in skin, hair and nails and until recently was used widely in veterinary medicine for the treatment of fungal infections, mainly against ringworm infections (Knasmuller *et al.*, 1997; Russel and Russel, 1992).

Older studies showed it to have low acute and repeat dose toxicity in rodents and cats, and there were apparently no effects on reproduction in limited studies in rats (Sharpe and Tomich, 1960). However, studies in mice demonstrated that griseofulvin was hepatocarcinogenic in mice after oral dosing and resulted in thyroid tumours in rats (Rustia and Shubik, 1978). Dietary administration to mice resulted in hepatotoxicity, disruption of hepatic architecture and lesions which had the appearance of liver tumours (DeMatteis *et al.*, 1966). Parenteral administration of griseofulvin to infant mice resulted in a high incidence of liver tumours (Epstein *et al.*, 1967). The mechanism of carcinogenicity is unclear (Williams, 1997a). The International Agency for Research on Cancer (IARC) concluded that griseofulvin was hepatocarcinogenic in mice and that there were inadequate data to assess the evidence for carcinogenicity in humans but that the substance was possibly carcinogenic to humans (IARC, 1974, 2002).

Griseofulvin has been tested in a number of assays for genotoxicity. In general, it has given negative results in tests for point mutations in bacterial systems, including the Ames test with strains of *Salmonella typhimurium*, and in a number of mammalian cell lines (De Carli and Larizza, 1988; Kuczuk *et al.*, 1978, Leonard *et al.*, 1979; Zeiger *et al.*, 1992; Zimmerman *et al.*, 1984). There is some limited evidence that griseofulvin is mutagenic in the mouse lymphoma (TK^+/TK^-) L5178Y assay (Sofuni *et al.*, 1996). Results in the micronucleus test have generally been negative (Heddle *et al.*, 1983; Kersten *et al.*, 1999; Labay *et al.*, 2001) although positive results were obtained in V79 cells and in a gut micronucleus test system (Kalweit *et al.*, 1999; Vanhauwaert *et al.*, 2001). Griseofulvin gave negative results in a test for DNA repair using rat and mouse hepatocytes (Mori *et al.*, 1984) and in bacterial systems (Leifer *et al.*, 1981).

However, in a number of studies for aneuploidy and other tests for chromosomal damage arising during mitosis and meiosis, clear positive results were seen (Bourner *et al.*, 1998; Curry *et al.*, 1984; De Carli *et al.*, 1973; Fahmy and Hassan, 1996; Grant, 1982; Inoue *et al.*, 1995; Kolachana and Smith, 1994; Larizza *et al.*, 1974; LeBoeuf *et al.*, 1996; Mailhes *et al.*, 1993; Marchetti *et al.*, 1992, 1996; Migliore *et al.*, 1999; Parry *et al.*, 1996; Qinghua *et al.*, 1999; Tiveron *et al.*, 1992; Waters *et al.*, 1986). The evidence demonstrates that griseofulvin is a potent aneugen in somatic cells and in germ cells. This may lead to loss of chromosomes and altered gene expression (Knassmuller *et al.*, 1997). The results demonstrate that griseofulvin is an antimitotic agent. The mechanism is unclear since it does not disrupt microtubules like some other spindle poisons but it does appear to bind to tubulin or at least to microtubule-associated proteins (De Carli and Larizza, 1988; Grisham *et al.*, 1973; Ueno, 1985; Wehland *et al.*, 1977). Aneuploidy is regarded as an important change in the process of carcinogenesis (Oshimura and Barrett, 1986) and this, taken with the results in animal studies, confirms griseofulvin's status as a carcinogen. For such indirect carcinogens, it should be possible to determine a threshold dose or concentration (Kirsch-Volders *et al.*, 2003; Parry *et al.*, 1994), but the question arises as to which study to employ to determine this as the drug gives different responses depending on the test system chosen (Kirkland, 1998).

The problems for griseofulvin do not end there. The drug was found to produce teratogenic effects in rats when given oral doses of 250 mg/kg per day from days 6 to 15 after mating. No malformations were noted with 125 mg/kg per day (Klein and Beall, 1972). Similar results were noted in other studies in rats (Aujezdska *et al.*, 1978; Steelman and Kocsis, 1978). An *in vitro* study with rat embryos also suggested teratogenic potential (Bechter and Schmid, 1987).

Therapeutic treatment of pregnant cats for ringworm resulted in malformations in the offspring including cleft palate, exencephaly, caudal displacement and hydrocephaly, along with multiple skeletal abnormalities including cranium bifidium, spina bifida and abnormal vertebrae. Cyclops and anophthalmia also occurred (Scott *et al.*, 1975). Similar cases have been reported in cats treated therapeutically with griseofulvin (Gillick and Bulmer, 1972; Gruffydd-Jones and Wright, 1977; Turner, 1977). Cats appear to be more susceptible to the toxic effects of griseofulvin (Kunkle and Meyer, 1987), but it is not known if this species is also more susceptible to the teratogenic effects of the drug.

In humans, griseofulvin has produced CNS toxicity and disturbances of porphyrin metabolism. There are also numerous reports of dermatological effects ranging from eczema to fatal toxic epidermal necrolysis (Boudghene-Stambouli and Merad-Boudia, 1989; Kojima *et al.*, 1988; Mahboob and Haroon, 1998; Mion *et al.*, 1989, 1990; Perfect *et al.*, 1992; Savage, 1977; Shimoyama and Nonaka, 1987; Taylor and Duffill, 1988; Thami *et al.*, 2001; Thyagarajan *et al.*, 1981;Vassileva *et al.*, 1998).

With this catalogue of adverse effects, it is perhaps not surprising that griseofulvin has not been supported through either the EU or JECFA MRL systems. The teratogenic effects are almost certainly due to the antimitotic effects described earlier, and hence it should be possible to determine thresholds for these too and eventually identify NOELs. However, faced with the research costs involved, and with no guarantee of success, it was always unlikely that companies would choose to defend the drug, particularly when newer antifungal drugs, with MRLs, are now available. Griseofulvin, without MRLs, is no longer permitted for use in food-producing animals in the EU.

8.3 β-Lactam antibiotics: penicillins and cephalosporins

8.3.1 Penicillins

The term penicillin was given to an antibacterial substance derived from a mould of the genus *Penicillium* by Sir Alexander Fleming in 1929 (Fleming, 1946). The drug soon found its way into human clinical use, and into veterinary medicine (Lovell, 1946). The most common members of the family used in veterinary practice are benzyl penicillin, amoxycillin, ampicillin and penicillin

G, the latter with benethamine, benzathine or procaine as the commonly used counter ion (Bishop, 1998; Wright and Wilkowske, 1991).

Penicillin drugs have been used widely since those pioneering days in both human and veterinary medicine (Black, 1984; Neu, 1977; Wright and Wilkowske, 1991; Wright, 1999). They are generally non-toxic in animals and in humans during clinical use (Bush *et al.*, 1995; Campbell and Cox, 1992; Gentry, 1992; Stewart, 1967, Wilkowske, 1977) and are relatively non-hepatotoxic (George and Crawford, 1996; Hautekeete, 1995). They are also of low potential for nephrotoxicity except after very high doses (Geller *et al.*, 1986; Morin *et al.*, 1984). However, for benzyl penicillin, there are virtually no published results of conventional toxicology studies (JECFA, 1991a). Along with other penicillins, it is known to be neurotoxic after intravenous injection in humans and animals but only after very large doses (Currie *et al.*, 1971; Johnson, 1971; Lerner *et al.*, 1967; Schliamser, 1988; Schliamser *et al.*, 1988a,b,c, 1991; Weiss *et al.*, 1974). It appears not to be a problem after oral administration, the route where consumers will be exposed to residues of the drug. In fact, benzyl penicillin only appears to be acutely toxic in animals when given at high doses to rats given high sugar diets (Boyd *et al.*, 1966). Amoxicillin has a low order of toxicity in animals (Jones and Hill, 1974), and this is also the case for temocillin (Cockburn *et al.*, 1985). There was no evidence of carcinogenicity for ampicillin either in a conventional gavage carcinogenicity study of 2 years duration in rats and mice, or in a 26-week experimental system in Tg-rasH2 mice (Adachi *et al.*, 2002; National Toxicology Program (NTP), 1987; Dunnick *et al.*, 1989). Penicillin VK gave negative results in rodent bioassays (Dunnick *et al.*, 1989). Ampicillin gave negative results in a range of genotoxicity studies (NTP, 1987).

Overall, therefore, the toxicological profile with regard to consumer safety is very reassuring. However, and as the 1991 JECFA Monograph notes, '[benzyl penicillin] may induce all possible clinical forms of allergic reactions depending on dose, route, frequency of exposure, genetic predisposition and other factors' (JECFA, 1991a). Penicillins are low molecular weight substances and are not by themselves immunogenic. In fact they are haptens, substances that bind irreversibly to tissue macromolecules such as proteins to produce immunogenic materials. In the case of penicillins, the hapten is a metabolite of penicillin, the β-lactam ring or, more precisely, the penicilloyl moiety arising from cleavage of the β-lactam ring (Ahlstedt *et al.*, 1980; Davis, 1984; Erffmeyer, 1981, 1986; Mitchell *et al.*, 1990; Rosenblum, 1968; Wright, 1999).

As a result, penicillins may elicit a variety of allergic reactions ranging from mild skin rashes to potentially fatal anaphylaxis (Idsoe *et al.*, 1968). It has been estimated that penicillin may account for up to 75% of deaths due to anaphylaxis in the United States (Delage and Irey, 1972). The frequency of allergic reactions to penicillins ranges from 0.7 to 10% of patients treated (Anderson and Adkinson, 1987; Idsoe *et al.*, 1968; Van Ardsel, 1965). Even within the skin reactions, these may be mild to severe and life threatening; penicillins can cause mild urticaria and erythema, rashes, erythema multiforme and toxic epidermal necrolysis (Alanis and Weinstein, 1983; Adcock and Rodman, 1996; Arias *et al.*, 1995; Chopra *et al.*, 1989; de Haan *et al.*, 1986; Egawa, 1994; Fellner, 1976, 1986; Gastaminza *et al.*, 2000; Herman and Jick, 1979; Herold *et al.*, 1983; Hoffman *et al.*, 1989; Jiminez *et al.*, 1997; Johnson, 1971; Minguez *et al.*, 1998; Puavilai and Timpatanapong, 1989; Romano *et al.*, 1993, 1997; Rosenthal *et al.*, 1979; Russel and Lessof, 1971; Saenz de San Pedro Morera *et al.*, 1999; Staretz and DeBoom, 1990; Tagami *et al.*, 1983; Takahashi, 1976; Vega, 1994; Ward *et al.*, 1990). Contact dermatitis and urticaria, either as a result of systemic sensitisation or repeated dermal exposure, can also occur, for example, following ingestion of contaminated foods or due to occupational exposure to penicillin present as residues in milk or to penicillin itself (Borrie and Barret, 1961; Cany, 1977; Erskine, 1958; Girard, 1978; Kautz, 1959; Lindemayr *et al.*, 1981; Lisi *et al.*, 1997; Mauranges, 1972; Minkin and Lynch, 1969; Olson and Sanders, 1975; Pigatto *et al.*, 1986; Reisman and Arbesman, 1968; Rudzki and Rebandel, 1985; Stewart, 1967, 1969; Vickers, 1964; Vickers *et al.*, 1958; Wicher *et al.*, 1969; Woodward, 1991; Zimmerman, 1959).

There has been a report of a patient who experienced an anaphylactic reaction after a steak dinner. The patient, known to be sensitised to penicillin, developed generalised pruritis, difficulty in swallowing and speaking, and dyspnoea within 20 minutes of eating. The meat was later found to contain penicillin or penicilloyl moieties (Schwartz and Sher, 1984). A similar event occurred after pork consumption (Tscheuschner, 1972). There has even been a report of anaphylaxis in a patient after the consumption of a soft drink (Wicher and Reisman, 1980). Although penicillin was detected in the drink, its origins were obscure. Although there are some limited animal models for penicillin hypersensitivity, including cutaneous anaphylaxis (Hattori *et al.*, 1997; Kornbrust *et al.*, 1989; Kristofferson and Ahlstedt, 1982; Kubo *et al.*, 1989), it is not possible at present to predict which patients will react, and in which way.

As others have noted, it is difficult to quantify the public health risks of penicillin residues in foods (Dewdney and Edwards, 1984). Several factors combine to make the risk of adverse reactions to penicillin residues in food very low, including the dose received, oral intake and the low density of antigenic determinants (Dewdney *et al.*, 1991), and indeed, the literature supports this view; allergic reactions to antibiotic residues are very rare (Dayan, 1993). In the establishment of MRLs, the CVMP in the EU and JECFA have addressed this problem. In fact, the CVMP estimated that 10 International Units (IU; 1 IU benzyl penicillin = 0.6 μg) of penicillin were required to evoke an allergic response, presumably in sensitised individuals. However, it concluded that concentrations as low as 0.01 could inhibit dairy starter cultures, and hence aspects of food processing, and recommended that residues of penicillin in milk should not exceed 0.005 IU. In order to protect both the consumer and dairy processing, the MRLs for a range of penicillins were established at between 50 (benzyl penicillin, ampicillin and amoxicillin) ppb for tissues and 4 ppb for milk, and 300 (oxacillin, cloxacillin and dicloxacillin) ppb for tissues and 30 ppb for milk. (CVMP, Penicillins, Summary Report). JECFA on the other hand, which only considers safety and not food processing, considered that intake of benzyl penicillin should be kept below 30 μg of the drug. In practice, this resulted in MRLs for benzyl penicillin that are the same as those established by the EU, namely 50 ppb for tissues and 4 ppb for milk (JECFA, 1990).

8.3.2 Cephalosporins

The cephalosporins are chemically related to the penicillins and both share the β-lactam ring structure. However, in place of the thiazolidine ring of the penicillins, cephalosporins possess the six-membered dihydrothiazine ring (Abraham, 1987; Gustaferro and Steckelberg, 1991; Klein and Cunha, 1995; Van Heyningen, 1967). A number of cephalosporins, including cefalonium, cefalexin, cefuroxime, ceftiofur, cefquinome, cefoperazone, cefazolin, cefapirin and cefacetrile are used in veterinary medicine in food animals. Like the penicillins, cephalosporins have low toxicity in mammalian toxicity tests and indeed in humans (Birkhead *et al.*, 1973; Capel-Edwards *et al.*, 1979; Esposti *et al.*, 1986; Fekety, 1990; Gerber and Craig, 1981; Grassi, 1995; Griffith and Black, 1970; Gustaferro and Steckelberg, 1991; Klein and Cunha, 1995; Kradolfer *et al.*, 1974; Meyers, 1985; Norrby, 1987; Norrby and Alestig, 1981; Parker and Park, 1984; Smith and LeFrock, 1983; Speight *et al.*, 1972; Spurling *et al.*, 1986; Tauchi *et al.*, 1979a,b,c,d,e,f,g; Thompson and Jacobs, 1993; Welles *et al.*, 1968; Yoneda *et al.*, 1980). Cefuroxime and ceftiofur have a low order of toxicity (JECFA, 1996a, 2002a).

Cephalosporins, like penicillins can be neurotoxic but usually after direct application to the brain surface or after high doses, particularly to renally compromised patients (Fekety, 1990; Norrby, 1987; Schliamser *et al.*, 1991; Thompson and Jacobs, 1993; Weiss *et al.*, 1974). Hepatotoxicity is rare (George and Crawford, 1996; Hautekeete, 1995). However, cephalosporins can cause renal damage through hypersensitivity-induced interstitial nephritis or through direct toxicity on the renal tubules. Again, this is rare, especially with the third generation compounds and when nephrotoxicity does occur, it is generally at high doses (Barza, 1978; Cojocel *et al.*, 1988; Fekety, 1990; Norrby, 1987; Preziosi, 1981; Sack *et al.*, 1977; Tune *et al.*, 1996; Yilmaz *et al.*, 1999). In general there is no evidence of genotoxicity in the cephalosporins group but one compound used in veterinary medicine, ceftiofur, produced positive results in an *in vitro* cytogenetics assay (Aaron *et al.*, 1995a) suggesting that it might have clastogenic potential. However, further investigations revealed this to be reversible, casting doubt on whether or not this was a true genotoxic effect. Furthermore, the drug had a major effect on the cell cycle kinetics and the effects thus appeared to be due to a prolongation of the cell cycle (Aaron *et al.*, 1995b). *In vivo* studies for clastogenicity gave negative results (Aaron *et al.*, 1995c). Hence, it can be concluded that ceftiofur is not a clastogen.

Like the penicillins, cephalosporins can induce hypersensitivity reactions leading to a skin rashes, urticaria, contact dermatitis, and toxic epidermal necrolysis, but anaphylaxis is very rare as are severe skin reactions (Blanco, 1994; Christ, 1991; Dave *et al.*, 1991; Hogan and Rooney, 1987; Jick and Derby, 1995, Kelmar and Li, 2001; McCloskey and Massa, 1997; Milligan and Douglas, 1986; Romano *et al.*, 1992, 2000, 2001; Speight *et al.*, 1972). Occupational dermatitis has been reported (Foti *et al.*, 1997; Straube *et al.*, 2000). There is some degree of cross-reactivity between penicillins and cephalosporins, but the degree and mechanisms are not clear although the actual incidence appears low (Audicana *et al.*, 1994; Beam and Spooner, 1984; Dhar and Kulkarni, 1994; Igea *et al.*, 1992, Kelmar and Li, 2001). One study suggested that up to 10% of those sensitised to penicillin might have serious adverse events due to cross-reactivity if exposed to cephalosporins (Herbert *et al.*, 2000) although this might not be true in respect of anaphylaxis (Goodman *et al.*, 2001). In general, the adverse hypersensitivity reactions with cephalosporins appear to be less frequent and less severe than those seen with the penicillins.

The CVMP has set ADIs for the cephalosporins based on microbiological effects on the gut microflora. In all instances, these are lower than the toxicological ADIs. The MRL for cefalonium was based on effects on dairy starter cultures, the NOEL for this being significantly lower than both those for the toxicological and microbiological ADI values. JECFA used the microbiological end-points to establish ADIs for ceftiofur and cefuroxime (JECFA, 1996b, 2002b).

8.4 Macrolide antibiotics: spiramycin, tylosin and tilmicosin

Macrolide antibiotics possess a macrocyclic lactone ring to which are attached one or more deoxy sugar residues. Erythromycin is the major macrolide antibiotic used in human medicine (Kapusnik-Uner *et al.*, 1996). In veterinary medicine, the major macrolides are spiramycin, tylosin and tilmicosin.

8.4.1 Spiramycin

Spiramycin has low acute oral toxicity in mice, rats and dogs although some evidence of hepatotoxicity was observed at very high doses. It also had low toxicity after repeated oral administration to rats and dogs (Boyd and Price-Jones, 1960). There was no evidence of teratogenic effects in mice and rabbits, although embryotoxicity, probably due to toxic effects on the pregnant females, did occur at higher doses. It was not genotoxic in a range of *in vitro* and *in vivo* genotoxicity studies and no evidence of carcinogenicity was seen in a two-year study in rats (Boyd, 1958; Boyd *et al.*, 1958; Boyd and Brown, 1958; Dubost *et al.*, 1956; JECFA, 1991b). There is a paucity of data following use in humans. There are isolated reports referring to effects on gastric motility and an ulcerated oesophagus (Perreard and Klotz, 1989; Qin *et al.*, 1987); macrolides are known to reduce gastric motility when given in high doses (Kapusik-Uner *et al.*, 1996; Pilot and Qin, 1988). There are no data to suggest that spiramycin has significant toxicity in humans when used therapeutically and adverse effects are limited to occasional nausea, vomiting and allergic skin reactions. There has been a single report of allergic vasculitis following the use of spiramycin (Galland *et al.*, 1987).

Following occupational exposure, there have been a few reports of dermatitis and bronchial asthma (Davis and Pepys, 1975; Moscato *et al.*, 1984; Paggiaro *et al.*, 1979; Veien *et al.*, 1980, 1983), including reports of occupational asthma in pharmaceutical company workers exposed to spiramycin (Malo and Cartier, 1988; Nava, 1976). It is evident that the adverse event profile for spiramycin is significantly lower than that for the penicillins.

The most sensitive studies were those of effects on the gastrointestinal flora where both *in vitro* and *in vivo* methods had been employed, and JECFA established the ADI for spiramycin on this basis (JECFA, 1991c, 1995a). A similar approach was adopted in calculating the ADI by the CVMP.

8.4.2 Tylosin

Like spiramycin, tylosin has very low mammalian toxicity after oral administration, is not carcinogenic or genotoxic and shows no evidence of adverse effects in reproduction or teratology studies (Aiso *et al.*, 1966; Anderson *et al.*, 1966; JECFA, 1991c). Like spiramycin also, there have been occasional reports of contact dermatitis and asthma in those occupationally exposed (Barbera and de la Cuadra, 1989; Caraffini *et al.*, 1994; Danese *et al.*, 1994; Gollins, 1989; Jung, 1983; Lee *et al.*, 1989; Pirkis *et al.*, 1997; Tuomi and Rasanen, 1995; Veien *et al.*, 1980; Verbov, 1983).

Like spiramycin, the most sensitive end-point for the calculation of the ADI was microbiological rather than toxicological, and the EU established the ADI for tylosin on this basis. Almost certainly, the same approach would have been taken up by JECFA, but the initial report required further data (JECFA, 1991c) and it seems the MRL was not pursued.

8.4.3 Tilmicosin

Tilmicosin is structurally closely related to tylosin. It appears to have higher acute toxicity than either spiramycin or tylosin after oral administration to mammalian species. However, this higher toxicity was only seen in fasted animals; when given to non-fasted animals, the toxicity was similar to that of spiramycin and tylosin. Dogs given oral doses of tilmicosin for three months showed increased heart rates and 50% of animals given 70 mg/kg body weight per day died (Main *et al.*, 1996). The NOEL was 6 mg/kg per day. In a one-year study in dogs, heart rates were increased at oral doses of 12 or 36 mg/kg per day and cardiac enlargement occurred at the higher dose. The NOEL was 4 mg/kg per day. There were no notable adverse effects in a reproductive study in rats, or in teratogenicity studies in rats and rabbits. There was no evidence of genotoxicity in a range of *in vitro* and *in vivo* studies (Altunok *et al.*, 2002;

JECFA, 1996c; Jordan *et al.*, 1993). No carcinogenicity study was conducted, and JECFA felt that this was not necessary in view of the results from genotoxicity studies, the lack of any indication that carcinogenicity might be an issue in other studies and the fact that the closely-related macrolide tylosin was not carcinogenic.

Unlike the other macrolides, there have been no significant reports of occupational exposure and allergy although there have been several reports of adverse effects in workers who have accidentally suffered a needle stick injury on a needle contaminated with the drug. The majority of these were minor local effects resulting from needle punctures (McGuigan, 1994). However, there have been reports of cardiac effects in workers who have accidentally injected themselves with significant quantities of the medicine. These have included chest pains, electrocardiographic abnormalities and intraventricular conduction delays (Crown and Smith, 1999; Von Essen *et al.*, 2003). There has been a report of a death following accidental intravenous injection (Kuffner and Dart, 1996) and a fatality in an 18–year-old woman (reported in Von Essen *et al.*, 2003). Similar toxicity has been noted with erythromycin, including torsades de pointes (Brandriss *et al.*, 1994; Farrar *et al.*, 1993; Nattel *et al.*, 1990; Orban *et al.*, 1995; Regan *et al.*, 1969). Experimental studies in dogs show that a negative inotropic effect developed after intravenous administration of tilmicosin, with reductions in left ventricular systolic pressure and electrocardiographic abnormalities. These studies indicate that tilmicosin might pose an occupational risk when administered by injection, but the quantities required orally to exert cardiac effects are too great for residues to pose a risk.

JECFA chose the NOEL of 4 mg/kg per day from the 12–month study in dogs as the toxicological ADI (JECFA, 1998a). The drug had little microbiological effect on the gut microflora of rats in an *in vivo* study. Consequently, JECFA on this occasion used the NOEL from the toxicological studies and a safety factor of 100, to calculate the ADI. The CVMP took a different strategy. It chose an NOEL from a study in germ-free rats, infected with human gut flora, treated with tilmicosin. This NOEL was lower than the toxicological NOEL and so the ADI was based on microbiological effects.

8.5 Aminoglycosides

The aminoglycosides share a common structure of amino sugars linked to an amino hexose (aminocyclitol – a derivative of cyclitol, hexahydroxy-cyclohexane) moiety, via glycosidic bonds; hence the use of the term aminoglycoside. The most common examples used in veterinary medicine are neomycin, streptomycin, gentamicin and dihydrostreptomycin although kanamycin and aminosidine are also used. Spectinomycin is a related compound; it is an aminocyclitol without the amino sugar residues (Burrows, 1980; Chambers and Sande, 1996; Houdeshell *et al.*, 1982).

The two major adverse effects of the aminoglycosides are ototoxicity and nephrotoxicity, both of which have been reported in animals and humans.

8.5.1 Ototoxicity

Studies in cats with oral doses of 300 mg/kg dihydrostreptomycin for 21 days or 100 mg/kg for 60 days showed loss of hair cells in the cochlea, and damage to the sensorimotor epithelium. Dogs given 50 or 100 mg/kg streptomycin for 20 days showed auditory impairment. Degeneration of the nerve cells of the central nuclei, primarily the vestibular and cochlear nuclei was seen in guinea-pigs given 100–400 mg/kg per day streptomycin for 3 to 6 weeks. Ototoxicity has also been noted in cats with gentamicin and neomycin in mammals, including primates and this may be exaggerated by co-administration of loop diuretics (Brummett, 1981a, b; Christensen *et al.*, 1951; Erlanson and Lundgren, 1964; Ernst *et al.*, 1994; Hawkins and Lurie, 1953; Hodges *et al.*, 1985; Leake *et al.*, 1997; McGee and Olszewski, 1962; Riskaer *et al.*, 1952, 1956; Tsang and Chin, 1963; Waitz *et al.*, 1971; Webster *et al.*, 1971; Yakota *et al.*, 1984). Hearing loss and auditory and vestibular damage has been reported in humans treated with aminoglycoside antibiotics, including gentamicin, neomycin and streptomycin (Chambers and Sande, 1996; Dayal *et al.*, 1979; Erlandson and Lundgren, 1964; Gailiunas *et al.*, 1978; Greenberg and Momary, 1965; Halpern and Heller, 1961; Lerner *et al.*, 1986; Lindsay *et al.*, 1960; Meyers, 1970; Waisbren and Spink, 1950). Ototoxicity has been reported in the children of mothers treated with streptomycin and dihydrostreptomycin during pregnancy (Davies, 1991; Erlanson and Lundgren, 1964; Matz, 1993; Robinson and Cambon, 1964; Snider *et al.*, 1980; Varpela *et al.*, 1969; Warkany, 1979).

8.5.2 Nephrotoxicity

The aminoglycoside antibiotics have been shown to be nephrotoxic in experimental animals including mice (JECFA, 1995a; Molitor *et al.*, 1946; Nelson *et al.*, 1951; Waitz *et al.*, 1971). Nephrotoxicity is relatively common in patients treated with aminoglycosides (Chambers and Sande, 1996; Greenberg and Momary, 1965; Hewitt, 1974; Masur, *et al.*, 1976; Noone *et al.*, 1978; Powell and Hooker, 1956; Pratt and Fekety, 1986; Solgaard *et al.*, 2000) and neonates may be particularly susceptible (Heimann, 1983; Khoory *et al.*, 1996). The incidence is relatively high; in patients given aminoglycosides for more than a few days, around 10 to 25% will develop mild renal impairment, and in those exposed for longer or to relatively high doses, ultimately cellular necrosis of the proximal tubules (Chambers and Sande, 1996; Fillastre *et al.*, 1989). The effects are usually reversible.

8.5.3 Other adverse effects

The only other common adverse effect associated with the use of aminoglycosides is contact dermatitis and this has been reported following neomycin and gentamicin treatment, largely following dermal application (Baer and Ludwig, 1952; Bigby *et al.*, 1989; Calnan and Sarkany, 1958; Epstein, 1956, 1965; Epstein and Wenzel, 1962; Gette *et al.*, 1992; Ghadially and Ramsay, 1988; Goh, 1989; Hannuksela *et al.*, 1981). Streptomycin has been associated with anaphylaxis (Tinkelman and Bock, 1984).

The CVMP established ADIs for aminosidine, dihydrostreptomycin and streptomycin on the basis of conventional toxicity as the toxicological ADI was below that of the microbiological ADI. For gentamicin, the lowest ADI was the microbiological ADI and this served as the basis for the MRLs. Only with neomycin was the toxicological ADI the lowest *and* based on ototoxicity. A similar qualitative approach was taken by JECFA with the ADI values for streptomycin and dihydrostreptomycin, gentamicin and neomycin being established on the basis of toxicology, microbiology and ototoxicity (JECFA, 1995a).

8.5.4 Aminocyclitol – spectinomycin

Unlike its close relatives in the aminoglycosides group, spectinomycin is not ototoxic, nor is it nephrotoxic (Holloway, 1982; JECFA, 1994; Novak *et al.*, 1974). Both JECFA and the CVMP based the ADI values on microbiological effects.

8.6 Fluoroquinolones

The earliest quinolone antimicrobial drugs, the so-called first generation quinolones, are represented by oxolinic and nalidixic acids. However, the second generation drugs, the fluoroquinolones are typified by ciprofloxacin and enrofloxacin (Mitscher *et al.*, 1993). The important fluoroquinolones used in veterinary medicine are flumequine, enrofloxacin, sarafloxacin, danofloxacin, orbifloxacin, ibafloxacin and marbofloxacin (Greene and Budsberg, 1993; NOAH, 2001), while the major fluoroquinolone used in food animals is enrofloxacin.

The most significant major toxic effect of fluoroquinolones is on the articular cartilages, and several fluoroquinolones have been shown to have the ability to cause juvenile arthropathies in a number of species including rats, dogs and birds (Burkhardt *et al.*, 1990; Crist *et al.*, 1988; Hayem and Carbon, 1995; Kappel *et al.*, 2002; Kashida and Kato, 1997; Nagai *et al.*, 2002; Patterson, 1991; Peters *et al.*, 2002; Schluter, 1987; Stahlmann and Lode, 1999; Stahlmann, 1990; Stahlmann *et al.*, 2000; Takizawa *et al.*, 1999a,b). Grepafloxacin seems to have low toxicity in this respect (Leone *et al.*, 2003; Takizawa *et al.*, 1999a). They are associated with a low incidence of tendonitis in humans (Leone *et al.*, 2003; van der Linden *et al.*, 2001), and there have been no reports of arthritis or other major diseases of joints in paediatric populations exposed to fluoroquinolones (Camp *et al.*, 1994; Jick, 1997; Warren, 1997) although arthralgias and minor changes in cartilage have been noted (Gendrel and Moulin, 2001; Hooper and Wolfson, 1993).

The only other notable toxic effect is prolongation of the QT interval in human patients, and this appears to be a class effect. Such effects are seen at therapeutic doses (Hooper and Wolfson, 1993; Leone *et al.*, 2003).

In the EU, the ADI values calculated by the CVMP were based on microbiological effects for enrofloxacin, sarafloxacin, difloxacin and marbofloxacin, as these were substantially below the toxicological ADI values. However, for danofloxacin, the toxicological ADI, was based on an NOEL for arthropathy in dogs. A safety factor of 100 was used in the calculation of the ADI as the evidence suggests that these effects are rare in humans.

8.7 Sulfadimidine (sulfamethazine)

Sulfadimidine is a sulphonamide antimicrobial drug which has been widely used in food animal veterinary medicine, often potentiated with trimethoprim (Spoo and Riviere, 2001). Administration of sulfadimidine to rats, but not to mice for 90 days induced thyroid hyperplasia (Heath and Littlefield, 1984a,b). Administration to mice for up to 24 months resulted in follicular cell adenomas of the thyroid (Littlefield *et al.*, 1989). In rats, adenocarcinomas of the thyroid developed after exposure for up to 24 months in a two-generation study (Littlefield *et al.*, 1990). Thus the data suggested that sulfadimidine was carcinogenic in rats, and possibly carcinogenic in mice.

However, sulfadimidine has been shown to be goitrogenic in rodents resulting in constant stimulation of the thyroid by thyroid-stimulating hormone (TSH); humans are insensitive to this mechanism of thyroid-induced neoplasia (Fullerton *et al.*, 1987; Hill *et al.*, 1996, 1998; McClain, 1995; Poirier *et al.*, 1999). Hence, the tumours noted in rodents have no relevance to human risk assessment and are not predictive for human safety assessment (Galer and Monro, 1998b; Poirier *et al.*, 1999).

JECFA, taking a precautionary approach, established an NOEL based on thyroid changes in rats and pigs and calculated the ADI using a safety factor of 100. The CVMP took a similar approach. The MRL value was established at 100 μg/kg as this accounted not only for the toxicological ADI but also any potential allergic and microbiological effects (JECFA, 1995b).

8.8 Carbadox and olaquindox

Carbadox and olaquindox are quinoxaline-1,4–di-N-oxide derivatives with antimicrobial activity. They were used as growth promoting agents in pigs and were also used in the prevention and treatment of swine dysentery (Bronsch *et al.*, 1976; Holder and Sinclair, 1972; Kornegay *et al.*, 1968; Nabuurs and van der Molen, 1989; Nabuurs *et al.*, 1990; Rainier *et al.*, 1973; Schneider *et al.*, 1976).

In the EU, carbadox and olaquindox were registered as feed additives under Directive 70/524/EEC and were not authorised as veterinary medicines, and so were not subject to the requirements for the establishment of MRLs. However, both drugs have been assessed by JECFA.

The most relevant aspect of the toxicity of carbadox is its carcinogenic potential. Carbadox was examined in several studies in rats, and doses in excess of 1 mg/kg per day were associated with an increased incidence of benign and malignant liver tumours. Tumours were even noted in a very limited study of only 11 months duration and in a second study where rats were dosed by the intraperitoneal route prior to weaning for 8 to 20 days, and/or in the feed at 300 ppm, for one year (JECFA, 1991d; Sykora and Vortel, 1986). A range of in *vitro* and *in vivo* mutagenicity studies with a variety of end-points has provided positive results (Beutin *et al.*, 1981; Cihak and Srb, 1983; Cihak and Vontorkova, 1983, 1985; JECFA, 1991d; Negishi *et al.*, 1980; Ohta *et al.*, 1980; Oud *et al.*, 1979; Scheutwinkel-Reich and von der Hude, 1984; Voogd *et al.*, 1980; Yoshimura *et al.*, 1981). Hence, it is evident that carbadox is a genotoxic carcinogen, and this might be considered to have signalled its demise as a drug in food animals.

However, the major metabolites of carbadox in the pig, methyl carbazate, quinoline-2-carboxylic acid and desoxycarbadox gave negative results in carcinogenicity studies and in genotoxicity studies (JECFA, 1991d; Truhaut *et al.*, 1981). Relay toxicity studies were also employed to demonstrate the safety of carbadox residues. Relay toxicity studies are investigations whereby food containing residues of a drug is administered to experimental animals rather than the parent drug itself. Thus, the drug is administered to a food animal such as a pig, and the tissues of that animal are then used as the test substance in toxicity studies, including carcinogenicity studies (Boisseau, 1990; Craine, 1977; Ferrando and Truhaut, 1982; Galer and Munro, 1998a; Gallo-Torres, 1977, 1990; Truhaut and Ferrando, 1975, 1976).

While this methodology is useful in demonstrating the lability of residues bound to macromolecules, its usefulness in toxicity testing has been doubted. For example, it has been criticised because the doses of residues that are likely to be received in this way are too low to elicit a toxicological response, that in carcinogenicity studies the dose is far from the maximum tolerated dose usually employed, and the metabolites present as residues are usually unknown (Arnold, 1990; Boisseau, 1990; Guest and Fitzpatrick, 1990). Nevertheless, it can be argued for carcinogens at least that the doses likely to occur are somewhere towards the lower slope of a dose-response curve, and that in the case of drugs like carbadox, the metabolites in the rat are reasonably well characterised qualitatively and quantitatively. Hence, relay carcinogenicity studies have some validity, as part of a suite of toxicity studies and so they could complement standard studies, but not replace them (Arnold, 1990; Boisseau, 1990).

The relay carcinogenicity studies conducted with carbadox were of two years' duration in rats and 7.5 years' duration in dogs. There was no evidence of an increased incidence of tumours (Ferrando *et al.*, 1977, 1978). Taken together with metabolism studies in various species including pigs, the data suggest that only carbadox itself is genotoxic and carcinogenic, and that its metabolites present as residues pose no risk to the consumer. As carbadox was a genotoxic carcinogen, JECFA was unable to identify an NOEL or establish an ADI, but it elaborated MRLs for the drug, as it recognised that its residues did not pose a consumer risk (JECFA, 1990).

Olaquindox has similar genotoxic properties to carbadox (Beutin *et al.*, 1981, Cihak and Vontorkova, 1983; Nunoshiba and Nishioka, 1989; Pokorna, 1986; Scheutwinkel-Reich and von der Hude, 1984; Sram *et al.*, 1986a,b,c; Suter *et al.*, 1978; von der Hude *et al.*, 1988; Voogd *et al.*, 1980; Yoshimura *et al.*, 1981). It has been tested in a number of carcinogenicity studies in rodents, some of them inadequate to assess carcinogenic potential. However, it has been investigated in two adequate carcinogenicity studies, one in rats and the other in mice and there was no evidence of carcinogenic effects. Hence, it is a potent genotoxic agent but appears to lack carcinogenic activity. JECFA concluded that, like carbadox, it was unable to calculate an ADI because the drug was genotoxic, but provisionally concluded that the residues were acceptable (JECFA, 1991d).

Both carbadox and olaquindox were prohibited in the EU in 1998, not because of concerns over the safety of residues, but due to the hazards posed to those occupationally exposed to the substances (Anon, 1998).

8.9 Furazolidone and related compounds

Furazolidone is a member of the nitrofuran group of drugs which have been widely used as antimicrobials in veterinary medicine. A chemically related group, the nitroimidazoles, has also been used as antimicrobials and antiprotozoals; specifically, dimetridazole has been widely used in the treatment of histomoniasis in poultry (Brander *et al.*, 1982; Papich and Riviere, 2001).

The nitrofurans and nitroimidazoles are genotoxic and some of them, including furazolidone and nitrofurazone, have been shown to be carcinogenic (JECFA, 1993a,b; NTP, 1988). Such properties would make them unacceptable for use in food animals unless, like carbadox, they could be shown to be converted to innocuous metabolites by the treated animals so that consumers were not exposed to potentially toxic residues. Unfortunately, some of the residues of these drugs were shown to be bound to macromolecules *in vivo*. At first this might seem reassuring. If their residues are firmly bound to macromolecules, then this would suggest that they are safe. However, two questions arise from this observation. Are the residues 'lightly' bound so that toxic substances might easily be released? Are they firmly bound but with the potential for toxic substances to be released under severe conditions, for example when the macromolecules to which they are bound are digested in the human gastrointestinal tract? To put both these questions more simply: how bioavailable are the bound residues and how toxic/genotoxic/carcinogenic are they if they are bioavailable?

Various schemes have been put forward to address this question. One approach involves examining the effects of weak acid and alkalis, then strong acids and alkalis on the bound material to see what exactly is released under various conditions. A natural progression from this is then to look at the effects of digestive enzymes to determine what might then be released. In the case of genotoxic and carcinogenic drugs, the release of reactive moieties would be of significance and further tests (e.g. genotoxicity studies) on these would be justified (Frazier, 1990; Jaglan *et al.*, 1977; Lu *et al.*, 1987, 1990; Matula, 1990; Weiss, 1990; Yong, 1990). Another strategy would be to conduct relay toxicity tests, as described for carbadox, above.

Unfortunately for the nitroimidazoles and nitrofurans, and unlike carbadox, these approaches have proved inconclusive. Furazolidone and ronidazole (a nitroimidazole) produce a number of metabolites, and there is significant binding to macromolecules, particularly proteins (Alvaro *et al.*, 1992; De Angelis *et al.*, 1999; Hoogenboom, 1991; Hoogenboom *et al.*, 1992, 1994; Lu *et al.*, 1984, 1988; Miwa *et al.*, 1986; Sved and Foster, 1990; Vroomen *et al.*, 1990 a,b; Wislocki and Lu, 1990; Wislocki *et al.*, 1984). Some evidence suggests that bound furazolidone residues are degraded to non-toxic metabolites (Klee *et al.*, 1999) but in general, for both classes of drugs, there are insufficient data to state with certainty that the nitrofurans and nitroimidazoles do not pose a genotoxic or carcinogenic threat to the consumer, by way of their metabolites or from the release of bound residues from tissue macromolecules after consumption of food of animal origin. Consequently, the CVMP recommended the entry of nitrofurans (including furazolidone) and the nitroimidazoles ronidazole, dimetridazole and metronidazole into Annex IV of Regulation (EEC) No. 2377/90, and this was adopted by the European Commission in 1977. As a result, these drugs may no longer be administered to food-producing animals in the EU.

8.10 Chloramphenicol

Chloramphenicol is a relatively simple antibiotic substance produced by *Streptomyces venezulae.* It is now made synthetically. It was first used for the treatment of epidemic typhus in South America, and scrub typhus in Asia in the late 1940s, and it produced dramatic results. However, chloramphenicol was found to produce blood dyscrasias in humans. In fact it produces two distinct types of myelotoxicity. The less serious of these is a reversible bone marrow suppression due to mitochondrial damage which produces a mild anaemia (Chaplin, 1986; Holt *et al.*, 1993; Keiser and Buchegger, 1973; Nijhof and Kroon, 1974). The more serious effect is bone marrow aplasia or aplastic anaemia with pancytopenia and acellular bone marrow. In fact aplastic anaemia has been estimated to occur in 1 in 500 to 1 in 100 000 cases treated, and it is often fatal (Aksoy *et al.*, 1984; Al-Moudhiry, 1978; Baumelou and Najean, 1983; Benestad, 1979; Bottiger, 1979; Hausman and Skrandies, 1974; Keiser and Buchegger, 1973; Modan *et al.*, 1975; Najean and Baumelou, 1984; Perez *et al.*, 1981; Polak *et al.*, 1972; Sharp, 1963; Venning, 1983; Wallerstein *et al.*, 1969; Widayat *et al.*, 1983). These effects are not limited to adults and aplastic anaemia has been reported in children treated with the drug (Awaad *et al.*, 1975; Leiken *et al.*, 1961; Lepow, 1986; White *et al.*, 1986; Young *et al.*, 1979).

There is no firm correlation with dose administered and the development of aplastic anaemia, although total doses are often high and of the order of 4 to 80 grams (Hellriegel and Cross, 1974; Hodgkinson, 1971). However, cases of aplastic anaemia have been reported after topical administration (where the systemic dose may have been low), and after the application of ophthalmic drops (where the dose would have been low) (Abrams *et al.*, 1980; Carpenter, 1975; Fraunfelder and Bagby, 1982; Issaragrisil and Piankijagum, 1985; Korting and Kifle, 1985; Plaut and Best, 1982; Rosenthal and Blackman, 1965), although the risk associated with the use of eye drops or topical application is probably very small (Lancaster *et al.*, 1998; Walker *et al.*, 1998). There has been one report of aplastic anaemia in a shepherd occupationally exposed to an aerosol spray containing the drug, for the treatment of infections in sheep (Del Giacco *et al.*, 1981).

The mechanism of induction of aplastic anaemia is not fully understood. However, because of the lack of correlation with dose or duration of treatment, its seemingly random occurrence in treated populations, and its occurrence in identical twins, it possibly has a genetic background (Yunis and Bloomberg, 1964; Yunis, 1984, 1989). Although it has been possible to develop animal models of reversible bone marrow depression (Festing *et al.*, 2001; Holt *et al.*, 1997, 1998; Turton *et al.*, 1999, 2000, 2002a, b), the same success has not been achieved with aplastic anaemia. It has been proposed that chloramphenicol is toxic due to the activation of the *p*-nitro group to give a toxic nitroso compound in susceptible individuals (Yunis and Bloomberg, 1964; Yunis, 1984, 1989) and *in vitro* the nitroso compound does appear to be more toxic than chloramphenicol or thiamphenicol. However, at the present time the mechanism of aplastic anaemia induction remains obscure (Holt *et al.*, 1993; Malkin *et al.*, 1990).

Not only is chloramphenicol-induced aplastic anaemia often fatal in its own right, it can be the precursor to leukaemia (Krakoff *et al.*, 1955; Scott *et al.*, 1965; Yunis and Bloomberg, 1964). Leukaemia has been reported to follow chloramphenicol-associated aplastic anaemia in those who recover (Awaad *et al.*, 1975; Brauer and Dameshek, 1967; Forni and Vigliani, 1974; Fraumeni, 1967; Gadner *et al.*, 1973; Humphries, 1968; Kapusnik-Uner *et al.*, 1996; Meyer and Boxer, 1973; Meyler *et al.*, 1974; Scheres *et al.*, 1985, Schmitt-Graff, 1981; Seaman, 1969).

JECFA considered chloramphenicol in 1987 and considered that as it could not identify an NOEL for aplastic anaemia, then it could not calculate an ADI (JECFA, 1988). It considered the drug again in 1994. There were no new data to address the NOEL for aplastic anaemia, and several genotoxicity studies carried out since JECFA's last review in 1987, using different end-points, gave positive results. Positive results were noted with three mammalian metabolites of chloramphenicol. Consequently, JECFA remained unable to identify an NOEL, particularly now that the drug and some of its metabolites had been identified as being genotoxic (JECFA, 1995b; Robbana-Barnat *et al.*, 1997). Hence, an ADI could not be calculated, and MRLs were not elaborated.

The same conclusions were reached by the CVMP. In fact, the CVMP went further and concluded that it could not calculate an ADI, not only because of the lack of a threshold for aplastic anaemia and the genotoxicity of the drug, but additionally because there was no adequate carcinogenicity study, an NOEL could not be identified for foetotoxicity and there was no adequate reproductive study. In addition, there were a number of omissions from the residues file and the CVMP recommended its inclusion into Annex IV of Regulation No. (EEC) 2377/90, thus prohibiting its use in food animals in the EU.

The related drug thiamphenicol lacks the *p*-nitro group of chloramphenicol and in its place it has a methylsulphonyl group. Hence, based on the premise of Yunis (1988), it is less likely to be myelotoxic than chloramphenicol. This certainly seems to be the case. Although it can induce the reversible bone marrow suppression seen with chloramphenicol, it appears to have less of a preponderance to induce aplastic anaemia (Ando *et al.*, 1997; Frohli *et al.*, 1984; Kaltwasser *et al.*, 1974; Keiser and Burchegger, 1973; Turton *et al.*, 2000, 2002a,b; Yunis, 1984, 1988, 1989) and any bone marrow aplasia is rare (De Renzo *et al.*, 1981; Gluckman, 1971). Unlike chloramphenicol, there is an adequate carcinogenicity study available and this gave negative results (Kitamura *et al.*, 1997) and it does not induce DNA damage (Skolimowski *et al.*, 1983). JECFA was able to identify a toxicological ADI for thiamphenicol but the ADI for microbiological effects on the gut flora was lower, and this was used as the basis for the MRL (JECFA, 2000). The CVMP also took a similar view and the MRL was eventually elaborated on the basis of a microbiological ADI.

8.11 Ivermectin and related compounds

Ivermectin belongs to a group of substances known as the avermectins. These are compounds that have as their central structure a macrocyclic lactone ring that adjoins a spiroketal structure. Since ivermectin was first introduced, a series of related compounds has become available including abamectin, doramectin, emamectin and eprinomectin for use in veterinary medicine. A related compound, moxidectin, a milbemycin (an avermectin macrocycle lacking a bisoleandrosyloxy substituent at the C-13 position) has also been introduced. They are used as endectocides in sheep and cattle except for emamectin which is used as a parasiticide in farmed salmon. Many also have applications in companion animal medicine (McKellar and Benchaoui, 1996; Shoop *et al.*, 1995; Sutherland and Campbell, 1990; Williams, 1997b).

Ivermectin has moderate acute toxicity when given orally to experimental animals. No major adverse effects were noted in subchronic studies, and there was no evidence that ivermectin was genotoxic or teratogenic at doses which were not toxic to the maternal animals; at doses which were maternally toxic, cleft palates in mice and clubbed fore-paws in rabbits were noted (Burkhart, 2000; Campbell and Benz, 1984; JECFA, 1991d; Lankas *et al.*, 1989) and in veterinary medicine, toxicosis usually arises from overdosage, particularly when small animals are treated with large animal formulations (Roder and Stair, 1998). Ivermectin has been safely used in humans for the treatment of onchocerciasis, filariasis due to *Wucheria bancrofti*, loiasis and strongyloidiasis (Aziz *et al.*, 1982; Cartel *et al.*, 1992; Diallo *et al.*, 1984; Kumuraswami *et al.*, 1988; Lariviere *et al.*, 1985; Naquira *et al.*, 1989; Richard-Lenoble *et al.*, 1988). Adverse reactions in humans to ivermectin are usually rare and generally mild (Burnham, 1993; Chippaux *et al.*, 1993; Guzzo *et al.*, 2002). Deaths have been reported after patients in a nursing home were treated for scabies (Barkwell and Shields, 1997), but these findings were not duplicated in a later study (Alexander *et al.*, 1998), and the patients had been treated with other potentially toxic drugs including lindane, crotamiton and psychoactive drugs (Burkhart *et al.*, 1997). The major adverse reaction to ivermectin in humans appears to be the Mazzoti reaction, caused by an immune response to dead parasites, possibly through the activation of neutrophilic granules (Ackerman *et al.*, 1990; Njoo *et al.*, 1993).

Ivermectin is neurotoxic and its mode of action appears to be through binding of the drug to glutamate-gated chloride channels leading to increased chloride ion permeability, and eventually to hyperpolarisation of nerve and muscle cells. It may also interfere with γ-aminobutyric acid (GABA) mediated transmission of nerve impulses; the overall consequence is paralysis and death of the parasite, the therapeutic aim of the drug (Dawson *et al.*, 2000; Martin, 1996; Schaeffer and Haines, 1989). It is not generally neurotoxic in mammals as the blood-brain barrier protects the central nervous system. However, ivermectin had been studied in toxicity tests using the CF_1 mouse. This strain is deficient in P-glycoprotein, a protein which is a constituent of cell membranes that determines their permeability (Didier and Loor, 1995; Laffont *et al.*, 2002; Sharom, 1997; Schinkel *et al.*, 1996). Hence, the CF_1 mouse, and neonatal animals, which are also deficient in P-glycoprotein, are more sensitive to the toxic effects of ivermectin, including its neurotoxic effects (Kwei *et al.*, 1999; Lankas and Gordon, 1989; Lankas *et al.*, 1997, 1998; Marques-Santos, 1999; Schinkel *et al.*, 1994; Skopets *et al.*, 1996; Umbenhauer *et al.*, 1997). This extra sensitivity is seen in acute toxicity, subchronic toxicity, reproductive toxicity and teratology studies with CF_1 mice, and for the teratology results in NOELs that are five to ten times lower than those noted with rats or rabbits (JECFA, 1993c). Some Collie dogs and Murray Grey cattle are also more sensitive to the toxic effects of ivermectin (Fassler *et al.*, 1991; Hopper *et al.*, 2002; Seaman *et al.*, 1987). This may be due to decreased P-glycoprotein or to increased permeability due to other concomitant drugs (Hopper *et al.*, 2002).

JECFA eventually established an ADI based on an NOEL from a reproductive study in CF_1 mice. It intended to use a very high safety factor in the calculation of the ADI because of the implications of the neurotoxic and other effects seen in animals, for health assessment in humans. However, because the data in humans treated with ivermectin were reassuring, and showed no evidence of neurotoxicity, the safety factor was reduced to 500. It later reconsidered this opinion in the light of further reassuring data from use in humans, and data to show that the drug produced developmental toxicity rather than being a frank teratogen. It also concluded that the CF_1 mouse was an extremely sensitive model. It continued to use the NOEL based on the data from the CF_1 mouse but reduced the safety factor to 100 (JECFA, 1993c). In evaluating other drugs in this class, doramectin, eprinomectin and moxidectin, JECFA based its decisions largely on neurotoxicity in dogs, and safety factors of 200. However, as more evidence became available on the safety of ivermectin in humans, the size of the safety factor used in the calculation of the ADI has been reduced to 100 (for eprinomectin).

A similar approach has been adopted by the CVMP in the EU where the extensive experience with ivermectin contributed to the decisions on the related compounds, including doramectin, eprinomectin, emamectin and moxidectin. With the latter compound, the safety factor was reduced after a re-evaluation. The Joint FAO/WHO Meeting on Pesticide Residues (JMPR), a body that reviews pesticide residues in a similar manner to the way that JECFA deals with veterinary drugs, concluded that the CF_1 mouse was an inappropriate model for studying the toxicity of avermectins and instead used an NOEL from a reproductive study in rats to establish the ADI for abamectin. However, because it recognised that rats are extremely sensitive to the reproductive effects of avermectins, it used a safety factor of only 50 in calculating the ADI (JMPR, 1998).

8.12 Tranquillisers: xylazine and azaperone

8.12.1 Xylazine

Xylazine is a veterinary tranquillising agent. It is a thiazine derivative structurally closely related to clonidine and it acts by stimulation of α_2-receptors in the nervous system. Its effects include strong sedation and respiratory depression and it is used in both small and large animal veterinary medicines (Bishop, 1998; Bongso, 1980; Hoffmann *et al.*, 2001). It can result in hypotension, coma and death in overdose in both animals and in humans (Arnbjerg, 1979; Carruthers *et al.*, 1979; Fyffe, 1994; Gallanosa *et al.*, 1981; Hoffmann *et al.*, 2001; Mittleman *et al.*, 1998; Samanta *et al.*, 1990; Spoerke *et al.*, 1986; van Metre, 1992).

JECFA concluded that one of the metabolites of xylazine might be genotoxic and carcinogenic and so was unable to calculate an ADI (JECFA, 1996d). However, the CVMP concluded that as the drug was given to small numbers of animals, and as these were unlikely to be sent for slaughter (as they had probably undergone surgery or other treatment), and in view of its extremely rapid metabolism and depletion of its residues, that no MRL was necessary, and that xylazine should be entered into Annex II of Council Regulation (EEC) No. 2377/90 (no MRL required to protect public health) for cattle and horses.

8.12.2 Azaperone

Azaperone is a tranquilliser used in both small and large animals, either alone or in combination with other drugs (Henrikson *et al.*, 1995; Lees and Serrano, 1976; Radcliffe *et al.*, 2000; Serrano and Lees, 1976; Still *et al.*, 1996). However, it is also used as a sedative for pigs during transport prior to slaughter; this use can prevent economic losses which otherwise arise from stress and aggressiveness (Callear and van Gestel, 1973; Symoens and van den Brande, 1969; Symoens, 1970). Such uses have given rise to concern over the possible presence of pharmacologically active residues in the pigs and their meat products at slaughter.

JECFA concluded that pharmacological effects, rather than toxicological effects were the most relevant from the point of view of safety assessment, and identified an NOEL based on neurobehavioural effects in dogs and a safety factor of 100 (JECFA, 1998b). The CVMP considered the dog to be a relatively insensitive model for the effects of azaperone and instead, concluded that norepinephrine antagonism in a rat study was more suitable, presumably because it gave a much lower NOEL. It then calculated an ADI based on a 100-fold safety factor.

8.13 Carazolol

Carazolol is a β-receptor blocking agent used in obstetrics in pigs and in the treatment of tachycardia in this species (Bishop, 1996; Kadir *et al.*, 1990; Mejean *et al.*, 1995). High, prolonged doses in pigs can result in cardiac failure and this has been suggested as an experimental model (Petzold *et al.*, 1999).

The pharmacological effects of carazolol were considered by JECFA to be more relevant for consumer safety assessment than the toxicological effects, and the Committee established a temporary ADI of 0.1 μg/kg body weight using an NOEL based on inhibition of isoprenaline-induced tachycardia in rabbits and a safety factor of 200. Later, data from human patients became available. These were patients with chronic bronchitis or asthma. JECFA considered these to be an extreme group and an NOEL of 0.5 μg/kg body weight was identified. An NOEL of 10 μg/kg body weight was identified for healthy subjects. JECFA concluded that a safety factor of 100 applied to the NOEL for healthy subjects was in accord with the previous NOEL derived from the rabbit study, and it offered an extra safety margin of five-fold for patients with respiratory disease (JECFA, 1995c). An identical ADI, using similar reasoning, was calculated by the CVMP.

Summary reports, which give brief details of the data considered by the CVMP and its opinion, can be found on the EMEA's website.

8.14 Conclusions

The examples reviewed above demonstrate many of the principles of safety assessment of veterinary drugs reviewed in the previous chapter. It is evident that a significant amount of subjective judgement is used in the evaluation of the scientific facts generated in safety studies, and that for some issues there is no clear scientific answer to a particular issue; instead the evaluation process is dependent on the views of both individuals and scientific committees involved, and their own rules of procedure. Despite this, it is significant that the resulting evaluations are often remarkably similar and may, for example, differ only in the quantitative value ascribed to MRL values. In general, the overall processes involved lead to convergences of opinions and what is perhaps surprising is not that different evaluations occur occasionally, but that they tend to be very much in agreement.

8.15 References

AARON CS, YU RL, HARBACH PR, MAZUREK JM, SWENSON DH, KIRKLAND D, MARSHALL R and MCENANEY S. (1995a). Comparative mutagenicity testing of Ceftiofur sodium: I. Positive results in in vitro cytogenetics. *Mutat Res*, **345**, 27–35.

AARON CS, YU RL, BACON JA, KIRKLAND D, MCENANEY S and MARSHALL R. (1995b). Comparative mutagenicity testing of Ceftiofur sodium II. Cytogenetic damage induced in vitro by ceftiofur is reversible and is due to cell cycle delay. *Mutat Res*, **345**, 37–47.

AARON CS, YU RL, JAGLAN PS, ROOF RD, HAMILTON C, SORG R, GUDI R and THILAGAR A. (1995c). Comparative mutagenicity testing of Ceftiofur sodium. III. Ceftiofur sodium is not an in vivo clastogen. *Mutat Res*, **345**, 49–56.

ABRAHAM EP. (1987). Cephalosporins 1945–1986. *Drugs*, **34** (Suppl. 2), 1–14.

ABRAMS SM, DEGNAN TJ and VINCIGUERRA V. (1980). Marrow aplasia following topical application of chloramphenicol eye ointment. *Arch Intern Med*, **140**, 576–577.

ACKERMAN SJ, KEPHART GM, FRANCIS H, AWADZI K, GLEICH GJ and OTTESTEN EA. (1990). Eosinophils deregulation. An immunologic determinant in the pathogenesis of the Mazotti reaction in human onchocerciasis. *J Immunol*, **144**, 3961–3969.

ADACHI T, KUWAMURA Y, FUJIWARA T, TANIMOTO N, NISHIMURA T, KOGUCHI A, KOBAYASHI K, SASAKI Y, YAMAGUCHI C, HONDA T, KAWASHIMA K, YUASA H, YAMAMURA T and INUI T. (2002). Twenty-six week carcinogenicity study of ampicillin in CB61 TgrasH2 mice. *J Toxicol Sci*, **27**, 147–163.

ADCOCK BB and RODMAN DP. (1996). Ampicillin-specific rashes. *Arch Fam Med*, **5**, 301–304.

AHLSTEDT S, EKSTROM B, SVARD PO, SJOBERG B, KRISTOFFERSON A and ORTEN B. (1980). New aspects on antigens to penicillin allergy. *Crit Rev Toxicol*, **7**, 219–277.

AISO K, KANISAWA M, OKAMOTO T, OKITA M and CHUJO T. (1966). Tylosin. Chronic oral toxicity of tylosin. *Nippon Eiseigaku Zasshi*, **20**, 383–397.

AKSOY M, ERDEM S, DINCOL G, BAKIOGLU I and KUTLAR A. (1984). Aplastic anaemia due to chemicals and drugs: a study of 108 patients. *Sex Transm Dis*, **11**, 347–350.

ALANIS A and WEINSTEIN AJ. (1983). Adverse reactions associated with the use of oral penicillins and cephalosporins. *Med Clin North Am.*, **67**, 113–129.

ALEXANDER NDE, BOCKARIE MJ, KASTENS WA, KAZURA JW and ALPERS MP. (1998). Absence of ivermectin-associated excess deaths. *Trans R Soc Trop Med Hyg*, **92**, 342.

AL-MOUDHIRY HAB. (1978). Aplastic anaemia in Iraq. A prospective study. *Haematologia*, **12**, 159–164.

ALTUNOK V, YAZAR E, ELMAS M, TRAS B, BAS AL and COL R. (2002). Investigation of the haematological and biochemical side effects of tilmicosin in healthy New Zealand rabbits. *J Vet Med B Infect Dis Vet Public Health*, **49**, 68–70.

ALVARO RF, WISLOCKI PG, MIWA GT and LU AY. (1992). Drug residue formation from ronidazole , a 5–nitroimidazole. VIII. Identification of the 2–methylene position as a site of protein alkylation. *Chem Biol Interact*, **82**, 21–30.

ANDERSON JA and ADKINSON, NF. (1987). Allergic reactions to drugs and biologic agents. *JAMA,* **258**, 2891–2899.

ANDERSON RC, WORTH HM, SMALL RM and HARRIS PN. (1966). Toxicological studies on tylosin: Its safety as a feed additive. *Food Cosmet Toxicol*, **4**, 1–15.

ANDO J, ISHIWARA R, IMAI S, TAKANO S, KITAMURA T, TAKAHASHI M, YOSHIDA M and MAEKAWA A. (1997). Thirteen-week subchronic toxicity study of thiamphenicol in F344 rats. *Toxicol Lett*, **91**, 137–146.

ANON. (1998). Commission Regulation (EC) No 2788/98 of 22 December 1998 amending Council Directive 70/524/EEC concerning additives in Feedingstuffs as regards the withdrawal of authorisation for certain growth promoters. *Official Journal of the European Union*, **L347**, 31–32.

ARIAS J, FERNANDEZ-RIVAS M and PANADERO P. (1995). Selective fixed skin eruption to amoxycillin. *Clin Exp Dermatol*, **20**, 339–340.

ARNBJERG J. (1979). Clinical manifestations of overdose of ketamine-xylazine in the cat. *Nord Vet Med*, **31**, 155–161.

ARNOLD D. (1990). EEC perspectives on relay toxicity and bioavailability studies. *Drug Metab Rev*, **22**, 699–705.

AUDICANA M, BERNAOLA G, URRUTIA I, ECHECHIPIA S, GASTAMINZA G, MUNOZ D, FERNANDEZ E and FERNANDEZ DE CORRES L. (1994). Allergic reactions to betalactams: studies in a group of patients allergic to penicillin and evaluation of cross-reactivity with cephalosporin. *Allergy*, **49**, 108–113.

AUJEZDSKA A, JINDRA J and JANOUSEK V. (1978). Influence of griseofulvin on the mouse fetal skeleton. *Cesk Hygiena*, **23**, 55–58.

AWAAD S, KHALIFA AS and KAMEL K. (1975). Vacuolization of leukocytes and bone-marrow aplasia due to chloramphenicol toxicity. *Clin Pediatr*, **14**, 499–506.

AZIZ MA, DIALLO S, DIOP IM, LARIVIERE M and PORTA M. (1982). Efficacy and tolerance of ivermectin in human onchocerciasis. *Lancet*, **ii**, 171–173.

BAER RL and LUDWIG JS. (1952). Allergic eczematous sensitization to neomycin. *Ann Allergy*, (March–April), 136–137.

BARBERA E and DE LA CUADRA J. (1989). Occupational airborne allergic contact dermatitis from tylosin. *Contact Dermatitis*, **20**, 308–309.

BARKWELL R and SHIELDS S. (1997). Deaths associated with ivermectin treatment in scabies. *Lancet*, **349**, 1144–1145.

BARZA M. (1978). The nephrotoxicity of cephalosporins: an overview. *J Infect Dis*, **137** (Suppl), S60–S73.

BAUMELOU E and NAJEAN Y. (1983). Why still prescribe chloramphenicol in 1983? *Blut*, **47**, 317–320.

BEAM TR and SPOONER J. (1984). Cross allergenicity between penicillins and cephalosporins. *Chemioterapia*, **3**, 390–393.

BECHTER R and SCHMID BP. (1987). Teratogenicity *in vitro* – a comparative study of four antimycotic drugs using the whole-embryo culture system. *Toxicol in Vitro*, **1**, 11–15.

BENESTAD HB. (1979). Drug mechanism in marrow aplasia. In Geary GC (ed.), *Aplastic Anaemia*, Balliere Tindall, London, 26–42.

BEUTIN L, PRELLER E and KOWALSKI B. (1981). Mutagenicity of quindoxin, its metabolites, and two substituted quinoxaline-di-N-oxides. *Antimicrob Agents Chemother*, **20**, 336–343.

BIGBY M, STERN RS and ARNDT KA. (1989). Allergic cutaneous reactions to drugs. *Prim Care*, **16**, 713–727.

BIRKHEAD HA, BRIGGS GB and SAUNDERS LZ. (1973). Toxicology of cefazolin in laboratory animals. *J Infect Dis*, **128** (Suppl), S379–S381.

BISHOP Y. (ed.). (1996). *The Veterinary Formulary*. British Veterinary Association and Royal Pharmaceutical Society, London.

BISHOP Y. (ed.). (1998). *The Veterinary Formulary*. Pharmaceutical Press, London.

BLACK, WDE. (1984). The use of antimicrobial drugs in agriculture. *Can J Physiol Pharmacol,* **62**, 1044–1048.

BLANCO M. (1994). The contribution of the side chain of penicillins in the induction of allergic reactions. *J Allergy Clin Immunol*, **94**, 562–563.

BOISSEAU J. (1990). Relay toxicity. *Drug Metab Rev*, **22**, 685–697.

BONGSO TA. (1980). Use of xylazine for transport of elephants by air. *Vet Rec*, **107**, 492.

BORRIE P and BARRET J. (1961). Dermatitis caused by penicillin in bulked milk samples. *BMJ*, **ii**, 1267.

BOTTIGER LE. (1979). Epidemiology and aetiology of aplastic anaemia. *Haematol Blood Transfus*, **24**, 27–37.

BOUDGHENE-STAMBOULI O and MERAD-BOUDIA A. (1989). Fixed drug eruption induced by griseofulvin. *Dermatologica*, **179**, 92–93.

BOURNER RD, PARRY EM and PARRY JM. (1998). Chemically induced aneuploidy: investigations into chromosome specific effects in mitosis. *Mutat Res*, **404**, 191–197.

BOYD EM. (1958). The acute oral toxicity of spiramycin. *Can J Biochem Physiol*, **36**, 103–110.

BOYD EM and BROWN TMD. (1958). The chronic subcutaneous toxicity of spiramycin adipate. *CMAJ*, **78**, 671–674.

BOYD EM and PRICE-JONES MA. (1960). The comparative oral acute toxicity of spiramycin adipate in mice, rats, guinea-pigs and rabbits. *Antibiot Chemother*, **10**, 273–284.

BOYD EM, JARZYLO S, BODY CE and CASSELL WA. (1958). The chronic oral toxicity of spiramycin in dogs. *Arch Int Pharmacodyn*, **CVX**, 360–371.

BOYD EM, COVERT EL and PITMAN CA. (1966). Benzylpenicillin toxicity in albino rats fed synthetic high sugar diets. *Chemotherapia,* **11**, 320–330.

BRANDER GC, PUGH DM and BYWATER RJ. (1982). *Veterinary and Applied Pharmacology and Therapeutics*, 4th edn. Ballière Tindall, London, 525–533.

BRANDRISS MW, RICHARDSON WS and BAROLD SS. (1994). Erythromycin-induced QT prolongation and polymorphic ventricular tachycardia (torsades de pointes): case report and review. *Clin Infect Dis*, **18**, 995–998.

BRAUER MJ and DAMESHEK W. (1967). Hypoplastic anemia and myeloblastic leukaemia following chloramphenicol therapy. Report of three cases. *New Engl J Med*, **277**, 1003–1005.

BRONSCH K, SCHNEIDER D and RIGAL-ANTONELLI F. (1976). Olaquindox – a new growth promoting feed additive. I. Effectiveness in raising piglets. *Z Tierphsiol Tierernahr Futtermittelelkd*, **36**, 211–221.

BRUMMETT RE. (1981a). Ototoxicity resulting from the combined administration of potent diuretics and other agents. *Scand Audiol* **14** (Suppl.), 214–224.

BRUMMETT RE. (1981b). Effects of antibiotic-diuretic interactions in the guinea-pig model of ototoxicity. *Rev Infect Dis.*, **3** (Suppl.), S216–S223.

BURKHART CN. (2000). Ivermectin: an assessment of its pharmacology, microbiology and safety. *Vet Hum Toxicol*, **42**, 30–35.

BURKHARDT JE, HILL MA, CARLTON WW and KESTERTON JW. (1990). Ultrastructural changes in articular cartilages of immature beagle dogs dosed with difloxacin, a fluoroquinolone. *Vet Pathol*, **29**, 230–238.

BURKHART KM, BURKHART CN and BURKHART CG. (1997). Comparing topical scabietic treatments will soon become extinct. *Arch Dermatol*, **133**, 1314.

BURNHAM GM. (1993). Adverse reactions to ivermectin treatment for onchocerciasis. Results of a placebo-controlled, double blind-trial in Malawi. *Trans R Soc Trop Med Hyg*, **87**, 313–317.

BURROWS GE. (1980). Aminocyclitol antibiotics. *J Am Vet Med Assoc*, **176**, 1289–1281.

BUSH LM, CALMON J and JOHNSON CC. (1995). Newer penicillins and beta-lactamase inhibitors. *Infect Dis Clin North Am*, **9**, 653–686.

CALLEAR JFF and VAN GESTEL JFE. (1973). An analysis of the results of field experiments in pigs in the UK and Eire with the combination-anaesthetic azaperone and metomidate. *Vet Rec*, **92**, 284–287.

CALNAN CD and SARKANY I. (1958). Contact dermatitis from neomycin. *Br J Dermatol*, **70**, 435–445.

CAMP KA, MIYAGI SL and SCHROEDER DJ. (1994). Potential quinolone-induced cartilage toxicity in children. *Ann Pharmacother*, **28**, 336–338.

CAMPBELL BA and COX SM. (1992). The penicillins. *Obstet Gynecol Clin North Am*, **19**, 435–447.

CAMPBELL WC and BENZ GW. (1984). Ivermectin: a review of efficacy and safety. *J Pharmacol Vet Ther*, **7**, 1–16.

CANY J. (1977). A hidden source of allergic reactions by sensitisation to penicillin; food pollution. *Rev Franc Allergol,* **17**, 133–136.

CAPEL-EDWARDS K, ATKINSON RM and PRATT DA. (1979). Toxicological studies on cefuroxime. *Toxicology*, **13**, 1–5.

CARAFFINI S, ASSALVE D, STINGENI L and LISI P. (1994). Tylosin, an airborne contact allergen in veterinarians. *Contact Dermatitis*, **31**, 327–328.

CARPENTER G. (1975). Chloramphenicol eye-drops and marrow aplasia. *Lancet,* **i**, 326–327.

CARRUTHERS SG, NELSON M, WEXLER HR and STILLER CR. (1979). Xylazine hydrochloride (Rompun) overdose in man. *Clin Toxicol*, **15**, 281–285.

CARTEL J-L, NGUYEN NL, MOULIA-PELAT J-P, PLICHART R, MARTIN PMV and SPIEGEL A. (1992). Mass chemoprophylaxis of lymphatic filariasis with a single dose of ivermectin in a polynesian community with a high *Wuchereria bancrofti* infection rate. *Trans R Soc Trop Med Hyg*, **86**, 537–540.

CHAMBERS HF and SANDE MA. (1996). Antimicrobial agents. The aminoglycosides. In

Hardman JG, Limbird LE, Molinoff PB, Ruddon RW, and Gilman AG (eds), *Goodman and Gilman's The Pharmacological Basis of Therapeutics*, 9th edn, McGraw-Hill, London, 1103–1121.

CHAPLIN S. (1986). Bone marrow depression due to mianserin, phenylbutazone, oxyphenazone and chloramphenicol – Part II. *Adverse Drug React Poisoning Rev*, **3**, 181–196.

CHIPPAUX, J-P, GARDON-WENDEL N, GARDON J and ERNOULD J-C. (1993). Absence of any adverse effect of inadvertent ivermectin treatment during pregnancy. *Trans R Soc Trop Med Hyg*, **87**, 318.

CHOPRA R, ROBERTS J and WARRINGTON RJ. (1989). Severe delayed-onset hypersensitivity reactions to amoxicillin in children. *CMAJ*, **140**, 921–926.

CHRIST W. (1991). Pharmacological properties of cephalosporins. *Infection*, **19** (Suppl 5), S244–S252.

CHRISTENSEN E, HERTZ H, RISKAER N and VRA-JENSEN, G (1951). Histological investigations in chronic streptomycin poisoning in guinea-pigs. *Ann Otol*, **60**, 343–349.

CIHAK R and SRB V. (1983). Cytogenetic effects of quinoxaline-1,4–dioxide-type growth promoting agents. I. micronucleus test in rats. *Mutat Res*, **116**, 129–135.

CIHAK R and VONTORKOVA M. (1983). Cytogenetic effects of quinoxaline-1,4–dioxide-type growth promoting agents. II. Metaphase analysis in mice. *Mutat Res*, **117**, 311–316.

CIHAK R and VONTORKOVA M. (1985). Cytogenetic effects of quinoxaline-1,4–dioxide-type growth promoting agents. III. Transplacental micronucleus test in rats. *Mutat Res*, **144**, 81–84.

COCKBURN A, MELLOWS, G, JACKSON D and WHITE DJ. (1985). Temocillin. Summary of safety studies. *Drugs*, **29** (Suppl. 5), 103–105.

COJOCEL C, GOTTSCHE U, TOLLE KL and BAUMANN K. (1988). Nephrotoxic potential of first-, second-, and third-generation cephalosporins. *Arch Toxicol*, **62**, 458–464.

CRAINE E. (1977). Relay toxicity studies: a modification of the relay toxicity approach. *J Toxicol Environ Health*, **2**, 905–907.

CRIST W, LEHERT T and ULBRICH B. (1988). Specific toxicologic aspects of the quinolones. *Rev Infect Dis*, **10** (Suppl), 141–146.

CROWN LA and SMITH RB. (1999). Accidental veterinary antibiotic injection into a farm worker. *Tenn Med,* **92**, 339–340.

CURRIE TT, HAYWARD NJ, WESTLAKE G and WILLIAMS J. (1971). Epilepsy in cardiopulmonary bypass patients receiving large intravenous doses of penicillin. *J Thorac Cardiovasc Surg*, **62**, 1–6.

CURRY PT, REED RN, MARTINO RM and KITCHIN RM. (1984). Induction of sister-chromatid exchanges in vivo in mice by the mycotoxins sterigmatocystin and griseofulvin. *Mutat Res*, **137**, 111–115.

DANESE P, ZANCA A and BERTAZZONI MG. (1994). Occupational contact dermatitis from tylosin. *Contact Dermatitis*, **30**, 122–123.

DAVE J, HEATHCOCK R, FENELON L, BIHARI DJ and SIMMONS NA. (1991). Cephalexin induced toxic epidermal necrolysis. *J Antimicrob Chemother*, **28**, 477–478.

DAVIES DM. (1991). *Textbook of Adverse Drug Reactions.* 4th edn., Oxford University Press, London, 51.

DAVIS, LE. (1984). Hypersensitivity reactions induced by antimicrobial drugs. *J Am Vet Med Assoc*, **185**, 1131–1136.

DAVIS RJ and PEPYS J. (1975). Asthma due to inhaled chemical agents – the macrolide antibiotic Spiramycin. *Clin Allergy*, **1**, 99–107.

DAWSON GR, WAFFORD KA, SMITH A, MARSHALL GR, BAYLEY PJ, SCHAEFFER JM, MEINKE PT and RM MCKERNAN. (2000). Anticonvulsant and adverse effects of avermectin analogues are mediated through the γ-aminobutyric $acid_A$ receptor. *J Pharmacol Exp Ther*, **295**, 1051–1060.

DAYAL VS, CHAIT GE and FENTON SS. (1979). Gentamicin vestibulotoxicity. Long term disability. *Ann Otol Rhinol Laryngol*, **88**, 36–39.

DAYAN AD. (1993). Allergy to antimicrobial residues in food: an assessment of the risk to man. *Vet Microbiol.*, **35**, 213–226.

DE ANGELIS I, ROSSI L, PEDERSEN JZ, VIGNOLI AL, VINCENTINI O, HOOGENBOOM LA, POLMAN TH, STAMMATI A and ZUCCO F. (1999). Metabolism of furazolidone: alternative pathways and modes of toxicity in different cell lines. *Xenobiotica*, **29**, 1157–1169.

DE CARLI L and LARIZZA L. (1988). Griseofulvin. *Mutat Res*, **195**, 91–126.

DE CARLI L, LARIZZA G, SIMONI G, DI LERNIA R and TREDICI F. (1973). Effect of griseofulvin on chromosomal complements of human diploid and heteroploid cell cultures. *Mutat Res*, **21**, 27–28.

DE HAAN P, BRUYNZEEL DP and VAN KETEL, WG. (1986). Onset of penicillin rashes: relation between type of penicillin administered and type of immune reactivity. *Allergy*, **41**, 75–78.

DELAGE C and IREY NS. (1972). Anaphylactic deaths. A clinical pathologic study of 43 cases. *J Forensic Sci*, **17**, 525–540.

DEL GIACCO GS, PETRINI MT, JANNELLI S and CARCASI U. (1981). Fatal bone marrow hypoplasia in a shepherd using chloramphenicol spray. *Lancet*, **i**, 945.

DE MATTEIS F, DONNELLY AJ and RUNGE WJ. (1966). The effect of prolonged administration of griseofulvin in mice with references to sex differences. *Cancer Res*, **26**, 721–726.

DE RENZO A, FORMISANO S and ROTOLI B. (1981). Bone marrow aplasia and thiamphenicol. *Haematologica*, **66**, 98–104.

DEWDNEY JM and EDWARDS RG. (1984). Penicillin hypersensitivity – is milk a significant hazard?: A review. *J R Soc Med*, **77**, 866–867.

DEWDNEY JM, MAES L, RAYNAUD JP, BLANC F, SCHEID JP, JACKSON T, LENS S and VERSCHEUREN C. (1991). Risk assessment of antibiotic residues of beta-lactams and macrolides in food products with regard to immuno-allergic potential. *Food Chem Toxicol*, **29**, 477–483.

DHAR HL and KULKARNI DN. (1994). Cross reactivity of cephalosporins with penicillin. *Indian J Physiol Pharmacol.*, **38**, 303–305.

DIALLO S, LARIVIERE M, DIOP-MAR I, N'DIR O, N'DIAYE R, BADIANE S, PORTA M and AZIZ M. (1984). Conduct in Senegal of first studies on efficacy and safety of ivermectin (MK 993) in human onchocerciasis. *Bull Soc Pathol Exot Filiales*, **77**, 196–205.

DIDIER AD and LOOR F. (1995). Decreased biotolerability for ivermectin and cyclosporin A in mice exposed to potent P-glycoprotein inhibitors. *Int J Cancer*, **63**, 263–267.

DUBOST P, DUCROT R and KOLSKY M. (1956). Chronic toxicity and local tolerance of spiramycin. *Therapie*, **ii**, 329–336.

DUNNICK JK, EUSTIS SL, HUFF JE and HASEMAN JK. (1989). Two-year toxicity and carcinogenicity studies of ampicillin trihydrate and penicillin VK in rodents. *Fundam Appl Toxicol*, **12**, 252–257.

EGAWA Y. (1994). Use of patch-scratch tests to determine penicillin and cephalosporins allergies. *Nippon Ika Daigaku Zasshi*, **61**, 389–404.

EPSTEIN S. (1956). Contact dermatitis from neomycin due to dermal delayed (tuberculin-type) sensitivity. Report of 10 cases. *Dermatologica*, **113**, 191–201.

EPSTEIN S. (1965). Neomycin sensitivity and atopy. *Dermatologica*, **130**, 280–286.

EPSTEIN S and WENZEL FJ. (1962). Cross-sensitivity to various 'mycins'. *Arch Dermatol*, **86**, 183–194.

EPSTEIN SS, ANDREA J, JOSHI S and MANTEL N. (1967). Hepatocarcinogenicity of griseofulvin following parenteral administration to infant mice. *Cancer Res*, **27**, 1900–1906.

ERFFMEYER, JE. (1981). Adverse reactions to penicillin. *Ann Allergy*, **47**, 294–300.

ERFFMEYER, JE. (1986). Penicillin allergy. *Clin Rev Allergy*, **4**, 171–188.

ERLANSON P and LUNDGREN A. (1964). Ototoxic side effects following treatment with streptomycin, dihydrostreptomycin, and kanamycin. Connection with dosage and renal function; preventative medicine. *Acta Med Scand,* **176**, 147–163.

ERNST A, REUTER G, ZIMMERMAN U and ZENNEER HP. (1994). Acute gentamicin ototoxicity in cochlear cells of the guinea pig. *Brain Res*, **636**, 153–156.

ERSKINE D. (1958). Dermatitis caused by penicillin in milk. *Lancet*, **i**, 431–432.

ESPOSTI G, ESPOSTI D, GUERINO G, BICIIISAO E and FRASCHINI F. (1986). Effects of cephacetrile on reproduction cycle. *Arzneimittelforschung*, **36**, 484–486.

FAHMY MA and HASSAN NH. (1996). Cytogenetic effects of griseofulvin in mouse spermatocytes. *J Appl Toxicol*, **16**, 177–183.

FARRAR HC, WALSH-SUKYS MC, KYLLONEN K and BLUMER JL. (1993). Cardiac toxicity associated with intravenous erythromycin lactobionate: two case reports and a review of the literature. *Pediatr Infect Dis*, **12**, 688–691.

FASSLER PE, TRANQUILLI WJ, PAUL AJ, SOLL MD, DIPIETRO JA and TODD KS. (1991). Evaluation of the safety of ivermectin in beef-based formulation to ivermectin-sensitive Collies. *J Am Vet Med Assoc*, **199**, 457–460.

FEKETY FR. (1990). Safety of parenteral third-generation cephalosporins. *Am J Med*, **88** (Suppl 4A), 4A-38S–4A-44S.

FELLNER MJ. (1976). Penicillin allergy 1976: a review of reactions, detection and current management. *Int J Dermatol*, **15**, 497–504.

FELLNER M. (1986). Adverse reactions to penicillin and related drugs. *Clin Dermatol*, **4**, 133–141.

FERRANDO R and TRUHAUT R. (1982). General aspects of relay toxicity: its applications. *Toxicol Europ Res*, **IV**, 221–228.

FERRANDO R, TRUHAUT R and RAYNAUD J-P. (1977). Principles of a full relay toxicity experiment and results conducted with carbadox a feed additive used as a growth promoter for growing swine. *Folia Vet Lat*, **7**, 333–340.

FERRANDO R, TRUHAUT R, RAYNAUD J-P and SPANOGUE J-P. (1978). Relay toxicity III. Safety in use for the human consumer of carbadox, a feed additive for swine, as estimated by a 7 year relay toxicity on dogs. *Toxicology*, **11**, 167–183.

FESTING MFW, DIAMANTI P and TURTON JA. (2001). Strain differences in haematological response to chloramphenicol succinate in mice: implications for toxicological research. *Food Chem Toxicol*, **39**, 375–383.

FILLASTRE JP, MOULIN B and JOSSE S. (1989). Aetiology of nephrotoxic damage to the renal interstitium and tubuli. *Toxicol Lett*, **46**, 45–54.

FLEMING A. (1946). Introduction. In Fleming A (ed.), *Penicillin*, Butterworth, London, 1–23.

FORNI A and VIGLIANI EC. (1974). Chemical leukemogenesis in man. *Ser Haematol*, **7**, 211–213.

FOTI C, BONAMONTE D, TRENTI R, VENA GA and ANGELINI G. (1997). Occupational contact allergy to cephalosporins. *Contact Dermatitis*, **36**, 104–105.

FRAUMENI JF. (1967). Bone-marrow depression induced by chloramphenicol or phenylbutazone. *JAMA*, **201**, 150–156.

FRAUNFELDER ET and BAGBY GC. (1982). Fatal aplastic anemia following topical administration of ophthalmic chloramphenicol. *Am J Ophthalmol*, **93**, 356–360.

FRAZIER JM. (1990). Application of the basic toxicological screening process to problems in bound residue toxicity. *Drug Metab Rev*, **22**, 821–827.

FROHLI P, GRAF CH and RHYNER K. (1984). Thiamphenicol induced bone marrow suppression as a therapy of myeloproliferative diseases. *Blut*, **49**, 457–463.

FULLERTON FR, KUSHMAUL RJ, SUBER RL and LITTLEFIELD NA. (1987). Influence of oral administration of sulfamethazine on thyroid hormone levels in Fischer 344 rats. *J Toxicol Environ Health*, **22**, 175–185.

FYFFE JJ. (1994). Effects of xylazine on humans: a review. *Aust Vet J*, 294–295.

GADNER H, GETHMANN U, JESSENBERGER K and RIEHM H. (1973). Acute leukaemia following exposure to chloramphenicol? Three case reports and review of the literature. *Monatsschr Kinderheilk*, **121**, 590–594.

GAILIUNAS P, DOMINGUEZ-MORENO M, LAZARUS M, LOWRIE EG AND GOTTLIEB MN and MERRILL JP. (1978). Vestibular toxicity of gentamicin. Incidence in patients receiving long-term haemodialysis therapy. *Arch Intern Med*, **138**, 1621–1624.

GALER DM and MONRO AM. (1998a). Veterinary drugs no longer need testing for carcinogenicity in rodent bioassays. *Regul Toxicol Pharmacol*, **28**, 115–123.

GALER DM and MONRO AM. (1998b). Evaluation of the toxicity of drug residues in food: the case for 'relay' toxicity studies. *Food Add Contam*, **15**, 494–500.

GALLAND MC, RODOR F and JOUGLARD J. (1987). Spiramycin and allergic toxidermy-like vasculitis. *Therapie*, **42**, 227–229.

GALLANOSA AG, SPYKER DA, SHIPE JR and MORRIS DL. (1981). Human xylazine overdose: A comparative review with clonidine, phenothiazines, and tricyclic antidepressants. *Clin Toxicol*, **18**, 663–678.

GALLO-TORRES H. (1977). Methodology for the determination of bioavailability of labelled residues. *J Toxicol Environ Health*, **2**, 827–845.

GALLO-TORRES H. (1990). The rat as a drug residue bioavailability model. *Drug Metab Rev*, **22**, 707–751.

GASTAMINZA G, AUDICANA MT, FERNANDEZ E, ANDA M and ANSOTEGUI IJ. (2000). *Allergy*, **55**, 510–511.

GELLER RJ, CHEVALIER RL and SPYKER DA. (1986). Acute amoxicillin nephrotoxicity following an overdose. *J Toxicol Clin Toxicol*, **24**, 175–182.

GENDREL D and MOULIN F. (2001). Fluoroquinolones in paediatrics. *Paediatr Drugs*, **3**, 365–377.

GENTRY LO. (1992). Therapy with newer oral beta-lactam and quinolones agents for infections of the skin and skin structures: A review. *Clin Infect Dis*, **14**, 285–297.

GEORGE DK and CRAWFORD DHG. (1996). Antibacterial-induced hepatotoxicity. Incidence, prevention and management. *Drug Saf*, **15**, 79–85.

GERBER AU and CRAIG WA. (1981). Worldwide clinical experience with cefoperazone. *Drugs*, **22** (Suppl 1), 108–118.

GETTE MT, MARKS JG and MALONEY ME. (1992). Frequency of postoperative allergic contact dermatitis to topical antibiotics. *Arch Dermatol*, **128**, 365–367.

GHADIALLY R and RAMSAY CA. (1988). Gentamicin: systemic exposure to a contact allergen. *J Am Acad Dermatol* **19**, 428–430.

GILLICK A and BULMER WS. (1972). Griseofulvin, a possible teratogen. *Can Vet J*, **13**, 244.

GIRARD JP. (1978). Recurrent angioneurotic oedema and contact dermatitis due to penicillin. *Contact Dermatitis*, **4**, 309.

GLUCKMAN E, VEYSSIER P, SULTAN C and DREYFUS B. (1971). Adverse effects on the blood of thiamphenicol. Report of 3 cases of aplastic anemia. *Presse Med*, **79**, 1385–1388.

GOH CL. (1989). Contact sensitivity to topical medicaments. *Int J Dermatol*, **28**, 25–28.

GOLLINS WJF. (1989). Occupational asthma to tylosin tartrate. *Br J Ind Med*, **46**, 894.

GOODMAN EJ, MORGAN MJ, JOHNSON PA, NICHOLS BA, DENK N and GOLD BB. (2001). Cephalosporins can be given to penicillin-allergic patients who do not exhibit an anaphylactic response. *Clin Anesth*, **13**, 561–564.

GRANT WF. (1982). Chromosome aberration in Alium. A report of the US Environmental Protection Agency. *Mutat Res.*, **99**, 273–291.

GRASSI GG. (1995). Pharmacology and toxicology of oral cephalosporins. *Antibiot Chemother*, **47**, 8–33.

GREENBERG LH and MOMARY H. (1965). Audiotoxicity and nephrotoxicity due to orally administered neomycin. *JAMA*, **194**, 827–828.

GREENE CE and BUDSBERG SC. (1993). Veterinary use of quinolones. In Hooper DC and Wolfson JS (eds), *Quinolone Antimicrobial Agents*, American Society for Microbiology, Washington, DC, 473–488.

GRIFFITH RS and BLACK HR. (1970). Cephalexin. *Med Clin North Am*, **54**, 1229–1244.

GRISHAM LM, WILSON L and BENSCH KG. (1973). Antimitotic action of griseofulvin does not involve disruption of microtubules. *Nature*, **244**, 294–296.

GRUFFYDD-JONES TJ and WRIGHT AI. (1977). Deformed kittens. *Vet Rec*, **100**, 206.

GUEST GB and FITZPATRICK SC. (1990). Overview on bound residue issue – regulatory aspects. *Drug Metab Rev*, **22**, 595–599.

GUSTAFERRO CA and STECKELBERG JM. (1991). Cephalosporin antimicrobial agents and related compounds. *Mayo Clin Proc*, **66**, 1064–1073.

GUZZO CA, FURTEK CI, PORRAS AG, CHEN C, TIPPING R, CLINESCHMIDT CM, SCIBBERAS DG, HSIEH JY-K and LASSETER KC. (2002). Safety, tolerability and pharmacokinetics of escalating high doses of ivermectin in healthy adult subjects. *J Clin Pharmacol*, **42**, 1122–1133.

HALPERN EB and HELLER MF (1961). Ototoxicity of orally administered neomycin. *Arch Ototlaryngol*, **73**, 675–677.

HANNUKSELA M, SUHONEN R and FORSTROM L. (1981). Delayed contact dermatitis in patients with photosensitivity dermatitis. *Acta Derm Venereol*, **61**, 303–306.

HATTORI H, YAMAGUCHI F, WAGAI N, KATO M and NOMURA M. (1997). An assessment of antigenic potential of beta-lactam antibiotics, low molecular weight drugs, using guinea pig models. *Toxicology*, **123**, 149–160.

HAUSMAN K and SKRANDIES G. (1974). Aplastic anaemia following chloramphenicol therapy in Hamburg and surrounding districts. *Postgrad Med J*, **50**, 136–142.

HAUTEKEETE ML. (1995). Hepatotoxicity of antibiotics. *Acta Gastroenterol Belg*, **LVIII**, 290–296.

HAWKINS JE and LURIE MH. (1953). The ototoxicity of dihydrostreptomycin and neomycin in the cat. *Ann Otol Rhinol Laryngol*, **62**, 1128–1148.

HAYEM G and CARBON C. (1995). A reappraisal of quinolone tolerability. The experience of the musculoskeletal effects. *Drug Saf*, **13**, 338–342.

HEATH JE and LITTLEFIELD NA. (1984a). Effects of subchronic oral sulfamethazine administration on Fischer 344 rats and B6C3F1 mice. *J Environ Pathol Toxicol Oncol*, **5**, 201–214.

HEATH JE and LITTLEFIELD NA. (1984b). Morphological effects of subchronic oral sulfamethazine administration on Fischer 344 rats and B6C3F1 mice. *Toxicol Pathol*, **12**, 3–9.

HEDDLE JA, HITE M, KIRKHART B, MAVOURIN K, MACGREGOR JT, NEWELL GW and SALAMONE MF. (1983). The induction of micronuclei as a measure of genotoxicity. A report of the US Environmental Protection Gene-Tox Program. *Mutat Res*, **123**, 61–118.

HEIMANN G. (1983). Renal toxicity of aminoglycosides in the neonatal period. *Pediatr Pharmacol.*, **3**, 251–257.

HELLRIEGEL KP and CROSS R. (1974). Follow-up studies in chloramphenicol-induced aplastic anaemia. *Postgrad Med J*, **50** (Suppl 5), 136–142.

HENRIKSON H, JENSEN-WAERN M and MYMAN G. (1995). Anaesthetics for general anaesthesia in growing pigs. *Acta Vet Scand*, **36**, 401–411.

HERBERT ME, BREWSTER GS and LANCTOT-HERBERT M. (2000). Ten percent of patients who are allergic to penicillin will have serious reactions if exposed to cephalosporins. *West J Med*, **172**, 341.

HERMAN R and JICK H. (1979). Cutaneous reaction rates to penicillins oral versus parenteral. *Cutis*, **24**, 232–234.

HEROLD M, OLTMANNS G, DUCK HJ and MARU M. (1983). Severe cutaneous drug reactions: case reports. *Ethiop Med J*, **21**, 227–232.

HEWITT WL. (1974). Gentamicin: toxicity in perspective. *Postgrad Med J*, (Suppl 7), 55–59.

HILL RN, CRISP TM, HURLEY PM, ROSENTHAL SL and SINGH DV. (1996). Thyroid follicular cell carcinogenesis. *Fundam Appl Toxicol.*, **12**, 627–697.

HILL RN, CRISP TM, HURLEY PM, ROSENTHAL SL and SINGH DV. (1998). Risk assessment of thyroid follicular cell tumors. *Environ Health Perspect*, **106**, 447–457.

HODGES GR, WATANABE IS, SINGER P, RENGACHARY S, BRUMMETT RE, REEVES D, JUSTESEN DR, WORLEY SE and GEPHARDT EP. (1985). Ototoxicity of intraventricularly administered gentamicin in adult rabbits. *Res Commun Chem Pathol Pharmacol*, **50**, 337–347.

HODGKINSON R. (1971). Infectious hepatitis and aplastic anaemia. *Lancet*, **i**, 1014.

HOFFMAN DR, HUDSON P, CARLYLE SJ and MASSELLO W. (1989). *Ann Allergy*, **62**, 91–93.

HOFFMANN U, MEISTER CM, GOLLE K and ZSCHIESCHE M. (2001). Severe intoxication with the veterinary tranquilizer xylazine in humans. *J Anal Toxicol*, **25**, 245–249.

HOGAN DJ and ROONEY ME. (1987). Toxic epidermal necrolysis due to cephalexin. *J Am Acad Dermatol*, **17**, 852–853.

HOLDER JM and SINCLAIR AN. (1972). Carbadox: a new feed additive for pigs. *Aust Vet J*, **48**, 579.

HOLLOWAY WJ. (1982). Spectinomycin. *Med Clin North Am*, **66**, 169–173.

HOLT D, HARVEY D and HURLEY R. (1993). Chloramphenicol toxicity. *Adv Drug React Toxicol Rev*, **12**, 83–95.

HOLT DE, RYDER TA, FAIRBAIRN A, HURLEY R and HARVEY D. (1997). The myelotoxicity of chloramphenicol *in vitro* and *in vivo* studies: I. *In vitro* effects on cells in culture. *Hum Exp Toxicol*, **16**, 570–576.

HOLT DE, ANDREWS CM, PAYNE JP, WILLIAMS TC and TURTON JA. (1998). The myelotoxicity of chloramphenicol *in vitro* and *in vivo* studies: II. *In vivo* myelotoxicity in the $B6C3F_1$ mouse. *Hum Exp Toxicol*, **17**, 8–17.

HOOGENBOOM LAP. (1991). The use of pig hepatocytes for biotransformation and toxicity studies. Thesis, Landbouwuniversiteit te Wageningen, Netherlands.

HOOGENBOOM LAP, BERGHMANS MC, POLMAN TH, PARKER R and SHAW IC. (1992). Depletion of protein-bound furazolidone metabolise containing the 3-amino-2-oxazolidinone side-chain from liver, kidney and muscle tissues from pigs. *Food Addit Contam*, **9**, 623–630.

HOOGENBOOM LAP, POLMAN TH, LOMMEN A, HUVENEERS MB and VAN RHIJN J. (1994). Biotransformation of furaltadone by pig hepatocytes and *Salmonella typhimurium* TA 100 bacteria, and the formation of protein bound metabolites. *Xenobiotica*, **24**, 713–727.

HOOPER DC and WOLFSON JS. (1993). Adverse effects. In Hooper DC and Wolfson JS (eds), *Quinolone Antimicrobial Agents*, American Society for Microbiology, Washington, DC, 489–512.

HOPPER K, ALDRICH J and HASKINS SC. (2002). Ivermectin toxicity in 17 collies. *J Vet Intern Med*, **16**, 89–94.

HOUDESHELL JW, LAMENDOLA JF and MCCRACKEN JS. (1982). Clinical pharmacology of aminoglycosides. *Mod Vet Pract*, **63**, 707–710.

HUMPHRIES KR. (1968). Acute myelomonocytic leukaemia following chloramphenicol therapy. *N Z Med J*, **68**, 248–249.

IARC. (1974). IARC Monographs on the evaluation of the carcinogenic risk of chemicals to man: Some naturally occurring substances, **10**, 153–161.

IARC. (2002). IARC Monographs on the evaluation of the carcinogenic risk of chemicals to humans, **79**, 291–315.

IDSOE O, GUTHE T, WILCOX RR and DE WECK AL. (1968). Nature and extent of penicillin side-reactions, with particular reference to fatalities from anaphylactic shock. *Bull World Health Organ*, **38**, 159–188.

IGEA JM, FRAJ J, DAVILA I, CUEVAS M, CUESTA J and HINOJOSA M. (1992). Allergy to cefazolin: study of in vivo cross reactivity with other betalactams. *Ann Allergy*, **68**, 515–519.

INOUE H, BABA H, AWANO K and YOSHIKAWA K. (1995). Genotoxic effect of griseofulvin in somatic cells of Drosophila melanogaster. *Mutat Res*, **343**, 229–234.

ISSARAGRISIL S and PIANKIJAGUM A. (1985). Aplastic anaemia following topical administration of ophthalmic chloramphenicol: report of a case and review of the literature. *J Med Assoc Thai*, **88**, 309–312.

JAGLAN PS, GLENN MW and NEFF AW. (1977). Experiences in dealing with drug-related bound residues. *J Toxicol Environ Health*, **2**, 815–826.

JECFA. (1988). Chloramphenicol. Toxicological evaluation of certain veterinary drug residues in food, WHO Food Additives Series 23, WHO, Geneva, 1–71.

JECFA. (1990). Evaluation of certain veterinary drug residues in food. Thirty-sixth report of the Joint FAO/WHO Expert Committee on Food Additives. Technical Report Series 799, WHO, Geneva.

JECFA. (1991a). Benzylpenicillin. Toxicological evaluation of certain veterinary drug residues in food, WHO Food Additives Series 27, WHO, Geneva, 105–116.

JECFA. (1991b). Spiramycin. Toxicological evaluation of certain veterinary drug residues in food, WHO Food Additives Series 29, WHO, Geneva, 109–138.

JECFA. (1991c). Evaluation of certain veterinary drug residues in food. Thirty-eighth report of the Joint FAO/WHO Expert Committee on Food Additives. Technical Report Series 815, WHO, Geneva.

JECFA. (1991d). Ivermectin. Toxicological evaluation of certain veterinary drug residues in food, WHO Food Additives Series 27, WHO, Geneva, 27–73.

JECFA. (1993a). Furazolidone. Toxicological evaluation of certain veterinary drug residues. WHO Food Additives Series 31. International programme on Chemical Safety, WHO, Geneva, 85–123.

JECFA. (1993b). Nitrofural. Toxicological evaluation of certain veterinary drug residues. WHO Food Additives Series 31. International programme on Chemical Safety, WHO, Geneva, 125–145.

JECFA. (1993c). Ivermectin. Toxicological evaluation of certain veterinary drug residues in food, WHO Food Additives Series 31, WHO, Geneva, 23–36.

JECFA. (1994). Spectinomycin. Toxicological evaluation of certain veterinary drug residues in food, WHO Food Additives Series 33, WHO, Geneva, 59–89.

JECFA. (1995a). Evaluation of certain veterinary drug residues in food. Forty-third report of the Joint FAO/WHO Expert Committee on Food Additives. Technical Report Series 855, WHO, Geneva.

JECFA. (1995b). Sulfadimidine. Toxicological evaluation of certain veterinary drug residues. WHO Food Additives Series 33. International programme on Chemical Safety, WHO, Geneva, 91–103.

JECFA. (1995c). Carazolol. Toxicological evaluation of certain veterinary drug residues. WHO Food Additives Series 34. International programme on Chemical Safety, WHO, Geneva, 3–7.

JECFA. (1996a). Ceftiofur. Toxicological evaluation of certain veterinary drug residues in food, WHO Food Additives Series 36, WHO, Geneva, 61–84.

JECFA. (1996b). Evaluation of certain veterinary drug residues in food. Forty-fifth report of the Joint FAO/WHO Expert Committee on Food Additives. Technical Report Series 864, WHO, Geneva.

JECFA. (1996c). Tilmicosin. Toxicological evaluation of certain veterinary drug residues in food, WHO Food Additives Series 38, WHO, Geneva, 109–130.

JECFA. (1996d). Xylazine. Toxicological evaluation of certain veterinary drug residues. WHO Food Additives Series 38. International programme on Chemical Safety, WHO, Geneva, 45–75.

JECFA. (1998a). Evaluation of certain veterinary drug residues in food. Forty-seventh report of the Joint FAO/WHO Expert Committee on Food Additives. Technical Report Series 876, WHO, Geneva.

JECFA. (1998b). Azaperone. Toxicological evaluation of certain veterinary drug residues. WHO Food Additives Series 41. International programme on Chemical Safety, WHO, Geneva, 149–152.

JECFA. (2000). Thiamphenicol. Toxicological evaluation of certain veterinary drug residues in food, WHO Food Additives Series 43, WHO, Geneva, 7–12.

JECFA. (2002a). Cefuroxime. Toxicological evaluation of certain veterinary drug residues in food, WHO Food Additives Series 49, WHO, Geneva, 27–62.

JECFA. (2002b). Evaluation of certain veterinary drug residues in food. Fifty-eighth report of the Joint FAO/WHO Expert Committee on Food Additives. Technical Report Series 911, WHO, Geneva.

JICK H and DERBY LE. (1995). A large population-based follow-up study of trimethoprim-sulphamethoxazole, trimethoprim, and cephalexin for uncommon serious drug toxicity. *Pharmacotherapy*, **15**, 428–432.

JICK S. (1997). Ciprofloxacin safety in a paediatric population. *Pediatr Infect Dis J*, **16**, 130–133.

JIMINEZ I, ANTON E, PICANS I, SANCHEZ I, QUINONES MD and JEREZ J. (1997). Fixed drug eruption from amoxycillin. *Allergol Immunopathol*, **25**, 247–248.

JMPR. (1998). Pesticide residues in food – 1997. Evaluations 1997. Part II. Toxicological and Environmental. International Programme on Chemical Safety, WHO, Geneva, 3–19.

JOHNSON AH. (1971). Antibiotic toxicity. *J S C Med Assoc*, **67**, 351–352.

JONES KH and HILL SA. (1974). The toxicology, absorption and pharmacokinetics of amoxicillin. *Adv Clin Pharmacol*, **7**, 20–27.

JORDAN WH, BYRD RA, COCHRANE RL, HANASOMO GK, HOYT JA, MAIN MS, MEYERHOFF RD and SARAZAN RD. (1993). A review of the toxicology of the antibiotic Micotil 300. *Vet Hum Toxicol*, **35**, 151–158.

JUNG HD. (1983). Occupationally-induced contact eczema by tylosin (Tylan). *Dermatol Monatsschr*, **169**, 235–237.

KADIR F, ZUIDEMA J, PIJPERS A, MELENDEZ R, VULTO A and VERHEIJDEN JHM. (1990). Pharmacokinetics of intravenously, intramuscularly and intra-adiposely administered carazolol in pigs. *J Vet Pharmacol Ther*, **13**, 350–355.

KALTWASSER JP, WERNER E, SIMON B, BELLENBERG U and BECKER HJ. (1974). The effect of thiamphenicol on normal and activated erythropoieis in the rabbit. *Postgrad Med J*, **50** (Suppl 5), 118–122.

KALWEIT S, UTESCH D, VON DER HUDE and MADLE S. (1999). Chemically induced micronucleus formation in V79 – cells comparison of three different test approaches. *Mutat Res*, **439**, 183–190.

KAPPEL EM, SHAKIBAEI M, BELLO A and STAHLMAN R. (2002). Effects of the Des-F(6)-quinolone garenoxacin (BMS-284756) in comparison to those of ciprofloxacin and ofloxacin, on joint cartilage in immature rats. *Antimicrob Agents Chemother*, **46**, 3320–3322.

KAPUSNIK-UNER JE, SANDE MA and CHAMBERS HF. (1996). Antimicrobial agents. Tetracyclines, chloramphenicol, erythromycin, and miscellaneous antibacterial agents. In Hardman JG, Limbird LE, Molinoff PB, Ruddon RW, and Gilman AG (eds), *Goodman and Gilman's The Pharmacological Basis of Therapeutics*, 9th edn, McGraw-Hill, London, 1123–1153.

KASHIDA Y and KATO M. (1997). Characterization of fluoroquinolone-induced Achilles tendon toxicity in rats: Comparison of toxicities of 10 fluoroquinolones and effects of anti-inflammatory compounds. *Antimicrob Agents Chemother*, **41**, 2389–2393.

KAUTZ HD. (1959). Penicillin and other antibiotics in milk. *JAMA*, **171**, 135–137.

KEISER G and BUCHEGGER U. (1973). Haematological side effects of chloramphenicol and thiamphenicol. *Helv Med Acta*, **37**, 265–278.

KELMAR PS and LI T-C. (2001). Cephalosporin allergy. *New Engl J Med*, **345**, 804–809.

KERSTEN B, ZHANG J, BRENDLER-SCHWAAB SY, KASPER P and MULLER L. (1999). The application of the micronucleus test in Chinese hamster cell to detect drug-induced photogenotoxicity. *Mutat Res*, **445**, 55–71.

KHOORY BJ, FANOS V, DALL'AGNOLA A and CATALDI L. (1996). Aminoglycosides, risk factors and neonatal kidney. *Pediatr Med Chir*, **18**, 495–499.

KIRKLAND D. (1998). Chromosome aberration testing in genetic toxicology past, present and future. *Mutat Res*, **404**, 173–185.

KIRSCH-VOLDERS M, VANHAUWAERT A, EICHENLAUB-RITTER U and DECORDIER I. (2003). Indirect mechanisms of genotoxicity, *Toxicol Lett*, **140–141**, 63–74.

KITAMURA T, ANDO J, ISHIHARA R, TAKANO S, IJIMA T, NISHIMURA S, YOSHIDA M, TAKAHASHI M and MAEKAWA A. (1997). Lack of carcinogenicity of thiamphenicol in F344 rats. *Food Chem Toxicol*, **35**, 1075–1080.

KLEE S, BAUMUNG I, KLUGE K, UNGEMACH, FR, HORNE E, O'KEEFE M, DE ANGELIS I, VIGNOLI AL, ZUCCO F and STAMMATI A. (1999). A contribution to safety assessment of veterinary drug residues: *in vivo/ex vivo* studies on the intestinal toxicity and transport of covalently bound residues. *Xenobiotica*, **29**, 641–654.

KLEIN MF and BEALL JR. (1972). Griseofulvin: a teratogenic study. *Science*, **175**, 1483–1484.

KLEIN NC and CUNHA BA. (1995). The selection and use of cephalosporins: A review. *Adv Therap*, **12**, 83–101.

KNASMULLER S, PARZEFALL W, HELMA C, KASSIE F, ECKER S and SCHULTE-HERMANN R. (1997). Toxic effects of Griseofulvin: Disease models, mechanisms, and risk assessment. *Crit Rev Toxicol*, **27**, 495–537.

KOJIMA T, HASEWAGA T, ISHIDA H, FUJITA M and OKAMOTO S. (1988). Griseofulvin-induced photodermatitis – a report of six cases. *J Dermatol*, **15**, 76–82.

KOLACHANA P and SMITH MT. (1994). Induction of kinetochore-positive micronuclei in human lymphocytes by the anti-fungal drug griseofulvin. *Mutat Res*, **322**, 151–159.

KORNBRUST D, EYDELLOTH R and GARRATTY G. (1989). Investigations of the potential for 5 beta-lactam antibiotics to elicit type II hypersensitivity reactions in rats and monkeys. *Fundam Appl Toxicol*, **12**, 558–566.

KORNEGAY ET, DAVIS JW and THOMAS HR. (1968). Evaluation of carbadox in prevention of swine dysentery. *Vet Med Small Anim Clin*, **63**, 1076–1077.

KORTING GW and KIFLE H. (1985). Systemic side-effects from external application of chloramphenicol. *Hautarzt*, **36**, 181–183.

KRADOLFER F, SACKMANN W, ZAK O, BRUNNER H, HESS R, KONOPOKA EA and GELZER J. (1974). Cephacetrile: chemotherapy and toxicology in laboratory animals. *Arzneim Forsch*, **24**, 1459–1462.

KRAKOFF IH, KARNOFSKY DA and BURCHENAL JH. (1955). Effects of large doses of chloramphenicol on human subjects. *New Engl J Med*, **253**, 7–10.

KRISTOFFERSON A and AHLSTEDT S. (1982). Mice do not respond with delayed hypersensitivity to penicillin derived determinants. *Immunology*, **45**, 537–543.

KUBO K, NAGATAHIRA R, YOSHIDA J, OKUDA T, YOSHINAKA I and KURIYAMA K. (1989). Penicillin G-induced cutaneous anaphylaxis in the guinea pig. *J Toxicol Sci.*, **14**, 269–277.

KUCZUK MH, BENSON PM, HEATH H and HAYES AW. (1978). Evaluation of the mutagenic potential of mycotoxins using *Salmonella typhimurium* and *Saccharomyces cerevisiae. Mutat Res*, **53**, 11–20.

KUFFNER EK AND DART RC. (1996). Death following intravenous injection of Micotil 300. *J Toxicol Clin Toxicol*, **34**, 574.

KUMARASWAMI V, OTTESEN EA, VIJAYASEKARAN V, DEVI U, SWAMINATHAN M, AZIZ MA, SARMA GR, PRABHAKAR R and TRIPATHY SP. (1988). Ivermectin for the treatment of *Wuchereria bancroftii* filariasis. *JAMA*, **259**, 3105–3153.

KUNKLE GA AND MEYER DJ. (1987). Toxicity of high doses of griseofulvin to cats. *J Am Vet Med Assoc*, **191**, 322–323.

KWEI GY, ALVARO RF, CHEN Q, JENKINS HJ, HOP CEAC, KEOHANE CA, LY VT, STRAUSS JR, WANG RW, WANG Z, PIPPERT TR and UMBENHAUER DR. (1999). Disposition of ivermectin and cyclosporin A in CF-1 mice deficient in *mdr1a* P-glycoprotein. *Drug Metab Dispos*, **27**, 581–587.

LABAY K, OULD-ELHKIM M, KLES V, GUFFROY M, POUL JM and SANDERS P. (2001). Effects of griseofulvin in medium-term liver carcinogenesis and peripheral blood micronucleus test in rat. *Teratog Carcinog Mutagen*, **21**, 441–451.

LAFFONT CM, TOUTAIN P-L, ALVINERIE M and BOUSQUET-MELOU A. (2002). Intestinal secretion is a major route for parent ivermectin elimination in the rat. *Drug Metab Dispos*, **30**, 626–630.

LANCASTER T, SWART AM and JICK H. (1998). Risk of serious haematological toxicity with use of chloramphenicol eye drops in British general practice database. *BMJ*, **316**, 667.

LANKAS GR and GORDON LR. (1989). Toxicology. In Campbell WC (ed.), *Ivermectin and Abamectin*. Springer-Verlag, New York, 89–112.

LANKAS GR, MINSKER DH and ROBERTSON RT. (1989). Effects of ivermectin on reproduction and neonatal toxicity in rats. *Food Chem Toxicol*, **27**, 523–529.

LANKAS GR, CARTWRIGHT ME and UMBENHAUER DR. (1997). P-Glycoprotein deficiency in a subpopulation of CF-1 mice enhances avermectin-induced neurotoxicity. *Toxicol Appl Pharmacol*, **143**, 357–365.

LANKAS GR, CARTWRIGHT ME, PIPPERT T and UMBENHAUER DR. (1998). Placental P-glycoprotein deficiency enhances susceptibility to chemically induced birth defects in mice. *Reprod Toxicol*, **12**, 457–463.

LARIVIERE M, VINGTAIN P, AZIZ M, BEAUVAIS B, WEIMANN D, DEROUIN F, GINOUX J, SCHULZ-KEY H, GAXOTTE P and BASSET D. (1985). Double-blind study of ivermectin and diethylcarbamazine in African onchocerciasis patients with ocular involvement. *Lancet*, **2**, 174–177.

LARIZZA L, SIMONI G, TREDICI F and DE CARLI L. (1974). Griseofulvin: A potential agent of chromosomal segregation in cultured cells. *Mutat Res*, **25**, 123–130.

LEAKE PA, KUNTZ AL, MOORE CM and CHAMBERS PL. (1997). Cochlear pathology induced by aminoglycoside ototoxicity during maturation in cats. *Hear Res*, **113**, 117–132.

LEBOEUF RA, KERCKAERT GA, AAREMA MJ, GIBSON DP, BRAUNINGER R and ISFORT RJ. (1996). The pH 6.7 Syrian hamster embryo cell transformation assay for assessing the carcinogenic potential of chemicals. *Mutat Res*, **356**, 85–127.

LEE HS, WANG YT, YEO CT, TAN KT and RATNAM KV. (1989). Occupational asthma due to tylosin tartrate. *Br J Ind Med*, **46**, 498–499.

LEES P AND SERRANO L. (1976). Effects of azaperone on cardiovascular and respiratory functions in the horse. *Br J Pharmacol*, **56**, 263–269.

LEIFER Z, KADA T, MANDEL M, ZEIGER E, STAFFORD R and ROSENKRANZ HS. (1981). An evaluation of tests using DNA repair-deficient bacteria for predicting genotoxicity and carcinogenicity. *Mutat Res*, **87**, 211–297.

LEIKEN SL, WELCH H and GUIN GH. (1961). Aplastic anaemia due to chloramphenicol. *Clin Proc Child Hosp*, **17**, 171–180.

LEONARD A, PONCELET F, GRUTMAN G, CARBONELLE E and FABRY L. (1979). Mutagenicity tests with griseofulvin. *Mutat Res*, **68**, 225–234.

LEONE R, VENEGONI M, MOTOLA D, MORETTI U, PIAZZETTA V, COCCI A, RESI D, MOZZO F, VELO G, BURZILLERI L, MONTANARO N and CONFORTI A. (2003). Adverse drug reactions related to the use of fluoroquinolone antimicrobials. An analysis of spontaneous reports and fluoroquinolone consumption data from three Italian regions. *Drug Saf*, **26**, 109–120.

LEPOW ML. (1986). Aplastic anaemia following chloramphenicol therapy still happens! *Pediatr*, **77**, 932–933.

LERNER PI, SMITH H and WEINSTEIN L. (1967). Penicillin neurotoxicity. *Ann NY Acad Sci*, **145**, 310–318.

LERNER SA, SCHMITT BA, SELIGSOHN R and MATZ GJ. (1986). Comparative study of ototoxicity and nephrotoxicity in patients randomly assigned to treatment with amikacin or gentamicin. *Am J Med*, **80** (6B), 98–104.

LINDEMAYR H, KNOBLER R, KRAFT D and BAUMGARTNER W. (1981). Challenge of penicillin-allergic volunteers with penicillin-contaminated meat. *Allergy*, **36**, 471–478.

LINDSAY JR, PROCTOR LR and WORK WP. (1960). Histopathological inner ear changes in deafness due to neomycin in a human. *Laryngoscope*, **70**, 382–392.

LISI, P, LAPOMARDA V, STINGENI L, ASSALVE D, HANSEL K, CARAFFINI S and AGOSTINELLI. (1997). Skin tests in the diagnosis of eruptions caused by betalactams. *Contact Dermatitis*, **37**, 151–154.

LITTLEFIELD NA, GAYLOR DW, BLACKWELL BN and ALLEN RR. (1989). *Food Chem Toxicol*, **27**, 455–463.

LITTLEFIELD NA, SHELDON WG, ALLEN R and GAYLOR DW. (1990). Chronic toxicity/carcinogenicity studies of sulphamethazine in Fischer 344/N rats: two-generation exposure. *Food Chem Toxicol*, **28**, 156–167.

LOVELL R. (1946). Penicillin in animal diseases. In Fleming A (ed.), *Penicillin*, Butterworth, 337–349.

LU AYH, WISLOCKI PG, BAGAN ES, WANG RW, WALSH JS and MIWA GT. (1984). Mechanism of metabolic activation of ronidazole, a 5–nitroimidazole. *Biochem Soc Trans*, **12**, 7–9.

LU AYH, WISLOCKI PG, CHIU S-HL and MIWA GT. (1987). Tissue drug residues and their toxicological significance. *Drug Metab Rev*, **18**, 363–378.

LU AYH, MIWA GT and WISLOCKI PG. (1988). Toxicological significance of covalently bound drug residues. *Rev Biochem Toxicol*, **9**, 1–27.

LU AYH, CHIU S-HL and WISLOCKI PG. (1990). Development of a unified approach to evaluate the toxicological potential of bound residues. *Drug Metab Rev*, **22**, 891–904.

MACNEIL JD and ELLIS RL. (1995). Regulatory overview of antibiotic use in food-producing animals in North America and current methods of detection and analysis. In Oka H, Nakazawa H, Harada K-I and MacNeil JD (eds), *Chemical Analysis for Antibiotics Used in Agriculture.* AOAC International, Arlington, 1–29.

MAHBOOB A and HAROON TS. (1998). Drugs causing fixed eruptions: a study of 450 cases. *Int J Dermatol*, **37**, 833–838.

MAILHES JB, MARCHETTI F and AARDEMA MJ. (1993). Griseofulvin-induced aneuploidy and meiotic delay in mouse oocytes: effect of dose and harvest time. *Mutat Res*, **300**, 155–163.

MAIN BW, MEANS JR, RINKEMA LE, SMITH WC and SARAZAN RD. (1996). Cardiovascular effects of the macrolide antibiotic tilmicosin, administered alone and in combination with propranolol or dobutamine, in conscious unrestrained dogs. *J Vet Pharmacol Ther*, **19**, 225–232.

MALKIN D, KOREN G and SAUNDERS EF. (1990). Drug-induced aplastic anaemia: pathogenesis and clinical aspects. *Am J Pediatr Hematol Oncol*, **12**, 402–410.

MALO J-L AND CARTIER A. (1988). Occupational asthma in workers of a pharmaceutical company. *Thorax*, **43**, 371–377.

MARCHETTI F, TIVERON C, BASSANI B and PACCHIEROTTI F. (1992). Griseofulvin-induced aneuploidy and meiotic delay in female mouse germ cells. II. Cytogenetic analysis of one cell zygotes. *Mutat Res*, **266**, 151–162.

MARCHETTI F, MAILHES JB, BAIRNSFATHER L, NANDY I and LONDON SN. (1996). Dose-response study and threshold estimation of griseofulvin-induced aneuploidy during female mouse meiosis I and II. *Mutagenesis*, **11**, 195–200.

MARQUES-SANTOS LF, BERNARDO RR, DE PAULA EF and RUMJANEK VM. (1999). Cyclosporin A and trifluoperazine, two resistance-modulating agents, increase ivermectin neurotoxicity to mice. *Pharmacol Toxicol*, **84**, 125–129.

MARTIN RJ. (1996). An electrophysiological preparation of Ascaris suum pharyngeal muscle reveals a glutamate-gated chloride channel sensitive to the avermectin analogue, Milbemycin D. *Parasitology*, **112**, 247–252.

MASUR H, WHELTON PK and WHELTON A. (1976). Neomycin toxicity revisited. *Arch Surg,* **111**, 822–825.

MATULA TI (1990). Validity of *in vitro* testing. *Drug Metab Rev*, **22**, 777–787.

MATZ GJ. (1993). Aminoglycoside cochlear ototoxicity. *Otolaryngol Clin North Amer*, **26**, 705–712.

MAURANGES P. (1972). Antibiotics and animal feed: Allergic accidents to residues. *Econ Med Animal*, **13**, 131–135.

MCCLAIN RM. (1995). Mechanistic considerations for the relevance of animal data on thyroid neoplasia to human risk assessment. *Mutat Res.*, **333**, 131–142.

MCCLOSKEY GL and MASSA MC. (1997). Cephalexin rash in infectious nucleosis. *Cutis*, **59**, 251–254.

MCGEE TM and OLSZEWSKI J. (1962). Streptomycin sulphate and dihydrostreptomycin toxicity. *Arch Otolaryngol*, **75**, 295–311.

MCGUIGAN MA. (1994). Human exposures to tilmicosin (Micotil). *Vet Hum Toxicol*, **36**, 306–308.

MCKELLAR QA and BENCHAOUI HA. (1996). Avermectins and milbemycins. *J Vet Pharmacol Ther*, **19**, 331–351.

MEJEAN A, GUILLAUME J-L and STROSBERG AD. (1995). Carazolol: a potent, selective β_3-adrenoceptor agonist. *Eur J Pharmacol*, **291**, 359–366.

MEYER JS and BOXER M. (1973). Leukemic thrombi in pulmonary blood vessels. Subleukemic myelogenous leukaemia following chloramphenicol-induced aplastic anaemia. *Cancer*, **32**, 363–372.

MEYERS BR. (1985). Comparative toxicities of third-generation cephalosporins. *Am J Med*, **79** (2A), 96–103.

MEYERS RM. (1970). Ototoxic effects of gentamicin. *Arch Otolaryngol*, **92**, 160–162.

MEYLER L, POLAK BCP, SCHUT D, WESSELING H and HERXHEIMER A. (1974). Blood dyscrasias attributed to chloramphenicol. A review of 64 published and unpublished cases. *Postgrad Med J*, **50** (Suppl 5), 123–126.

MIGLIORE L, ZOTTI-MARTELLI L and SCARPATO R. (1999). Detection of chromosome loss and gain induced by griseofulvin, estramustine and vanadate in binucleated lymphocytes using FISH analysis. *Environ Mol Mutagen*, **34**, 64–68.

MILLIGAN A and DOUGLAS WS. (1986). Contact dermatitis to cephalexin. *Contact Dermatitis*, **15**, 91.

MINGUEZ MA, ZAPATERO L, CALOTO M and MARTINEZ-MOLERO MI. (1998). A study of allergy to penicillin antibiotics in the Child Allergy Department of the Gregorio Maranon University. *Allergol Immunopathol*, **26**, 43–46.

MINKIN W and LYNCH PJ. (1969). Allergic reaction to penicillin in milk. *JAMA,* **209**, 1089–1090.

MION G, VERDON R, LE GULLUCHE Y, CARSIN H, GARCIA A and GUILBAUD J. (1989). Fatal toxic epidermal necrolysis after griseofulvin. *Lancet*, **ii**, 1331.

MION G, LE GULLUCHE Y, CARSIN H, VERDON R and PAULET R. (1990). Fatal Lyell's syndrome caused by griseofulvin. *Ann Fr Anesth Reanim*, **9**, 305–308.

MITCHELL JA, GILLAM, EMJ, STANLEY, LA and SIM, E. (1990). Immunotoxic side-effects of drug therapy. *Drug Saf*, **5**, 168–178.

MITSCHER LA, DEVASTHALE P and ZAVOD R. (1993). Structure activity relationships. In Hooper DC and Wolfson JS (eds), *Quinolone Antimicrobial Agents*, American Society for Microbiology, Washington, DC, 3–51.

MITTLEMAN RE, HEARN WL and HIME GW. (1998). Xylazine toxicity – Literature review and report of two cases. *J Forensic Sci*, **43**, 400–402.

MIWA GT, WISLOCKI P, BAGAN E, WANG R, WALSH JS and LU AY. (1986). Studies on the activation and the mutagenicity of ronidazole, a 5–nitroimidazole. *Chem Biol Interact*, **197**, 527–535.

MODAN B, SEGAL S, SHAM M and SHEBA C. (1975). Aplastic anaemia in Israel: evaluation of the etiological role of chloramphenicol on a community-wide basis. *Am J Med Sci*, **270**, 441–445.

MOLITOR H, GRAESSLE OE, KUNA S, MUSHETT CW and SILBER RH. (1946). Some toxicological and pharmacological properties of streptomycin. *J Pharm Exp Ther*, **86**, 151–173.

MORI H, KAWAI K, OHBAYASHI F, KUNIYASU T, YAMAKAZI M, HAMASAKI T and WILLIAMS GM. (1984). Genotoxicity of a variety of mycotoxins in the hepatocytes primary culture /DNA repair test using rat and mouse hepatocytes. *Cancer Res*, **44**, 2918–2923.

MORIN JP, FILLASTRE JP and OLIER B. (1984). Antibiotic nephrotoxicity. *Chemioterapia*, **3**, 33–40.

MOSCATO G, NALDI L and CANDURA F. (1984). Bronchial asthma due to spiramycin and adipic acid. *Clin Allergy*, **14**, 355–361.

NABUURS MJA and VAN DER MOLEN ER. (1989). Clinical signs and performance of pigs during the administration of different levels of carbadox and after withdrawal. *J Vet Med*, **36A**, 209–217.

NABUURS MJ, VAN DER MOLEN EJ, DE GRAAF GJ and JAGER LP. (1990). Clinical signs and performance of pigs treated with different doses of carbadox, cyadox and olaquindox. *Zentralbl Veterinarmed A*, **37**, 68–76.

NAGAI A, MIYAZAKI M, MORITA T, FURUBO S, KIZAWA K, FUKUMOTO H, SANZEN T, HAYAKAWA H and KAWAMURA Y. (2002). Comparative articular cartilage of garenoxacin, a novel quinolone antimicrobial agent, in juvenile beagle dogs. *J Toxicol Sci*, **27**, 219–228.

NAJEAN Y and BAUMELOU E. (1984). Toxic epidemiology of aplastic anaemia. *Sex Transm Dis*, **11**, 343–346.

NAQUIRA C, JIMINEZ G, GUERRA JG, BERNAL R, NALIN DR, NEU D and AZIZ M. (1989). Ivermectin for human strongyloidiasis and other intestinal helminths. *Am J Trop Med Hyg*, **40**, 304–309.

NATTEL S, RANGER S, TALAJIC M, LEMERY R and ROY D. (1990). Erythromycin-induced long QT syndrome: concordance with quinidine and underlying cellular electrophysiologic mechanism. *Am J Med*, **89**, 235–238.

NAVA C. (1976). Work risks from antibiotics: contribution to the study of occupational disease from spiramycin. *Securitas*, **61**, 275–280.

NEGISHI T, TANAKA K and HAYATSU H. (1980). Mutagenicity of carbadox and several quinoxaline 1,4–dioxide derivatives. *Chem Pharm Bull*, **28**, 1347–1349.

NELSON AA, RADOWSKI JL and HAGAN EC. (1951). Renal and other lesions in dogs and rats from intramuscular injection of neomycin. *Fed Proc*, **10**, 366–367.

NEU HC. (1977). The penicillins. Overview of pharmacology, toxicology, and clinical use. *N Y State J Med.*, **77**, 962–967.

NIJHOF W and KROON AM. (1974). The interference of chloramphenicol and thiamphenicol with the biogenesis of mitochondria in animal tissues. A possible clue to the toxic action. *Postgrad Med J*, **50** (Suppl 5), 53–59.

NJOO FL, FLACK CE, OOSTING J, STILMA JS and KIJLSTRA A. (1993). Neutrophil activation in ivermectin-treated onchocerciasis patients. *Clin Exp Immunol*, **94**, 330–333.

NOAH (NATIONAL OFFICE OF ANIMAL HEALTH). (2001). Compendium of Data Sheets for

Veterinary Products 2002–2003, NOAH, Enfield, Middlesex.

NOONE P, BEALE DF, POLLOCK SS, PERRERA MR, AMIRAK ID, FERNANDO ON and MOORHEAD JF. (1978). Monitoring aminoglycoside use in patients with severely impaired renal function. *BMJ*, **ii**, 470–473.

NORRBY R and ALESTIG K. (1981). Gastrointestinal reactions to cefoperazone. *Lancet*, **ii**, 1417.

NORRBY SR. (1987). Side effects of cephalosporins. *Drugs*, **34** (Suppl 2), 105–120.

NOVAK E, SCHAGEL CA, LEZOTTE LA and PFEIFER RT. (1974). The tolerance of high dose intravenous spectinomycin therapy in man. *J Clin Pharmacol*, **14**, 442–447.

NTP (1987). NTP Toxicology and carcinogenesis studies of ampicillin trihydrate (CAS No. 7177–48–2) in F344/N rats and B6C3F1 mice (gavage studies). Natl Toxicol Program Tech Rep Service, **318**, 1–190.

NTP. (1988).Toxicology and carcinogenesis studies of nitrofurazone (CAS No. 59–87–0) in F344 rats and $B_6C_3F_1$ mice. Technical Report Series No. 337. US Department of Health and Human Services, Public Health Service/National Institutes of Health National Toxicology Program.

NUNOSHIBA T and NISHIOKA H. (1989). Genotoxicity of quinoxaline 1,4–dioxide derivatives in *Escherichia coli* and *Salmonella typhimurium*. *Mutat Res*, **217**, 23–28.

OHTA T, MORIYA M, KANEDA Y, WATANABE K, MIYAZAWA T, SUGIYAMA F and SHIRASU Y. (1980). Mutagenicity screening of feed additives in the microbial system. *Mutat Res*, **77**, 21–30.

OLSON JC and SANDERS AC. (1975). Penicillin in milk and milk products: Some regulatory and public health considerations. *J Milk Food Technol*, **38**, 630–633.

ORBAN Z, MACDONALD LL, PETERS MA and GUSLITS B. (1995). Erythromycin-induced cardiac toxicity. *Am J Cardiol*, **75**, 859–861.

OSHIMURA M and BARRETT JC. (1986). Chemically induced aneuploidy in mammalian cells: Mechanisms and biological significance in cancer. *Environ Mutagen*, **8**, 129–159.

OUD JL, REUTLINGER, AH and BRANGER J. (1979). An investigation into the cytogenetic damage induced by the coccidiostatic agents amprolium, carbadox, dimetridazole and ronidazole. *Mutat Res*, **68**, 179–182.

PAGGIARO PL, LOI AM and TOMA G. (1979). Bronchial asthma and dermatitis due to spiramycin in a chick breeder. *Clin Allergy*, **9**, 571–574.

PAPICH MG and RIVIERE JE. (2001). Chloramphenicol and derivatives, macrolides, lincosamides, and miscellaneous antimicrobials. In Adams HR (ed.), *Veterinary Pharmacology and Therapeutics*. 8th edn, Iowa State Press, Ames, 868–897.

PARKER RH and PARK S. (1984). Safety of cefuroxime and other new beta-lactam antibiotics. *J Antimicrob Chemother*, **14** (Suppl B), 331–335.

PARRY JM, FIELDER RJ and MCDONALD A. (1994). Thresholds for aneuploidy-inducing chemicals. *Mutagenesis*, **9**, 503–504.

PARRY JM, PARRY EM, BOURNER R, DOHERTY A, ELLARD S, O'DONOVAN J, HOEBEE B, STOPPELAAR JM, MOHN GR, ONFELT A, RENGLIN A, SCHULTZ N, SODERPALM-BERNDES C, JENSEN KG, KIRSCH-VOLDERS M, ELHAJOUJI A, VAN HUMMELEN P, DEGRASSI F, ANTOCCIA A, CIMINI D, IZZO M, TANZARELLA C, ADLER I-D, KLIESCH U, SCHRIEVER-SCHWEMMER G, GASSER P, CREBELLI R, CARERE A, ANDREOLI C, BENIGNI R, LEOPARDI P, MARCON F, ZINJO Z, NATARAJAN AT, BOEI JJWA, KAPPAS A, VOUTSINAS G, ZARANI FE, PATRINELLI A, PACHIEROTTI F, TIVERON C and HESS P. (1996). The detection and evaluation of aneugenic chemicals. *Mutat Res*, **353**, 11–46.

PATTERSON DR. (1991). Quinolone toxicity: methods of assessment. *Am J Med*, **91** (Suppl 6A), 35–37.

PEREZ RP, PUIG ML, SANCHEZ JLA and TORRES EL. (1981). Aplastic anaemia and drugs as causal factors. *Rev Cub Farm*, **15**, 97–103.

PERFECT JR, LINDSAY MH and DREW RH. (1992). Adverse drug reactions to systemic antifungals. Prevention and management. *Drug Saf*, **7**, 323–363.

PERREARD M and KLOTZ F. (1989). Ulcerated oesophagus after taking spiramycin. *Ann Gastroenterol Hepatol*, **25**, 313–314.

PETERS TL, FULTON RM, ROBERSON KD and ORTH MW. (2002). Effects of antibiotics on in vitro and in vivo avian cartilage degradation. *Avian Dis*, **46**, 75–86.

PETZOLD T, FEINDT P, MENGER MD and GAMS E. (1999). Beta-adrenoceptor inhibition for induction of acute cardiac failure in pigs. *Lab Anim*, **33**, 366–371.

PIGATTO PD, DE BLASIO A, ALTOMARE GF and GIACCHETI A. (1986). Contact sensitivity from systemic ampicillin. *Contact Dermatitis*, **14**, 196.

PILOT MA and QIN XY. (1988). Macrolides and gastrointestinal motility. *J Antimicrob Chemother*, **22** (Suppl B), 201–206.

PIRKIS JE, O'REGAN K and BAILIE R. (1997). Contact dermatitis and in-feed exposure to antibiotics among pig feed handlers. *Aust J Rural Health*, **5**, 76–79.

PLAUT ME and BEST WR. (1982). Aplastic anemia after parenteral chloramphenicol: warning renewed. *New Engl J Med*, **306**, 1486.

POIRIER LA, DOERGE DR, GAYLOR DW, MILLER MA, LORENTZEN RJ, CASCIANO DA, KADLUBAR FF and SCHWETZ BA. (1999). An FDA review of sulfamethazine toxicity. *Regul Toxicol Pharmacol*, **30**, 217–222.

POKORNA D. (1986). Cytogenetic analysis of bone marrow cells in Chinese hamster after the administration of cyadox and olaquindox. *Biol Chem Vet (*Prague), **22**, 23–28.

POLAK BCP, WESSELING H, SCHUT D, HERXHEIMER A and MEYLER L. (1972). Blood dyscrasias attributed to chloramphenicol. A review of 576 published and unpublished cases. *Acta Med Scand*, **192**, 409–414.

POULSEN E. (1995). René Truhaut and the acceptable daily intake: A personal note. *Teratog Carcinog Mutagen*, **15**, 273–275.

POWELL LW and HOOKER JW. (1956). Neomycin nephropathy. *JAMA*, **160**, 557–560.

PRATT WB and FEKETY R. (1986). Bactericidal inhibitors of protein synthesis, the aminoglycosides. In *The Antimicrobial Drugs*, Oxford University Press, Oxford, 153–183.

PREZIOSI P. (1981). Nephrotoxicity of first generation cephalosporins: consideration on experimental and clinical pharmacology. *Clin Ter*, **15**, 241–260.

PUAVILAI S and TIMPATANAPONG P. (1989). Prospective study of cutaneous drug reactions. *J Med Assoc Thai*, **72**, 167–171.

QIN X, PILOT M, THOMSON H and MASKELL J. (1987). Effects of spiramycin on gastrointestinal motility. *Chemoterapia*, **2** (Suppl), 319–320.

QINGHUA S, SCHMID TE and ADLER I-D. (1999). Griseofulvin-induced aneuploidy and meiotic delay in male mouse germ cells: detected by using conventional cytogenetics and three-color FISH. *Mutat Res*, **441**, 181–190.

RADCLIFFE RW, FERRELL ST and CHILDS SE. (2000). Butorphanol and azaperone as a safer alternative for repeated chemical restraint in captive white rhinoceros (*Ceratoterium simum*). *J Zoo Wildl Med*, **31**, 196–200.

RAINIER RH, CHALQUEST RR, BABCOCK WE and THRASHER GW. (1973). Therapeutic efficiency of carbadox in field outbreaks of swine dysentery. *Vet Med Small Anim Clin*, **68**, 272–276.

REGAN TJ, KHAN MI, OLDEWURTEL HA and PASSANNANTE AJ. (1969). Antibiotic effect on myocardial K^+ transport and the production of ventricular tachycardia. *J Clin Invest*, **48**, 68a.

REISMAN RE and ARBESMAN CE. (1968). Systemic allergic reactions due to inhalation of penicillin. *JAMA*, **203**, 184–185.

RENWICK AG. (1991). Safety factors and establishment of acceptable daily intakes. *Food Add Contam*, **8**, 135–150.

RICHARD-LENOBLE D, KOMBILA M, RUPP EA, PAPPAYLIOU ES, GAXOTTE P, NGUIRI C and AZIZ MA. (1988). Ivermectin in loiasis and concomitant *O. volvulus* and *M. perstans* infections. *Am J Trop Med Hyg*, **39**, 480–483.

RISKAER N, CHRISTENSEN E and HERTZ H. (1952). The toxic effects of streptomycin and dihydrostreptomycin in pregnancy, illustrated experimentally. *Acta Tuber Pneumol Scand*, **27**, 211–216.

RISKAER N, CHRISTENSEN E, PETERSEN E and WEIDMAN H. (1956). The ototoxicity of neomycin. Experimental investigations. *Acta Otolaryngol*, **46**, 137–152.

ROBBANA-BARNAT S, DECLOITRE F, FRAYSSINET C, SEIGNEURIN JM, TOUCAS L and LAFARGE-FRAYSSINET C. (1997). Use of human lymphoblastoid cells to detect the toxic effect of chloramphenicol and metabolites possibly involved in aplastic anaemia in man. *Drug Chem Toxicol*, **20**, 239–253.

ROBINSON CG and CAMBON KG. (1964). Hearing loss in infants of tuberculous mothers treated with streptomycin during pregnancy. *New Engl J Med*, **271**, 949–951.

RODER JD and STAIR EL. (1998). An overview of ivermectin toxicosis. *Vet Hum Toxicol*, **40**, 369–370.

ROMANO A, PIETANTONIO F, DI FONSO M and VENUTI A. (1992). Delayed hypersensitivity to cefuroxime. *Contact Dermatitis*, 27, 270–271.

ROMANO A, DI FONSO M, POCOBELLI D, GIANNARINI L, VENUTI A and GARCOVICH A. (1993). Two cases of toxic epidermal necrolysis caused by delayed hypersensitivity to beta-lactam antibiotics. *J Investig Allergol Clin Immunol,* **3**, 53–55.

ROMANO A, QUARATINO D, PAPA G, DI FONSO M and VENUTI A. (1997). Aminopenicillin allergy. *Arch Dis Child*, **76**, 513–517.

ROMANO A, MAYORGA C, TORRES MJ, ARTESANI MC, SUAU R, SANCHEZ PEREZ E, VENUTI A and BLANCA M. (2000). Immediate allergic reactions to cephalosporins: cross reactivity and selective responses. *J Allergy Clin Immunol*, **106**, 1177–1183.

ROMANO A, TORRES MJ, DI FONSO M, LEYVA L, ANDRIOLO M, PETTINATO R and BLANCA M. (2001). Delayed hypersensitivity to cefazolin: report on a case involving lymphocyte transformation studies with different cephalosporins. *Ann Allergy Asthma Immunol*, **87**, 238–242.

ROSENBLUM, A H. (1968). Penicillin allergy. *J Allergy*, **42**, 309–318.

ROSENTHAL AL, BINNICK S, PANZER P and PIROZZI DJ. (1979). Drug-induced toxic epidermal necrolysis in children. Report of two cases. *Cutis,* **24**, 437–440.

ROSENTHAL RL and BLACKMAN A. (1965). Bone marrow hypoplasia following use of chloramphenicol eye drops. *JAMA*, **191**, 148–149.

RUDZKI E and REBANDEL P. (1985). Occupational contact urticaria from penicillin. *Contact Dermatitis*, **13**, 192.

RUSSEL AS and LESSOF MH. (1971). Hypersensitivity to drugs. *Clin Allergy*, **1**, 179–187.

RUSSEL D and RUSSEL AD. (1992). Treatment of ringworm: old remedy versus new. *J Infect*, **24**, 333.

RUSTIA M and SHUBIK P. (1978). Thyroid tumours in rats and hepatomas in mice after griseofulvin treatment. *Br J Cancer*, **38**, 237–249.

SACK K, KAISER U and ZULLICH B. (1977). Experimental studies on the renal tolerance of cefuroxime. *Infection*, **5**, 92–94.

SAENZ DE SAN PEDRO MORERA B, ENRIQUEZ JQ and LOPEZ JF. (1999). Fixed drug eruptions due to betalactams and other chemically unrelated antibiotics. *Contact Dermatitis*, **40**, 220–221.

SAMANTA A, ROFFE C and WOODS KL. (1990). Accidental self administration of xylazine in a veterinary nurse. *Postgrad Med J*, **66**, 244–245.

SAVAGE J. (1977). Fixed drug eruptions to griseofulvin. *Br J Dermatol*, **97**, 107–108

SCHAEFFER JM and HAINES HW. (1989). Avermectin binding in *Caenorhabditis elegans*. A two-state model for the avermectin binding site. *Biochem Pharmacol*, **38**, 2329–2338.

SCHERES JMJC, HUSTINX TWJ, GERAEDTS JPM, LEEKSMA CHW and MELTZER PS. (1985). Translocation 1:7 in hematologic disorders. A brief review of 22 cases. *Cancer Genet Cytogenet*, **18**, 207–213.

SCHEUTWINKEL-REICH M and VON DER HUDE W. (1984). Sister-chromatid exchange in Chinese hamster V79 cells exposed to quindoxin, carbadox and olaquindox. *Mutat Res*, **139**, 199–202.

SCHINKEL AH, SMIT JJM, VAN TELLINGEN O, BEIJNEN JH, WAGENAAR E, VAN DEEMTER L, MOL CAAM, VAN DER VALK MA, ROBANUS-MAANDAG EC, TE RIELE HPJ, BERNS AJM and BORST P. (1994). Disruption of the mouse *mdr1a* P-glycoprotein gene leads to a deficiency in the blood-brain barrier and to increased sensitivity to drugs. *Cell*, **77**, 491–502.

SCHINKEL AH, WAGENAAR E, MOL CAAM and VAN DEEMTER L. (1996). P-glycoprotein in the blood-brain barrier of mice influences the brain penetration and pharmacological activity of many drugs. *J Clin Invest*, **97**, 2517–2524.

SCHLIAMSER SE. (1988). Neurotoxicity of beta-lactam antibiotics. Experimental kinetics and neurophysiological studies. *Scand J Infect Dis*, Suppl., **55**, 1–61.

SCHLIAMSER SE, BROHOLM K-A, LILJEDAHL A-M and NORRBY, SR. (1988a). Comparative neurotoxicity of benzylpenicillin, imipen/cilastatin and FCE 22101, a new injectable penem. *J Antimicrob Chemother*, **22**, 687–695.

SCHLIAMSER SE, BOLANDER H, KOURTOPOULOS H and NORRBY SR. (1988b). Neurotoxicity of benzylpenicillin: correlation to concentrations in serum, cerebrospinal fluid and brain tissue in rabbits. *J Antimicrob Chemother*, **21**, 365–372.

SCHLIAMSER SE, BOLANDER H, KOURTOPOULOS H, SIGAARDJ and NORRBY SR. (1988c). Neurotoxicity of benzylpenicillin in experimental *Escherichia coli* meningitis. *J Antimicrob Chemother*, **22**, 521–528.

SCHLIAMSER SE, CARS O and NORRBY SR. (1991). Nephrotoxicity of beta-lactam antibiotics: predisposing factors and pathogenesis. *J Antimicrob Chemother*, **27**, 405–425.

SCHLUTER G. (1987). Ciprofloxacin: Review of potential toxicologic effects. *Am J Med.*, **82** (Suppl 4A), 91–93.

SCHMITT-GRAFF A. (1981). Chloramphenicol-induced aplastic anemia terminating with acute nonlymphocytic leukaemia. *Acta Haematol*, **66**, 267–268.

SCHNEIDER D, BRONSCH K and RICHTER L. (1976). Olaquindox a new growth promoting feed additive. II. Effects on the performance in swine fattening. *Z Tierphsiol Tierernahr Futtermittelelkd*, **36**, 241–248.

SCHWARTZ HJ and SHER TH. (1984). Anaphylaxis to penicillin in a frozen dinner. *Ann Allergy*, **52**, 342–343.

SCOTT FW, DE LAHUNTA A, SCHULTZ RD, BISTNER SI and RIIS RC. (1975). Teratogenesis in a cat associated with griseofulvin therapy. *Teratology*, **11**, 79–86.

SCOTT JL, FINEGOLD SM, BELKIN GA and LAWRENCE JS. (1965). A controlled double blind study of the haematologic toxicity of chloramphenicol. *New Engl J Med*, **272**, 1137–1142.

SEAMAN AJ. (1969). Sequels to chloramphenicol aplastic anemia: Acute leukaemia and paroxysmal nocturnal hemoglobinuria. *Northwest Med*, **68**, 831–834.

SEAMAN JT, EAGLESON JS, CARRIGAN MJ and WEBB RF. (1987). Avermectin B_1 toxicity in a herd of Murray Grey cattle. *Aust Vet J*, **64**, 284–285.

SERRANO L and LEES P. (1976). The applied pharmacology of azaperone in ponies. *Res Vet Sci*, **20**, 316–323.

SHAROM FJ. (1997). The P-glycoprotein efflux pump: how does it transport drugs. *J Membr Biol* 160, 161–175.

SHARP AA. (1963). Chloramphenicol-induced blood dyscrasias. Analysis of 40 cases. *Br Med J*, **284**, 1331.

SHARPE HM and TOMICH EG. (1960). Studies in the toxicology of griseofulvin. *Toxicol Appl Pharmacol*, **2**, 44–53.

SHIMOYAMA T and NONAKA S. (1987). Biochemical studies on griseofulvin-induced protoporphyrias. *Ann NY Acad Sci*, **514**, 160–169.

SHOOP WL, MROZIK H and FISHER MH. (1995). Structure and activity of avermectins and milbemycins in animal health. *Vet Parasitol*, **59**, 139–156.

SKOLIMOWSKI IM, KNIGHT RC and EDWARDS DI. (1983). Molecular basis of chloramphenicol and thiamphenicol toxicity to DNA *in vitro*. *J Antimicrob Chemother*, **12**, 535–542.

SKOPETS B, WILSON RP, GRIFFITH JW and LANG CM. (1996). Ivermectin toxicity in young animals. *Lab Animal Sci*, **46**, 111–112.

SMITH BR and LE FROCK JL. (1983). Cefuroxime: antimicrobial activity, pharmacology and clinical efficacy. *Ther Drug Monit*, **5**, 149–160.

SNIDER DE, LAYDE PM, JOHNSON MW and LYLE MA. (1980). Treatment of tuberculosis during pregnancy. *Am Rev Resp Dis*, **122**, 65–79.

SOFUNI T, HONMA M, HAYASHI M, SHIMADA H, TANAKA N, WAKURI S, AWOGI T, YAMAMOTO KI, NISHI Y and NAKADATE M. (1996). Detection of in vitro clastogens and spindle poisons by the mouse lymphoma assay using the microwell method: Interim report of an international collaborative study. *Mutagenesis*, **11**, 349–355.

SOLGAARD L, TUXOE JI, MAFI M, DUE OLSEN S and TOFTGAARD JENSEN T. (2000). Nephrotoxicity by dicloxacillin and gentamicin in 163 patients with intertrochanteric hip fractures. *Int Orthop*, **24**, 155–157.

SPEIGHT TM, BROGDEN RN and AVERY GS. (1972). Cephalexin: A review of its antibacterial, pharmacological and therapeutic properties. *Drugs*, **3**, 9–78.

SPOERKE DG, HALL AH, GRIMES MJ, HONEA BN and RUMACK BH. (1986). Human overdose with the veterinary tranquilizer xylazine. *Am J Emerg Med*, **3**, 222–224.

SPOO JW AND RIVIERE JE. (2001). Sulfonamides. In Adams HR (ed.), *Veterinary Pharmacology and Therapeutics*, 8th edn, Iowa State Press, Ames, 796–817.

SPURLING NW, HARCOURT RA and HYDE JJ. (1986). An evaluation of the safety of cefuroxime axetil during six months oral administration to beagle dogs. *J Toxicol Sci*, **11**, 237–277.

SRAM RJ, FERNANDEZ RODRIGUEZ SF and KOCISOVA J. (1986a). Chromosomal aberration in the bone marrow of mice after long-continued administration of cyadox and olaquindox. *Biol Chem Vet* (Prague), **22**, 17–22.

SRAM RJ, FERNANDEZ RODRIGUEZ SF and KOCISOVA J. (1986b). Effect of long-term oral administration of cyadox and olaquindox on the frequency of dominant lethal mutations and sperm abnormalities in mice. *Biol Chem Vet* (Prague), **22**, 37–45

SRAM RJ, FERNANDEZ RODRIGUEZ SF and KOCISOVA J. (1986c). Dominant lethal mutation in female mice following the oral application of cyadox and olaquindox. *Biol Chem Vet* (Prague), **22**, 29–35.

STAHLMANN R. (1990). Safety profile of the quinolones. *J Antimicrob Chemother*, **26** (Suppl. D), 31–44.

STAHLMAN R and LODE H. (1999). Toxicity of quinolones. *Drugs*, **58** (Suppl. 2), 37–42.

STAHLMAN R, KUHNER S, SHAKIBAEI M, SCHWABE R, FLORES J, EVANDER SA and VAN SICKLE DC. (2000). Chondrotoxicity of ciprofloxacin in immature Beagle dogs: Immunohistochemistry, electron microscopy and drug plasma concentrations. *Arch Toxicol*, **73**, 564–572.

STARETZ LR and DEBOOM GW. (1990). Multiple oral and skin lesions occurring after treatment with penicillin. *J Am Dent Assoc*, **121**, 436–437.

STEELMAN RL and KOCSIS JJ. (1978). Determination of the teratogenic and mutagenic potential of griseofulvin. *Toxicol Appl Pharmacol*, **45**, 343–344.

STEWART GT. (1967). Hypersensitivity and toxicity of the β-lactam antibiotics. *Postgrad Med J*, **43** (Suppl. 43), 31–36.

STEWART GT. (1969). Allergenic residues in penicillins. *Lancet*, **i**, 117–1183.

STILL J, RAATH JP and MATZNER L. (1996). Respiratory and circulatory parameters of African elephants (*Loxodonta africana*) anaesthetised with etorphine and azaperone. *J S Afr Vet Assoc*, **67**, 123–127.

STRAUBE MD, FREITAG M, ALTMEYER P and SZLISKA C. (2000). Occupational airborne contact dermatitis from cefazolin. *Contact Dermatitis*, **42**, 44–45.

SUTER W, ROSSELET A and KNUSEL F. (1978). Mode of action of quindoxin and substituted quinoxaline-di-N-oxides on *Escherichia coli*. *Antimicrob Agents Chemother*, **13**, 770–783.

SUTHERLAND IH and CAMPBELL WC. (1990). Development, pharmacokinetics and mode of action of ivermectin. *Acta Leiden*, **59**, 161–168.

SVED S and FOSTER B. (1990). Nitroimidazoles: Proposed studies on the toxicity of bound residues. *Drug Metab Res*, **22**, 849–861.

SYKORA I and VORTEL V. (1986). Post-natal study of the carcinogenicity of cyadox and carbadox. *Biol Vet Praha*, **22**, 52–62.

SYMOENS J. (1970). Prevention and treatment of aggression and stress in pigs with the neuroleptic azaperone. *Dtsch Tierarztl Wochenschr*, **77** 144–148.

SYMOENS J and VAN DEN BRANDE M. (1969). Prevention and cure of aggressiveness in pigs using the sedative azaperone. *Vet Rec*, **85**, 64–67.

TAGAMI H, TATSUTA K, IWATSKI K and YAMADA M. (1983). Delayed hypersensitivity in ampicillin-induced toxic epidermal necrolysis. *Arch Dermatol*, **119**, 910–913.

TAKAHASHI H. (1976). Drug toxicity. 8. Penicillin hypersensitivity. *Kansesshogaku Zasshi*, **40**, 863.

TAKIZAWA T, HASHIMOTO K, ITOH N, YAMASHITA S and OWEN K. (1999a). A comparative study of the repeat dose toxicity of grepafloxacin and a number of other fluoroquinolones in rats. *Hum Exp Toxicol*, **18**, 38–45.

TAKIZAWA T, HASHIMOTO K, MINAMI T, YAMASHITA S and OWEN K. (1999b). The comparative arthropathy of fluoroquinolones in dogs. *Hum Exp Toxicol*, **18**, 392–399.

TAUCHI K, KAWANISHI H, IGARASHI N, MAEDA Y, MAEYAMA Y, EBINO K, SUZUKI K and IMAMICHI T. (1979a). Studies on toxicity of cephadroxil (S-578). I. Acute toxicity. *Jpn J Antibiot*, **32**, 1230–1232.

TAUCHI K, KAWANISHI H, IGARASHI N, MAEDA Y, MAEYAMA Y, EBINO K, SUZUKI K and IMAMICHI T. (1979b). Studies on toxicity of cephadroxil (S-578). II. Subacute toxicity in rats. *Jpn J Antibiot*, **32**, 1233–1257.

TAUCHI K, KAWANISHI H, IGARASHI N, MAEDA Y, MAEYAMA Y, EBINO K, SUZUKI K and IMAMICHI T. (1979c). Studies on toxicity of cephadroxil (S-578). III. Chronic toxicity in rats. *Jpn J Antibiot*, **32**, 1259–1287.

TAUCHI K, KAWANISHI H, IGARASHI N, MAEDA Y, MAEYAMA Y, EBINO K, SUZUKI K and IMAMICHI T. (1979d). Studies on toxicity of cephadroxil (S-578). IV. Subacute and chronic toxicity in dogs. *Japan J Antibiot*, **32**, 1289–334.

TAUCHI K, KAWANISHI H, IGARASHI N, MAEDA Y, MAEYAMA Y, EBINO K, SUZUKI K and IMAMICHI T. (1979e). Studies on toxicity of cephadroxil (S-578). VI. Teratogenicity study in rats. *Jpn J Antibiot*, **33**, 487–496.

TAUCHI K, KAWANISHI H, IGARASHI N, MAEDA Y, MAEYAMA Y, EBINO K, SUZUKI K and IMAMICHI T. (1979f). Studies on toxicity of cephadroxil (S-578). VII. Teratogenicity study in dogs. *Jpn J Antibiot*, **33**, 497–502.

TAUCHI K, KAWANISHI H, IGARASHI N, MAEDA Y, MAEYAMA Y, EBINO K, SUZUKI K and IMAMICHI T. (1979g). Studies on toxicity of cephadroxil (S-578). VIII. Peri- and post-natal development study in rats. *Jpn J Antibiot*, **33**, 503–509.

TAYLOR B and DUFFILL M. (1988). Toxic epidermal necrolysis from griseofulvin. *J Am Acad Dermatol*, **19**, 565–567.

THAMI GP, KAUR S and KANWAR AJ. (2001). Erythema multiforme due to griseofulvin with positive re-exposure test,. *Dermatology*, **203**, 84–85.

THOMPSON JW and JACOBS RF. (1993). Adverse effects of newer cephalosporins. *Drug Saf*, **9**, 132–142.

THYAGARAJAN K, KAMALAN A and THAMBIAH AS. (1981). Fixed drug eruption to griseofulvin. *Mykosen*, **24**, 482–484.

TINKELMAN DG and BOCK SA. (1984). Anaphylaxis presumed to be caused by beef containing streptomycin. *Ann Allergy*, **53**, 243–244.

TIVERON C, MARCHETTI F, BASSANI B and PACCHIEROTTI F. (1992). Griseofulvin-induced aneuploidy and meiotic delay in female mouse germ cells. I. Cytogenetic analysis of metaphase II. *Mutat Res*, **266**, 143–150.

TRUHAUT R and FERRANDO R. (1975). Relay toxicity. General principles for a new methodological approach for the toxicologic evaluation of additives to food of animal origin. *Toxicology*, 3, 361–368.

TRUHAUT R and FERRANDO R. (1976). Results of 8 years of research on the toxicologic evaluation of additives for animal feeding stuffs by the method known as relay toxicology. *Europ J Toxicol*, **9**, 413–422.

TRUHAUT R, FERRANDO R, FACCINI JM and MONRO AM. (1981). Negative results of carcinogenicity bioassay of methyl carbazate in rats: significance for the toxicological evaluation of carbadox. *Toxicology*, **22**, 219–221.

TSANG YC and CHIN TC. (1963). Neurotoxicity of streptomycin. *Scientia Sinica*, **12**, 1019–1040.

TSCHEUSCHNER I. (1972). Penicillin anaphylaxis following pork consumption. *Z Haut Geschlechtskr*, **47**, 591–592.

TUNE BM, HSU CY and FRAVERT D. (1996). Cephalosporin and carbacephem nephrotoxicity. Roles of tubular cell uptake and acylating potential. *Biochem Pharmacol*, **51**, 557–561.

TUOMI ML and RASANEN L. (1995). Contact allergy to tylosin and cobalt in a pig-farmer. *Contact Dermatitis*, **33**, 285.

TURNER MC. (1977). Deformed kittens. *Vet Rec*, **100**, 391.

TURTON JA, YALLOP D, ANDREWS CM, FAGG R, YORK M and WILLIAMS TC. (1999). Haematotoxicity of chloramphenicol succinate in the CD-1 mouse and Wistar Hanover rat. *Hum Exp Toxicol*, **18**, 566–576.

TURTON JA, HAVARD AC, ROBINSON S, HOLT DE, ANDREWS CM, FAGG R and WILLIAMS TC. (2000). An assessment of chloramphenicol and thiamphenicol in the induction of aplastic anaemia in the BALB/c mouse. *Food Chem Toxicol*, **38**, 925–938.

TURTON JA, ANDREWS CM, HAVARD AC, ROBINSON S, YORK M, WILLIAMS TC and GIBSON FM. (2002a). Haemotoxicity of thiamphenicol in the BALB/c mouse and Wistar Hanover rat. *Food Chem Toxicol*, **40**, 1849–1861.

TURTON JA, ANDREWS CM, HAVARD AC and WILLIAMS TC. (2002b). Studies on the haemotoxicity of chloramphenicol succinate in the Dunkin Hartley guinea pig. *Int J Exp Pathol*, **83**, 225–238.

UENO Y. (1985). The toxicology of mycotoxins. *Crit Rev Toxicol*, **14**, 99–132.

UMBENHAUER DR, LANKAS GR, PIPPERT TR, WISE LD, CARTWRIGHT M, HALL SJ and BEARE CM. (1997). Identification of a P-glycoprotein-deficient subpopulation in CF-1 mouse strain using a restriction fragment length polymorphism. *Toxicol Appl Pharmacol*, **146**, 88–94.

VAN ARDSEL PP. (1965). Allergic reactions to penicillin. *JAMA*, **191**, 172–173.

VAN DER LINDEN PD, VAN PUIJENBROEK EP, FEENSTRA J, VELD BA, STURKENBOOM MC, HERINGS RM, LEUFKENS HG and STRICKER BH. (2001). Tendon disorders attributed to fluoroquinolones: a study on spontaneous reports in the period 1988 to 1998. *Arthritis Rheum*, **45**, 235–239.

VANHAUWAERT A, VANPARYS P, and KIRSCH-VOLDERS M. (2001). The in vivo gut micronucleus test detects clastogens and aneugens given by gavage. *Mutagenesis*, **16**, 39–50.

VAN HEYNINGEN E. (1967). Cephalosporins. *Adv Drug Res*, **4**, 1–70.

VAN METRE DC. (1992). A case report of the treatment of an overdose of xylazine in a cow. *Cornell Vet*, **82**, 287–291.

VARPELA E, HIETLAHTI J and ARO MJT. (1969). Streptomycin and dihydrostreptomycin medication during pregnancy and their effect on the child's inner ear. *Scand J Resp Dis*, **50**, 101–109.

VASSILEVA SG, MATEEV G and PARISH LC. (1998). Antimicrobial photosensitive reactions. *Arch Intern Med*, **158**, 1993–2000.

VEGA JM, BLANCA M, GARCIA JJ, CARMONA MJ, MIRANDA A, PEREZ-ESTRADA M, FERNANDEZ S, ACEBES JM and TERRADOS S. (1994). Immediate allergic reactions to amoxicillin. *Allergy*, **49**, 317–322.

VEIEN NK, HATTEL T, JUSTESEN O and NORHOLM A. (1980). Occupational contact dermatitis due to spiramycin and/or tylosin among farmers. *Contact Dermatitis*, **6**, 410–413.

VEIEN NK, HATTEL T, JUSTESEN O and NORHOLM A. (1983). Patch testing with substances not included in the standard series. *Contact Dermatitis*, **9**, 304–308.

VENNING GR. (1983). Identification of adverse reactions to new drugs. II – How were 18 important adverse reactions discovered and with what delays. *BMJ*, **286**, 289–292.

VERBOV J. (1983). Tylosin dermatitis. *Contact Dermatitis*, **9**, 325–326.

VICKERS HR. (1964). Dermatological hazards of the presence of penicillin in milk. *Proc R Soc Med*, 1091–1092.

VICKERS HR, BAGRATUNI L and ALEXANDER S. (1958). Dermatitis caused by penicillin in milk. *Lancet*, **i**, 351–352.

VON DER HUDE W, BEHM C, GURTLER R and BASLER A. (1988). Evaluation of the SOS chromotest. *Mutat Res*, **203**, 81–94.

VON ESSEN S, SPENCER J, HASS B, LIST P and SEIFERT SA. (2003). Unintentional human exposure to tilmicosin (Micotil 300). *Clin Toxicol,* **41**, 229–233.

VOOGD CF, VAN DER STEL JJ and JACOBS JJ. (1980). The mutagenic action of quindoxin, carbadox, olaquindox and some other N-oxides on bacteria and yeast. *Mutat Res*, **78**, 233–242.

VROOMEN LHM, BERGHMANS MCJ, VAN BLADEREN PJ, GROTEN JP, WISSINK CJ and KUIPER HA. (1990a). *In vivo* and *in vitro* metabolic studies of furazolidone: A risk evaluation. *Drug Metab Rev*, **22**, 663–676.

VROOMEN LHM, BERGHMANS MCJ, VAN BLADEREN PJ, GROTEN JP, WISSINK CJ and KUIPER HA. (1990b). Bound residues of furazolidone, a potential risk for the consumer. In Simon F, Lees P and Semjen G (eds), *Veterinary Pharmacology and Therapy in Food Producing Animals*, Unipharma, Budapest, 257–266.

WAISBREN BA and SPINK WW. (1950). A clinical appraisal of neomycin. *Ann Int Med*, **33**, 1099–1119.

WAITZ JA, MOSS EL and WEINSTEIN MJ. (1971). Aspects of the chronic toxicity of gentamicin sulfate in cats. *J Infect Dis*, **124** (Suppl), S125–S129.

WALKER S, DIAPER CJM, BOWMAN R, SWEENEY G, SEAL DV and KIRKNESS CM. (1998). Lack of evidence for systemic toxicity following topical chloramphenicol use. *Eye*, **12**, 875–879.

WALLERSTEIN RO, CANDIT PK, KASPER CK, BROWN JW and MORRISON FR. (1969). Statewide study of chloramphenicol therapy and fatal aplastic anemia. *JAMA*, **208**, 2045–2050.

WARD DJ, KRZEMINSKA EC and TANNER NS. (1990). Treatment of toxic epidermal necrolysis and a review of six cases. *Burns*, **16**, 97–104.

WARKANY J. (1979). Antituberculous drugs. *Teratology*, **20**, 133–138.

WARREN RW. (1997). Rheumatologic aspects of pediatric cystic fibrosis patients treated with fluoroquinolones. *Pediatr Infect Dis J*, **16**, 118–122.

WATERS MD, STACH HF, MAVOURNIN KH and DELLARCO VL. (1986). Genetic activity profiles of chemicals selected from the aneuploidy database. *Mutat Res*, **167**, 171–188.

WEBSTER JC, CARROLL R, BENITEZ JT and MCGEE TM. (1971). *J Infect Dis*, **124** (Suppl.), S139–S144.

WEHLAND J, HERZOG W and WEBER K. (1977). Interaction of griseofulvin with microtubules, microtubule protein and tubulin. *J Mol Biol*, **111**, 329–342.

WEISS G. (1990). The integration of pharmacological and toxicological testing of tissue residues in the evaluation of their human food safety. *Drug Metab Rev*, **22**, 829–848.

WEISS MH, KURZE T and NULSEN FE. (1974). Acute neurotoxicity. Laboratory and clinical study. *J Neurosurg*, **41**, 486–489.

WELLES JS, FROMAN RO, GIBSON WR, OWEN NV and ANDERSON RC. (1968). Toxicology and pharmacology of cephalexin in laboratory animals. *Antimicrob Agents Chemother.*, **8**, 489–496.

WHITE MP, HABOUSH HW and ALROOMI LG. (1986). Fatal bone marrow aplasia due to chloramphenicol in a baby. *Lancet,* **i**, 555–556.

WICHER K and REISMAN RE. (1980). Anaphylactic reaction to penicillin (or penicillin-like substance) in a soft drink. *J Allergy Clin Immunol*, **66**, 155–157.

WICHER K, REISMAN RE and ARBESMAN CE. (1969). Allergic reactions to penicillin in milk. *JAMA*, **208**, 143–145.

WIDAYAT, SUNARTO, SUTARYO, ZURGHIBAN M and ISMANGOEN. (1983). Aplastic anaemia in children. *Paediatr Indones*, **23**, 183–191.

WILKOWSKE CJ. (1977). The penicillins. *Mayo Clin Proc*, **52**, 616–624.

WILLIAMS GM. (1997a). Chemicals with carcinogenic activity in the rodent liver; mechanistic evaluation of human risk. *Cancer Lett*, **117**, 175–188.

WILLIAMS JC. (1997b). Anthelmintic treatment strategies: current status and future. *Vet Parasitol*, **72**, 461–470.

WINGFIELD J and APPELBE GE. (1984). Controls on the use of antibiotics in animal husbandry. *Pharm J*, **233**, 717–720.

WISLOCKI P and LU AY. (1990). Formation and biological evaluation of ronidazole bound residues. *Drug Metab Res*, **22**, 649–661.

WISLOCKI PG, BAGAN ES, VANDENHEUVEL WJ, WALKER RW, ALVARO RF, ARISON BH, LU AY and WOLF FJ. (1984). Drug residue formation from ronidazole, a 5-nitroimidazole. Cysteine adducts formed upon reduction of ronidazole by dithionite or rat liver enzymes in the presence of cysteine. *Chem Biol Interact*, **49**, 13–25.

WOODWARD KN. (1991). Hypersensitivity in humans and exposure to veterinary drugs. *Hum Vet Toxicol,* **33**, 168–172.

WOODWARD KN and SHEARER G. (1995). Antibiotic use in animal production in the European Union – Regulation and current methods for Residue Detection. In Oka H, Nakazawa H, Harada K-I and MacNeil JD (eds), *Chemical Analysis for Antibiotics Used in Agriculture.* AOAC International, Arlington, 47–76.

WRIGHT, AJ. (1999). The penicillins. *Mayo Clin Proc*, **74**, 290–307.

WRIGHT, AJ and WILKOWSKE CJ. (1991). The penicillins. *Mayo Clin Proc*, **66**, 1047–1063.

YAKOTA M, TAKEDA U, SAKAMOTO K, SETO N and IGARASHI M. (1984). The comparative ototoxicities of panimycin and gentamicin in cynomolgus monkeys (*Maccaca fascicularis). Chemotherapy*, **30**, 248–254.

YILMAZ O, CABALAR M and OZBILGIN S. (1999). The in vivo and in vitro comparative nephrotoxicity of cefazolin and gentamicin. *Vet Hum Toxicol*, **41**, 222–225.

YONEDA T, MASATANI H, SHIBATA T, KAWAMURA Y, SATO S, IWASAKI S, TAKIMOTO Y, NAGASAWA M and TAKAI A. (1980). Subacute toxicity test of cefoperazone in beagle dogs with the intravenous administration for 3 months. *Jpn J Antibiot*, **33**, 1028–1055.

YONG MS. (1990). Potential use of isolated organ or tissue preparations in the assessment of biological activities of bound residues. *Drug Metab Res*, **22**, 753–763.

YOSHIMURA H, NAKAMURA M, KOEDA T and YOSHIKAWA K. (1981). Mutagenicities of carbadox and olaquindox – growth promoters for pigs. *Mutat Res*, **90**, 49–55.

YOUNG LW, MITNICK JS, YANKUS WA and GENIESER NB. (1979). Radiological case of the month. *Am J Dis Child*, **133**, 545–546.

YUNIS AA. (1984). Differential in vitro toxicity of chloramphenicol, nitroso-chloramphenicol, and thiamphenicol. *Sex Transm Dis*, **11**, 340–342.

YUNIS AA. (1988). Chloramphenicol: relation of structure to activity and toxicity. *Annu Rev Pharmacol Toxicol*, **28**, 83–100.

YUNIS AA. (1989). Chloramphenicol toxicity: 25 years of research. *Am J Med*, **87**, 3-44N–3-48N.

YUNIS AA and BLOOMBERG GR. (1964). Chloramphenicol toxicity: clinical features and pathogenesis. *Prog Hematol*, **4**, 138–159.

ZEIGER E, ANDERSON B, HAWORTH S, LAWLORT and MORTELMANS K. (1992). Salmonella mutagenicity tests. V. Results from the testing of 311 chemicals. *Environ Mol Mutagen*, **19** (Suppl 21), 2–141.

ZIMMERMAN FK, VON BORSTAL RC, VON HALLE ES, PARRY JM, SIEBERT D, ZETTERBERG G,

BARALE R and LOPRIENO N. (1984). Testing of chemicals for genetic activity with *Saccharomyces cerevisiae*: a report of the U.S. Environmental Protection Agency Gene-Tox Program. *Mutat Res*, **133**, 199–244.

ZIMMERMAN MC. (1959). Chronic penicillin urticaria from dairy products, proved by penicillinase cures. *Arch Dermatol*, **79**, 1–6.

ZIV G. (1986). Therapeutic use of antibiotics in farm animals. In Moats WA (ed.), *Agricultural Uses of Antibiotics*. American Chemical Society Symposium Series 320, American Chemical Society, Washington DC, 8–22.

9

The rapid detection of veterinary drug residues

N. van Hoof, K. de Wasch, H. Noppe, S. Poelmans and H. F. de Brabander, University of Ghent, Belgium

9.1 Introduction

An increase in education and consumer awareness has led to an evolution or revolution in the demand for safe and healthy food. One of the challenges in the food industry is to meet the requirements and demands of the consumer. Consumers want to know what they eat, it has to be healthy and not harmful. Objective information has to be passed on to the consumer. The confidence of the consumer has been tested several times over the last few years. After the dioxin crisis, BSE, foot and mouth disease, the nitrophen crisis, MPA crisis, to name just a few. Consumers have become very critical when it comes to their food. Also the attitude of the consumer towards the intense use of antibiotics is not positive. A wide range of veterinary medicinal products (VMP) such as antibiotics is administered legitimately to farm animals to treat outbreaks of disease or prevent disease from spreading. Necessary medication should be applied in the prescribed dose and carefully recorded. These records must be traceable by government inspection services. In order to reduce the likelihood of harmful levels of these substances reaching the human food chain, the European Union and many other countries have set maximum residue limits (MRLs). Regulatory bodies are required to enforce and verify these requirements. Laboratory testing of food products has to ensure that regulations are met.

Official samples taken at the slaughterhouse or the farm are analysed for forbidden substances but also for registered veterinary medicinal products, legally or illegally applied. The results of these analyses are used as part of a holistic approach in food quality assurance. Both violative and compliant results are reported. The criteria that are used for generating the results, i.e. for identification and quantification of the analytes, meet the strict internationally required standards. In residue analysis, uncompromising quality is not an option – it is an obligation. It is not a vague goal – it is standard operating procedure.

Quality begins in the farms where every aspect of good working practice should ensure the quality of the end product. Assurance of the different aspects of the quality is also given by laboratory results. Therefore residue laboratories working for the government have to be accredited (ISO 17025). Every step, from the incoming sample to the outgoing result, is traceable. Quality control in every step of the procedure assures trustworthy results. By maintaining this intense level of quality control, by developing new methods and using highly technological equipment operated by well trained personnel, laboratories will maintain their important position as part of the chain of food quality assurance.

A wide range of different groups of veterinary medicinal products is used in practice. Since every group requires a specific extraction and detection procedure, it has become too expensive to check every sample for a whole batch of different groups. Screening methods are developed to eliminate a large number of false positive samples and give an indication of the specific group of veterinary medicinal products. Only the truly 'suspect' samples are transferred for confirmation. This confirmation procedure is more expensive than the screening but at this stage a positive identification of an analyte can be combined with a quantification. A quantification compares the concentration of the analyte with the MRL value prescribed by law.

9.2 Veterinary medicinal products

9.2.1 Definition

A 'medicinal product' is defined in Article 1 of Directive 65/65/EEC as any substance or combination of substances presented for treating or preventing diseases in human beings or animals. Any substance or combination of substances which may be administered to human beings or animals with a view to making a medicinal diagnosis or to restoring, correcting or modifying physiological functions in human beings or animals is likewise considered a medicinal product. A veterinary medicinal product is used to mean any product within the above definition that is subject to Article 1 of Directive 81/851/EEC.

The major goal of the animal health industry is to make veterinary medicinal products available which improve the health, welfare and productivity of animals whilst ensuring food and environmental safety (Council Directive 65/65/EEC, 1965).

9.2.2 Legislation

The evaluation of the safety of residues is based on the determination of the acceptable daily intake (ADI) on which in turn maximum residue limits (MRL) are based. The ADI is an estimate of the residue that can be ingested daily over a lifetime without a health risk to the consumer. The ADI is determined following the evaluation of pharmacological and toxicological studies. The basis for the calculation of the ADI is the no-observed-effect-level (NOEL) and the calculation includes an extremely large safety factor. In addition, to derive MRLs from the ADI it is assumed that the average person consumes, on a daily basis, 500 g of meat, 1.5 l of milk and 100 g of eggs or egg products (Grein, 2000).

Veterinary medicinal products having a pharmacological action, as defined by the European Union (EU), are 'substances capable of pharmacological action in the context of Article 4 of Directive 81/851/EEC and should be interpreted as substances which are pharmacologically active at the dose at which they are administered to the target animal by means of the veterinary medicinal product in which they are included'. (EMEA/CVMP/046/00-Rev. 3, 17 April 2002). Residues of veterinary medicinal products are 'pharmacologically active substances (whether active principles, excipients or degradation products) and their metabolites which remain in foodstuffs obtained from animals to which the veterinary medicinal product in question has been administered' (Council Regulation (EEC) No. 2377/90, 1990).

An MRL means the maximum concentration of residue resulting from the use of a veterinary medicinal product (expressed in mg/kg or μg/kg on a fresh weight basis) which may be accepted by the Community to be legally permitted or recognised as acceptable in food (Council Regulation (EEC) No. 2377/90, 1990). Once the MRL has been allocated it is necessary to determine the withdrawal period. This is the period after administration of the veterinary medicinal product during which the target animal must not be slaughtered or during which milk or eggs must not be taken for human consumption. This ensures that residues from the product concerned will not exceed the MRL (Grein, 2000). The responsibility for keeping residues under the MRL lies with veterinary surgeons and farmers using licensed animal medicines. Regulatory bodies and laboratories testing food products are required to ensure that regulations are met.

Official samples taken by inspection services in the slaughterhouse or the farm need to be analysed in official laboratories for forbidden substances and for legally used veterinary drugs. In Belgium, if residues of a veterinary medicine are detected in a concentration higher than the MRL then the farm receives an R-status. This means that for eight weeks there will be one analysis for every ten slaughtered animals at the cost of the owner. If residues are found of a forbidden substance the consequences are more severe and the farm will receive an H-status (Okerman *et al.*, 1999). This is implemented for 52 weeks. A sample from one of every ten animals slaughtered will be analysed at the cost of the owner.

9.3 Methods for detecting residues

9.3.1 Screening methods

A screening test is an analytical method which will give a strong indication if there is some form of drug residue present in a sample. The residue present may be in the form of parent drug or metabolite. Screening tests are generally expected to provide inexpensive, qualitative and sometimes semi-quantitative test responses. Various rapid tests for detecting veterinary drugs in foods have been reported. They are classified as either microbiological and electrophoretic methods or immunological methods and receptor tests (Watanabe *et al.*, 1998). Microbiological tests are considered as multi-residue screening tests, while immunological and receptor tests are more specific and can detect one substance or a group of related chemicals (De Wasch *et al.*, 1998b; Okerman *et al.*, 1998).

Microbiological identification tests use bacterial strains with varying sensitivities to antibiotics on media of varying pH values and supplemented with substances blocking or enhancing the action of certain antibiotics or antibiotic groups (Myllyniemi *et al.*, 2001). An example of such an inhibition test is the four plate test (FPT). As the name infers four plates are required with three using the organism *Bacillus subtilis* at different pH values and the fourth using *Micrococcus luteus* (Woodward and Shearer, 1995). The addition of a plate seeded with *Escherichia coli* to the system will facilitate the detection of quinolones (Okerman *et al.*, 1998). From the size and the pattern of the annular zone on the various plates an idea can be formed of the identity and the concentration of the analyte (Woodward and Shearer, 1995). The composition and the properties of the medium used in a microbiological inhibition test influence the detection limits of antibiotics; in particular, the pH of the medium is an important factor. It is therefore possible that tissue components such as proteins change the composition of the medium and influence the inhibitory zone produced by an antibiotic residue present in the sample (Okerman *et al.*, 1998).

Next to the microbiological inhibition tests, electrophoretic systems can be used as an aid in identifying antibiotics. Discs of meat are placed on a gel nutrient media and high voltage electrophoresis is carried out after a short diffusion time. Depending on the pH and the nature of the gel, antibiotics have differing mobilities. After applying the voltage, the gel is overlaid with an organism-containing gel and incubated. Zones of inhibition indicate the presence of antibiotics and the position on the plate could indicate the nature of the antibiotic (Woodward and Shearer, 1995).

The purpose of microbiological and electrophoretic tests is to select samples, which probably contain one or more analytes and which should be investigated with more sophisticated immunochemical and/or chromatographic methods. Microbiological tests should be simple, cheap, easy and fast. Multi-residue screening methods are preferred to methods detecting only one analyte (Okerman *et al.*, 1998, 1999).

Immunological (radioimmunoassay (RIA) and enzyme-linked immunosorbent assay (ELISA)) and receptor tests have similar working mechanisms. In both cases there is a reaction between an analyte and an antibody. Immunological tests are based on the competition between a labelled antigen (tracer) and an analyte. First a carrier is coated with a monoclonal or polyclonal antibody that recognises both the tracer and the analyte. The carrier is then brought in contact with the labelled antigen as well as with an extract of a sample. If the extract is residue free only the tracer will bind to the antibody. If some analyte is present in the extract some of the spaces on the carrier will be occupied with unlabelled analyte. The antigen is labelled with a radioactive isotope (RIA) or with an enzyme (ELISA). The reaction in ELISA is made visible afterwards by adding a substrate, which will be converted into a coloured product through reaction with the enzyme. So for both RIA and ELISA qualitative and quantitative results are obtained (De Wasch *et al.*, 1998b; Okerman *et al.*, 1999; Woodward and Shearer, 1995; Haasnoot and Schilt, 2000).

Receptor tests make use of the reaction between an antibacterial compound and a bacterial receptor. Receptors are isolated from sensitive organisms and they are able to bind antibiotics (Okerman *et al.*, 1999). Immunological and receptor tests are more specific than inhibition tests and provide faster results but the kits cost more and the reagents are not stable for a long time (De Wasch *et al.*, 1998b).

The objective of a qualitative screening method is to check whether a sample contains antibiotics. It is not the intensity of the signal, but the sensitivity that is important (Arts *et al.*, 1998). Screening tests can only be used if no false-negative results are possible, because negative samples are accepted without further confirmation analysis (Okerman *et al.*, 1998). The semi-quantitative screening methods can often be used more efficiently and hence at lower cost than the more sophisticated quantitative chromatographic methods. Nevertheless the latter are necessary for confirmation of suspected samples obtained during screening (Arts *et al.*, 1998).

9.3.2 Confirmation methods

Numerous confirmation methods have been described for the detection of veterinary drugs in various matrices. Most techniques comprise a chromatographic separation and a detection method. A chromatographic system on its own does not provide unambiguous confirmation of the identities of the components because the signal obtained is devoid of structural information. The only criterion of identity is the retention time. Unfortunately any one of a given number of substances can have the same retention time (Rose, 1990). Liquid chromatography (LC) is often combined with ultraviolet detection (UV), fluorescence detection and mass spectrometry (MS) (Mellon, 1991). Gas chromatography (GC) can be combined with electron capture detection (ECD), infrared detection (IR) and mass spectrometry (Rose, 1990).

The hyphenation of gas chromatography and mass spectrometry was first introduced in 1952. Because some products (with a molecular mass higher than 1500 and thermolabile molecules) cannot be separated with GC, the development of LC-MS technologies and applications started almost 20 years ago (De Brabander *et al.*, 1998). To obtain better detection limits MS-MS was developed. MS-MS methods offer great advantages in three areas: structural studies, the characterisation of mixture compounds and trace analysis. The use of LC-MS^n has led to a reduction of the sample extraction and clean-up (Scrivens and Rollins, 1990).

Confirmation methods can be both qualitative and quantitative. Quantitative methods are necessary to detect veterinary products that are permitted in some matrices in a maximum concentration. The methods need to confirm if the concentration of an analyte is below or above this limit. Therefore such confirmation methods need to have a quantification limit lower than the MRL. The quantification limit should be approximately 0.5 times the MRL (see Section 9.4.3).

Qualitative methods are used for forbidden substances and violative use of veterinary medicinal products. These methods are always semi-quantitative. To determine if an analyte is present or absent an action limit (AL) is used. An action limit separates a signal from the background noise. An action limit is not a legal value; it is an agreement between the laboratories and the inspection services and depends on the analytical possibilities at that moment. There are three main differences between an MRL and an AL:

1. MRLs are situated in a higher concentration level than ALs
2. MRLs are only used for registered veterinary drugs in edible products whereas ALs are used for forbidden substances
3. MRL has a legal implementation, whereas AL is a convention between laboratories and inspection services (De Brabander *et al.*, 1998).

9.4 Validating detection methods

9.4.1 Method validation

Every regulatory analytical method should be validated for different parameters. The most important parameters are recovery, detection and quantification limits. Recovery means 'the percentage of the true concentration of a substance recovered during the analytical procedure'. The limit of detection means 'the smallest content of the analyte that may be detected in a sample after applying the appropriate identification criteria'. The limit of quantification means 'the smallest measured content of the identified analyte in a sample that can be quantified with a specified degree of accuracy and precision' (Council Directive 96/23/EC, 1996).

9.4.2 Identification

Every confirmation method requires a 'standard injection protocol' (SIP) to guarantee the quality of the detection and quantification. An SIP is a logical succession of standards, blanks and samples (Table 9.1).

When a sample reveals a 'suspected' mass spectrum, quality criteria are necessary for the qualification and quantification. These criteria are determined by the EU, but are constantly evaluated. Quality criteria for the identification of organic residues and contaminants are based on the use of identification points

Table 9.1 The 'standard injection protocol' (SIP) for the detection and quantification of veterinary drugs

Detection	Quantification
1. standard	1. standard
2. blank (mobile phase)	2. blank (mobile phase)
3. samples in positive mode	3. sample
4. blank	4. blank (mobile phase)
5. samples in negative mode	5. blank
6. blank (mobile phase)	6. spike at MRL connection
7. standard	7. spike at 10 × MRL concentration
	8. blank (mobile phase)
	9. standard

(IP). The system of identification points balances the identification power of the different analytical techniques and moreover has the advantage that new techniques may easily be incorporated in the procedure. The minimum number of IPs for forbidden compounds is set to four, for compounds with an MRL a minimum of three IPs are required for the confirmation of the compound's identity. The most important limitations of these criteria are: they are not applicable to all compounds and they are ambiguous. Not all forbidden substances generate four IPs and diagnostic ions that appear at relatively high concentration may disappear when the concentration of the analyte decreases.

All diagnostic ions must have a signal-to-noise ratio of at least 3:1. The relative intensities of the detected ions expressed as a percentage of the intensity of the most intense ion must correspond to those of the standard analyte or spiked matrix at comparable concentrations and measured under the same conditions, within the tolerances given in Table 9.2.

If mass fragments are measured the system of identification points shall be used to interpret the data. LC-MS^n precursor ions earn 1 IP, LC-MS^n transition products earn 1.5 IP. Moreover at least one ion ratio must be measured and all measured ion ratios must meet the criteria described above. The criteria for identification are based on precursor and diagnostic ions, which give structural information. Retention time is another parameter that gives an indication of the identity of an analyte, but it contains no structural information. Moreover various substances have the same retention time (André *et al.*, 2001).

Table 9.2 The allowed margins for the relative ion intensities for LC-MS-MS

Relative intensity	Maximum permitted tolerance
>50%	±20%
>20–50%	±25%
>10–20%	±30%
<10%	±50%

9.4.3 Quantification

The identification of compounds has to be completed before their quantification. A quantitative validation is required for each sample containing a permitted veterinary drug. Such a validation consists of determining the required validation parameters at three levels: ½MRL, MRL and 2MRL. This validation approach is very elaborate and time consuming.

Because of the high concentrations of VMPs in injection sites an alternative validation is proposed for that matrix. De Wasch *et al.* (2002) described an alternative validation consisting of a comparison of the analyte concentration in the sample with the spike at MRL and 10 times MRL concentration. The alternative approach is performed as a mini-validation. A mini-validation consists of five blank matrices fortified with the MRL concentration of the analyte, five blank matrices fortified with 10 times the MRL concentration of the analyte and one blank matrix. This approach allows the analyst to meet the needs and requirements of the customer awaiting the results. The analysis is accurate, fast and the total cost of this approach is minimised in comparison with a traditional validation and analysis. In Section 9.5.2 this alternative validation is illustrated by the example of sulfadimethoxine. The conditions that need to be fulfilled before reporting a sample as violative are described by De Wasch *et al.* (2002).

Traditional validation procedures require extensive studies to obtain all necessary data. Such a validation is time consuming and expensive. It is, however, not practical or necessary that all analytical methods are assessed at this ideal level. The alternative validation gives a rapid reporting to the customer and the costs are lower than for a traditional analysis. Identification can be performed within 48 hours and an extra 24 hours are necessary for the quantification. The choice between a traditional validation and an alternative validation depends on the analytical purpose and method.

9.5 Rapid on-line confirmation of different veterinary residues

9.5.1 General

A Belgian research project financed by the Federal Ministry of Agriculture and the Institute of Veterinary Inspection started in January 2001 in which injection sites were collected at the slaughterhouse. In analysing these samples, an overview could be given of what is frequently used nowadays in practice. Another important aspect to consider is that injection sites very often contain high concentrations of the administered product. Injection sites are considered as meat by inspection services and therefore the MRL for meat applies, especially because of the possible consumption of an injection site. To develop and to use very specific confirmation methods takes time and is expensive. Because of the high concentrations there is no demand for the registered VMPs to be quantified in the concentration range of the MRL. A different validation can be used (Section 9.4.3).

Since the beginning of 2001 different injectable or standard solutions of registered veterinary medicine products were collected. These solutions were subjected to infusion-MS^n and LC-MS^n. The collected data will function as a database for the identification of analytes present in an injection site. Injectable solutions are not the active compounds but the VMPs as used in veterinary practice. Additional impurities can therefore obscure the chromatogram and the spectrum, but this can also be expected in injection sites. The use of an ointment base such as polyethyleneglycol can mask the pure product when using direct infusion (De Wasch *et al.*, 2002).

9.5.2 Examples

For the identification of 'unknown analytes' two approaches can be used: infusion-MS^n (example: flunixine) and LC-MS^n (example: sulfadimethoxine). Electrospray ionisation is preferred for both because it is a soft ionisation technique and fragmentation of the pseudo-molecular ion in full scan MS is not as intense as when using APCI. Possible molecular masses are calculated from MH^+ or MH^- ions, Na^+, $NH4^+$ or Ac^- adducts. There are different identification strategies. It is possible to derive the molecular weight of the unknown analyte by complementary data from the positive and negative ions (MH^+ and MH^- ions). Sometimes there appears only one pseudo-molecular ion either in positive or negative ion mode and an adduct in the other mode. Adducts are formed by reaction between the analyte and the solvent used in the mobile phase. Knowledge of the solvents used is therefore very important. For example when an acid is added to methanol or water acetate, adducts can be formed in negative ion mode, ammoniumacetate leads to $NH4^+$ adducts. It is also possible to detect only adducts in both ion modes. Some analytes, depending on their functional groups, cannot form positive or negative ions or adducts. The absence of ions in one ion mode also gives structural information about the analyte. In the presence of a second compound (a veterinary drug or a chemical product) different combinations can be formed leading to mass spectra in which these different combinations can be recognised. Different masses will appear in the spectrum at different retention times. De Wasch *et al.* (2002) demonstrated this with the example Penicillin G – benzathin. These different strategies demonstrate that some knowledge is required for the interpretation of mass spectra. First, knowledge about the chromatographic system, the mobile phase in particular. This mobile phase can lead to the formation of an adduct in positive or negative ion mode. Second, knowledge about the mass spectrometer. Electrospray ionisation is a soft ionisation technique and gives rise to the pseudo-molecular ion without extensive fragmentation.

Using the collected data of the different injectable or standard solutions and the database of the Merck index the identity of the analyte can be elucidated. All possible compounds from the database are filtered based on their therapeutic category or intended use. Ion traces of 'known' compounds (collected injectable and standard solutions of registered veterinary medicinal products) can be more easily detected using LC-MS^n by applying a layout. A layout is an option in the software in which mass traces of pseudo-molecular ions of injectable solutions are combined in a window. A layout can be added depending on the knowledge of injectable analytes at that time.

In the next examples the identification of some veterinary medicinal products is described using infusion-MS^n or LC-MS^n. The identity of the analyte can be elucidated using the mass spectra in MS-full scan and/or MS-full scan and the collected data of different injectable or standard solutions and the database of the Merck index. The alternative validation consisting of a comparison of the analyte concentration in the sample with the spike at MRL and 10 times MRL concentration is illustrated in the first example of sulfadimethoxine. Such a validation is comparable for each compound.

Identification of sulfadimethoxine

Sulfadimethoxine (Fig. 9.1) is a sulfonamide antibiotic used in veterinary medicine to treat susceptible bacterial and coccidial infections. It is recommended in cattle for the treatment of bovine respiratory disease complex, bacterial pneumonia associated with *Pasteurella* spp., necrotic pododermatitis (foot rot) and calf diphtheria caused by *Fusobacterium necrophorum*. Sulphonamides are antibacterial agents widely used in veterinary practice to prevent infections in livestock. They have also been used in animal feeds to promote growth and to treat disease. Residues are often found in meat and milk

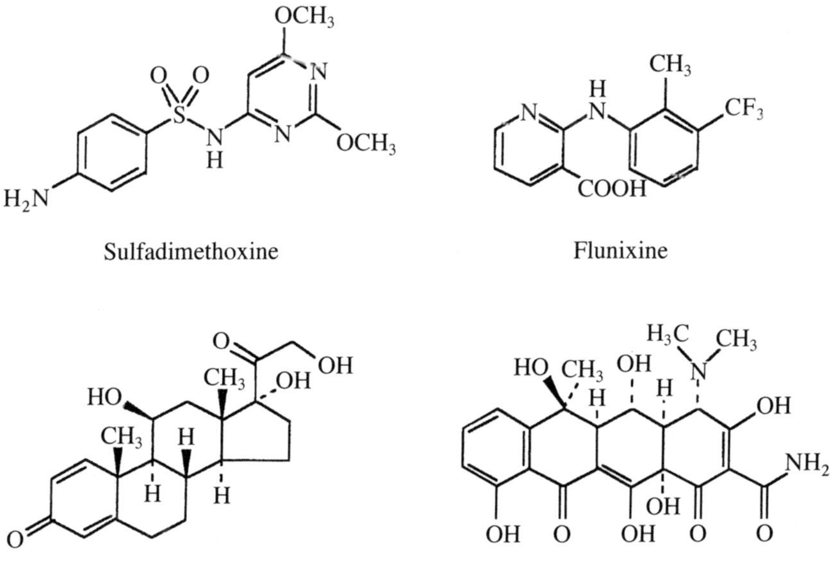

Fig. 9.1 Structural formulas of sulfadimethoxine, flunixine, prednisolone and oxytetracycline.

Table 9.3 Identity and percentage of the analytes present in injection sites in 2002

Analyte	Group of VMPs	Number of violations	Percentage
Penicillin G	β-lactam	26	7.6
Flunixin	NSAID	19	5.6
Oxytetracycline	tetracycline	10	2.9
Sulfadimethoxine	sulfonamide	6	1.8
Enrofloxacin	quinolone	5	1.5
Trimethoprim	diamine derivatives	5	1.5
Prednisolone	corticosteroid	4	1.2
Erythromycine	macrolide	4	1.2
Tilmycosine	macrolide	4	1.2
Tylosine	macrolide	4	1.2
Florfenicol	florfenicol	3	0.9
Tolfenamic acid	NSAID	3	0.9
Lincomycin	lincosamide	2	0.6
Dexamethasone	corticosteroid	2	0.6
Tetracycline	tetracycline	2	0.6
Sulfadoxine	sulfonamide	1	0.3
Meloxicam	NSAID	1	0.3

products where they enter the human food chain. The presence of sulphonamide residues in food is of concern because some of the compounds are carcinogenic and they enhance the risk of developing bacterial resistance, which makes the therapeutic use of this medicine inefficient (Dost *et al.*, 2000) Most of the sulphonamides are combined with trimethoprim that potentiates the antibacterial effects of the sulphonamide. These combinations are believed to act synergistically on specific targets in bacterial DNA synthesis (Woodward and Shearer, 1995). Table 9.3 shows that trimethoprim was detected in five samples and this always in combination with sulfadimethoxine. Sulfadimethoxine has an MRL of 100 μg/kg in muscle. Because injection sites are considered as meat by inspection services, the MRL for meat applies.

Injection of an extract of an injection site revealed in MS-full scan an intensive negative ion with m/z 309 and an intensive positive ion with m/z 311. An analyte with molecular mass 310 can be expected from the complementary information of the positive and negative ion spectra. Using the Merck index a search is performed in the molecular weight range 309–311. Different possibilities were found: altrenogestagen (prostagen), mepazine (tranquilliser), methoprene (ectoparasiticide), sulfadoxine (antibacterial) and sulfadimethoxine (antibacterial). Mass spectra of the injectable and standard solutions of some of these compounds revealed that both sulfadoxine and sulfadimethoxine (MM 310.33) produce the same pseudo-molecular ions as the 'unknown' sample. There are no differences between the two components in MS-full scan, but the ion ratio in MS is different (sulfadoxine: 108 (±15%), 156 (100%), 218 (±2%), 245 (±20%); sulfadimethoxine: 108 (±10%), 156 (100%), 218 (±40%), 245

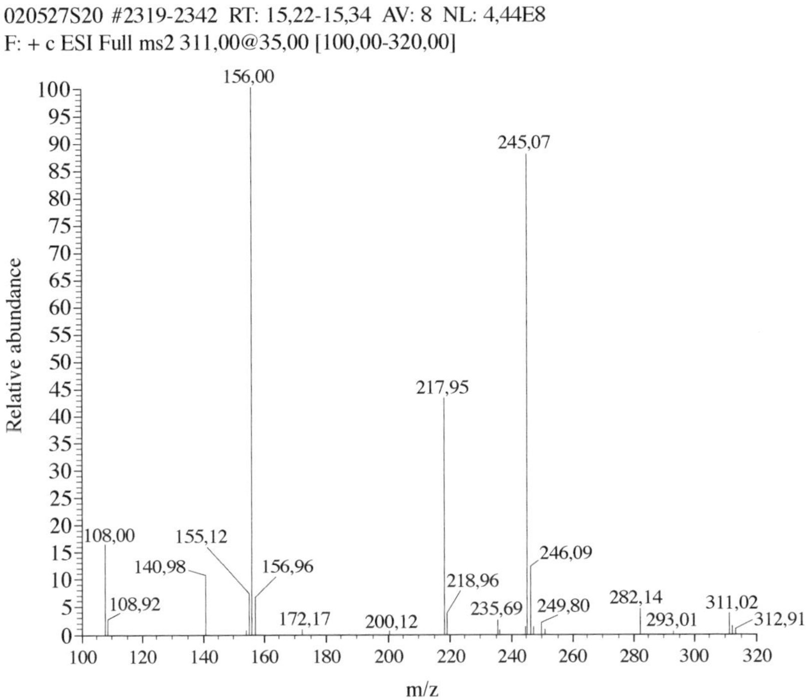

Fig. 9.2 MS^2 fragmentation of the ion with m/z 311 in positive mode.

(±90%)). Therefore a second injection of the extract is performed in the positive ion mode, both in MS-full scan and MS^2-full scan (Fig. 9.2). Also the standard solutions of sulfadoxine and sulfadimethoxine are injected (Fig. 9.3). Not only the ion ratio in MS is different, but also the retention time (sulfadoxine elutes around 10 min and sulfadimethoxine around 14 min). It can be concluded that the injection site contains sulfadimethoxine.

Because sulfadimethoxine is a legally used veterinary medicinal product with an MRL of 100 μg/kg a quantification is required (Fig. 9.4). This is performed by comparing the analyte concentration in the sample with the spike at MRL and 10× MRL concentration. The area ratio is calculated by dividing the area of sulfadimethoxine by the area of the internal standard desoximethasone. The area ratio of the sample is 34.732, the one of the spike at MRL concentration is 0.0066 and the one at 10× MRL concentration is 0.0618. Subsequently the conditions described by De Wasch *et al.* (2002) on which violation is based, are calculated. The ratio of the area ratio of the spike at 10 × MRL concentration and the area ratio of the spike at MRL concentration is 9.36 (the prescribed ratio is 4) and the ratio of the area ratio of the sample and the area ratio of the spike at MRL concentration is 5262 (the prescribed ratio is 10). The sample is thus clearly violative for sulfadimethoxine, with a concentration higher than the MRL concentration.

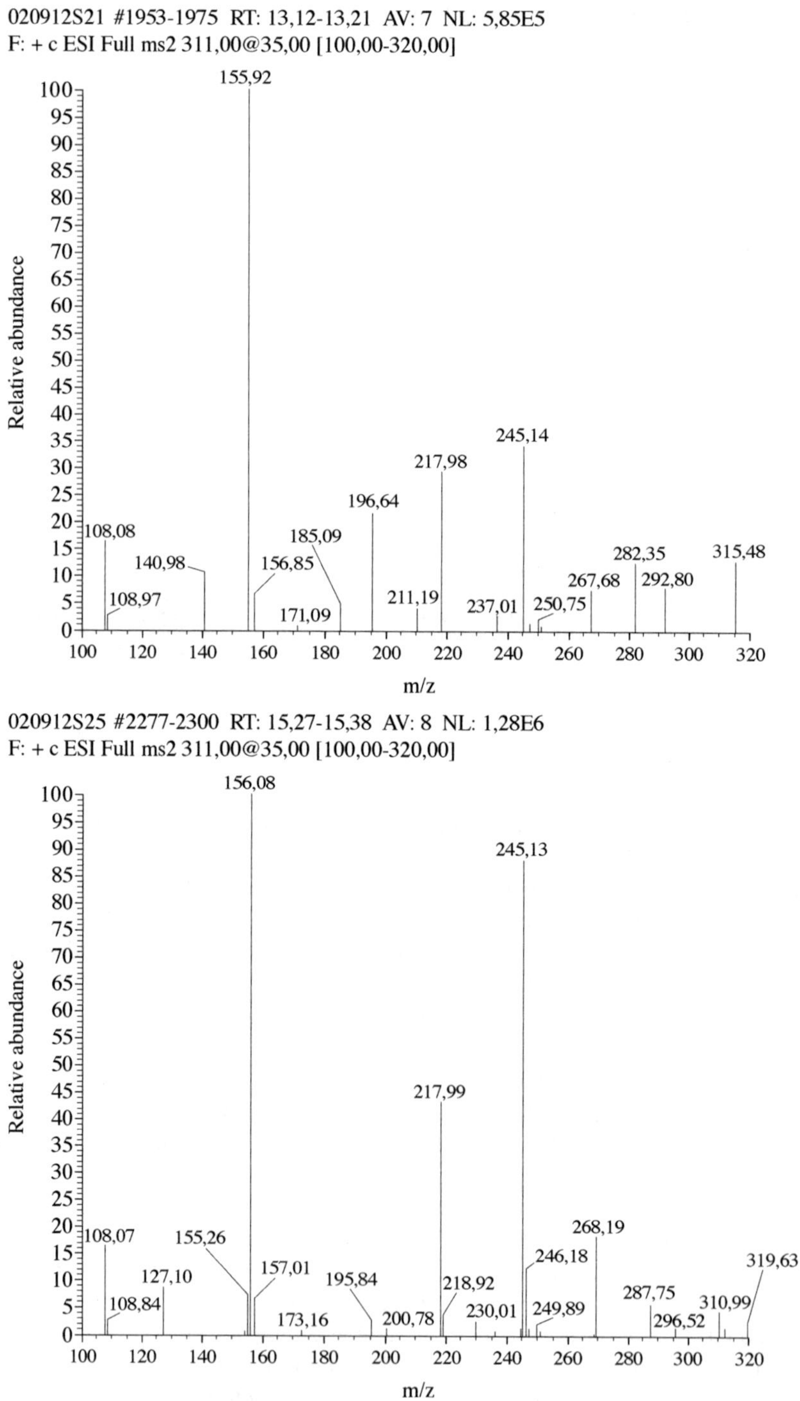

Fig. 9.3 MS²-full scan spectrum of sulfadoxine (top) and sulfadimethoxine (bottom).

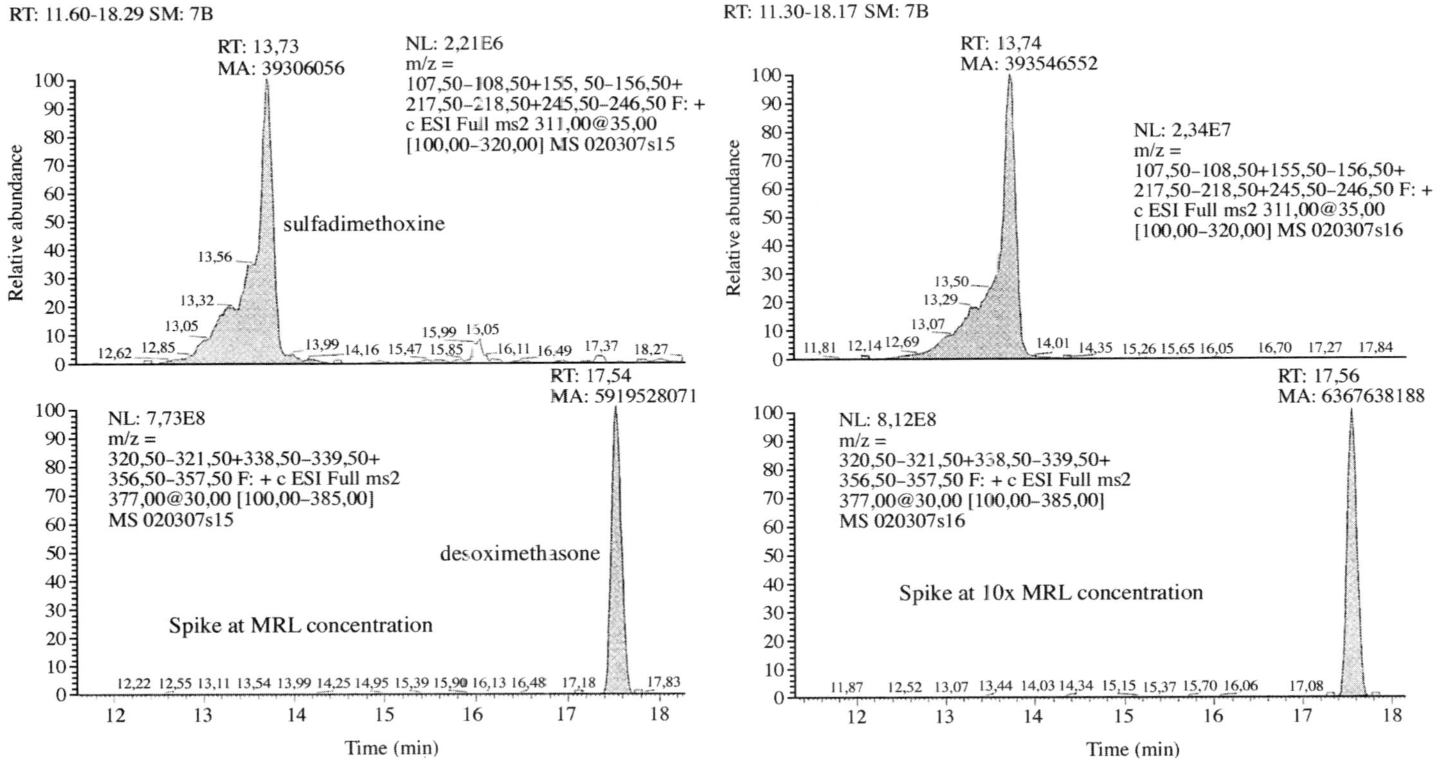

Fig. 9.4 The chromatograms of sulfadimethoxine and desoximethasone (IS), each with the retention time and the area, of a spike at MRL concentration, a spike at 10× MRL concentration and the extract of an injection site. The calculation of the conditions for violation.

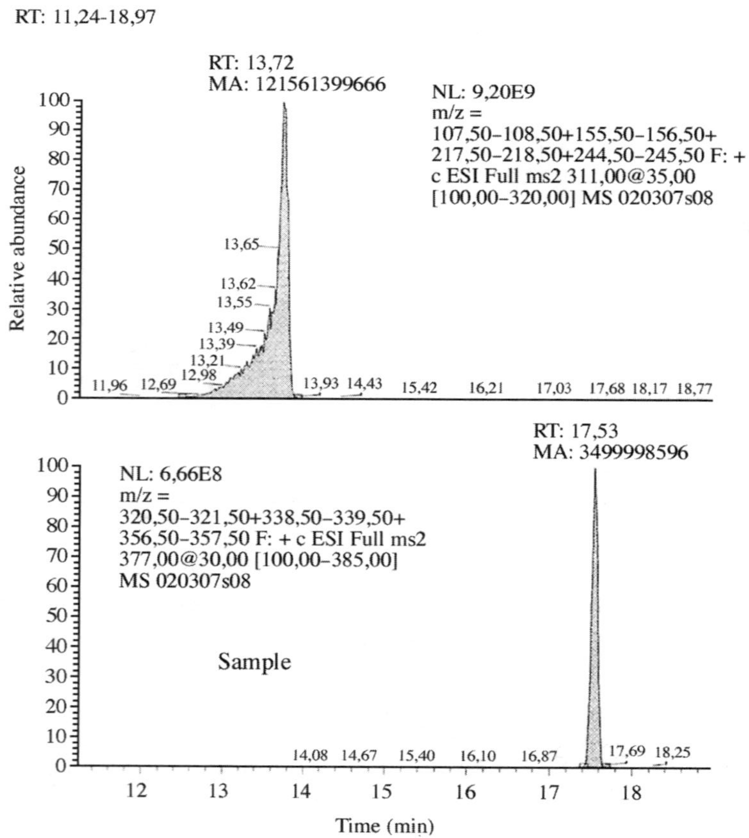

MRL:
Area sulfadimethoxine = 39 306 056
Area desoximethasone (IS) = 5 919 528 071
Area ratio 0,0066

10 MRL:
Area sulfadimethoxine = 393 546 552
Area desoximethasone (IS) = 6 367 638 188
Area ratio 0,0618

Sample
Area sulfadimethoxine = 121 561 399 666
Area desoximethasone (IS) = 3 499 998 596
Area ratio 34,732

Area ratio MRL/area ratio 10MRL = 9,36 > 4
Area ratio sample/area ratio MRL = 5262 > 10

Fig. 9.4 Continued

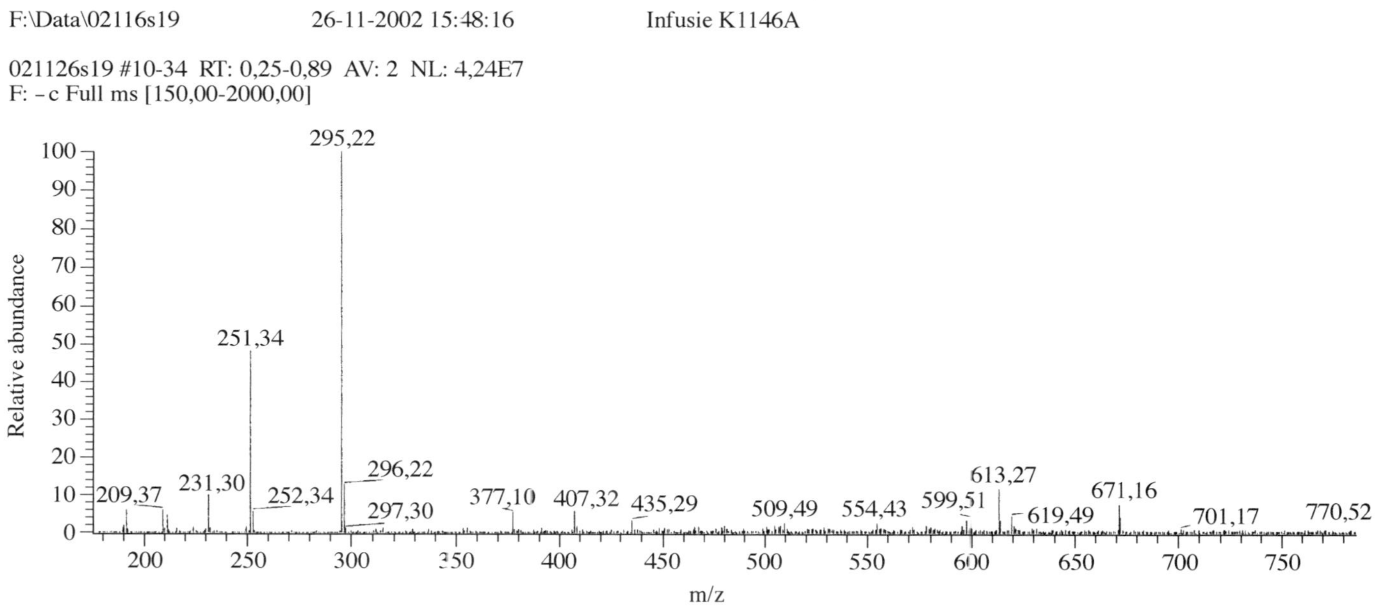

Fig. 9.5 MS-full scan of an injection site in positive and negative mode.

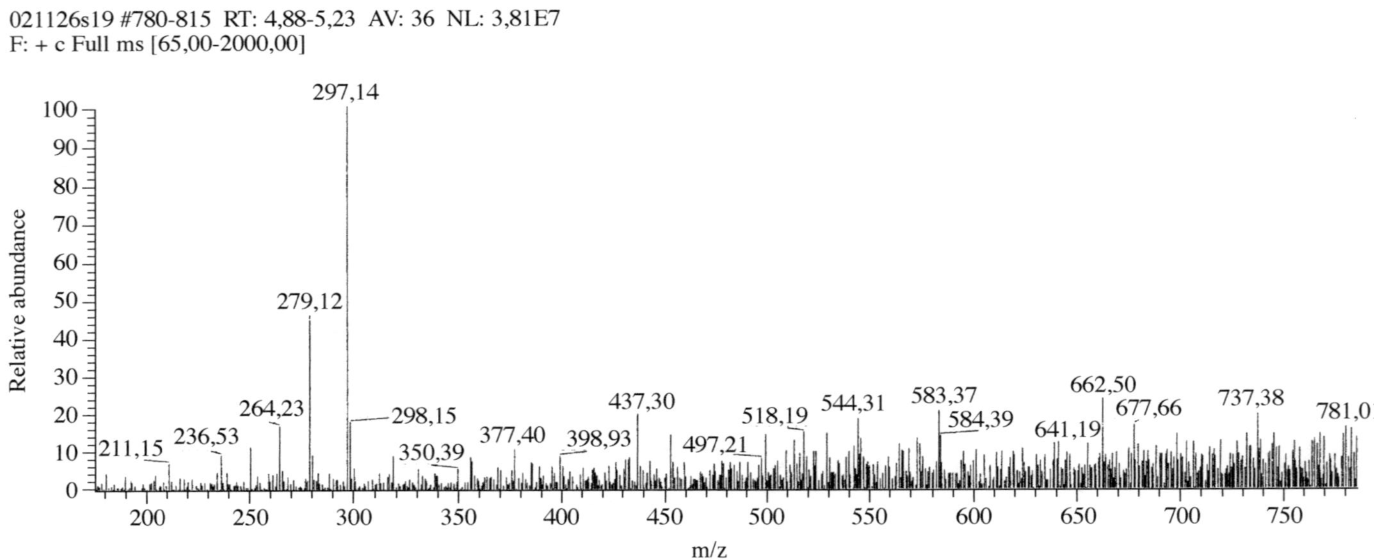

Fig. 9.5 Continued

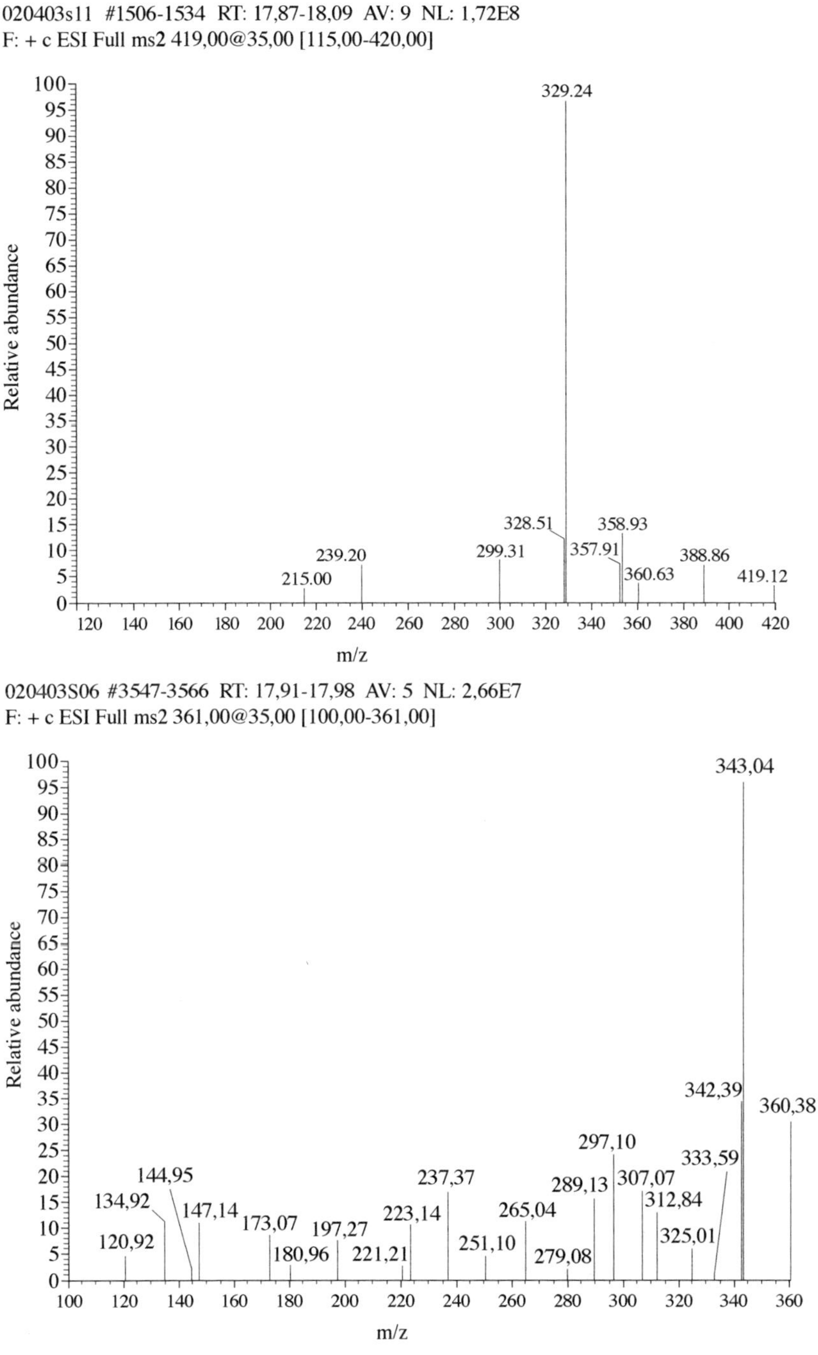

Fig. 9.6 MS^2 fragmentation of the ion with m/z 419 in negative mode (top) and MS^2 fragmentation of the ion with m/z 361 in positive mode (bottom).

Identification of flunixine

Flunixine (Fig. 9.1) is a nonsteroidal anti-inflammatory drug (NSAID) used to alleviate inflammation and pain in veterinary medicine. NSAIDs are used either alone or in combination with approved antibiotics to treat food-producing animals. Flunixine is a legally used veterinary medicinal product with an MRL of 20 μg/kg in muscle.

An extract of an injection site was infused in the mass spectrometer through a T-piece. In positive ion mode, ions with m/z 297 and 279 were observed, in negative ion mode, ions with m/z 295 and 251 (Fig. 9.5). The molecular mass 296 can be derived from the complementary information of positive and negative ions. MS fragmentation of the ion with m/z 297 in positive mode and the ion with m/z 295 in negative mode indicates that the other two ions observed after infusion are fragments of the pseudo-molecular ion. Using the Merck index the compounds with molecular weight 296 are filtered based on their use in veterinary medicine. Even then still a lot of possibilities remained. Making use of our database of mass spectra of injectable solutions of registered veterinary medicine products it can be concluded that the analyte present in the injection site was flunixine (MW 296.25).

Identification of prednisolone

Prednisolone (Fig. 9.1) is a glucocorticoid used for the suppression of inflammatory and allergic disorders in veterinary medicine. Besides the therapeutic use of glucocorticoids research demonstrated that these compounds are capable of increasing weight gain and reducing feed conversion, and they have a synergetic effect when combined with other molecules like β-agonists or anabolic steroids. Thus corticosteroids are illegally used as growth promoters in cattle, administered through livestock food or by injection (Antignac *et al.*, 2001). Prednisolone has an MRL of 4 μg/kg in muscle.

Injection of the extract of an injection site showed in MS-full scan in negative ion mode the ions with m/z 419 and 359 and in positive mode the ion with m/z 361. The molecular weight 360 can be derived from the positive and negative ions (positive ions: $361 - 1 = 360$ and negative ions: $359 + 1 = 360$, $419 - 60$ (acetate adduct) $= 359$).

In MS^2-full scan in positive mode of the ion with m/z 361 a specific spectrum was revealed. A large number of product ions is observed decreasing in intensity with decreasing m/z. This pattern of decreasing ion peaks is typical for glucocorticoids (De Wasch *et al.*, 1998a). In negative mode the spectrum in MS-full scan of the ion with m/z 419 reveals a loss of 60 due to the acetate, followed by a loss of 30 (Fig. 9.6). Using the Merck index a search is performed in the molecular weight range 359–361. Two glucocorticoids were found: cortisone and prednisolone. MS fragmentation of the extract corresponds to the standard of prednisolone (MW 360.44) that was already acquired in a different application.

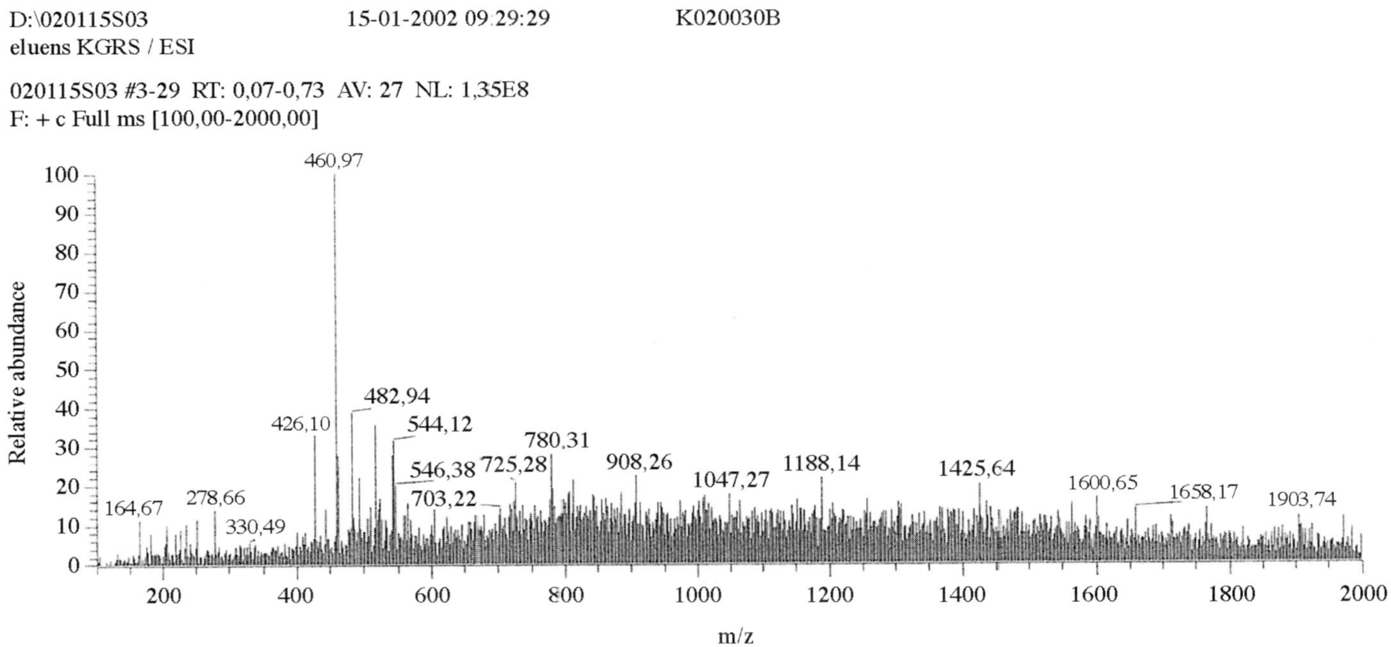

Fig 9.7 MS-full scan of an injection site in positive and negative ion mode.

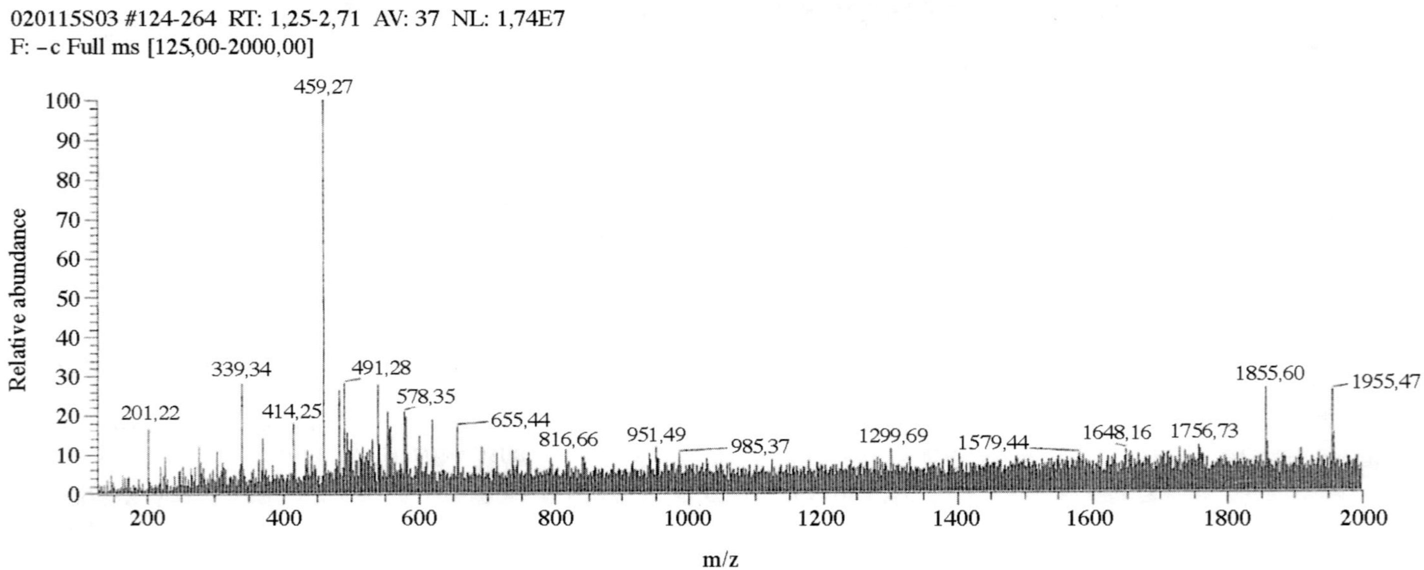

Fig. 9.7 Continued

Identification of oxytetracycline
Tetracyclines are broad spectrum antibiotics, used to treat respiratory disease in cattle, sheep, pigs and chicken and they may be given in feed or drinking water. Oxytetracycline (Fig. 9.1) is used to treat enteric disease in a number of species. It is a legally used veterinary medicinal product with an MRL of 100 μg/kg in muscle.

Infusion of an extract of an injection site showed in positive mode especially the ion with m/z 461 and in negative the ion with m/z 459 (Fig. 9.7). A search was performed in the Merck index for the molecular weight 460 (range 459–461). There was only one compound that is used in veterinary practice: oxytetracycline. The spectrum of MS of the extract in positive mode corresponds to that of the standard solution of oxytetracycline collected in our database.

9.5.3 Conclusion

In 2002, 342 injection sites were analysed for 'unknown analytes', 101 of them (29.5%) were reported violative with a concentration higher than the MRL. Table 9.3 gives a summary of the identity and the percentage of these analytes. In 17 injection sites (5%) the identity of a veterinary drug could be demonstrated, but with a concentration lower than the MRL. Penicillin G and flunixine are the most commonly used veterinary medicines in this study. Also oxytetracycline and sulfadimethoxin are frequently used.

9.6 Future trends

This chapter illustrates the advantages of using infusion-MS^n and/or LC-MS^n to detect and confirm the presence of highly concentrated compounds in injection sites. It is a multi-residue approach which is able to detect a wide range of administered products.

Injection sites can contain a wide range of analytes in high concentrations. To develop specific confirmation methods and switching instruments to different applications for only one sample, is time consuming and expensive. An alternative approach was therefore necessary. For the examples illustrated in this chapter no specific method development for extraction or clean-up or confirmation was performed. There is no need for quantification of the registered VMPs in the concentration range of the MRL. An alternative validation is used comparing the analyte concentration in the sample with the spike at MRL and 10 times MRL concentration. The alternative approach is performed as a mini-validation. Identification is based on the collected data of the different injectable and standard solutions of registered VMPs and the database of the Merck index.

Extraction and identification can be performed within 48 hours. If the identified compound needs to be quantified, an extra 24 hours are necessary before the result can be reported. To create a faster method the clean-up can be performed on-line. Due to the simplicity of the extraction and clean-up (only SPE) an online procedure should be possible. Extraction and clean-up is necessary because the injection sites are rather dirty. Such an on-line method will lead to faster and more homogeneous results. The detection method itself cannot be shortened because then there is a chance that some veterinary medicinal products would not be detected. The interpretation of the mass spectra can also be very time consuming. It is therefore important to collect as much mass spectra as possible of injectable and standard solutions of VMPs. Then the interpretation can be more automated using a library. A library contains all mass spectra of injectable and standard solutions and can be correlated to the interpretation of the data. The interpretation can so be simplified and even automated.

There is a continuing need for reliable analytical methods for use in determining compliance with national regulations as well as international requirements in all areas of food quality and safety. The reliability of a method is determined by some form of validation procedure. Method validation needs to be carried out under an appropriate quality system. The final goal is to produce correct results, by means of a reliable quantitative validation, and minimise the costs and time doing so. This will lead to specialisation of laboratories and to alternative validations if the analytical goal permits it. It is important that correct results can be produced within a reasonable period of time.

9.7 Acknowledgements

This work was supported financially by the Belgian Federal Ministry of Agriculture and the Institute of Veterinary Inspection (S6044/S3).

9.8 References

ANDRÉ F, DE WASCH K K G, DE BRABANDER H F, IMPENS S R, STOLKER L A M, VAN GINKEL L, STEPHANY R W, SCHILT R, COURTHEYN D, BONNAIRE Y, FÜRST P, GOWIK P, KENNEDY G, KUHN T, MORETAIN JP and SAUER M (2001), 'Trends in the identification of organic residues and contaminants: EC regulations under revision', *Trends Anal Chem*, 20 (8), 435–445.

ANTIGNAC JP, LE BIZEC B, MONTEAU F, POULAIN F and ANDRÉ F (2001), 'Multi-residue extraction-purification procedure for corticosteroids in biological samples for efficient control of their misuse in livestock production', *J Chrom B, Biomed Appl*, 757 (1), 11–19.

ARTS C J M, VAN BAAK M J, ELLIOT C J, HEWITT A, COOPER J, VAN DE VELDE-FASE K and WITKAMP R F (1998), 'Comparison of conventional immunoassays and the oestrogen radioreceptor assay for screening for the presence of oestrogenic anabolic compounds in urine samples', *Analyst*, 123, 2579–2583.

COUNCIL DIRECTIVE 65/65/EEC OF 26 JANUARY 1965 OF PROVISIONS LAID DOWN BY LAW, REGULATION OR ADMINISTRATIVE ACTION RELATING TO MEDICINAL PRODUCTS (1965)

Official Journal of the European Communities, no. L 22 of 9.2., 369.

COUNCIL REGULATION (EEC) NO. 2377/90 OF JUNE 1990 LAYING DOWN A COMMUNITY PROCEDURE FOR THE ESTABLISHMENT OF MAXIMUM RESIDUE LIMITS OF VETERINARY MEDICINAL PRODUCTS IN FOODSTUFFS OF ANIMAL ORIGIN (1990), *Official Journal of the European Communities*, no. L 67 of 7.3, 1.

COUNCIL DIRECTIVE 96/23/EC OF 29 APRIL 1996 ON MEASURES TO MONITOR CERTAIN SUBSTANCES AND RESIDUES THEREOF IN LIVE ANIMALS AND ANIMAL PRODUCTS AND REPEALING DIRECTIVES 85/358/EEC AND 86/469/EEC AND DECISION 89/187/EEC AND 91/664/EEC (1996), *Official Journal of the European Communities*, no. L 125, 32–45.

DE BRABANDER H F, DE WASCH K, OKERMAN L and BATJOENS P (1998), 'Moderne analysemethodes voor additieven, contaminanten en residuen', *Vlaams Diergeneeskundig Tijdschrift*, 67, 96–105.

DE WASCH K, DE BRABANDER H, COURTHEYN D and VAN PETEGHEM C (1998a), 'Identification of corticosteroids in injection sites and cocktails by MS^n', *Analyst*, 123, 2415–2422.

DE WASCH K, OKERMAN L, CROUBELS S, DE BRABANDER H, VAN HOOF J and DE BACKER P (1998b), 'Detection of residues of tetracycline antibiotics in pork and chicken meat: correlation between results of screening and confirmatory tests', *Analyst*, 123, 2737–2741.

DE WASCH K, VAN HOOF N, POELMANS S, OKERMAN L, COURTHEYN D, ERMENS A, CORNELIS M and DE BRABANDER H F (2002), 'Identification of "unknown analytes" in injection sites: a semi-quantitative interpretation', *Anal Chim Acta*, accepted.

DOST K, JONES D C and DAVIDSON G (2000), 'Determination of sulfonamides by packed column supercritical fluid chromatography with atmospheric pressure chemical ionization mass spectrometric detection', *Analyst*, 125, 1243–1247.

GREIN K (2000), 'The safe use of veterinary medicines and the need of residue surveillance', in van Ginkel L A and Ruiter A, *Proceedings of the Euroresidue IV conference*, Veldhoven, The Netherlands.

HAASNOOT W and SCHILT R (2000), 'Immunochemical and receptor technologies', in O'Keeffe M, *Residue analysis in food – principles and applications*, Singapore, Harwood Academic Publishers, 107–144.

MELLON F A (1991), 'Liquid chromatography/mass spectrometry', in *VG Monographs in Mass Spectrometry*, 2 (1).

MYLLYNIEMI A L NUOTIO L, LINDFORS E, RANNIKKO R, NIEMI A and BÄCKMAN C (2001), 'A microbiological six-plate method for the identification of certain antibiotic groups in incurred kidney and muscle samples', *Analyst*, 126, 641–646.

OKERMAN L, DE WASCH K and VAN HOOF J (1998), 'Detection of antibiotics in muscle tissue with microbiological inhibition tests: effects of the matrix', *Analyst*, 123, 2361–2365.

OKERMAN L, DE WASCH K, DE BRABANDER H, ABRAMS R, VAN HOOF J, CORNELIS M and LAURIER L (1999), 'Oude en nieuwe opsporingstechnieken voor antibioticaresiduen in het kader van de huidige Belgische en Europese wetgeving', *Vlaams Diergeneeskundig Tijdschrift*, 68, 216–223.

ROSE M E (1990), 'Modern practice of gas chromatography/mass spectrometry', in *VG Monographs in Mass Spectrometry*, 1 (1).

SCRIVENS J H and ROLLINS K (1990), 'Tandem mass spectrometry', in *VG Monographs in Mass Spectrometry*.

WATANABE H, SATAKE A, MATSUMOTO M, KIDO Y, TSUJI A, ITO K and MAEDA M (1998), 'Monoclonal-based enzyme-linked immunosorbent assay and immuno-

chromatographic rapid assay for monesin', *Analyst*, 123, 2573–2578.
WOODWARD K N and SHEARER G (1995), 'Antibiotic use in animal production in the European Union – Regulations and current methods for residue detection', in Oka H, Nakazawa H, Harada K I and Macneil J D, *Chemical Analysis for Antibiotics used in Agriculture*, Arlington, AOAC International, 47–76.

10

New techniques for the rapid detection of growth promoters in farm animals

E. Magner and M. Jamal, University of Limerick, Ireland

10.1 Introduction: detecting the use of growth promoters

Current measurement techniques for the detection of growth promoters rely on random sampling, primarily at the point of slaughter, with specific tissue (muscle, liver, fat) or fluid (bile, urine) samples being taken to a centralised laboratory for analysis. The procedures involved in analysis can be relatively complex, and do not lend themselves to rapid (few minutes) measurements. Current testing methods are not in widespread use due to the inherent cost involved (€20–25 per sample), the *ex situ* nature of the analysis technique employed, the time lag involved (typically 24–36 hours) and the relatively complex techniques used which require skilled laboratory personnel.

Rapid testing would enable the implementation of a screening programme allowing regulatory bodies to monitor animals continuously prior to slaughter and thus identify animals with enhanced levels of hormone residues for detailed analysis of biological fluids. An effective screening system could allow on the spot decisions to be made regarding the androgen residue status of an animal, enabling meat entering the food chain to be certified free from residues of the particular androgens tested. Implementation of such a system would help allay consumer fears regarding the presence of potentially dangerous residues of androgen hormones.

The most promising format for the rapid and inexpensive determination of growth promoters relies on using a biosensor. According to the IUPAC definition 'biosensors are analytical devices incorporating a biological material (e.g. tissue, microorganisms, organelles, cell receptors, enzymes, antibodies, nucleic acids, etc.), a biologically derived material or biomimic intimately associated with or integrated within a physiochemical transducer or transducing microsystem, which may be optical, electrochemical, thermometric, piezoelectric or magnetic.'[1]

Of currently available biosensors, glucose biosensors[2] represent the only commercially successful example. It is worth examining the reasons for this success in order to ascertain the attributes necessary for a successful detection system for growth promoters.

A range of factors ensured the commercial viability of glucose biosensors:

- a demonstrable need for such testing (due to the complications caused by diabetes)
- a sensor that is relatively easy to use and which requires a small sample volume of 5 μl or less (the smaller the volume the less painful the test)
- a disposable, single use sensor that uses whole blood, requiring no dilution or addition of reagents
- a stable and cheap biorecognition element (glucose oxidase)
- a reasonably high analyte concentration (*ca.* 5 mM), and
- the ability to mass-produce the sensors at low cost on a large scale (10^6 units/day).

A successful test for growth promoters should

- be relatively small, cheap and portable
- be stable, with a shelf-life of at least six months in a refrigerator
- possess stable calibration
- be easy to use and as far as possible, have all required components incorporated, to ensure ease of use by the end user who may not have experience in running an assay
- be capable of mass production
- be low in cost, and
- be relatively immune to environmental factors, such as fluctuations in temperature and humidity.

A reliable and rapid test for growth promoters faces a number of technical challenges, which include a much smaller concentration of analyte (nM versus mM), and a requirement to detect a range of analytes rather than one single analyte. In addition the number of analytes will continue to increase as testing regimes for commonly used growth promoters are implemented.

10.2 Existing detection techniques and their limitations

A range of techniques has been applied to detect growth promoters in biological fluids, including: radioimmunoassay (RIA),[3] enzyme immunoassay (EIA),[4] high performance liquid chromatography (HPLC),[5] gas chromatography-mass spectrometry (GC-MS), dissociation enhanced lanthanide fluorescence immunoassay (DELFIA),[3] liquid chromatography-mass spectrometry-mass spectrometry (LC-MS-MS),[6] androgen receptor-luciferase expression (AR-

LUX) bioassay,[7] and liquid chromatography-electrospray ionisation-mass spectrometry (LC-ESI-MS).[8]

RIA is an extremely sensitive method[9] but suffers greatly from the requirement for radioactive materials. GC-MS is a reliable, sensitive and suitable technique for the assay of growth promoters (GP), but is time consuming, as it requires derivatisation due to the polarity and thermal instability of the analytes. Some growth promoters can be difficult to derivatise or may be unstable under the conditions used for derivatisation. Alternatives to GC-MS are HPLC-MS and HPLC-MS-MS in SRM (selected reaction monitoring) mode,[10] which have acceptable detection limits of 2 ppb, the limit of decision fixed by the EU.[11] Recently several steroids (from bovine kidney) have been analysed by LC-MS-MS using atmospheric pressure chemical ionisation in SRM mode[12] with a limit of detection (Table 10.1). Buiarelli *et al.*[10] determined the amount of the synthetic androgen trenbolone in calf urine and serum by LC-MS-MS with atmospheric pressure ionisation (API in SRM mode). A detection limit of 2 ng/ml was obtained.

With increasing enforcement of regulations governing the use of growth promoting agents, producers are rapidly changing the compounds used and the amounts administered, making detection of illicitly administered agents much more difficult. This is particularly so when individual compounds are used at very low levels and as components of cocktails which may contain masking agents. Barry *et al.*[7] have developed an assay, which is capable of measuring the integrated effect of cocktails (mixtures of all compounds). The assay is based on a human cell line featuring a luciferase reporter gene and can detect the presence of growth promoters in various different cocktails, which were not detected by GC-MS or LC-MS based methods. However, as with all currently available detection methods, the assay is laboratory based, and does not lend itself to rapid, simple analysis. A thorough screening technique requires assays that are portable, reliable and cost effective.

As immunoassays show good sensitivity with a low limit of detection, efforts have focused on sensors based on antibodies (immunosensor), aptamers, molecular imprinited polymer, receptor etc. combined with different detection techniques.

Table 10.1 Limits of detection for laboratory based methods

Method	Limit of detection ng/ml	Hormone
RIA	0.07	Progesterone[6]
EIA	0.08	Testosterone
DELFIA	0.2	Testosterone
GC-MS	1.0	Corticosteroid[7]
LC-MS-MS	1.0	Trenbolone/metabolites[8]
LC-ESI-MS	$\leq$1.0	Corticosteroid

10.3 The use of immunosensors to detect growth promoters

An immunosensor contains an antibody as the biorecognition element. In electrochemical asssays, the immunoassay step takes place at the surface of a modified electrode, to which antibodies have been chemically or physically adsorbed. In the competitive immunoassays (Fig. 10.1(a)), a small analyte

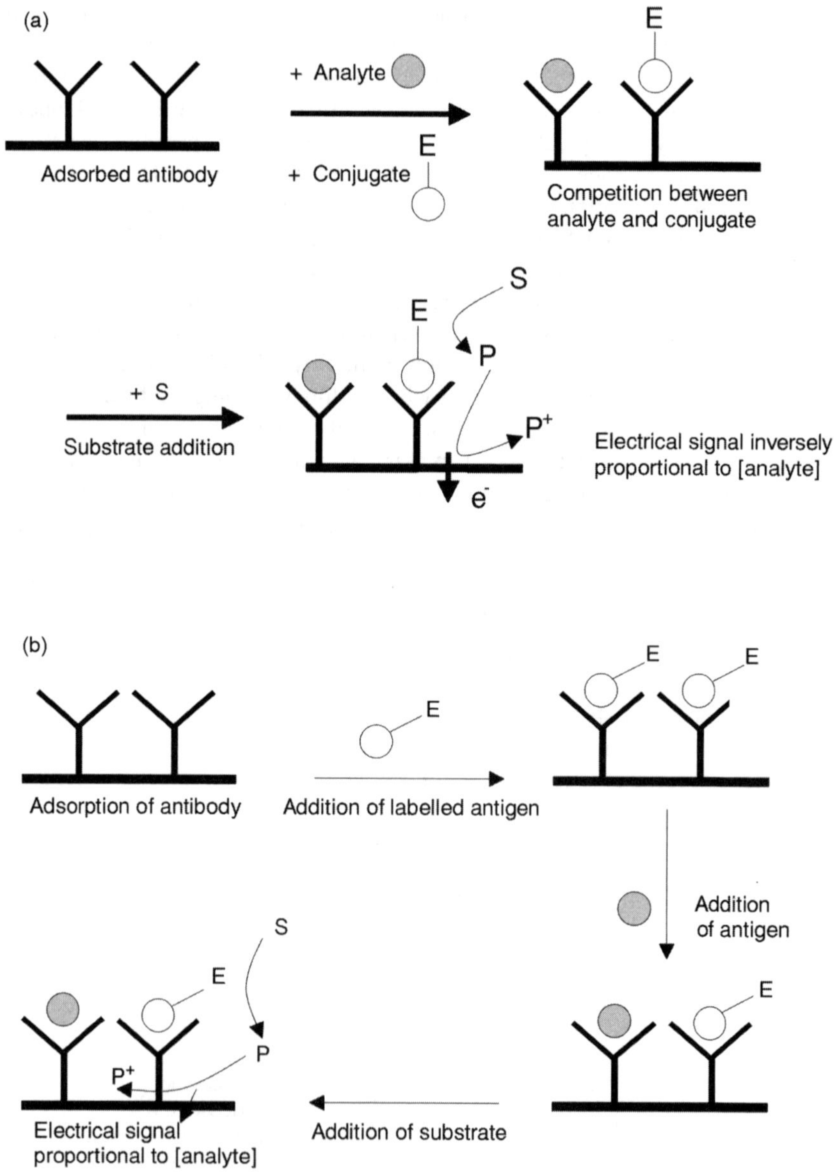

Fig. 10.1 (a) Competition immunoassay; (b) displacement immunoassay.

(hapten) and enzyme-labelled analyte compete with one another to bind to the antibody. When the labelled analyte is bound, it will result in a catalytic current, generally via oxidation of a mediator at the electrode surface. As the concentration of hapten is increased the amount of labelled antibody at the surface of the electrode will decrease, resulting in a diminished signal. By measuring this current, which is inversely proportional to the amount of antigen in the sample, it is possible to measure the concentration of analyte in the sample. In displacement assays (Fig. 10.1(b)), the antibody is bound to labelled antigen. On exposure to unlabelled antigen, the labelled antigen is displaced, resulting in a decrease in signal.

10.3.1 Antibody

An antibody (Ab) is a substance produced by the body in response to an antigen (Ag) that specifically reacts with the antigen. The body produces antibodies as a defence against foreign substances. Antibodies may be identified and quantified to determine whether an individual has been infected by a pathogen. Antibody molecules are highly specific for their corresponding antigen, making them relatively easy to isolate and study and invaluable as probes of biological processes.

Initially, enzyme-based electrochemical biosensors required the separation of bound and unbound species. This separation and the removal of background signals results in increased complexity of the assay format, making it unsuitable for rapid sensor analysis. In 2000 Killard *et al.*[13] developed an electrochemical immunosensor for the pesticide atrazine in buffer that did not require the separation of bound and unbound molecules in a competition immunoassay format. This allowed single step immunoassays to be performed using an Ab-based system, and also allowed for the real-time monitoring of Ab–Ag interactions. Killard *et al.* also showed that this type of assay was possible in both batch and flow injection formats. Recently it has been shown that the measurement of real-time interactions was possible using electrochemical immunoassay systems. This opened the way for rapid, real time immunoassay using simple, inexpensive electrochemical devices.[14] However, problems associated with the use of antibodies remain, such as the difficulty and expense of producing Ab molecules. In addition, the results for this type of immunosensor were obtained in buffer,[13] not in the matrix of interest. It is essential that any immunosensor for growth promoters be capable of obtaining results from biological samples. In addition given that the range of known growth promoters is expanding, a large number of antibodies would be required in order to have a realistic chance of detecting and identifying an unknown agent.[15]

Much work has been done to decrease the limit of detection of enzyme immunoassays (EIAs). Initially for many analytes, it was necessary to extract biological samples with an organic solvent.[16] The sensitivity of the method however, suffers in this case and could be improved by avoiding this solvent

Table 10.2 Limits of detection for different immunoassays

Analyte	Assay	Limit of detection pg/mL	UK legal limit pg/mL
Testosterone	EIA	84	500
	DELFIA	225	
Estradiol	RIA	10	500
	DELFIA	10	
Progesterone	RIA	71	40
	DELFIA	314	

extraction step. To liberate hormones from proteins, samples were heated to 70° C in alkaline buffer.[17] Inclusion of this type of step necessary for accurate measurement, does not lend itself to rapid screening. To detect testosterone, antibody (Ab) was raised using dimeric testosterone derivatives, which improved the sensitivity and specificity. Different combinations of Ab and enzyme-labelled hormone derivatives influenced the sensitivity and specificity of immunoassays.[18] Also homologous EIA proved less sensitive compared to heterologous immunoassay. In steroid EIAs the association of hapten-enzyme conjugate with the antibody varied from that of the hapten itself. In homologous assays, both types of haptens (Ab produced against hapten and Ab mixed with hapten-enzyme conjugates) are similar. In heterologous assay, they are different.

Paleologo *et al.* examined porcine urine as a sample matrix.[19] In urine, the concentration of hormones is usually higher than in serum and remains high for several weeks if the sample is properly stored. On the basis of 57 samples, it was concluded that, employing immunoassay and solid phase extraction as the sample clean-up method, it was not possible to measure residues down to 2 ppb. Elliot has developed DELFIA kits with improved performance, which are capable of producing results within 2–3 hours of the sample being submitted for analysis. The detection limits for a range of immunoassays are shown in Table 10.2.

The most important element in the development of any biosensor is its molecular recognition component. It is possible to use recognition elements other than antibodies. Improvement in the affinity, specificity and the ability to mass-produce the molecular recognition component(s) may ultimately dictate the success or failure of detection technologies in both a technical and commercial sense. There have been fewer reports on such recognition elements, e.g. molecular imprinted polymer (MIP), aptamers and synthetic receptors. These are described briefly below.

10.3.2 Imprinted polymer

An artificial antibody can be constructed by synthesising a polymer in the presence of a template molecule. When the template is removed, the polymer is imprinted with the shape of the template and with complementary functional groups that can

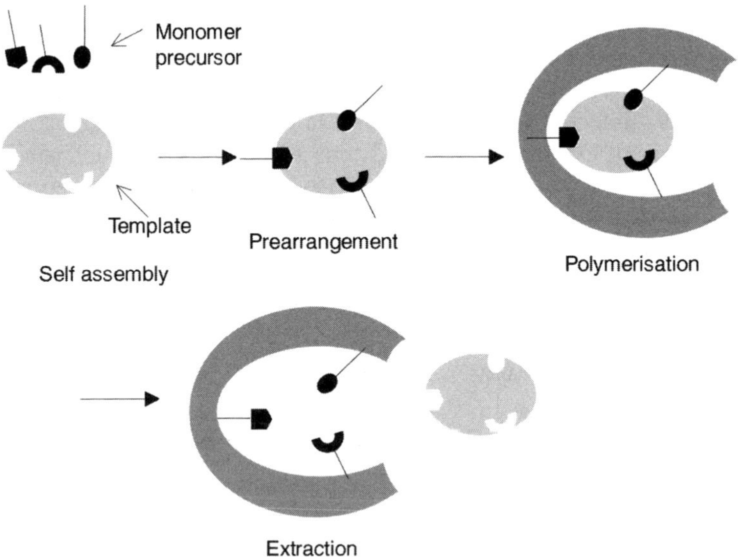

Fig. 10.2 Formation of imprinted polymer.

bind to the template (Fig. 10.2). The imprinted polymer can be used as a stationary phase in affinity chromatography or a recognition element in a chemical sensor, because the polymer preferentially binds the template molecule.

Although the concept of molecular imprinting has existed for 60 years, interest was stimulated by a recent report on 'plastic antibodies'.[20] Molecular imprinting (MIP) is approached in two ways, the self-assembly[21] and pre-organised[22] approaches. The former method utilises host–guest complexes that are produced from weak intermolecular interactions (such as ionic or hydrophobic interactions, hydrogen bonding and metal coordination) between the analyte and the monomer precursors. Conversely, the pre-organised molecular imprinting approach involves the formation of strong, reversible, covalent arrangements (e.g. boronate esters, imines and ketals) of the monomers with the print molecules before polymerisation. In some cases, the binding affinities of some of these MIPs (also referred to as antibody binding mimics) have been comparable with the binding of some natural monoclonal Abs.[23]

One of the advantages of molecular imprinting is that imprints can be made of compounds against which it is difficult, if not possible, to raise Abs. The use of animals, often necessary with Ab production, is avoided, and scale-up for bulk manufacture is easily done. Thus benefits are reaped from practical, ethical and economical points of view.

MIPs also possess long-term stability and resistance to chemically harsh environments. So far, MIPs had been used primarily as stationary phases in HPLC heterogeneous binding assays and in biomimetic affinity sensors. A MIP-based biosensor was first proposed in 1991,[24] but the results obtained were not quantitative. In 1997, Muldoon *et al.*[25] first used molecular imprinting technology for residue analysis in complex biological samples. They used an atrazine MIP as the solid phase in sample extraction columns. The columns were used to purify tissue sample extracts prior to analysis and quantification by reversed phase HPLC and ELISA. The time required for measurement with MIP-based sensors was *ca.* 15–60 min. By optimising the kinetics and selectivity of the polymers, it may be possible to reduce the time of analysis.

It is believed that the use of highly rigid polymers favours selectivity (at the expense of increased response time), because of the higher energy barriers, which are associated with entry and exit of the analyte. Similarly, polymer porosity can increase polymer-binding capacity and response time.[26] Although the current generation of MIP biomimetric sensors is 100 to 1000-fold less sensitive than other types of sensor, it has been shown to have superior sensitivity to affinity-based biosensors and in some cases may prove useful in hormone analysis.

10.3.3 Receptors

A receptor is a macromolecule or a macromolecular complex, which binds an analyte with high structural selectivity. It is difficult to present any coherent classification of the types of receptors. Neuroreceptors and hormonal receptors occur naturally. Synthetic receptors include materials such imprinted polymers (section 10.3.2). Biological receptors (neuroreceptors and hormonal receptors) tend to have an affinity for a range of structurally related compounds rather than one specific analyte, which is often an attractive feature for use in biosensors. Biological receptors are often used with labelled materials such as radioactive, fluorescence or enzyme labelled ligands. These receptor-based biosensors are broadly grouped into intact receptor-based and isolated receptor-based biosensors.

While isolated receptors may be suitable for the detection of growth promoters, no such sensor currently exists. Recently Scippo developed receptor assays based on competition between analytes present in the sample and radio-labelled ligands.[27] Receptors were isolated from bacterial or eukaryotic cells which were genetically modified to produce receptors for the determination of analogues of steroid hormone residues: human receptors of estrogens, androgens, progesterones and glucocorticoids. In comparison to receptors prepared from animal tissues, the use of DNA-recombinant receptors offers a number of advantages: an inexhaustible source of material, homogeneous binding proteins and stable binding properties. The main problem with this type of receptor is in interpretation of the results, as the sample contains, in addition to the analyte of interest, endogenous hormones at concentrations varying from minimal to high. Because of the presence of natural endogenous hormones, this background will have to be evaluated for each matrix by analysing a large number of 'blank' samples (collected from animals that have received no hormonal treatment). Still, it must be stressed that binding assays represent potential multi-analyte screening methods. One of the major advantages of using this type of receptor assay is it should detect all the members of a class of compounds sharing the same binding property. Such a survey strategy should result in the discovery of new compounds suspected of being used but not yet chemically identified.

Steroid hormone action is mediated by specific nuclear receptors, which are a member of a large family of ligand-dependent transcription factors.[28] In the absence of ligands, these steroid receptors are inactive and often form part of a multi-protein complex in the cell.[29] Upon binding of hormone to the receptor, the complex dissociates, the receptor dimerizes and binds specific steroid response elements (SREs) on target gene promoters and activates their transcription. Taking advantage of this series of events, stable reporter cell lines have been established recently, which can respond to the presence of gluco-corticoids, progesterone and androgens by inducing a bio-luminescence cellular signal with a limit of detection as low as 0.3 ng/g tissue.[29] Further work is required to produce receptor-based electrochemical biosensors.

10.3.4 Aptamers

Aptamers are artificial nucleic acid ligands that can be generated against amino acids, drugs, proteins and other molecules. As high affinity, high selectivity ligands, aptamers have potential use in detection systems including biosensors (Fig. 10.3). The first biosensor based on aptamers as the recognition element was reported by Kleinjung *et al.*[30] The nucleic acid selected by the SELEX (systematic evolution of ligands by exponential enrichment) method for binding L-adenosine was attached via an avidin-biotin bridge to the core of a multimode optical fibre. Binding of FITC-labelled L-adenosine and real-time measurement was performed by competition with unlabelled L-adenosine in the sample. This sensor also can determine kinetic and equilibrium constants, which may be of interest.

Aptamers[31] include RNA, single stranded deoxyribonucleic acid (ssDNA), chemically modified RNA or modified ssDNA isolated from large combinatorial

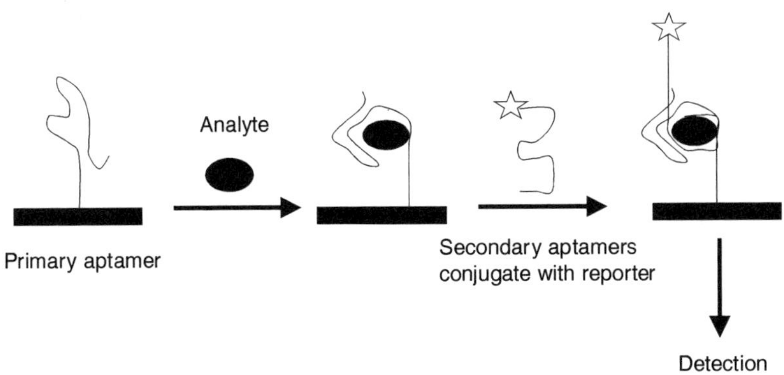

Fig. 10.3 Schematic diagram of aptamer sensor.

libraries of nucleic acid sequences by a technique called *in vitro* selection. Combinatorial nucleic acid libraries are mixtures of billions of different nucleic acid sequences, which can be screened for individual molecules with specific functions. These functions include catalytic activity, the specific molecular recognition of target molecules or the inhibition of enzymes. Their advantages over alternative approaches include the use of relatively simple techniques and apparatus for their isolation, the number of alternative molecules that can be screened (routinely in the order of 10^{15}) and their chemical simplicity. Disadvantages of aptamers include their polymorphism, their high molecular mass and the restricted range of target sites.

Aptamers have been used for 'sandwich' assays as with enzyme-linked immunoassay (ELISA).[32] Fluorescent-labelled aptamers have also been used to quantify the amount of immunoglobulin E and thrombin using a rapid method based on capillary electrophoresis laser induced fluorescence (CE/LIF), with a limit of detection of 50 pM. Recently, electrochemical detection was also developed by Kuhr.[33] Kuhr also pointed out the power and flexibility of electrochemical methods in combination with micro fabrication techniques, in order to provide high sensitivity and parallel analysis.

10.4 Key issues in developing new biosensors

The most sensitive assay can now reliably detect hormone concentrations in the low parts per billion range. Enzyme-linked immunoassay has been the most widely used method in recent years. Methods utilizing GC-MS and a recombinant yeast cell culture are being refined to yield even lower limits of detection. However, there is still significant variability among measurements reported by different laboratories. This variation may be due to differences in the antibody preparations used and to differences in extraction methods. The latter may be more or less efficient in recovering all the hormone molecules in a sample and in removing interfering substances[34]

Detection of growth promoters in matrices of biological origin can be difficult due to extensive metabolism of the compounds and/or the low dosages used. In addition, new substances and new classes of compounds are continually introduced in an attempt to evade detection by regulatory bodies. To improve the efficiency of residue testing programmes, it is necessary to study the kinetics and metabolism of substances in the target animal and to produce reference standards of compounds and metabolites.[35] In order to detect the use of new compounds, combined efforts are necessary, and not only between laboratories, but also between laboratories and inspection services. Until recently, only five or six steroids were used illegally. Nowadays, many more steroids are used, making it essential that a multianalyte sensor be developed which is capable of detecting classes of compounds. Such a device need not be highly accurate, since confirmatory testing can still be performed at a central laboratory.

10.4.1 Need for a new biosensor

Although immunoassay methods (EIA, RIA) can be effective when the use or abuse of a limited number of substances has to be controlled, the increase in the range of illegal growth promoting substances requires the development of a multianalyte sensor. Besides, the generally high specificity of antibody-based sensors precludes the sensitive detection of more than one substance, rendering their widespread use uneconomic. Thus, in order to develop rapid, inexpensive, multianalyte detection assays, receptor assays can be proposed, which allow the analysis of a large number of samples in a short time.[27] Currently, there is no such type of sensor available for field use, the development of which is crucial.

10.5 References

1. BRIAN E, *Biosensors: An Introduction*, Wiley & Teubner, 1996.
2. MAGNER E, 'Trends in electrochemical biosensors', *Analyst*, 1998 **123**(10) 1967–1970.
3. ELLIOTT C T, FRANCIS K S, SHORTT A D, MCCAUGHEY W J, 'Determination of the concentration of the steroids estradiol, progesterone and testosterone in bovine sera: comparison of commercial dissociation enhanced lanthanide fluorescence immunoassay kits with conventional radio and enzyme immunoassays', *Analyst*, 1995 **120** 1827–1830.
4. TATEISHI K, YAMAMOTO H, OGIHARA T, 'Enzyme immunoassay of serum testosterone', *Steroids*, 1977 **30**(1) 25–32.
5. MARTIN Y, 'Determination of three anabolic compounds in calf urine by liquid chromatography with photodiode-array detection', *Analyst*, 2000 **125** 2230–2235.
6. ROSA D, LUCA P, CAMILLA M, EMANUELE F, FERNANDA D Q, 'Confirmatory analysis of residues of stanozolol and its major metabolite in bovine urine by liquid chromatography-tandem mass spectrometry', *J of Chromatography A,* 2001 **926**(1) 69–77.
7. BARRY M G, BLANKVOORT JAC M M, AARTS J G, ROBERT S, PETER G, BERT S, RODENBURG R J T, 'Detection of hormonal anabolic compounds in calf urine and unverified growth-promoting preparations: application of the AR-LUX bioassay for screening and determination of androgen activity.' *The Analyst*, 2003 **128** 1373–1381.
8. HORIE M AND HIROYUKI N, 'Determination of trenbolone and zeranol in bovine muscle and liver by liquid chromatography-electrospray mass spectrometry', *Journal of Chromatography A*, 2000 **882**(1–2) 53–62.
9. CALBREATH D F, *A Fundamental Text Book of Clinical Chemistry,* USA, Saunders, 1996, p. 672.
10. BUIARELLI F, CARTONI G P, COCCIOLI F, ROSSI A D, NERI B, 'Determination of trenbolone and its metabolite in bovine fluids by liquid chromatography-tandem mass spectrometry', *Journal of Chromatography B*, 2003 **784**(1) 1–15.
11. COUNCIL DIRECTIVE 88/146/EEC OF 7 MARCH, *Official Journal L070, 16/03/1988, pp. 0016–0018*, 1988, Corrigendum: Official Journal N. L087, 02/04/1992, p. 0036.
12. JOOS P E, VAN RYCKEGHEN M, 'Liquid chromatography-tandem mass spectrometry of some anabolic steroids', *Anal. Chem.*, 1999 **71** 4701–4710.
13. KILLARD A J, SMYTH M R, GRENNAN K, MICHELI L, PALLESCHI G, 'Rapid antibody

biosensor assays for environmental analysis', *Biomedical Society Transactions*, 2000 **28**(2).

14. KILLARD A J, ZHANG S, ZHAO H, JOHN R, IWUOHA E I AND SMYTH M R, 'Development of an electrochemical flow injection immunoassay (FIIA) for the real-time monitoring of biospecific interactions', *Anal. Chim. Acta.*, 2000 **400** 109–119.
15. HASELEY S R, 'Carbohydrate recognition: a nascent technology for the detection of bioanalytes', *Anal. Chim. Acta.*, 2002 **457** 39–45.
16. RAJKOWSKI K M, HANQUEZ C, BAUZOUMOU A, CITTANOVA N, 'A competitive microtitre plate enzyme immunoassay for plasma testosterone using polyclonal antitestosterone immunoglobulin', *Clin. Chim. Acta.*, 1989 **183** 197–200.
17. TARUN K D AND ESAHAK A, 'Direct microtitre plate enzyme immunoassay of testosterone in unextracted serum', *J Immuno. Meth.*, 1992 **147** 167–72.
18. MOHAMMAD J R, KUMARI L G, RAO P N, SHRIVASTAV G T, PANDEY P H, 'Influence of different combinations of antibodies and penicillinase-labeled testosterone derivatives on sensitivity and specificity of immunoassays', *Steroids*, 1992 **57** 112–118.
19. PALEOLOGO O M, ANGELETTI R, BASTIANI E, NACHTMANN C, VAN OOSTHUYZE K E, PETEGHEM V C, 'Screening of calf urine for 19-nortestosterone: matrix effect in some immunoassays', *Analyst*, 1995 **120** 577–579.
20. VLATAKIS G, ANDERSSON L I, MULLER R, MOSBACH K, 'Drug assay using antibody mimics made by molecular imprinting', *Nature*, 1993 **361** 645-47.
21. LINDSEY J S, 'Self assembly in synthetic routes to molecular devices. Biological principles and chemical perspectives: a review', *New J. Chemistry*, 1991 **15** 153–80.
22. MOSBACH K, RAMSTRON O, 'The emerging technique of molecular imprinting and its future impact on biotechnology', *Bio. Technol.*, 1996 **14**(2) 163–170.
23. ANDERSON L I, MULLER R, VLATAKIS G, MOSBACH K, 'Mimics of the binding sites of opioid receptors obtained by molecular imprinting of enkephalin and morphine', *Proc. Natl. Acad. Sc. USA*, 1995 **92** 4788–92.
24. MOSBACH K., Swedish Patent App, 1991.
25. MULDOON T M, LARRY H S, Molecular imprinted solid phase extraction of atrazine from beef liver extracts', *Anal. Chem.*, 1997 **69** 803–808.
26. KRIZ D, RAMSTROM O, MOSBACH K, 'Molecular imprinting-based biomimetric sensors could provide an alternative to often unstable biosensors for industry, medicine and environmental analysis', *Analytical Chemistry*, 1997 **69** 345A–349A.
27. SCIPPO M L, CÉCILE V D, WEERDT P W, JEAN-MARIE F, FRANÇOISE R D, MARC M J, MARTIAL A, GUY M R, 'Detection of illegal growth promoters in biological samples using receptor binding assays', *Anal. Chim. Acta*, 2002 **473**(1–2) 135–141.
28. EVANS R M, 'The steroid and thyroid-hormone receptor superfamily', *Science*, 1988 **240**(4854) 889–895.
29. WILLEMSEN P, SCIPPO M L, ROGISTER G M, MARTIAL J A, MULLER M, 'Use of specific bioluminescent cell lines for the detection of steroid hormone (ant) agonists in meat producing animals', *Anal. Chim. Acta.*, 2002 **473** 119–226.
30. KLEINJUNG F, KLUSSMANN S, ERDMANN V A, SCHELLER F W, FÜRSTE J P, BIER F F, 'High-affinity RNA as a recognition element in a biosensor', *Anal. Chem.*, 1998 **70**(2) 328–331.
31. MEYERS R A (ed), *Encyclopaedia of Analitical Chemistry*, John Wiley & Sons Ltd.
32. DROLET D W, 'An enzyme linked oligonucleotide assay', *Nature Biotech.*, 1996 **14**(8) 1021–1027.

33. KUHR W G, 'Electrochemical DNA analysis comes of age', *Nat. Biotechnol.*, 2003 **18** 1042–1043.
34. COURTHEYN D, BIZEC B L, BRAMBILLA G, BRABANDER H F D, COBBAERT E, WIELE M V, VERCAMMEN J, WASCH K D, 'Recent developments in the use and abuse of growth promoters', *Anal. Chim. Acta.*, 2002 **473**(1–2) 71–82.
35. SANGIORGI E, CURATOLO M, ASSINI W, BOZZONI E, 'Application of neutral loss mode in liquid chromatography-mass spectrometry for the determination of corticosteroids in bovine urine', *Analytica Chim. Acta*, 2003 **483**(1–2) 259–267.

11

The rapid detection of coccidiostat drug residues in farm animals

M. Tuomola and T. Lövgren, University of Turku, Finland

11.1 Introduction

A wide range of veterinary medicines is administered to food-producing animals for treating and preventing disease and promoting growth. Surveillance schemes have been established to monitor the presence of veterinary drug residues in foods in order to ensure that consumers are not exposed to drug residues at potentially harmful concentrations. The task is very demanding because the list of chemical contaminants that may be present in foods is very long. Coccidiostats comprise one major group of medical compounds that are widely used especially in the poultry industry. It is now a mandatory requirement (Council Directive 96/23/EC) for members of the European Union and any country exporting to the EU to monitor coccidiostat residues in their residue programmes. However, implementation of the Directive has been compromised by the lack of suitable analytical methods. For some of the compounds methods have been lacking completely and the existing methods have been either too insensitive or very complex, and too slow to be carried out on a routine basis.

An efficient residue control system can be achieved by a combination of screening and confirmatory tests. Screening tests are simple, rapid, and high volume tests that are designed to select tentatively positive samples for confirmatory analysis. They are biased to produce no false negatives and to classify a large number of samples as being either 'negative' or 'potentially positive'. All samples in the latter category are subjected to a technically demanding, low volume, high cost confirmatory analysis that is typically based on mass spectrometry. Immunoassays are particularly suitable for sample screening and an increasing number of applications, mainly based on enzyme-linked immunosorbent assay (ELISA), have been published detailing methods for detecting food contaminants (for a review, see Stanker and Beier, 1996; Haasnoot and Schilt, 2000).

The advantages of immunoassays have also been noticed in the measurement of coccidiostat residues and several ELISA applications have been developed for this purpose (e.g., Elissalde *et al.*, 1993; Pauillac *et al.*, 1993; Godfrey *et al.*, 1997; Kennedy *et al.*, 1995a, 1995b, 1997; Beier *et al.*, 1998; Crooks *et al.*, 1998; Watanabe *et al.*, 2001). These methods have significantly improved the speed, sensitivity and the cost-efficiency of testing compared with more traditional methods based on gas chromatography, high-performance liquid chromatography and thin-layer chromatography. However, there is lack of uniformity between assay performance and for several analytes the specific immunochemical reagents are not even available. The current ELISA-based methods also require multiple assay steps and automation is lacking, which slows down the test throughput and makes the assays more prone to errors.

The need for improvement in the analytical capabilities with respect to the monitoring of coccidiostat residues is widely recognised (Elliott *et al.*, 1998). This chapter describes novel immunochemical technology that can provide efficient tools for coccidiostat analysis because it overcomes the above-mentioned limitations of the current methods. The screening system is based on the use of the dry reagent all-in-one immunoassay concept and time-resolved fluorescence. The fully automated immunoassay system is already available for human diagnostic applications and can, after some minor modifications, be applied for the rapid detection of harmful agents throughout the food chain.

11.2 The use of anticoccidial drugs in poultry farming

Anticoccidial drugs are used extensively in all countries where chickens are reared under intensive housing conditions. These drugs are used to control the infection of the single-cell protozoa of the genus *Eimeria*, which spend most of their lives in the intestinal tract of the host animal and damage the intestinal mucosa (Crosby, 1991). In its acute form coccidiosis causes high mortality. The sub-acute form causes interruption of feeding and digestive processes, dehydration, blood loss, and increased susceptibility to other disease agents. Much of the economic loss associated with this parasitic disease is incurred prior to diagnosis, which makes the prevention more important than treatment.

The widespread use of coccidiostats may present a potential risk to the consumer if residues enter the food chain. Provided that the drug is used in accordance with its product licence, and appropriate withdrawal periods are observed prior to slaughter of the animal, harmful drug residues should not occur in human food. In practice, however, the occurrence of coccidiostats in poultry tissues and eggs has been widely reported (Kennedy *et al.*, 1996, 1998, 2000; McEvoy, 2002). Violations may occur as a result of accidental contamination of feed or environment, accidental or deliberate contravention of withdrawal periods, or improper use of drugs (Kennedy *et al.*, 2000; McEvoy, 2002).

Controlling residues of coccidiostats presents a challenge not only to the regulatory authorities carrying out the residue monitoring programmes but also to the industry implementing an integrated 'from farm to fork' approach. New LC-MS methods have been developed for confirmatory analysis but suitable analytical methods are still lacking especially with respect to simple, high-throughput, and cost effective screening methods.

Coccidiostat drugs are not easy to analyse by traditional analytical methods because they are not volatile and most of them do not possess a fluorophore or chromophore structure which would facilitate the detection of the analyte. To circumvent these limitations, the methods have either been based on slow bioassays which measure the biological activity of the drug or they have employed complex derivatisation procedures in order to improve the chromatographic behaviour and detection sensitivity of the compound (Weiss and MacDonald, 1985; Elliott *et al.*, 1998). Immunoassays are, however, not affected by these factors. The EU research project 'Poultry-check' (QLK1-CT99-00313) has addressed the need for efficient screening methods by developing rapid tests based on time-resolved fluoroimmunoassays and dry chemistry and the results from this project will be used in this chapter as an example of the technology. So far novel tests have been developed for nicarbazin, halofuginone and for the group of nitroimidazole compounds (Fig. 11.1).

Nicarbazin is a coccidiostat composed of an equimolar complex of 4,4′-dinitrocarbanilide (DNC) and 2-hydroxy-4,6-dimethylpyrimidine. The compound does not have a EU maximum residue limit (MRL), but the Codex Alimentarius Commission has through its Joint Expert Committee on Food Additives (JECFA) set the MRL for DNC marker of 200 μg/kg in poultry liver, muscle, kidney and fat. Halofuginone (DL-*trans*-7-bromo-6-choloro-3[3-(hydroxyl-2-piperidyl)acetonyl]-4(3H)-quinazolinone) has MRLs of 10 and

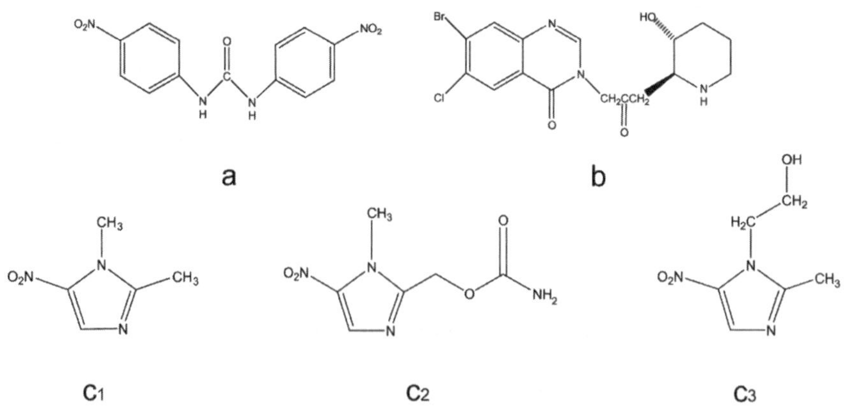

Fig. 11.1 Coccidiostat compounds included in the screening assays: a) dinitro-carbanilide (marker compound for nicarbazin), b) halofuginone, c1) dimetridazole, c2) ronidazole, c3) metronidazole.

30 μg/kg for bovine muscle and liver, respectively. However, the European Agency for the Evaluation of Medicinal Products has not yet established MRLs for residues in poultry. Nitroimidazoles such as dimetridazole (1,2-dimethyl-5-nitroimidazole), ronidazole (1-methyl-2-(carbamoylmethyl)-5-nitroimidazole) and metronidazole (1-(2-hydroxyethyl)-2-methyl-5-nitroimidazole) have previously been used to prevent and treat coccidiosis in poultry. They are now suspected of possessing carcinogenic and mutagenic properties and their use in food-producing animals has been banned (Council Regulation 2377/90, 2205/2001). As these drugs are considered unsafe on consumer health grounds, no MRLs can be set. No MRLs have been set for coccidiostat residues in eggs because these compounds are not even licensed for use in egg layers.

11.3 The use of time-resolved fluoroimmunoassays (TR-FIAs)

Time-resolved fluoroimmunoassays (TR-FIAs) based on the use of lanthanide chelates are well established in human *in vitro* diagnostics (Soini and Lövgren, 1987; Hemmilä and Mukkala, 2001). The technique combines the advantages of other nonradioisotopic assays (stability of the reagent and lack of radiation) with a substantial increase in sensitivity and assay range in comparison with conventional enzyme immunoassays and fluoroimmunoassays (FIAs). The use of fluorescent small molecules rather than enzymes as labels avoids problems associated with enzyme activity and stability. The assays are also simpler to perform because the extra steps needed for the enzymatic signal development, which have to be carefully controlled, are avoided. The sensitivity of ordinary FIAs is, however, compromised by inherent problems associated with high background interference, and quenching from sample matrices and other material used in the assays.

The fluorescence decay time of common fluorophores like fluorescein isothiocyanate (FITC) is very short (few nanoseconds) and in practice the light emitted has to be simultaneously measured with the excitation. Unfortunately, this will also include autofluorescence and scattering in the measurement. The background is further increased due to the fact that these labels exhibit only a small Stokes' shift (~25 nm for FITC), which means that the excitation and emission wavelengths are partially overlapping in the fluorescence spectrum. These background problems can be fully overcome by the use of lanthanide chelate labels and the measurement of fluorescence in a time-resolved mode. These labels have a very long fluorescence decay time (several hundred microseconds), very narrow emission spectra and an exceptionally large Stokes' shift (around 200–300 nm) (Soini and Lövgren, 1987; Lövgren and Pettersson, 2000). The long fluorescence decay time allows the user to measure fluorescence after the background fluorescence has fully subsided. A typical measurement lasts for one second during which the excitation pulse–delay–measurement cycle is repeated 1000 times (Fig. 11.2). High sensitivity and good precision are obtained both in competitive and non-competitive (immunometric)

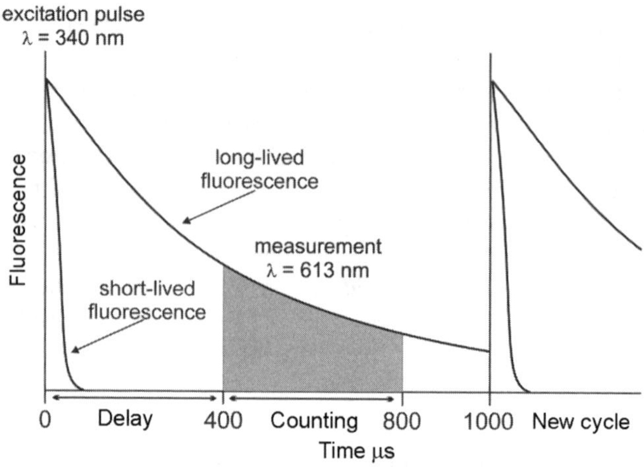

Fig. 11.2 The principle of measurement of time-resolved fluorescence. The flash excitation produces a short pulse of light and the measurement of long-lived fluorescence is performed after the short-lived fluorescence has dissipated to zero. The cycle is typically repeated 1000 times per second.

assays employing time-resolved fluorescence. Immunometric methods obviously benefit more extensively from the low background signal and high specific activity of the label. Very high signal-to-noise ratio can be achieved with the technique, and assays using europium chelate labels have reached sensitivities in the attomole (10^{-18} mol) range (Pettersson and Söderholm, 1990).

A number of TR-FIA methods have emerged in the field of food analysis since the mid-1990s and some applications have also been developed for veterinary drug residue analysis. To date, TR-FIA methods have been published for the measurement of medroxyprogesterone (Elliott *et al.*, 1994), beta-agonists (Bacigalupo *et al.*, 1995; Elliott *et al.*, 1996), monensin (Crooks *et al.*, 1998), ivermectin (Crooks *et al.*, 2000), and zeranol (Cooper *et al.*, 2002; Tuomola *et al.*, 2002a). The majority of TR-FIA methods so far developed have been based on the dissociation-enhanced lanthanide fluorescence immunoassay (Delfia®) technique. The Delfia® technology is based on a lanthanide (typically Eu^{3+}) bound to a non-fluorescent chelate. The chelate is covalently bound to the immunoreactant and it is carried quantitatively through the biospecific reaction. In the final step of the assay, europium fluorescence is developed after the ion is released by dissociation in the presence of an enhancement solution that contains the energy-absorbing ligands required for the formation of a new, strongly fluorescent chelate (Hemmilä *et al.*, 1984). The necessity of ligand exchange, however, makes the assays susceptible to contamination by exogenous lanthanides and interference by other chelators that may be present in the samples.

Alternative strategies have been developed (*e.g.*, Takalo *et al.*, 1994) that improve the situation by using stable, intrinsically fluorescent lanthanide chelates as labels. In these kinds of labels the binding constant of lanthanide ion to the chelate is very high and the excitation energy absorption, energy transfer and emission properties are built into the primary label structure. This enables the measurement to be done also by using a desorptive nondissociative enhancement which avoids the detection of free lanthanide ions and produces a signal that is proportional to the quantity of the chelator present (Mitrunen *et al.*, 1995). Furthermore, it has made it possible to measure the label signal directly from the dry surface of the microwells without any enhancement step (Meriö *et al.*, 1996). This simplifies the assay design and reduces the need for liquid handling to a minimum.

11.4 Screening for coccidiostat residues by automated TR-FIAs

The TR-FIAs employing lanthanide chelate labels have potential to be used in a simplified one-step all-in-one assay (AIO) format which significantly facilitates the automation of the methods (Lövgren *et al.*, 1996). In this format all the analyte specific reagents are predispensed into the microtitre wells and dried. At the time of analysis the biospecific reaction is started, simply by the addition of the sample (or calibrator) and a common assay buffer as all the assay components are already present in the wells. The technique is easy to automate either in a random access or a batch system because the use of stable, intrinsically fluorescent chelate labels and one-step procedure minimises the necessary assay steps, and the use of dry chemistry totally excludes the handling of assay-specific reagents. The concept is extremely simple to apply from the user's point of view and can be applied both for competitive and non-competitive immunoassays.

The concept of competitive one-step AIO dry reagent immunoassay is presented in Fig. 11.3. The analyte-specific primary antibody is immobilised onto the surface of the microtitre well either by using wells with secondary anti-species antibody coating or by biotinylating the primary antibodies and using streptavidin-coated wells. An insulating carbohydrate layer is added on top of the immobilised antibodies and dried. The dry layer also contains all the assay buffer reagents such as proteins and detergents that become solubilised at the time of analysis. Finally, the labelled analyte is added in a small volume on top of the insulating layer and instantly dried in order to keep the dry layer intact. The resultant all-in-one dry wells are stored in sealed packages that contain desiccant. The assay is started simply by opening the package and adding the samples and buffer to the wells. After a short incubation the wells are washed and the time-resolved fluorescence is measured either from the dry surface of the wells or from a signal enhancement solution (Lövgren *et al.*, 1996). The role of the insulating layer is important as it prohibits the premature binding of the labelled analyte to the specific antibody on the solid phase. It is also important in non-competitive assays where it controls the non-specific binding of the labelled

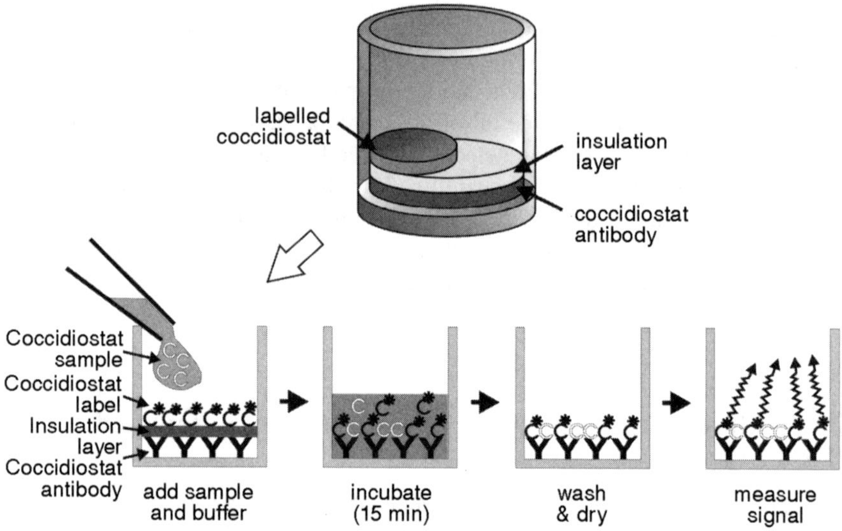

Fig. 11.3 Schematic principle of all-in-one dry chemistry immunoassay. All the assay steps in the reaction well are performed automatically by the immunoanalyser.

reagent. The components in the layer are optimised specifically for each analyte to provide the best sensitivity, kinetics and storage stability.

The AIO assay concept has also been applied for drug residue analysis (Crooks *et al.*, 1998; Tuomola *et al.*, 2002a, Cooper *et al.*, 2002). The use of dry chemistry has improved both the speed and simplicity of the assays but the sample throughput has been limited due to the lack of automation and the use of a fluorescence enhancement step at the end of the assay. In addition, the applications have adhered to the use of 'standard' 96-well plate format. This forces the end-users to work with a predetermined sample batch size because it is not economically feasible to use only part of the reagents of an assay kit. Handling of the microtitre plate also has to be carefully controlled in the assay in order to avoid the so-called 'edge effect', which may produce variation in the assay response in different locations of the plate. These issues can be addressed by using a fully automated Aio! immunoanalyser (Innotrac Diagnostics Oy, Turku, Finland), based on the use of single-well assays (Fig. 11.4). The Aio! analyser is a random-access machine designed specifically for the handling of dry chemistry assays and the primary application area is in clinical point-of-care testing (Pettersson *et al.*, 2000). A test-specific reagent pen used in the analyser contains 12 dry wells, and as many as 30 pens (each of which can potentially be a different test) can be stored inside the machine. The test pen is the only analyte-specific component of the kit, because only one 'universal' buffer solution is used in the analyser and the test protocol is the same for all of the assays. This gives the user total freedom for deciding which tests are run and in which order they are performed. The waste handling is also straightforward because the Aio! system produces only water-based buffer and empty assay

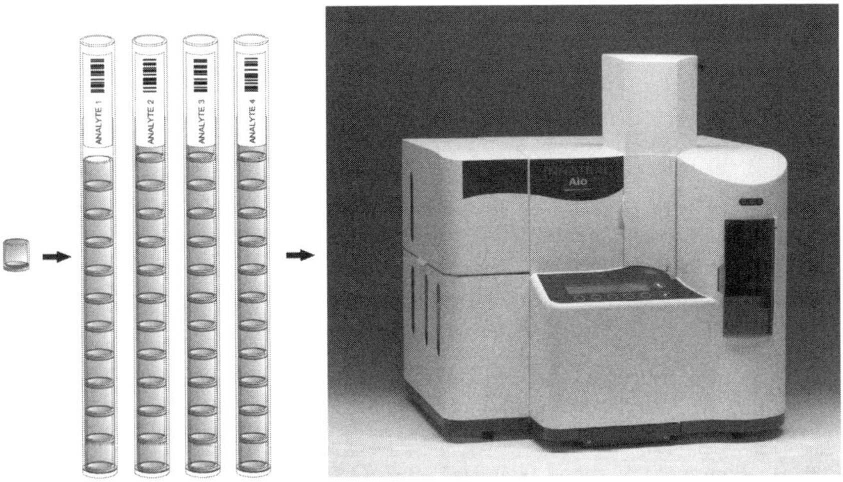

Fig. 11.4 Single-well immunoassays are based on the use of test-specific reagent pens containing 12 wells. The random-access immunoanalyser needs only the test pen and a common assay solution to run the assay.

wells as waste. The total processing time for each test is 18 minutes and the maximum sample throughput is 70 assays per hour.

The development of a coccidiostat residue screening assay can only be started if specific antibody has been obtained for the selected compound. The performance of any immunoassay is for the most part dependent on the binding properties of the analyte-specific antibody and success in the antibody production is ensured by paying special attention to the design of the immunogen structure. A number of analyte analogues, derivatives, attachment chemistries and carrier proteins have been used for the development of antibodies against different coccidiostat compounds. Polyclonal and monoclonal antibodies have been produced against polyether ionophoric coccidiostats such as monensin (Pauillac *et al.*, 1993; Godfrey *et al.*, 1997), salinomycin (Elissalde *et al.*, 1993; Kennedy *et al.*, 1995b; Watanabe *et al.*, 2001), lasalocid (Kennedy *et al.*, 1995a), and maduramicin (Kennedy *et al.*, 1997). Highly specific antibodies have also been produced for smaller analytes including the nicarbazin marker compound, dinitrocarbanilide (DNC) (Beier *et al.*, 2001; Connolly *et al.*, 2002), and for halofuginone (Rowe *et al.*, 1994). A successful strategy has also been developed for the production of a group-specific antibodies against nitroimidazole compounds (Fodey *et al.*, 2003) which allows screening for the presence of several compounds (metronidazole, hydroxymetronidazole, dimetridazole, hydroxydimetridazole, ronidazole, and ipronidazole) in a single bioaffinity reaction.

The label for the competitive TR-FIA can be synthesised by attaching the lanthanide chelate directly to the analyte or its derivative, but most often it is produced by coupling both the lanthanide chelate and homologous or heterologous drug analogue to a protein carrier (e.g., Crooks *et al.*, 1998, 2000; Tuomola *et al.*,

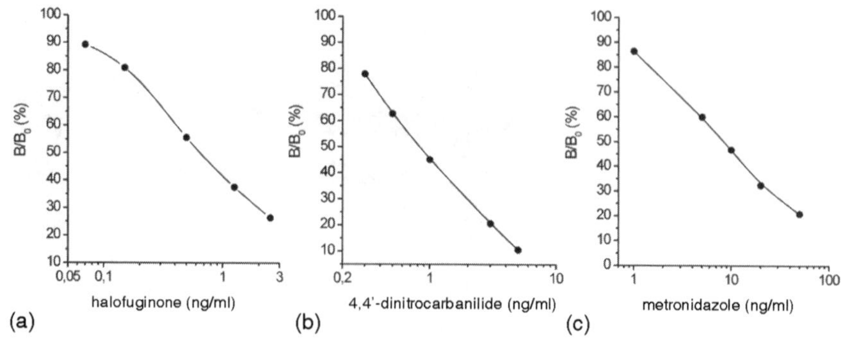

Fig. 11.5 Standard curves of the coccidiostat TR-FIA measurements: a) halofuginone, b) nicarbazin, c) nitroimidazoles (metronidazole).

2002a). Figure 11.5 shows standard curves for three coccidiostat TR-FIAs (halofuginone, nicarbazin and generic nitroimidazole assays) that have been created by using hapten-protein conjugates labelled with stable and intrinsically fluorescent Eu-chelates. The assays have subsequently been adapted to the dry chemistry format by introducing an optimised insulating layer to the wells. The labelled component is added on top of the dry layer in a small volume and the single wells are packed in the reagent pens after a drying step.

A major advantage of the immunoassays is their specificity, which makes it possible to develop direct assays that may not require sample preparation at all or need only simplified sample clean-up procedures. Some TR-FIA applications that have been developed for veterinary residue analysis have taken advantage of this possibility and allow the direct analysis of diluted urine (Bacigalupo *et al.*, 1995; Elliott *et al.*, 1996) and plasma (Crooks *et al.*, 1998). The use of stable lanthanide chelate labels has even enabled the direct measurement of whole blood samples (Pettersson *et al.*, 2000; Tuomola *et al.*, 2002b). Solid food matrices such as meat, liver and eggs naturally require some form of extraction, and if organic solvents are used they have to be exchanged for a buffer system that is compatible with the immunochemical assay system. In strict contrast to alternative techniques such as liquid- or thin-layer chromatography, the need for subsequent purification steps is minimal or does not exist. In the majority of coccidiostat residue assays sample pretreatment consists only of liquid extraction, evaporation to dryness and reconstitution in buffer system.

At the time of analysis the operator chooses which assays are going to be performed and inserts the respective test pens inside the Aio! analyser. Any combination of tests can be used and the continuous-access analyser also allows pens to be added later during the analysis. Sample pipetting and all the immunoassay steps are handled automatically by the analyser and the result is ready after 18 minutes of processing. Depending on the nature of the analytical need, either qualitative or quantitative results are produced. In the case of drug residue screening the need is usually qualitative (is the compound of interest present in the sample?) or semi-quantitative (does the concentration of the analyte exceed a given critical level, e.g., MRL concentration?). The all-in-one assays can also produce fully quantitative results if a standard curve is established for the analyte. This is useful, for example if the actual dose of the drug needs to be determined in the feedingstuffs. Different tests can be carried out in any desired order, which means that multi-residue screening can be achieved with no switch-over time between the analysis of different analytes. This is a major improvement compared with methods based on liquid chromatography where the equipment is typically dedicated to the measurement of a particular analyte, and it takes several hours or days to switch the system between different methods.

11.5 Future trends

Laboratories performing food analysis are constantly challenged with an ever increasing number of tests, more diverse testing needs, a requirement for shorter turnaround times and an increased emphasis on quality assurance. Analytical capabilities also have to be flexible so that services can be adapted to changing needs and different situations. Immunochemical methods will be increasingly used to meet these multiple needs. A growing number of tests will be based on new, simpler, and increasingly user-friendly assay formats and they will also include multi-residue methods.

Environmental considerations will direct method development towards the reduced use of solvents and waste production. More and more of the routine testing will be performed by dedicated analysers, which may be coupled with robotic sample pre-treatment systems. Random access systems will allow the laboratory to perform testing continuously and minimise the need for batching and scheduling of tests. In general, the higher degree of automation and system integration will enable higher analysis throughput, better cost-efficiency and more precise results. The test systems will also be adapted for on-site testing and connecting analytical instruments directly to the laboratory information system will facilitate data management.

The analytical technology, the regulatory climate, and economic outlook for food safety testing are moving in the same general direction, which leads to simpler, more cost-effective and more pragmatic food safety programmes. Success in achieving satisfactory consumer safety will rest with putting promising new technologies such as automated all-in-one dry chemistry immunoassays into practical use.

11.6 Acknowledgement

This work has been supported by the European Commission, Quality of Life and Management of Living Resources Programme, Key Action 1 on Food, Nutrition and Health – Contract No. QLK1-1999-00313.

11.7 References

BACIGALUPO M A, IUS A, MERONI G, DOVIS M, PETRUZZELLI E (1995), 'Comparison of time-resolved fluoroimmunoassay and immunoenzymometric assay for clenbuterol', *Analyst*, 120, 2269–2271.

BEIER R C, DUTKO T J, BUCKLEY S A, MULDOON M T, HOLTZAPPLE C K, STANKER L H (1998), 'Detection of halofuginone residues in chicken liver tissue by HPLC and a monoclonal-based immunoassay', *J. Agric. Food Chem.*, 46, 1049–1054.

BEIER R C, RIPLEY L H, YOUNG C R, KAISER C M (2001), 'Production, characterization, and cross-reactivity studies of monoclonal antibodies against the coccidiostat nicarbazin', *J Agric. Food Chem.*, 49, 4542–4552.

CONNOLLY L, FODEY T L, CROOKS S R H, DELAHAUT P, ELLIOTT C T (2002), 'The production and characterisation of dinitrocarbanilide antibodies raised using antigen mimics', *J Immunol. Methods*, 264, 45–51.

COOPER K M, TUOMOLA M, LAHDENPERÄ S, LÖVGREN T, ELLIOTT C T, KENNEDY D G (2002), 'The development and validation of dry reagent time-resolved fluoro-immunoassays for zeranol and α-zearalenol to assist in distinguishing zeranol abuse from *Fusarium* spp. toxin contamination in bovine urine', *Food Addit. Contam.*, 19, 1130–1137.

CROOKS S R H, FODEY T L, GILMORE G R, ELLIOTT C T (1998), 'Rapid screening for monensin residues in poultry plasma by a dry reagent dissociation enhanced lanthanide fluoroimmunoassays', *Analyst*, 123, 2493–2496.

CROOKS S R H, ROSS P, THOMPSON C S, HAGGAN S A, ELLIOTT C T (2000), 'Detection of unwanted residues of ivermectin in bovine milk by dissociation-enhanced lanthanide fluoroimmunoassay', *Luminescence*, 15, 371–376.

CROSBY N T (1991), *Determination of Veterinary Residues in Food*, Woodhead Publishing, Cambridge, UK, 123–147.

ELISSALDE M H, BEIER R C, ROWE L D, STANKER L H (1993), 'Development of a monoclonal-based enzyme-linked immunosorbent assay for the coccidiostat salinomycin', *J. Agric. Food Chem.*, 41, 2167–2171.

ELLIOTT C T, FRANCIS K S, MCCAUGHEY W J (1994), 'Investigation of dissociation enhanced lanthanide fluoroimmunoassay as an alternative screening test for veterinary drug residues', *Analyst*, 119, 2565–2569.

ELLIOTT C T, BAXTER A, HAASNOOT W, LOMMEN A, MCCAUGHEY W J (1996), 'Development of a dual label time-resolved fluoroimmunoassay for the detection of β-agonists in cattle urine', *Food Agric. Immunol.*, 8, 219–227.

ELLIOTT C T, KENNEDY D G, MCCAUGHEY W J (1998), 'Methods for the detection of polyether ionophores residues in poultry', *Analyst*, 123, 45R-56R.

FODEY T L, CONNOLLY L, CROOKS S R H, DELAHAUT P, ELLIOTT C T (2003), 'The production and characterisation of polyclonal antibodies to a range of Nitroimidazoles', *Anal. Chim. Acta*, 483, 193–200.

GODFREY M A J, LUCKEY M F, KWASOWSKI P (1997), 'IAC/cELISA detection of monensin elimination from chicken tissues, following oral therapeutic dosing', *Food Addit. Contam.*, 14, 281–286.

HAASNOOT W, SCHILT R (2000), 'Immunochemical and receptor technologies', in O'Keefe M (ed.), *Residue Analysis in Food*, Amsterdam, Harwood Academic Publishers, 107–144.

HEMMILÄ I, MUKKALA V-M (2001), 'Time-resolution in fluorometry technologies, labels, and applications in bioanalytical assays', *Crit. Rev. Clin. Lab. Sci.*, 38, 441–519.

HEMMILÄ I, DAKUBU S, MUKKALA V-M, SIITARI H, LÖVGREN T (1984), 'Europium as a label in time-resolved immunofluorometric assays', *Anal. Biochem.*, 137, 335–343.

KENNEDY D G, BLANCHFLOWER W J, O'DORNAN B C (1995a), 'Development of an ELISA for lasalocid and depletion kinetics of lasalocid residues in poultry', *Food Addit. Contam.*, 12, 83–92.

KENNEDY D G, BLANCHFLOWER W J, O'DORNAN B C (1995b), 'Development of an ELISA for salinomycin and depletion kinetics of salinomycin residues in poultry', *Food Addit. Contam.*, 12, 93–99.

KENNEDY D G, BLANCHFLOWER W J, HUGHES P J, MCCAUGHEY W J (1996), 'The incidence and cause of lasalocid residues in eggs in Northern Ireland', *Food Addit. Contam.*, 13, 787–794.

KENNEDY D G, BLANCHFLOWER W J, O'DORNAN B C (1997), 'Development of an ELISA for maduramicin and determination of the depletion kinetics of maduramicin residues in poultry', *Food Addit. Contam.*, 14, 27–33.

KENNEDY D G, HUGHES P J, BLANCHFLOWER W J (1998), 'Ionophore residues in eggs in Northern Ireland: incidence and cause', *Food Addit. Contam.*, 15, 535–541.

KENNEDY D G, CANNAVAN A, MCCRACKEN R J (2000), 'Regulatory problems caused by contamination, a frequently overlooked cause of veterinary drug residues', *J Chromatogr. A*, 882, 37–52.

LÖVGREN T, PETTERSSON K (2000), 'Time-resolved fluoroimmunoassay, advantages and limitations', in Van Dyke K, Van Dyke R (eds), *Luminescence Immunoassay and Molecular Applications*. Boca Raton, CRC Press, 233–253.

LÖVGREN T, MERIÖ L, MITRUNEN K, MÄKINEN M-L, MÄKELÄ M, BLOMBERG K, PALENIUS T, PETTERSSON K, (1996), 'One-step all-in-one dry reagent immunoassays with fluorescent europium chelate label and time-resolved fluorometry', *Clin. Chem.*, 42, 1196–1201.

MCEVOY J D G (2002), 'Contamination of animal feedingstuffs as a cause of residues in food: a review of regulatory aspects, incidence and control', *Anal. Chim. Acta*, 473, 3–26.

MERIÖ L, PETTERSSON K, LÖVGREN T (1996), 'Monoclonal antibody-based dual-label time-resolved fluorometric assays in a simplified one-step format', *Clin. Chem.*, 42, 1513–1517.

MITRUNEN K, PETTERSSON K, PIIRONEN T, BJÖRK T, LILJA H, LÖVGREN T (1995), 'Dual-label one-step immunoassay for simultaneous measurement of free and total prostate-specific antigen concentrations and ratios in serum', *Clin. Chem.*, 41, 1115–1120.

PAUILLAC S, HALMOS T, LABROUSSE J, ANTONAKIS K, AVRAMEAS S (1993), 'Production of highly specific monoclonal antibodies to monensin and development of a microELISA to detect this antibiotic', *J Immunol. Methods*, 164, 165–173.

PETTERSSON K S I, SÖDERHOLM J R-M (1990), 'Ultrasensitive two-site immunometric assay of human lutropin by time-resolved fluorometry', *Clin. Chem.*, 36, 1928–1933.

PETTERSSON K, KATAJAMÄKI T, IRJALA K, LEPPÖNEN V, MAJAMAA-VOLTTI K, LAITINEN P (2000), 'Time-resolved fluorometry (TRF)-based immunoassay concept for rapid and quantitative determination of biochemical myocardial infarction markers from whole blood, serum and plasma', *Luminescence*, 15, 399–407.

ROWE L D, BEIER, R C, ELISSALDE M H, STANKER L H (1994), 'Production and characterization of monoclonal antibodies against the poultry coccidiostat halofuginone', *J. Agric. Food Chem.*, 42, 1132–1137.

SOINI E, LÖVGREN T (1987), 'Time-resolved fluorescence of lanthanide probes and applications in biotechnology', *CRC Crit. Rev. Anal. Chem.*, 18, 105–154.

STANKER L H, BEIER R C (1996), 'Introduction to immunoassays for residue analysis', in Beier R C, Stanker L H (eds), *Immunoassays for Residue Analysis*, Washington, American Chemical Society, 2–16.

TAKALO H, MUKKALA V-M, MIKOLA H, LIITTI P, HEMMILÖ I (1994), 'Synthesis of europium(III) chelates suitable for labeling of bioactive molecules', *Bioconjugate Chem.*, 5, 278–282.

TUOMOLA M, COOPER K M, LAHDENPERÄ S, BAXTER G A, ELLIOTT C T, KENNEDY D G, LÖVGREN T (2002a), 'A specificity-enhanced time-resolved fluoroimmunoassay for zeranol employing the dry reagent all-in-one-well principle', *Analyst*, 127, 83–86.

TUOMOLA M, VAINIO J, LÖVGREN T (2002b), 'Rapid time-resolved immunofluorometric assay for the measurement of creatine kinase enabling the direct use of unprocessed whole blood samples', *J. Agric. Food Chem.*, 50, 6659–6662.

WATANABE H, SATAKE A, KIDO Y, TSUJI A (2001), 'Monoclonal-based enzyme-linked immunosorbent assay and immunochromatographic rapid assay for salinomycin', *Anal. Chim. Acta*, 437, 31–38.

WEISS G, MACDONALD R (1985), 'Methods for determination of ionophores-type antibiotic residues in animal tissues', *J. Assoc. Off. Anal. Chem.*, 68, 971–980.

Part III

Pesticides

12

Surveillance for pesticide residues

C. K. Winter, University of California – Davis, USA

12.1 Introduction

Pesticides used in agriculture to control pests, such as insects, weeds, and plant diseases, have been subject to considerable legislative, regulatory, and consumer scrutiny over the past few decades. Pesticides are, by their nature, toxic chemicals; since many pesticides may potentially leave residues on foods available for human consumption, there is much concern regarding the potential health risks of pesticides in the human diet. Concerns stem from possible risks of acute poisoning from exposure to large amounts of pesticides consumed in a short duration as well as from chronic risks from exposure to low levels of pesticide residues over extended periods of time. In the United States, particular concern has been raised as to the potential carcinogenic effects of pesticides consumed in the diet (NRC, 1987). More recent concerns have emerged regarding the potential of some pesticides to affect endocrine functions (Colburn *et al.*, 1996). Federal regulatory activities have also recently focused on ensuring that the risks faced by infants and children consuming pesticides are not excessive (Winter, 2001).

In addition to consumer concerns, pesticide use also presents risks to agricultural workers involved in the mixing, loading, or application of pesticides and to those working in fields treated with pesticides (California Department of Pesticide Regulation, 1999). Occupational illnesses and injuries resulting from pesticide use have been reported frequently and some epidemiological evidence has linked specific pesticides with increases in specific types of cancers among those exposed occupationally (Hoar *et al.*, 1986). Pesticides also present environmental concerns including water and soil contamination, air pollution, destruction of natural vegetation, reductions in natural pest populations, effects upon non-target organisms including fish, wildlife, and livestock, creation of secondary pest problems, and the evolution of pesticide resistance.

Advances in crop protection technology have actually resulted in a small decrease in overall pesticide use in the United States since 1979 (EPA, 1999). Much of this reduction may have resulted from widespread adoption of 'Integrated Pest Management' (IPM) techniques that stress the judicious use of pesticides in combination with other cultural, physical, and biological practices. Nevertheless, public concerns about pesticide residues in foods are still strong, with some surveys indicating that the vast majority of consumers consider pesticide residues in foods to represent a serious health threat (Bruhn *et al.*, 1998). Such consumer concern has led some retail outlets to work with private laboratories to certify that their produce is free of detectable pesticide residues, and has likely contributed to the dramatic growth of the organic foods industry.

While much attention has focused on the potential health and environmental risks posed by pesticides, the benefits of pesticides also require consideration. It is clear that pesticide use is frequently associated with increases in crop yield and reductions in crop loss. One estimate indicates that the economic benefits from the use of pesticides in developed countries range from $3.50 to $5.00 for every dollar spent on pesticides, and that 40% of the world's food supply would be at risk if pesticides were not available (Pimentel *et al.*, 1992). In a developed nation like the United States, the use of pesticides undoubtedly has resulted in a greater availability of fruits, vegetables, and grains at lower consumer costs.

This review focuses on the surveillance of pesticide residues in foods in the United States. Surveillance programs comprise one type of several different programs put in place by the US government and by US food producers in a comprehensive effort to regulate and manage pesticides; the results of such programs provide one indication of the effectiveness of such pesticide regulatory and management efforts.

12.2 Pesticide regulation in the United States

Regulation of pesticides at the US federal level involves three agencies: the Environmental Protection Agency (EPA), the Food and Drug Administration (FDA), and the Department of Agriculture (USDA). Individual states also have the authority to regulate pesticides and are allowed to apply pesticide use restrictions that are more stringent than those established federally. The most comprehensive state pesticide regulatory program is in California; other large state pesticide regulatory programs exist in Florida, Texas, Michigan, and New York.

12.2.1 Agency responsibilities

The primary law governing pesticide regulation in the United States is the Federal Insecticide, Fungicide, and Rodenticide Act (FIFRA) of 1947. FIFRA is primarily a risk/benefit balancing statute; if the benefits of specific uses of a pesticide are deemed to outweigh their risks, the pesticide is allowed for such specific uses. Some of the potential risks, as discussed above, include human health effects and environmental factors; benefits may include greater production efficiency, lower food costs, and public health protection (for example, mosquito abatement programs).

The USDA was initially assigned the responsibility of implementing FIFRA. When the EPA was created in the early 1970s, it assumed FIFRA responsibility for approving and/or revoking pesticide registrations.

Currently, the EPA spends much effort reviewing toxicological and environmental fate data submitted by a pesticide's manufacturer in a request to have the pesticide registered for use. A full battery of toxicological tests must be performed before a pesticide can be registered for use on a food crop; such studies investigate the pesticide's acute, subchronic, and chronic exposure, carcinogenicity, teratogenicity, mutagenicity, and metabolic fate, among other things. The manufacturer of the pesticide must also provide studies on the pesticide's potential effects on non-target organisms, food residue studies, and studies of the environmental behavior of the pesticide. It may take ten years or more for the studies to be conducted and submitted by the manufacturer and reviewed by the EPA; the cost of completing the studies may often exceed $30 million (Ecobichon, 1996).

If the use of the pesticide may have the potential to leave residues on foods, the EPA is also required to determine the maximum allowable residues on the crops (known as the tolerances, see section 12.2.2). Tolerances are pesticide and commodity specific; the same pesticide may have different tolerances established on different commodities while the same commodity may have several different tolerances established for various pesticides that are allowed for use on the commodity (Winter, 1992).

The FDA is the primary US federal agency involved in pesticide residue monitoring and in enforcing pesticide tolerances for domestic and imported foods shipped in interstate commerce. The FDA performs its regulatory monitoring program to enforce pesticide tolerances (FDA, 2003). In this program, sampling is not random as the FDA targets the types and origins of commodities considered most likely to present violative residues. Violative residues may occur when pesticide residues are found that exceed the established tolerances, but are more commonly associated with the finding of a residue of a pesticide on a commodity for which no tolerance has been established.

The FDA also performs its annual Total Diet Study, in which food samples are collected as 'market baskets' from four geographical regions in the United States and from three cities in each region (FDA, 2003). Each market basket comprises 257 or 258 different food items obtained from retail outlets and the food items are all prepared for consumption prior to analysis. Unlike the FDA's regulatory monitoring program, the Total Diet Study is not designed to enforce pesticide tolerances but rather to provide an estimate of dietary pesticide residue exposure to the general US population and to specific US population subgroups.

The USDA conducts two pesticide residue monitoring programs as well. USDA's National Residue Program obtains samples of meat, poultry, and raw eggs that are analyzed for pesticide residues as well as for animal drugs and environmental contaminants. The USDA initiated its Pesticide Data Program (PDP) in 1991. In contrast with FDA's regulatory monitoring programs that are designed primarily to enforce pesticide tolerances, PDP's sampling protocols are designed to more accurately reflect residue levels that reach consumers and, as such, provide a more reliable tool for assessing human dietary risk from exposure to pesticides. In 2001, ten states (California, Colorado, Florida, Maryland, Michigan, New York, Ohio, Texas, Washington, and Wisconsin) participated in collecting and analyzing samples in the PDP program (USDA, 2003).

12.2.2 Establishing pesticide tolerances

Since pesticide residue surveillance programs frequently are designed to enforce pesticide tolerances, it is critical to understand how pesticide tolerances are established and their significance with respect to human health and/or agricultural practices. Tolerances are frequently, and incorrectly, considered to represent safety standards while violative residues are frequently implied to represent unsafe residues. In actuality, tolerances have a valuable role as indicators of proper pesticide use but should not be considered as barometers of safety. The seemingly counterintuitive practices used to establish pesticide tolerances are described in detail by Winter (1992) and are summarized below.

In general, tolerances are established at levels that represent the maximum residues that might be expected on commodities resulting from 'worst-case' application conditions such as maximum allowed application rate, maximum number of applications per growing season, and harvest at the minimum legal interval following the final application. Pesticide manufacturers interested in obtaining tolerances for their pesticides on specific commodities perform a series of field studies in a variety of geographical locations. Once samples have been taken and the residues analyzed, the manufacturer petitions the EPA to establish a tolerance at or above the maximum residue detected from the 'worst-case' field studies. As a result, tolerances should be considered as enforcement tools to indicate whether pesticide application practices have been performed in accordance with directions; residues detected in excess of tolerances most likely would occur only in cases in which pesticide applications were not made properly.

While the tolerance values themselves are not health-based, it should not be implied that the potential health effects from exposure to pesticide residues are not considered. The EPA, before approving a pesticide tolerance, will perform its own risk assessment to ensure that exposure to the pesticide from its proposed use(s) as well as from its existing uses, is at acceptable levels to ensure a 'reasonable certainty of no harm.' If exposure is deemed to be acceptable, the EPA will accept the manufacturer's petition to establish the tolerance at or above the maximum level encountered from the field trials. If the expected exposure to the pesticide is determined to be excessive, the EPA will not approve the tolerance or will approve the tolerance only if other uses of the pesticide are eliminated to ensure that exposure is acceptable.

Prior to 1996, the risk assessments used to determine whether pesticide tolerances should be established considered individual pesticides on a case-by-case basis and considered only dietary exposure to pesticides. Passage of the 1996 Food Quality Protection Act (FQPA) expanded EPA's responsibility to consider the 'aggregate' exposure to the pesticide from food, water, and from residential sources. In addition, in cases where several different individual pesticides share a common mechanism of toxicological action, the risk assessments must include consideration of the 'cumulative' exposure to all of the pesticides sharing the common mechanism rather than just individual pesticides. Consideration of the potential increased susceptibility of infants and children to pesticides is also an important provision of FQPA. The EPA is required to consider all of these factors in its efforts to reassess all pesticide tolerances by August 2006; several pesticide tolerances have already been revoked resulting from the increased scrutiny required by FQPA. It should be emphasized, however, that the levels established for pesticide tolerances are still set to equal or slightly exceed the maximum residues found in the manufacturers' field trials. As such, the tolerances still represent enforcement tools and should not be confused as safety standards even though the EPA does consider possible health risks prior to establishing tolerances.

12.3 Sample collection, preparation, and analysis

As discussed previously, different pesticide residue surveillance programs use different sampling methods. The FDA's regulatory monitoring program is primarily developed to enforce tolerances; in this program, sampling is focused to provide analysis of samples most likely to contain violative residues based upon FDA intelligence and historical patterns. As such, particular commodities or commodity origins may be preferentially sampled and results from sample analysis may not be representative of the typical residue profiles that reach US consumers. Approximately two-thirds of all samples collected in FDA's 2001 regulatory monitoring program involved foods grown in other countries that were imported into the US (FDA, 2003). In contrast, samples collected and analyzed in USDA's PDP in 2001 were primarily (82 percent) from domestic sources, and thus the sampling was much more representative (USDA, 2003). As a result, findings from this program may be useful in assessing potential human dietary risks and are often used by the EPA to suit this purpose.

There are frequently large differences in residue levels between residues on raw agricultural commodities and those in a form actually consumed. The FDA's regulatory monitoring program focuses on the raw commodities while PDP samples are often washed, presumably just as typical consumers would do, prior to analysis. In FDA's Total Diet Study, foods are prepared in institutional kitchens to be 'ready for consumption' before analysis. Residues encountered following this approach more closely resemble residues to which consumers may be exposed, as this approach takes into account such factors as washing, cooking, peeling, processing, evaporation, and the passage of time.

Samples collected for pesticide residue analysis are subject to several laboratory steps before pesticides can be detected and the residue levels are determined. Food samples are usually subject to an initial blending step followed by extraction using organic solvents or newer solvent-minimizing steps to isolate the pesticides (analytes) from many other components in the foods. Additional unwanted components that may have been extracted along with the pesticides may be removed using clean-up procedures often involving column chromatography, volatilization, liquid-liquid partitioning, or chemical degradation. Such procedures often result in the 'fractionizing' of the analyte extract into different subgroups; the properties of the individual pesticides will determine the particular subgroup into which each pesticide will primarily reside (Seiber, 2001).

Chemical modification steps frequently follow the clean-up procedures and may result in the formation of pesticides modified to make them easier to separate, detect, or quantify.

Analytical instruments in the laboratory such as high performance liquid chromatographs and gas chromatographs are frequently used to separate individual pesticides found in the cleaned-up extracts from other pesticides and other components of the extract. At the end of the instrument is a detector that takes advantage of the properties of the analyte to detect its presence once it has been separated from other components in the extract. Both qualitative and quantitative detection measurements are used to identify the analyte and determine how much of the analyte is present (Seiber, 2001).

When violative residues are determined in tolerance enforcement programs, the commodities from which the violative residues reside are subject to seizure and possible destruction. To provide assurance that the samples are indeed violative, a second, independent analytical method is frequently used to confirm the findings of the original method.

While single residue methods (SRMs) for individual pesticides are frequently developed by the pesticide manufacturers and submitted to the EPA, US regulatory agencies normally use multi-residue methods (MRMs) capable of detection of a large number of different pesticides. Such methods frequently involve fractioning the original sample extract into many different subgroups and analyzing each subgroup separately. The MRM procedures used in FDA's regulatory monitoring program, for example, are capable of detecting more than 200 individual pesticides, representing approximately half of the pesticides with EPA tolerances and many others that have no tolerances (FDA, 2003). Occasionally, regulatory agencies must rely on other SRMs or MRMs capable of detecting pesticides that cannot be determined using the more common MRMs.

Analytical advances are leading to the development of more specific and more sensitive methods to separate, identify, and quantify pesticide residues from foods. The use of mass spectrometers, either alone or coupled to high performance liquid chromatographs and gas chromatographs, provides even greater sensitivity and analyte selectivity. In addition, a technique known as immunoassay, in which sensitive antibodies are developed from laboratory organisms and used to identify pesticide residues, is gaining widespread popularity due to its relatively low cost and low sample preparation requirements.

12.4 Results from pesticide surveillance programs

Results from various pesticide surveillance programs conducted in the United States are presented in this section. While results from many of the programs are similar, it is important to understand how each of the programs differs with respect to sampling strategies, sample preparation, and the types of pesticides analyzed.

12.4.1 FDA Regulatory Monitoring Program

The most recent FDA pesticide residue regulatory monitoring data are available for 2001 (FDA, 2003). During that year, FDA analyzed 6475 food samples for pesticide residues. More samples were taken from imported foods (4374 samples, or 67.6%) than from domestic foods (2101 samples, or 32.4%).

The results of FDA's 2001 monitoring of pesticide residues in imported foods are shown in Fig. 12.1. Overall, 72.0 percent of the samples showed no detected residues, and violations were identified in 4.8 percent of the samples. Figure 12.2 shows the comparable results from domestic foods where 60.2 percent of the samples showed no detectable residues, and violations were present in 1.1 percent of the samples.

As described previously, pesticide residue violations commonly take one of two forms. The most common form of residue violation occurs when residues of a pesticide are detected on a commodity for which a tolerance for that pesticide has not been established. Such a violation may occur from application of the pesticide to the wrong commodity, uptake from soil contaminated from a prior use of the pesticide on a different commodity, or drift of a pesticide applied to an adjacent field. The other type of violation occurs when residue levels exceed the tolerance established for the pesticide/commodity combination. In 2001, only 7.1 percent of the violative import samples involved residues detected above the tolerance levels while 92.9 percent of the import violations occurred when pesticides were detected on commodities for which no tolerance was established. A different pattern emerges from domestic samples where 11 samples were detected above tolerance levels and another 11 showed residues of pesticides not allowed on the commodities. Fruits and vegetables showed the highest percentages of both detected residues and violations.

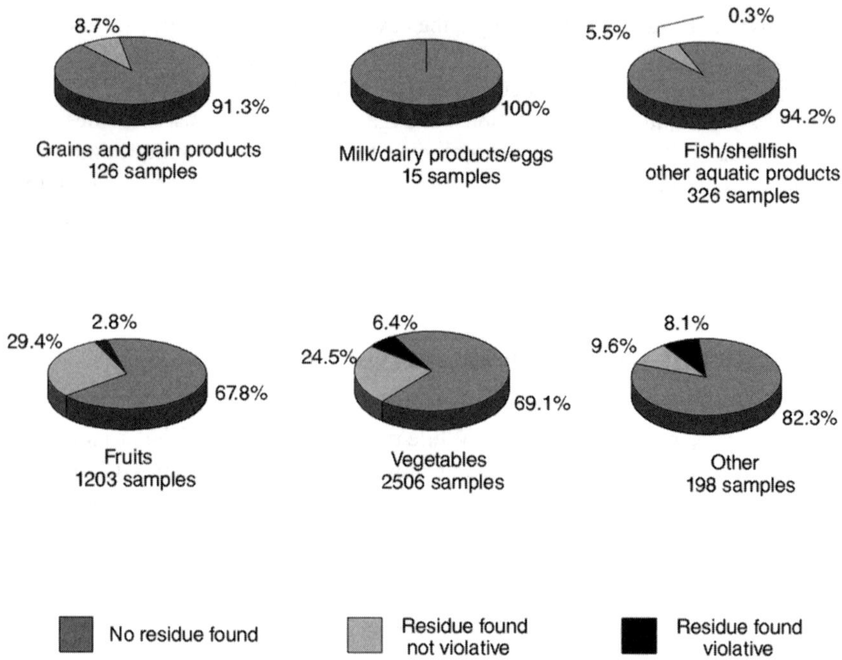

Fig. 12.1 US Food and Drug Administration Pesticide Residue Monitoring, 2001 – imported foods. *Source*: FDA (2003).

12.4.2 FDA Total Diet Study

As described previously, FDA's Total Diet Study determines pesticide residues in foods prepared for consumption (FDA, 2003). Since it is not primarily an enforcement program, the analytical methods used in the Total Diet Study are refined to permit measurement of residues at levels 5–10 times lower than those often used in enforcement programs, allowing, in some cases, detection at the one part per billion level.

The 19 most frequently found residues in FDA's 2001 Total Diet Study are shown in Table 12.1. The levels of these pesticides are well below regulatory limits. The five most frequently detected residues, DDT, chlorpyrifos-methyl, endosulfan, malathion, and dieldrin, have been shown over the past several years to represent the most commonly detected pesticides in the program.

By combining the results of FDA's Total Diet Study with crude estimates of human consumption of the food items sampled, it is possible to derive estimates of potential daily human dietary consumption of the pesticides detected in this program. Unfortunately, the FDA no longer makes such exposure estimates available. Results reported from the 1991 Total Diet Study did indicate that for most pesticides, the typical daily exposure estimates represented only a small fraction (often less than one percent), of the levels of regulatory concern, known as the reference doses or acceptable daily intakes (Winter, 2001). These levels of

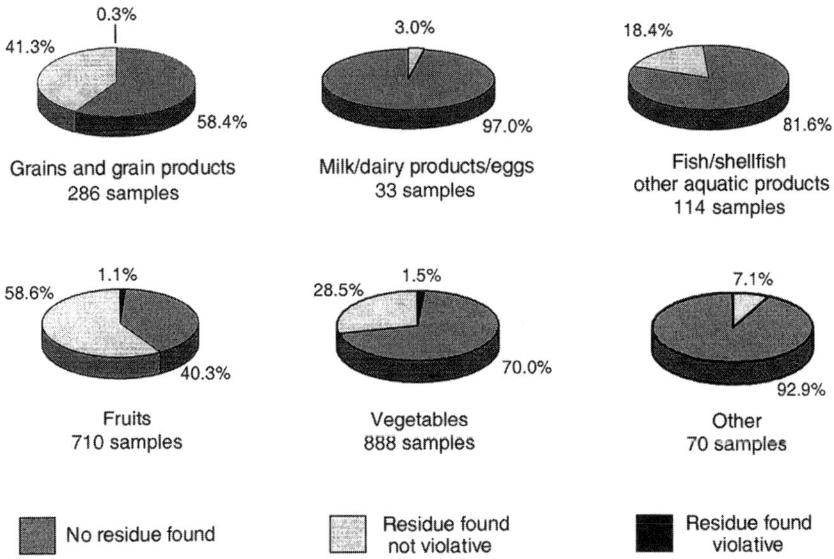

Fig. 12.2 US Food and Drug Administration Pesticide Residue Monitoring, 2001 – domestic foods. *Source*: FDA (2003)

regulatory concern are derived by first identifying, in laboratory animals, the highest level of exposure to the pesticide that causes no observed adverse effects, and then by dividing that level by an uncertainty factor (usually 100; typical range: 10–1,000) that presumably covers potential variability resulting from extrapolation of findings from animal to human populations and interhuman variability. Put another way, the levels estimated for daily human exposure to pesticides in FDA's 1991 Total Diet Study frequently correspond to levels 10,000 times or more below those administered to laboratory animals on a daily basis that do not produce any noticeable adverse effects in the animals (Winter, 2001).

12.4.3 USDA's National Residue Program

USDA's National Residue Program is similar to FDA's Regulatory Monitoring Program in that it is designed primarily to enforce pesticide tolerances and to maximize the chances of detecting violative residues. While the FDA has primary authority for enforcing tolerances on fruits, vegetables, and grains, USDA's jurisdiction extends to meat, poultry, and raw eggs.

Sampling in USDA's National Residue Program is quite focused and is specific for food product/pesticide class combinations. In 2000, this program proposed analyzing 2159 samples of imported food products and 8450 domestic

Table 12.1 Frequency of occurrence of pesticide residues found in total diet study foods in 2001 (FDA, 2003)[a]

Pesticide[b]	Total no. of findings	Occurrence (%)	Range (ppm)
DDT	234	23	0.0001 – 0.031
chlorpyrifos-methyl	201	20	0.0001 – 0.537
endosulfan	185	18	0.0001 – 0.266
malathion	164	16	0.0007 – 0.080
dieldrin	152	15	0.0001 – 0.020
chlorpropham	73	7	0.0006 – 1.029
chlorpyrifos	71	7	0.0001 – 0.058
permethrin	60	6	0.0004 – 1.856
carbaryl[c]	55	5	0.0004 – 1.459
iprodione	39	4	0.0003 – 3.541
dicloran	36	3	0.0002 – 0.197
heptachlor	35	3	0.0001 – 0.0005
lindane	28	3	0.0001 – 0.002
hexachlorobenze	28	3	0.0001 – 0.002
thiabendazole[d]	27	3	0.015 – 0.524
methamidophos	25	2	0.001 – 0.243
acephate	24	2	0.002 – 0.505
methoxychlor	24	2	0.0002 – 0.020
quintozene	22	2	0.0001 – 0.0043

[a] Based on four market baskets analyzed in 2001 consisting of 1030 total items. Only those found in >2% of the samples are shown.
[b] Isomers, metabolites, and related compounds are included with the 'parent' pesticide from which they arise.
[c] Reflects overall incidence; however, only 93–95 selected foods per market basket (i.e., 377 items total) were analyzed for N-methylcarbamates.
[d] Reflects overall incidence; however, only 67 selected foods per market basket (i.e., 268 items total) were analyzed for the benzimidazole fungicides thiabendazole and benomyl.

food products for chlorinated hydrocarbon and chlorinated organophosphate insecticides. Results of such analyses are not yet available (USDA, 2001).

12.4.4 USDA's Pesticide Data Program

In 2001, USDA's PDP collected and analyzed 12,264 samples of fresh and processed fruits and vegetables, rice, beef and poultry tissues, and drinking water (USDA, 2003). Specific fruits and vegetables analyzed included apples, bananas, broccoli, carrots, celery, cherries, grapes, green beans, lettuce, mushrooms, nectarines, oranges, peaches, pineapples, potatoes, canned sweet corn, canned sweet peas, and canned tomato paste. A total of 9903 samples were from fruit and vegetable commodities while 689 were from enriched milled rice, 464 were from poultry, 911 were from beef, and 297 drinking water samples were collected. As discussed previously, the majority (82 percent) of the samples taken in PDP was of domestic origin and sampling was based on a statistical design to ensure that the data are reliable for use in exposure assessments and can be used to guide conclusions about pesticide residues in the US food supply.

Results from USDA's 2001 PDP are summarized in Table 12.2. Overall, 44 percent of all samples contained no detectable residues while 24 percent contained one residue and 32 percent contained more than one residue. Residues exceeding an established tolerance were detected in 0.1 percent of the samples, while residues found on commodities for which no tolerance was established were detected in 1.8 percent of the samples.

12.4.5 California Department of Pesticide Regulation Residue Monitoring Program

Results from California's Residue Monitoring Program for 2001 are provided in Fig. 12.3. This program analyzed 7513 samples of fresh produce of both domestic and imported origin using MRMs capable of detecting residues of more than 200 pesticides and their breakdown products (California Department of Pesticide Regulation, 2003). No residues were detected in 68.2 percent of the samples while residues detected at levels below the tolerance were found in 30.3 percent of the samples and violations occurred in 1.5 percent of the samples. While the breakdown of violations between over-tolerance residues and residues detected on commodities for which no tolerance was established was not provided for 2001, the breakdown is likely to be similar to that reported by the California Department of Pesticide Regulation for 1999 when approximately 12 percent of the violations involved over-tolerance residues (Winter, 2001).

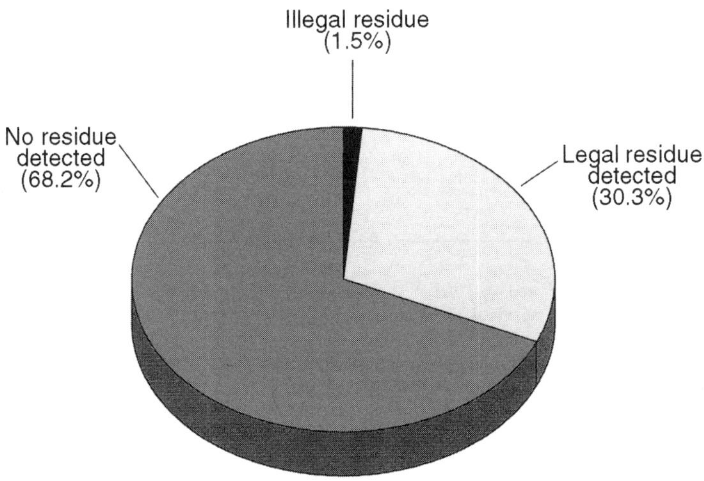

Fig. 12.3 California Department of Pesticide Regulation Pesticide Residue Monitoring, 2001. *Source*: California Department of Pesticide Regulation (2002)

Table 12.2 Number of samples and residues detected by commodity, 2001 pesticide data program (USDA, 2003)

	Total samples analyzed	Samples with residues detected	% of samples with detections	Different residues detected	Total residue detections
Fresh fruit and vegetables					
Apples	736	671	91	24	1,584
Bananas	702	317	45	3	334
Broccoli	720	209	29	22	265
Carrots	739	600	81	35	1,270
Celery	736	693	94	35	2,321
Cherries	286	254	89	37	828
Grapes	705	515	73	22	903
Green Beans	707	440	62	29	1,150
Lettuce	554	272	49	29	562
Mushrooms	184	121	66	12	192
Nectarines	362	351	97	25	1,171
Oranges	745	615	83	14	837
Peaches	529	522	99	38	2,318
Pineapples	730	54	7	6	57
Potatoes	733	601	82	18	795
Total fresh	9,168	6,235	68		14,587
Processed fruit and vegetables					
Sweet Corn, Canned	181	2	1	1	2
Sweet Peas, Canned	185	0	0	0	0
Tomato Paste, Canned	369	112	30	8	191
Total processed	735	114	15		193
Processed Grain product					
Rice	689	214	31	8	237
Water project					
Water, Drinking	297	145	49	17	455
Meat tissues					
Beef, Adipose	291	173	59	10	218
Beef, Liver	311	0	0	0	0
Beef, Muscle	309	1	<1		1
Poultry, Adipose	155	0	0	0	0
Poultry, Liver	155	0	0	0	0
Poultry, Muscle	154	0	0	0	0
Total meats	1375	174	13		219

Fruits and vegetables:
Number of Samples Analyzed = 9,903
Number of Samples with Residues Detected = 6,349
Percent Residue Detections = 64.1%
Total Number of Different Residues Detected = 100
Total Number of Residue Detections = 14,780
All commodities:
Number of Samples Analyzed = 12,264
Number of Samples with Residues Detected = 6,882
Percent with Residue Detections = 56.1%
Total Number of Different Residues Detected = 116
Total Number of Residue Detections = 15,691

12.4.6 Pesticides in organic foods

Although foods have been sold as 'organic' in the United States and elsewhere for more than a decade, the USDA adopted final identity standards for organic foods in 2000 to bring national consistency to several dozen pre-existing state and private standards. The standards do not generally allow the use of synthetic pesticides in the production of organic foods although several pesticides, primarily of natural origin, are allowed to be used when growing organic crops. A few synthetic pesticides including sulfur, oil sprays, and copper-based fungicides, are allowed for use in organic production. While many consumers may consider organic produce to represent 'pesticide-free' produce, it is also clear that many of them are unaware that pesticides can be, and are, commonly used in organic production. At the same time, it is logical to assume that pesticide residues in organic produce should differ considerably, both quantitatively and qualitatively, from those observed in conventional produce.

Using publicly-available data obtained from PDP and from the California Department of Pesticide Regulation, Baker *et al.* (2002) compared residue monitoring results of organic produce with that of produce for which no market claim (presumably conventional) was made. Results from this study are summarized in Table 12.3. PDP data obtained from 1994–1999 showed that 23 percent of 127 fresh food samples designated as organic had detectable residues while 73 percent of the 26,571 food samples for which no market claim had been made had detectable residues. Many of the residues detected on the organic produce were due to unavoidable contamination by persistent chlorinated hydrocarbon insecticides that had been banned from use many years ago. After eliminating the residues of these banned insecticides, pesticide residues from the foods designated as organic were detected in 13 percent of the samples.

Similar comparisons were made with results from pesticide monitoring by the California Department of Pesticide Regulation from 1989 to 1998. The analysis of 1097 samples of organic produce indicated residues in 6.5 percent of the samples, compared with residues in 30.9 percent of the 66,057 samples for which no market claim was made.

Table 12.3 Comparison of pesticide residue findings between organic produce and produce for which no market claim was made (Adapted from Baker *et al.*, 2002)

Source	Organic			No market claim		
	No. of samples	No. of positives	Percent positive	No. of samples	No. of positives	Percent positive
USDA Pesticide Data Program 1994–1999	127	29	23	26,571	19,485	73
California Department of Pesticide Regulation 1989–1998	1,097	71	6	66,057	20,410	31

Such results indicate that while residues of pesticides are less common in organic produce than in conventional produce, detection of residues in organics is still quite common. The presence of detectable residues in the organic samples is considered by Baker *et al.* (2002) to result from many factors such as product mislabeling, misidentification of the samples during data entry, post-harvest fungicide contamination, or inadvertent, unavoidable contamination from environmentally persistent pesticides or from drift from pesticide applications made to adjacent crops.

12.5 Interpreting the results of pesticide residue surveillance programs

Results of pesticide residue surveillance programs are commonly interpreted to indicate that either pesticide residues pose a significant risk to human health or that they do not. Frequently, analysis of the same data can yield different conclusions based upon the reader's perceptions, values, and background. As an example, the FDA's Residue Monitoring Program showed that 68.2 percent of the samples (combining both domestic and imported samples) showed no detectable residues and that 2.1 percent of the samples were violative (FDA, 2003). Some may conclude that the detection and violation rates for pesticide residues are low and that pesticides therefore do not constitute a serious health threat to consumers. Others, though, may conclude that such detection and violation rates are excessive and therefore provide little assurance that the risks posed by pesticide residues in the diet are at acceptable levels.

From a toxicological standpoint, expressing frequency of detection or violation rates provides little useful information on which to predict the risks posed by pesticide residues in foods. Of far greater concern among risk assessors is the actual amount of exposure to pesticide residues, which is determined by considering both the residue levels (not just the presence/absence of residues) and the amount of the food items consumed. Sophisticated models have been developed to predict both long-term exposure to pesticides in the diet as well as short-term exposure (Winter, 2003).

It should be emphasized again that violative residues should not be confused with 'unsafe' residues since tolerance levels are enforcement tools designed to determine whether pesticide applications have been made in accordance with directions rather than safety standards (Winter, 1992). While violative residues have been a source of unsafe residues in a tiny number of cases, most violations are of no health significance but rather result from the improper management of pesticides.

Much has been made of the marked differences in violation rates between imported and domestic produce in the US; according to the 2001 FDA Residue Monitoring Program, the violation rate for imported samples (4.8 percent) was more than four times higher than that for domestic samples (1.1 percent). Interestingly, the percentage of samples detected for which the tolerances were exceeded was greater for domestic samples (0.5 percent) than for imported samples (0.3 percent); this is also consistent with the finding of more detected residues on domestic samples (39.8 percent) than on imported samples (28.0 percent).

Imported samples showed a much higher occurrence of violations for which residues were detected that did not have a tolerance established on the commodity (4.5 percent) than did domestic samples (0.5 percent). A reasonable explanation for this finding is that food exporters distributing their products throughout the world may face a large number of different standards for pesticide residues in the countries to which they export. For a given pesticide/ commodity combination, for example, a Chilean fruit producer may face different standards in the United States, Canada, Europe, Japan, and Korea; the pesticide may be permitted on the commodity at different levels in some countries and not permitted at all in others. Unless the exporter has kept excellent records concerning pesticide use and has complete knowledge of how much residue is allowed and in which countries the pesticide is even permitted, it is likely that mistakes may be made and food containing residues that are legal in some countries may be exported to other countries for which the residues are not allowed. Foods produced in the United States for domestic consumption are not subject to such complications and this may explain the much lower relative violation rates. It would be interesting, though, to determine what percentage of food exported from the US contains violative residues upon arrival in the importing country. In all cases involving violations, however, it is important that one not assumes that the violative residues are of health significance.

12.6 Future trends

It is likely that pesticide residue monitoring programs in the United States will not change significantly in the next few years. They serve a role in demonstrating that most pesticide residues are not violative, suggesting that pesticide application and management practices have been made according to the legal directions.

One trend that may be identified in future pesticide residue monitoring programs is a decreased use of pesticides in agriculture due to improvements in non-pesticide control measures as well as more stringent pesticide regulation and public demand for foods containing lower residues. In addition, the development of new genetically-modified foods may also reduce pesticide use since such pesticidal properties may be engineered directly into the foods themselves. This could significantly reduce environmental and occupational risks resulting from pesticide use.

One recent concern is that of terrorism resulting from the intentional contamination of foods using pathogenic microorganisms, acutely toxic pesticides, or nerve toxins related to many common pesticides. There is a need to develop rapid, inexpensive, and sensitive analytical methods to test for the presence of such potential biological and chemical threats in the food supply. Developments in immunological methods of chemical and biological analysis will most likely aid in the development of such surveillance tools that can be rapidly applied to the analysis of a wide number of different food items.

12.7 Sources of further information and advice

As this manuscript has documented, there are several major US agencies involved in the surveillance of pesticide residues. Pesticide surveillance and regulation practices are dynamic and evolving; up-to-date information of agency activities is commonly available on their websites:

US Environmental Protection Agency – http://www.epa.gov
US Food and Drug Administration – http://www.fda.gov
US Department of Agriculture – http://www.usda.gov
California Department of Pesticide Regulation – http://www.cdpr.ca.gov

12.8 References

BAKER B P, BENBROOK C M, GROTH E and LUTZ BENBROOK K (2002), Pesticide residues in conventional, integrated pest management (IPM)-grown and organic foods: insights from three US data sets, *Food Additives and Contaminants* 19(5), 427–446.

BRUHN C M, WINTER C K, BEALL G A, BROWN S, HARWOOD J O, LAMP C L, STANFORD G, STEINBRING Y J and TURNER B (1998), Consumer response to pesticide/food safety risk statements: implications for consumer education, *Dairy Food Environ. Sanit.* 18(5), 278–287.

CALIFORNIA DEPARTMENT OF PESTICIDE REGULATION (1999), *Overview of the California Pesticide Illness Surveillance Program, 1996*, California Environmental Protection Agency, Sacramento, CA.

CALIFORNIA DEPARTMENT OF PESTICIDE REGULATION (2003), *Residues in Fresh Produce 2001*, California Environmental Protection Agency, Sacramento, CA.

COLBURN T, DUMANOSKI D and MYERS J P (1996), *Our Stolen Future: Are We Threatening Our Fertility, Intelligence, and Survival? A Scientific Detective Story*, Dutton Publishing, New York.

ECOBICHON D J (1996), Toxic effects of pesticides, in Klaasen, C D, *Casarett and Doull's Toxicology: The Basic Science of Poisons*, 5th edn, McGraw-Hill, New York, 643–685.

EPA (1999), *Pesticide Industry Sales and Usage, 1996 and 1997 Market Estimates*, US Environmental Protection Agency, Office of Prevention, Pesticides, and Toxic Substances, Washington, DC.

FDA (2003), *Food and Drug Administration Pesticide Program Residue Monitoring 2001*, US Food and Drug Administration, Washington, DC.

HOAR S K, BLAIR A, HOLMES F F, BOYSEN C D and ROBEL R J (1986), Agricultural herbicide use and risk of lymphoma and soft tissue sarcoma, *JAMA* 256(9), 1141–1147.

NRC (1987), *Regulating Pesticides in Food: The Delaney Paradox*, National Research

Council, National Academy of Sciences, National Academy Press, Washington, DC.

PIMENTEL D, ACQUAY H, BILTONEN M, RICE P, SILVA M, NELSON J, LIPNER V, GIORDANO S, HOROWITZ A and D'AMORE M (1992), Environmental and economic costs of pesticide use, *Bioscience* 42, 750–760.

SEIBER J N (2001), Analysis of chemical toxicants and contaminants in foods, in Helferich W G and Winter C K (eds), *Food Toxicology*, CRC Press, Boca Raton, FL, 203–218.

USDA (2001), *Food Safety and Inspection Service 2000 FSIS National Residue Program*, US Department of Agriculture Food Safety and Inspection Service, Washington, DC.

USDA (2003), *Pesticide Data Program Annual Summary Calendar Year 2001*, US Department of Agriculture, Agriculture and Marketing Service, Science and Technology, Washington, DC.

WINTER C K (1992), Pesticide tolerances and their relevance as safety standards, *Reg. Toxicol. Pharmacol.* 15, 137–150.

WINTER C K (2001), Pesticide residues in the food supply, in Helferich W G and Winter C K (eds), *Food Toxicology*, CRC Press, Boca Raton, FL, 163–186.

WINTER C K (2003), Exposure and dose-response modeling for food chemical risk assessment, in Schmidt R H and Rodrick G E (eds), *Food Safety Handbook*, Wiley Interscience, Hoboken, NJ, 73–88.

13

The rapid detection of pesticide residues

R. Luxton and J. Hart, University of the West of England, UK

13.1 Introduction

In today's world many different chemicals are used to protect food and our environment from spoilage by a range of pests such as rodents, weeds, insects and fungi. This has a great positive economic value by increasing the yield in the food supply chain. Despite having great benefit to society, the very nature of their use means that pesticides are highly toxic to humans and measures must be taken to prevent accidental exposure, whether from occupational exposure or more covertly via the food supply chain itself.

A wide range of compounds are used as pesticides such as the chlorinated hydrocarbons, which have been shown to be highly toxic and may have long-lasting effects on the environment. Research has shown that dichloro-diphenyltrichloroethane (DDT) has had a devastating effect on parts of the food chain. Another important group of pesticides is the organophosphate compounds, which are safer than chlorinated hydrocarbons but are still highly toxic. It is thought that the safest pesticides are those derived from plants, such as pyrethrum, but a disadvantage in using these compounds is that they require more frequent application. For the purpose of this chapter, further discussion will be focused on the detection and measurement of organophosphate compounds, although much of the discussion could be applied to other types of pesticides such as those mentioned above.

Organophosphates (OPs) are small molecules derived from phosphoric acid with the oxygen atoms being either replaced by other atoms, for example sulphur, and/or linked to aliphatic, aromatic, anhydrides or heterocyclic groups. Table 13.1 lists the more important categories of OP compounds with their particular side chains, and Fig. 13.1 shows the structure of three common OPs.

Table 13.1 Main side groups on different classes of organophosphate compounds

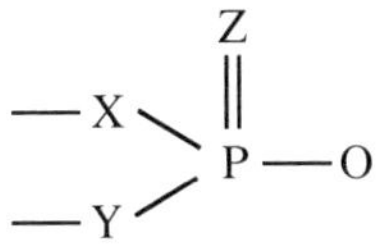

Class of organophosphorus	X	Y	Z
Phosphate	−O	−O	O
Phosphorothionate	−O	−O	S
Phosphorothiolate	−S	−O	O
Phosphorodithionothiolate	−S	−O	S
Phosphorodithiolate	−S	−S	O
Phosphoramidate	=N	−O	O
Phosphordiamidate	=N	=N	O
Phosphoramidothionate	=N	−O	S
Phosphoramidothiolate	=N	−S	O
Phosphonate	≡C	−O	O
Phosphonothionate	≡C	−O	S
Phosphonothionothiolate	≡C	−S	S

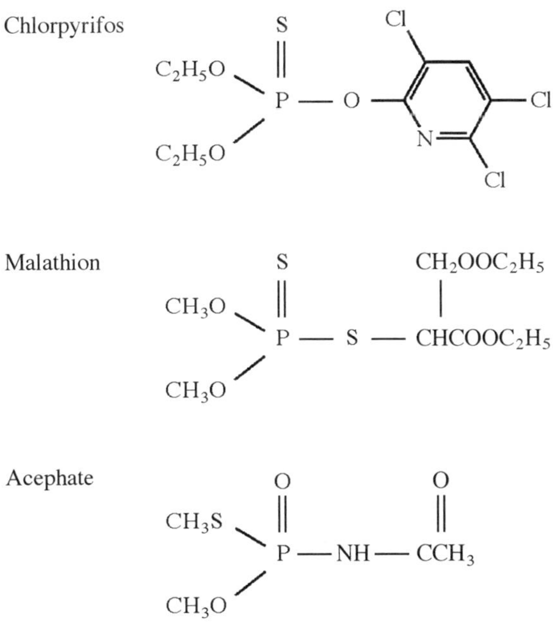

Fig. 13.1 Three examples of organophosphates.

For pesticide applications the sulphur containing compounds are more widely used than the other derivatives. However, all types of OPs are highly toxic to mammals, to differing extents; some are considered ‘relatively’ safe, such as malathion and dimethoate. OP compounds exert their toxic effects by their propensity to inhibit a number of important enzymes in particular the enzyme acetylcholine esterase. This enzyme is important in the inactivation of the fast-acting neurotransmitter acetylcholine found in the nerve synapses of the neuromuscular junction and brain nicotinic junctions. The inherent toxicity of OP compounds has been exploited by various nations in the production of chemical warfare nerve gas agents, such as sarin and tabun. Accidental occupational exposure to agricultural OP results in similar symptoms as being exposed to OP nerve gas agents. Symptoms include: nausea, vomiting, cramps, headache, dizziness, blurred vision, muscle twitches, difficulty in breathing, convulsions, respiratory paralysis and death

The widest application for OPs has been their use as insecticides, although they are also used as nematocides, helminthicides and have fungicidal and herbicidal properties. Due to the inherent toxicity of organophosphates, there is strict control over their use, particularly in their application to foodstuffs, which is supported by legislation. In many countries, the use of the most harmful compounds is banned but illegal application can still be a problem. From the results of a number of studies it has been estimated that, worldwide, pesticides are responsible for 10,000 deaths a year. The problems are associated with over-application to crops and spray drift with subsequent contamination of surrounding areas. To prevent harmful effects to the population in general, the use of agricultural pesticides is strictly regulated, and tables have been produced detailing the maximum permissible level of OP residue, known as the maximum residue limit (MRL) measured in ppm. MRL levels are set for different pesticides and different crops and additional variation is also seen between the different regulating authorities. In addition, only certain OPs are licensed, with many OPs being banned. Table 13.2 gives examples of MRLs for three different OP compounds and three different foods. Tenfold differences, or more, in the MRLs for particular crops are not uncommon.

For health and litigation considerations it is necessary to monitor the use of pesticides applied to crops, as the pesticide residues may find their way into the food chain. The technology available for measuring pesticide residues is becoming much more sophisticated and sensitive, and consequently MRL levels are now being set at much lower levels. The sophisticated analytical techniques used within laboratories tend to be expensive, relatively time consuming and require a sample of the foodstuff that is then transported to the laboratory where skilled personnel perform the analysis. Increasingly, there is a need for inexpensive, rapid tests to detect and measure levels of pesticides at, and below, ever reducing MRLs on raw food, which can be used on site by unskilled operatives. These new rapid tests may act as a preliminary screen giving assurance that there is no pesticide residue present on the food being tested, with a positive test being verified by traditional analytical techniques. In the near

Table 13.2 Maximum residue limits for three different crops and three different OP compounds

Organophosphate compound	Crop	Maximum residual limit (ppm)
Chlorpyrifos	Apples	0.50
Chlorpyrifos	Bananas	3.00
Chlorpyrifos	Cucumbers	0.05
Chlorpyrifos-methyl	Apples	0.50
Chlorpyrifos-methyl	Bananas	0.05
Chlorpyrifos-methyl	Cucumbers	0.05
Dichlorvos	Apples	0.10
Dichlorvos	Bananas	0.10
Dichlorvos	Cucumbers	0.50

future, as new rapid tests become more reliable, and are validated against 'gold standard' methods, the rapid test could replace expensive analytical technology.

13.2 Detecting pesticides: physicochemical methods

Traditionally, OPs have been measured by exploiting their chemical and physicochemical properties using a separation technique such as chromatography or electrophoresis. The spectral characteristics of pesticide residues have also been used in NMR techniques and mass spectroscopy to aid identification and measurement. In recent years, other approaches using the biochemical and immunological properties of pesticide residues have been developed and are now widely used; these are the immunoassay and enzyme inhibition techniques. In order to detect and measure pesticide residues at and below current MRL levels any method of analysis should demonstrate appropriate selectivity and sensitivity. For example, many chemical reactions are only specific for groups of compounds, and do not show selectivity, but when combined with separation techniques, individual compounds can be identified; an example of this approach is thin layer chromatography.

Conventional analysis of pesticide compounds is dominated by techniques employing a separation stage. This group of methods achieves selectivity by separating a mixture into individual components that are then identified by comparing the separation to pure standards. These approaches have the advantage that they can measure more than one compound simultaneously. Thin layer chromatography (TLC) and high performance thin layer chromatography (HPTLC) separate compounds according to their polarity and differential adsorption to silica gel. Visualisation of the separated OP compounds can be with direct ultraviolet irradiation or a chemical reaction to produce a coloured spot. These methods, although allowing a number of samples to be analysed simultaneously, are simple and relatively quick; however, they are only qualitative and involve the use of solvents. Recent studies have shown that quantitation can be achieved by measuring the density of the spots with detection limits being recorded from 0.05 μg to 1.0 μg of pesticide residue applied. These constraints limit the use of these methods to an analytical laboratory where skilled personnel perform them.

Quantification is more traditionally achieved using gas chromatography (GC) or high performance liquid chromatography (HPLC). In GC, the sample is heated to volatilise the OPs which are carried through a column by a flowing inert gas and separated by differential adsorption to a solid phase in the column. Newer instruments use a capillary column where adsorption takes place on the capillary wall rather than packing in the column, which leads to a faster separation and greater sensitivity. In some instances, called gas liquid chromatography (GLC), the solid phase may be covered with 'waxy' liquid to promote greater separation. OPs are measured as they come off the column by a thermionic emission or alkali-flame detector. Some OPs decompose at elevated temperatures resulting in misleading results. The technique is sensitive and relatively quick but uses expensive equipment that must have a gas supply, so is limited to laboratory use.

HPLC does not have the disadvantage of thermal degradation of the sample and is perhaps a preferred method for OP analysis. In this technique the sample is injected into a flowing solvent and is carried through a column containing a solid phase. Again, separation is due to differential adsorption to the solid phase and is determined to some extent by differing polarities of the OP compound in the sample. Detection is by UV absorption or refractive index change. As with the previous techniques described there are a number of limitations on its application; the equipment is expensive, uses solvents and requires trained operators and as such is limited to laboratory use.

Where identification is required, this can be achieved using spectral methods such as NMR and mass spectroscopy. NMR allows identification of a single pesticide residue whereas mass spectroscopy, when interfaced to either GC or HPLC, can identify a number of different pesticide residues. GC-MS is considered to be the gold standard for pesticide measurement and identification. Extremely low detection limits can be reached using tandem-mass spectroscopy with examples of 1300 ppt for dichlorvos and 0.1 ppt for trifluralin being quoted. These techniques are highly specialised, expensive and limited to laboratories where trained personnel perform the analysis.

As indicated in the above discussion, separation techniques do not lend themselves to rapid analysis times that are required for use in the field. Generally they rely on the use of expensive instrumentation, skilled personnel and are not easily transported.

13.3 Detecting pesticides: biological methods

These methods differ from the techniques described in the previous section as they depend on the interaction between a biological molecule and the pesticide residue. This interaction may be specific for a particular pesticide as in the interaction with an antibody, or non-specific as in the way a number of different pesticides interfere with an enzyme reaction.

13.3.1 Antibody methods

Antibodies are biological molecules formed as a part of a host response to foreign substances or microorganisms, for example toxins, viruses or bacteria. The substance to which an antibody is formed is called an antigen. Antibodies bind very specifically to the antigen they are directed against. Thus, methods that use antibodies are generally very specific for a particular pesticide but similar molecules may show some cross-reactivity. Antibodies are produced from animal cells either in a live animal or a cell culture. In both cases an immune response has to be initiated to start cells of the immune system synthesising specific antibody. In order to trigger the immune system to produce an antibody the antigen involved must be a large, complex molecule. Small molecules such as OP compounds do not generally trigger antibody production on their own. In order for small molecules to be recognised by the immune system and start antibody production, they have to be conjugated to a larger molecule such as a protein.

Antibodies are used in a group of techniques collectively called immunoassays. Here the antibody binds to a specific pesticide which it has been designed to recognise and forms an immune complex consisting of the antibody molecule binding with the pesticide residue. The higher the concentration of pesticide in the sample the more immune-complex formed. The immunoassay measures the amount of immune-complex formed and relates this to pesticide concentration.

As pesticides are small molecules, the immunoassay is designed to be a competitive technique where the pesticide in the sample is mixed with a fixed amount of labelled pesticide and then competes with it for a limited number of antibody binding sites. After an incubation period, the antibody has reacted to both the sample pesticide and the labelled pesticide. In order to make the measurement the unreacted label has to be removed leaving only the label associated with the antibody. In this competitive system, as the sample concentration increases the greater numbers of pesticide molecules from the sample will occupy more and more binding sites on the antibody. As a result there is less labelled pesticide in the antibody-binding sites. This gives rise to an inverse dose response curve with a high signal being seen with a low concentration of pesticide. Commonly the labels used in an immunoassay are enzyme labels, a fluorescent molecule, or sometimes a radioactive label. Enzyme labels can be used to generate a coloured product; a fluorescent product or an electroactive compound. The range of different end points of the immunoassay gives rise to a number of different measurement technologies that can be employed to detect the immune reaction.

Immunoassays are often performed in test tubes, 96 well plates and more recently by using lateral flow devices such as those used in pregnancy tests.

These lateral flow devices give a rapid answer, are convenient and can be easily used by non-skilled personnel in the field, but are only semi-quantitative and limited in sensitivity, thus only useful as a screening test. A positive result is seen as the absence or presence of a coloured line, depending on how the test has been devised. Recently equipment has been developed to measure the intensity of the coloured line making the test more quantifiable.

13.3.2 Enzyme methods

These methods rely on the fact that OP compounds inhibit the biological activity of particular enzymes preventing them forming their products from given substrates, in other words the enzyme is poisoned. As different OPs will inhibit the enzymes, these methods are not specific for a particular OP as are the antibody methods, but give an indication of total OP concentration. The most commonly used enzyme used in these methods is acetylcholine esterase (AChE) although butyrylcholine-esterase, organophosphorus hydrolase and ascorbate oxidase have been used.

The principle behind enzyme methods is that the organophosphate enters the active site of the enzyme and binds to the protein structure through a serine-hydroxyl group. This organophosphate binds strongly and is not released from the active site for many hours, in effect inactivating the enzyme. The natural substrate, acetylcholine, binds through the same serine-hydroxyl group. The natural substrate is cleaved by the enzyme, releasing choline and at the same time acetylating the serine-hydroxyl group. After only a few milliseconds the acetyl group is released returning the enzyme to its native state.

The amount of organophosphate that is required to inhibit enzyme activity by 50% is called the IC_{50} (inhibitory concentration-50%). It should be noted that different organophosphates have different IC_{50} values depending on both the particular organophosphate and the source of AChE. This is due to the particular side groups on the organophosphate causing steric hindrance and preventing the molecule entering the active site fully or at all. Secondly, AChE from different sources has an active site of differing sizes. Those enzymes possessing a small active site are not inhibited by larger organophosphates but only by smaller organophosphates. Conversely enzymes with large active sites are also inhibited by larger organophosphates. For example frogs, which tend to be resistant to acute organophosphate poisoning, have an AChE that has a smaller active site, and shows greater enzyme activity with acetylcholine compared with propionylcholine, a larger molecule. Conversely, in chickens, which are sensitive to acute organophosphate poisoning, AChE has a larger active site, and shows greater activity for propionylcholine compared to acetylcholine.

In addition to the size of the active site, susceptibility of a particular AChE to poisoning by organophosphate also depends on the hydrophobicity and electrophilicity of that organophosphate and the nucleophilic strength of the serine residue within the active site. For example, trout AChE shows greater inhibition of enzyme activity as the acidity of the phosphorus atom increases. In other types of AChE, such as from monkeys or rats, it is the nucleophilic strength of the active site that is more important in determining susceptibility of that enzyme to the organophosphate.

The enzyme assay depends on measuring the activity of the enzyme in the absence and presence of the sample. If organophosphate residues are present then there will be a decrease in enzyme activity noted. Enzyme activity is measured by monitoring the disappearance of substrate or the accumulation of product. This can be linked to a chemical reaction that produces a colour and the change in colour monitored.

In developing new and rapid detection methods for the detection and measurement of pesticides it is the biological technologies that have been exploited. In particular it has been the development of biosensor technology where the greatest advances have been made. Very sensitive instruments can be constructed to be light, portable, easy-to-use, inexpensive and can be operated by untrained personnel.

13.4 The principles of biosensors

Biosensors are analytical devices that use a biological molecule to interact with the analyte in question to produce a measurable output. Figure 13.2 shows a schematic of a biosensor device. The discussion below examines the parts of the biosensor that form the sensing element and briefly reviews the approaches that have been used in developing biosensors for pesticide analysis.

The unique feature of a biosensor is the biological layer, which is integral to the device and interacts with the analyte. The biological molecule is important for giving the device specificity and selectivity. Many different types of biological molecules exhibit selective or specific binding as part of their biological function. These include antibody molecules, enzymes, receptor molecules and lectins. In addition to these protein molecules, specific binding is also seen between complementary strands of nucleic acids. Nucleic acids are used to detect DNA from microbiological samples to detect bacteria or viruses. The great majority of biosensors for other analytes, including pesticides, use a protein molecule in the sensing element.

The biological molecules employed in the sensing element are immobilised on the surface of the transducer to form the sensing surface of the biosensor. Many different approaches have been employed to capture and hold biological molecules depending on the nature of the transducer surface and the biological molecule. These methods fall into three categories:

- adsorption type methods
- chemical coupling
- biological coupling.

The simplest of these is adsorption of the biological molecule to the transducer surface through the formation of non-covalent chemical bonds, such as

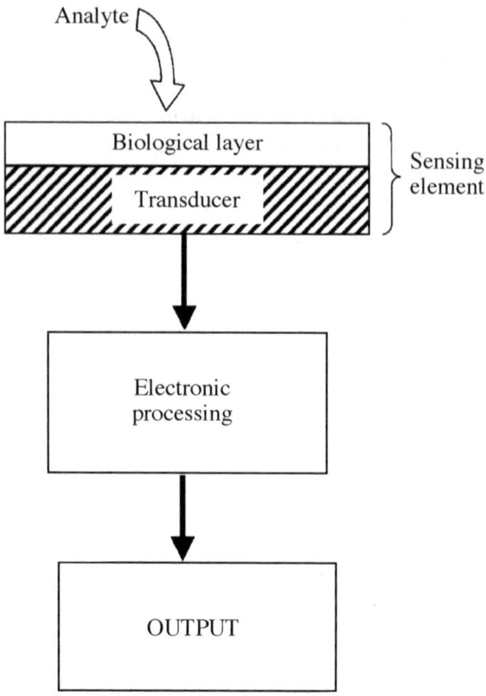

Fig. 13.2 Schematic diagram of a biosensor.

electrostatic and hydrophobic bonds. Electrostatic bonds can be formed between charges on the transducer surface and charged groups on the protein whereas hydrophobic bonds are formed between hydrophobic surfaces and hydrophobic domains of proteins. This type of immobilisation is simple and does not require any chemical reactions but has the disadvantage that the biological molecules are randomly orientated on the transducer surface. A proportion of the molecules will have parts of the molecule containing the reactive site for the analyte forming non-covalent bonds with the transducer surface and the reactive site will not be available to the analyte, leading to a loss of sensitivity; this is particularly true of antibodies. The other potentially major drawback of this type of immobilisation is that biological molecules can be lost from the surface during incubation and wash stages of the assay, again leading to loss of sensitivity.

Covalent coupling is achieved through chemical reactions between reactive groups on the surface of the transducer and the protein molecule. The principal groups used to cross-link proteins to a surface are amine, carboxyl and sulphydryl groups. A wide range of coupling chemistries using cross-linking agents is available for use with different reactive groups. The coupling or cross-linking agents can be broadly divided into those with homofunctional or heterofunctional activity. Homofunctional agents have the same reactive group at either end of the molecule and react with the same type of group on the transducer surface and protein molecule, such as an amino group. Glutaraldehyde is a good example of a homofunctional cross-linking agent. Heterofunctional agents have a different reactive site on either end of the cross-linking molecule and therefore can react with different reactive groups on the transducer surface and the protein, for example an amine group being coupled with a hydroxyl group. The advantage of chemically coupled biological molecules is the fact that they are not lost from the transducer surface during the assay and are necessary if a reusable biosensor is being developed. A potential disadvantage of chemical coupling is that if the chemistry could inactivate a percentage of the biological molecules thus reducing sensitivity. This depends somewhat on the harshness of the chemical reaction used. The advantage of covalent cross-linking is that biological molecules can be orientated on the transducer surface to present the reactive part of the molecule to the analyte, allowing greater sensitivity. This is particularly important in the orientation of antibodies on the transducer surface, where to gain maximum sensitivity the antigen-binding site should be orientated towards the sample.

As with covalent cross-linking biological coupling also ensures the correct orientation of the biological molecule interacting with the analyte. These methods are usually employed with antibody coated biosensors and use another protein that binds to an antibody by the non-specific Fc portion of the antibody. This leaves the antigen specific, antigen binding sites in the correct orientation to interact with the antigen.

The interaction between the biosensor and the analyte can be broadly grouped into three modes of action. Figure 13.3 shows these different modes of action. In the first mode of action, the direct mode (Fig. 13.3(a)), the analyte interacts directly with the biological layer on the surface of the transducer to produce a signal. Here, it is the analyte itself interacting with the biological layer that generates the change in signal measured by the transducer. The second mode (Fig 13.3(b)) of action involves competition between analyte and a labelled species for binding sites on the transducer surface. It is the label that is detected by the transducer. This competitive mode is a form of indirect detection, and commonly involves a fluorescent label or an enzyme label that produces the fluorescent or electroactive product. A third type of interaction is where the analyte binds to the biological layer on the transducer surface and causes a change in the biological activity or function (Fig. 13.3(c)). A good example of this is seen where enzyme is immobilised on the transducer surface, the reaction of pesticide to the biosensor inactivates the enzyme changing its biological activity.

The role of the transducer in a biosensor is to generate a measurable signal when the analyte interacts with the biological molecule associated with the transducer surface. The two common forms of transducers used for pesticide analysis are optical transducers and electrochemical transducers. Optical transducers generate a signal measured as a light intensity proportional to the concentration of pesticide in the sample; this may be an inverse relationship. Electrochemical transducers generate a current or voltage in proportion to the pesticide being measured; again this may be an inverse relationship.

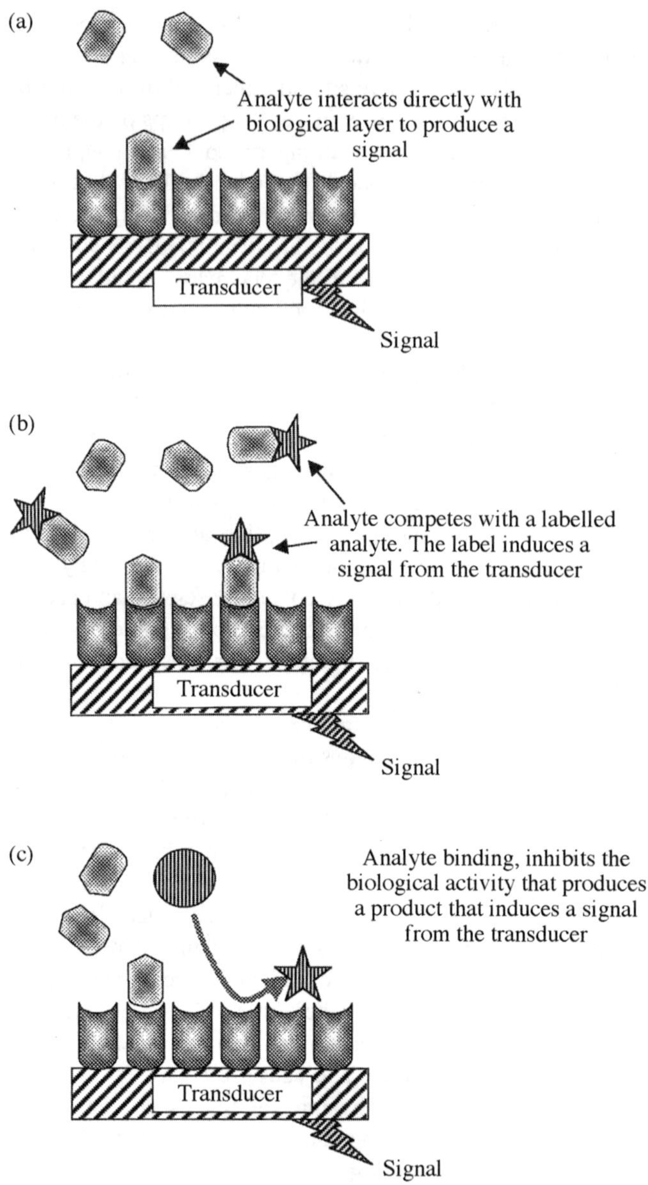

Fig. 13.3 Three modes of action for a biosensor determining pesticides: (a) direct mode, (b) competitive mode, (c) functional mode.

13.4.1 Optical biosensors

Optical transducers used in biosensors utilise the evanescent wave effect. The evanescent wave may interact directly with molecules on the surface of the transducer bringing about a change in signal, this is the principle behind surface plasmon resonance technologies. These devices measure a very small change in the refractive index at the surface of the transducer. As antigen binds to antibody immobilised to the transducer surface there is a mass change which in turn brings about a change in the refractive index measured. The greater the mass of the component binding to the immobilised biological layer the greater the signal generated. This has important implications when trying to detect small molecules using an antibody immobilised on the surface of the transducer. When small molecules bind there is only a small change in the mass on the surface, generating only a small signal. So for the detection and measurement of small molecules, such as pesticides, surface plasmon resonance type technologies can suffer from a lack of sensitivity. Typical detection limits quoted in the literature range from 0.05 to 5.0 μl/l, two specific examples for pesticide residues are atrazine and simazine, which have detection limits of 1.0 μl/l and 0.1 μl/l respectively. Instrumentation used for surface plasmon measurement is often large and not particularly portable and can be very expensive. New developments in this technology have seen surface plasmon resonance devices that utilise a capillary or fibre-optic rod that can be dipped manually into the sample. Using this type of technology a rapid handheld device is easily constructed, but is still expensive. Optical sensors suffer from the problem of non-specific binding, any interaction on the surface results in a change of the measured signal, so there is an issue of specificity. With high affinity antibodies immobilised on the transducer surface and for use of good blocking chemistry, non-specific interaction should be minimised.

In another type of optical transducer, the evanescent wave interacts with a fluorescent marker or label mixed with the sample as seen in Fig. 13.3(b). A fluorescently labelled antigen competes with antigen from the sample for antibody binding sites at the surface of the transducer. The evanescent wave penetrates into the sample interacting with the fluorescent label which absorbs light and emits its fluorescent signal which enters the wave guide and is measured. When high concentrations of antigen in the sample are found, only small amounts of labelled antigen can bind to the antibody, generating a small signal. Conversely, with a low concentration of antigen in the sample, greater numbers of antibody binding sides are occupied with fluorescently labelled antigen, giving rise to a larger signal.

13.4.2 Electrochemical biosensors

In recent years, there has been increasing interest in the construction and operation of organophosphate pesticide biosensors based on electrochemical transducers. One of the most common approaches has involved the use of acetylcholinesterase (AChE) as the biological recognition element, which has been integrated with a variety of carbon electrodes as transducers. Hart and co-workers have been investigating OP biosensors based on screen-printed carbon electrodes (SPCEs) which contain cobalt phthalocyanine (CoPC) as an electrocatalyst. In one approach, AChE (from electric eel) was immobilised

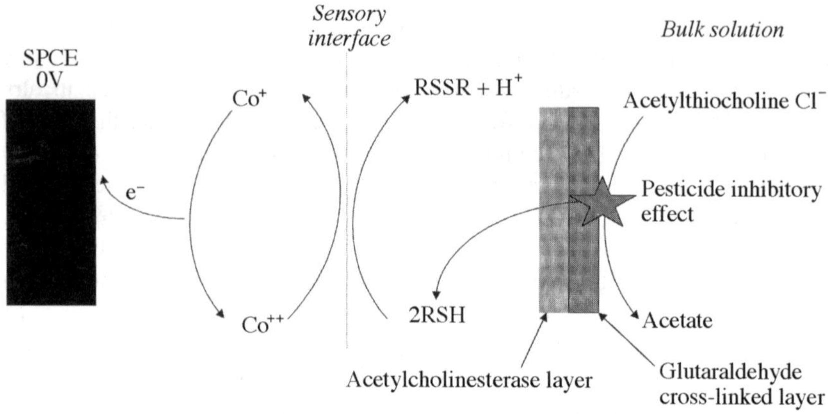

Fig. 13.4 Diagram to show the reactions taking place on the surface of a screen-printed carbon electrode (SPCE) biosensor using acetylcholinesterase as the biological layer. In the absence of an OP, acetyliocholine is enzymatically converted to thiocholine as it passes through the AChE layer; this species then chemically reduces the central cobalt ion, which is in the +2 state, to the +1 state. This latter ion is re-oxidised at the SPCE back to the +2 state by loss of an electron, and this current constitutes the analytical response. In the presence of an OP, the enzymatic conversion of acetylthiocholine to thiocholine is inhibited which results in less thiocholine being produced; consequently, the current is attenuated and this decrease is proportional to the OP concentration.

onto the CoPC-SPCE by simply drop coating a solution of this enzyme onto its surface, followed by a solution containing the cross-linking agent glutaraldehyde. Figure 13.4 shows a schematic diagram of the biosensor and the various reactions taking place during its operation.

Studies by Hart and co-workers have focused on optimisation of the OP biosensor for operation in several different modes. The first mode involved amperometry in stirred solution and two approaches were investigated. Initial studies were performed by transferring an aliquot of phosphate buffer pH 7.4 into a voltammetric cell at 37°C; the biosensor was then immersed in the solution and the potential applied. After nine minutes, 50 μl of acetylcholine was added to initiate the enzymatic reaction, giving a final concentration of 0.5 mM. When a steady state signal was achieved, the reaction was allowed to proceed for a further nine minutes before the addition of pesticides. Initial rates of decrease in current were measured and this data was used in the construction of calibration plots. It was found that plots of initial rates of current decrease vs log concentration of paraoxon were linear between 3.24×10^{-7} M and 3.24×10^{-6} M, the former representing the detection limit. Similarly for dichlorvos, the linear range was from 1.7×10^{-6} M to 1.4×10^{-5} M, the former representing the detection limit.

The second method utilising amperometry in stirred solution was performed by placing an OP biosensor into a solution containing buffer only, switching the cell on, then adding pesticide after three minutes; after a further ten minutes, acetylthiocholine was added and the resulting currents allowed to reach steady state (i_{ss}). The inhibition was calculated by measuring the difference between the

i_{ss} values in the absence, and presence, of pesticide and representing this difference as a percentage of the former value. Calibration plots were constructed by plotting percentage inhibition vs log pesticide concentration; in the case of dichlorvos the plot was linear from 7.1×10^{-7} to 5.6×10^{-6} M, the former representing the limit of detection. It should be mentioned that the sensitivity of this second approach could be improved by simply increasing the incubation time with pesticide before addition of the substrate.

The second mode of operation of the OP biosensor, investigated by Hart and co-workers, involved flow-injection analysis with amperometric detection. The biosensor was incorporated into a thin-layer flow cell and mobile phase allowed to flow over the surface at a rate of 1 ml min^{-1}. Pesticide determinations were carried out in three stages. First the amperometric response was recorded when a 20 μl aliquot of 1 mM acetylthiocholine was injected into the system. Next, the sample stream containing an OP was directed through the flow cell; thirdly, the flow was switched back to buffer only and the current measured after making an injection of 20 μl of substrate. The concentration of pesticide was determined from any decrease in the biosensor response. The detection limits obtained with an enzyme loading of 1.0 U per sensor were 6×10^{-9} M and 7×10^{-11} M for dichlorvos and paraoxon, respectively; with an enzyme loading of 0.05 U per sensor, a detection limit of 4.0×10^{-11} M was achieved for paraoxon. The use of a flow cell, in conjunction with amperometry, does seem to offer certain advantages, perhaps the most important being the possibility to produce a fully automated system. Further research is under way to develop an array of biosensors based on this technology for the identification and quantification of multiple OPs in a single food sample. In this case, mutations of AChE from drosophila are being investigated as the biorecognition elements of the proposed array; these are immobilised onto the SPCE array and interrogated using chronoamperometry. The goal of this research is to develop a fully automated system to determine OPs in a variety of raw food produce.

An alternative pesticide biorecognition system, for use with electrochemical transducers, has been developed by Wang and co-workers. The enzyme organophosphorus hydrolase (OPH) is reported to have broad substrate specificity and is able to hydrolyse a number of pesticides including parathion, methyl parathion, fenitrothion and paraoxon. In these cases, the enzyme catalyses hydrolysis of the OP compounds to generate p-nitrophenol, which is electroactive. Consequently biosensors could be constructed which were based on the direct oxidation of p-nitrophenol, and the magnitude of the response is directly proportional to the concentration of the pesticide. These workers constructed a remote OP biosensor by incorporating the device into a PVC housing tube attached to a 16 m long shielded cable via three-pin environmentally sealed rubber connections; Ag/AgCl reference electrode and platinum counter electrode completed the cell system. The biosensor was operated in the chronoamperometric mode by stepping from open circuit to +0.85 V vs Ag/AgCl. The response was found to be linear in the range 4.6–46 μM for paraoxon and up to 5 μM for methyl parathion; the limits of detection for these two pesticides were 0.9 μM and 0.4 μM respectively. It was reported that an advantage of this system is that the biosensors are reusable. However, they do not yet appear to possess the sensitivity achieved with the AChE based systems.

13.5 Developing low-cost biosensors

Biosensors are the ideal technology for developing rapid low-cost devices for measuring pesticides on the site of food production or food intake, alleviating the need to send a sample to a specialist laboratory. The sensor elements on which the biological layer is incorporated are small and can be built into a robust housing incorporated into the portable device. Ideally the measurement time will only be a few minutes, the incorporated electronics take the signal from the transducer, process the signal and present a result to the operator. The device should be easy to use enabling unskilled operators to make measurements. But the biggest factor in determining whether any such device will be a commercial success is the cost of the analysis.

Factors that influence the cost of analysis include choice of sensor, the nature of the biological material immobilised to the sensor surface and the number of units to be manufactured. For example, optical and surface plasmon resonance sensors are more expensive than screen-printed electrodes. The biological layer on the biosensor surface has to be from a reliable source ensuring consistency of purity and reactivity. The source of the biological material may have a significant impact on the price of the sensor particularly if genetically modified biological molecules are used. This in turn will influence the way the biosensor is used in practice.

There are two fundamentally different ways in which low-cost biosensors have been employed for pesticide analysis. The first approach is to use a reusable sensor where a number of different samples are applied to the same instrument, here the same sensor surface is regenerated between samples and can give a number of sequential readings. Obviously, this will reduce the cost of each analysis, recycling expensive biological molecules. The exact number of measurements that can be made from a single biosensor depends on the immobilisation chemistries, the nature of the biological molecule being used in the biosensor, the nature of the analyte being detected and other physical parameters such as the temperature. Typically, between 5 and 100 measurements have been described, but as the biosensor ages the sensitivity decreases. The second approach is to develop a sensor using a disposable chip, in this case a new sensor is used for each sample, with the loss of the biological material. The manufacturing process controls the reproducibility of these systems and the operator does not have to worry about the biosensor's performance slowly becoming degraded.

Whether using a reusable biosensor or a single-shot biosensor, sample presentation is a critical factor in the design of an instrument for the measurement of pesticides. Again there are two fundamentally different approaches to this.

Firstly, a system of fluidics or microfluidics can be used to present the sample to the sensor surface thereby necessitating the use of a sample entry port. The fluidics system delivers sample, wash buffer and regeneration solutions in turn. Ideally, as the sensor surface is regenerated there is no change in the activity and density of the biological layer so each subsequent reaction will occur under identical conditions. In practice, some of the biological layer is lost as a result of inactivation or being washed from the sensor surface during regeneration. The advantage of this type of system is that it can be self-contained with minimal user interaction. The second method of sample presentation is to design the biosensor in such a way as to enable it to be dipped into the sample. This has the advantage of not requiring any fluidics and keeping the device simple to operate and minimising costs. The big disadvantage of a dipping system is the potential problem of damage of the sensor surface.

Cost notwithstanding, the reliability and reproducibility of any biosensor device is vitally important for a commercial biosensor designed for unskilled use, whether it is has a reusable sensor or a disposable sensor. Although still in its infancy, biosensor systems designed for pesticide analysis more commonly employ a fluidics or microfluidics system that allows the reaction and the biosensor surface to be carefully controlled ensuring greater reproducibility for use by semi- or unskilled personnel at the point of sampling.

13.6 Using biosensors: pesticide residues in grain, fruit and vegetables

The detection and measurement of pesticide residues in water presents little problem in terms of sample presentation to the biosensor. On the other hand the analysis of foodstuffs such as grain, fruit and vegetables presents other problems. Pesticide residues have to be extracted from the food sample and then presented to the biosensor for the analytical measurement. In terms of developing a commercialised system for the detection and measurement of pesticide residues, the extraction and interfacing with the analytical module is a serious concern. Traditional extraction techniques are not applicable to portable devices; the use of solvents is incompatible with the technology and the environment in which the measurements are being made.

Pesticide residues are extracted from food samples and have been ground up, in the case of grain or mechanically homogenised in the case of fruit and vegetables. Solvent is added to extract the pesticide, the solid material has to be removed and the extract presented to the biosensor. Organic solvents are incompatible with the biological layer and thus have to be removed and the extracted pesticide re-dissolved in a solvent compatible with the biological layer of the biosensor.

Newer techniques such as supercritical fluid extraction (SFE) have been used to extract pesticide residue from food samples. Gas such as carbon dioxide is in a supercritical state when the pressure and temperature equals or exceeds the critical point (31°C and 73 atm for carbon dioxide). Supercritical fluids have been known for about 100 years and have both gas-like and liquid-like properties, with high solvation power making them ideal for rapid extractions with high recoveries. This also gives supercritical fluids lower viscosity and higher diffusivity than other liquid solvents, allowing them to penetrate into the sample more efficiently. By controlling the pressure or temperature the density and solvation power can be controlled thus simulating traditional organic solvents, for example for chloroform or hexane. By adjusting the solvation power targeted compounds can be preferentially extracted. Carbon dioxide has been greatly used in supercritical fluid extraction systems, as it is non-toxic, inexpensive, and can be obtained at high purity. As the extraction process is usually carried out at a low temperature this reduces decomposition of organic compounds and prevents other reactions. Supercritical carbon dioxide is very good for extracting hydrocarbons and nonpolar compounds, but in order to extract polar compounds a modifier can be added to the supercritical carbon dioxide. A range of different modifiers has been used but the most common is methanol although this is rather toxic for food applications. To alleviate this problem ethanol has been used as an alternative in a number of applications. The disadvantage of using supercritical carbon dioxide for extraction is that it involves expensive equipment operating at high pressures and puts additional costs onto the analytical procedure. Other gases have been used in supercritical fluid extraction methods including freons and nitrous oxide, which are particularly useful for the extraction of polar compounds. Due to environmental considerations these are rarely used.

Another new extraction technique is that involving the solvents containing phytosol, which is based on the compound 1,1,1,2-tetrafluoroethane. These solvents are non-flammable, non-toxic, have a neutral pH and are liquid at low temperatures and pressures such as those found in aerosol cans. The processed sample is placed into a heavy extraction vessel with a valve inlet that can take an aerosol can containing phytosol solvent. A measured quantity of solvent is added to the extraction vessel and allowed to mix with the food sample. This process is rather similar to using a supercritical fluid but does not involve the high pressures or temperatures. By releasing the valve on the extraction vessel the phytosol solvent is pushed into a second collection vessel under pressure. When the pressure is released the phytosol solvent evaporates leaving the pesticide residue in the collection vessel. In order to present the pesticide residue to the biosensor the residue must be dissolved in a small amount of solvent that is compatible with the biological layer of the biosensor. This may entail dissolving the residue in a small amount of solvent such as methanol or ethanol and then making the volume up with an aqueous buffer solution suitable for presenting the sample to the biosensor. This particular extraction procedure is simple, inexpensive and does not require complicated equipment and is easily adapted to interface with portable analytical biosensor modules.

For a rapid, low-cost, portable detection system for pesticide residues in food there has to be the amalgamation of an extraction process and an analytical device based on a biosensor. It is expected that the complete analytical process, from sample introduction to presentation of the result, should take less than 30 minutes with minimal intervention from the operator.

13.7 Future trends

As with all areas of technology, the field of biosensors is moving forward at a terrific pace. There are a range of new technologies being developed at the moment to enhance the performance of rapid detection and measurement of pesticides. We have seen in this chapter how technology ranges from expensive sophisticated instrumentation requiring highly skilled personnel and dedicated laboratory space, to small portable units that can be operated on-site by unskilled personnel. Using one biosensor, information about a single pesticide can be obtained if the biological layer has the specificity to that particular pesticide. By introducing more than one biosensor in the device, then multi-analyte detection and measurement is achievable. Using pattern recognition technologies, such as neural networks, the integration of many biosensors will lead to the simultaneous detection of a number of different pesticides. These technologies are being used for both antibody-based biosensors and enzyme-based biosensors.

The logical extension to having multiple biosensors in a device is to incorporate the active surfaces onto a single chip thereby reducing the amount of fluidics in the instrument. The challenge here is to develop isolated transducer elements on the chip to which the different biological layers are immobilised. With new techniques in nanotechnology and micro-engineered machines (MEM technology) this will soon be possible.

While array technology develops, new transducer technology is also being developed for use with biosensors. Magnetic technology is being developed in competition with optical, electrochemical and piezoelectric transducers. Magnetic biosensors will have the advantage that no chemistry or enzyme reaction is required nor is there any need for optical systems. The magnetic transducer will respond directly to magnetic or paramagnetic material associated with the biosensor surface. This has the advantage of potentially reducing the size and enhancing the portability of the device.

Looking further ahead it is possible to foresee the integration of other technologies such as radio telemetry being incorporated into biosensors that can be left on-site. For continuous and on-line monitoring of food in the manufacturing process, biosensors could also be incorporated with robotic technology. It can be seen that the development of biosensors has been an important technological advance in monitoring pesticide residues in food. This is a core technology that goes beyond the detection and measurement of pesticide residues but can be employed for the detection and measurement of any other compound where a biological interaction can be integrated into the biosensor.

13.8 Sources of further information and advice

There are many websites giving information and further details of pesticide related topics. The following websites are a small selection giving information regarding the measurement and the impact of pesticides in food and the environment.

http://www.pesticides.gov.uk/
http://www.defra.gov.uk/
http://www.environment-agency.gov.uk/
http://www.hgca.co.uk/
http://www.fsis.usda.gov/
http://www.epa.gov/pesticides
http://www.pesticideinfo.org/

13.9 Further reading

A selection of review articles and scientific papers relating to areas discussed in the text is given below for further information.

13.9.1 Selection of review articles

AL-SALEH, I A, Pesticides: a review article, *Journal of Environmental Pathology, Toxicology and Oncology: Official Organ of the International Society for Environmental Toxicology and Cancer*, Volume 13, Issue 3, 1994, pp. 151–161.

APREA, C, COLOSIO, C, MAMMONE, T, MINOIA, C and MARONI, M, Biological monitoring of pesticide exposure: a review of analytical methods, *Journal of Chromatography B: Analytical Technologies in the Biomedical and Life Sciences*, Volume 769, Issue 2, 5 April 2002, pp. 191–219.

GABALDÓN, J A, MAQUIEIRA, A, PUCHADES, R, Current trends in immunoassay-based kits for pesticide analysis, *Critical Reviews in Food Science and Nutrition*, Volume 39, Issue 6, November 1999, pp. 519–538.

HENNION, M-C and BARCELO D, Strengths and limitations of immunoassays for effective and efficient use for pesticide analysis in water samples: A review, *Analytica Chimica Acta*, Volume 362, Issue 1, 24 April 1998, pp. 3–34.

LANG, Q and WAI C M, Supercritical fluid extraction in herbal and natural product studies – a practical review, *Talanta*, Volume 53, Issue 4, 5 January 2001, pp. 771–782.

MULCHANDANI, A, CHEN, W, MULCHANDANI, P, WANG, J and ROGERS, K R, Biosensors for direct determination of organophosphate pesticides, *Biosensors and Bioelectronics*, Volume 16, Issues 4–5, June 2001, pp. 225–230.

REKHA, K, THAKUR, M S, KARANTH, N G, Biosensors for the detection of organophosphorous pesticides, *Critical Reviews in Biotechnology*, Volume 20, Issue 3, 2000, pp. 213–235.

SHERMA, J, Pesticide residue analysis (1999–2000): a review, *Journal of AOAC International*, Volume 84, Issue 5, September–October 2001, pp. 1303–1312.

13.9.2 Selected scientific papers

AGÜERA, A, CONTRERAS, M, CRESPO, J, FERNÁNDEZ-ALBA, A R, Multiresidue method for the analysis of multiclass pesticides in agricultural products by gas chromatography-tandem mass spectrometry, *The Analyst*, Volume 127, Issue 3, March 2002, pp. 347–354.

ANDREOU, V G, CLONIS, Y D, A portable fiber-optic pesticide biosensor based on immobilized cholinesterase and sol – gel entrapped bromcresol purple for in-field use, *Biosensors and Bioelectronics*, Volume 17, Issues 1–2, January 2002, pp. 61–69.

GULLA, K C, GOUDA, M D, THAKUR, M S, KARANTH, N G, Reactivation of immobilized acetyl cholinesterase in an amperometric biosensor for organophosphorus pesticide, *Biochimica et Biophysica Acta*, Volume 1597, Issue 1, May 20, 2002, pp. 133–139.

HARTLEY, I C, HART, J P, Amperometric Measurement of Organophosphate Pesticides using a Screen-printed Disposable Sensor and Biosensor Based on Cobalt Phthalocyanine, *Anal. Proceed.*, 1994, Volume 31, pp. 333–337.

HYE-SUNG LEE, YOUNG AH KIM, YOUNG AE CHO, YONG TAE LEE, Oxidation of organophosphorus pesticides for the sensitive detection by a cholinesterase-based biosensor, *Chemosphere*, Volume 46, Issue 4, January 2002, pp. 571–576.

KARCHER, A, EL RASSI, Z, Capillary electrophoresis and electrochromatography of pesticides and metabolites, *Electrophoresis*, Volume 20, Issue 15–16, October 1999, pp. 3280–3296.

LEHOTAY, S J, LIGHTFIELD, A R, HARMAN-FETCHO, J A, DONOGHUE, D J, Analysis of pesticide residues in eggs by direct sample introduction/gas chromatography/tandem mass spectrometry, *Journal of Agricultural and Food Chemistry*, Volume 49, Issue 10, October 2001, pp. 4589–4596.

MARTÍNEZ VIDAL, J L, ARREBOLA, F J and MATEU-SÁNCHEZ, M, Application of gas chromatography – tandem mass spectrometry to the analysis of pesticides in fruits and vegetables, *Journal of Chromatography A*, Volume 959, Issues 1–2, 14 June 2002, pp. 203–213.

MULCHANDANI, P, CHEN, W, MULCHANDANI, A, WANG J, CHEN L, Amperometric microbial biosensor for direct determination of organophosphate pesticides using recombinant microorganism with surface expressed organophosphorus hydrolase, *Biosensors and Bioelectronics*, Volume 16, Issues 7–8, September 2001, pp. 433–437.

RIPPETH, J J, GIBSON, T D, HART, J P, HARTLEY, I C and NELSON, G, Flow-injection Detector Incorporating a Screen-printed Disposable Amperometric Biosensor for Monitoring Organophosphate Pesticides, Analyst, 1997, Volume 122, pp. 1425–1429.

TEGELER, T, EL RASSI, Z, Capillary electrophoresis and electrochromatography of pesticides and metabolites, *Electrophoresis*, Volume 22, Issue 19, November 2001, pp. 4281–4293.

THURMAN, E M, AGA, D S, Detection of pesticides and pesticide metabolites using the cross reactivity of enzyme immunoassays, *Journal of AOAC International*, Volume 84, Issue 1, January–February 2001, pp. 162–167.

WANG, J, CHATRATHI, M P, MULCHANDANI, A, CHEN, W, Capillary electrophoresis microchips for separation and detection of organophosphate nerve agents, *Analytical Chemistry*, Volume 73, Issue 8, April, 2001, pp. 1804–1808.

14

Detecting residues of urea and carbamate pesticides

Y. Picó, G. Font and J. Mañes, University of Valencia, Spain

14.1 Introduction: key issues in detection

Urea and carbamate pesticides are widely used to control weeds, insects and fungus in different crops. Carbamates are substituted esters of carbamic acid (NH_2COOH) with aliphatic or aromatic substituents on the oxygen and nitrogen atoms. Urea pesticides derive from the replacement of hydrogen atoms on the urea molecule (H_2NCONH_2) by many diverse chemical groups.

The extraction, clean up, separation, identification and quantification of carbamate and urea residues in food are complex procedures that require different analytical strategies and can be accomplished by a number of immunochemical and chromatographic methods. Whereas immunochemical procedures play a predominant role in screening for the presence of pesticide residues in food products, the various existing chromatographic techniques are the most intensively used for confirmatory purposes. Capillary electrophoresis (CE) and liquid chromatography (LC) are the principal separation techniques prior to identification and determination, because most of these molecules are thermolabile and non-volatile, even after derivatization.

For pesticide residues occurring at sub mg/kg levels, specific detection can be achieved by either extensive sample preparation to separate the analyte from potential interferences or by using a less selective work-up but a more specific detector. As a direct consequence of the latter approach, increased specificity is pursued by the use of mass spectrometry.

This chapter reviews the latest developments in analytical techniques used for the determination of ureas and carbamates in food. It should be considered as an update to recently published comprehensive reviews on these pesticides. A number of analytical techniques has been employed to extract, purify and determine urea and carbamate residues since the early 1980s. These have already been covered in excellent review works that are listed in the sources of further information and advice (Nunes *et al.*, 1999a; Berrada *et al.*, 2003a; Picó *et al.*, 2000; Ahmed, 2001; Picó *et al.*, 2003). From these references the reader can obtain an overview of the classical methods used. This chapter summarizes the methods reported since 1998 to illustrate the trends in the analysis of these residues.

14.2 Sample preparation

Usually several sample pre-treatment steps are necessary between sampling and chromatography. Sample preparation can constitute the bottleneck in food analysis, occupying more than 60% of the analyst's time (Nunes *et al.*, 1999a; Berrada *et al.*, 2003a; Picó *et al.*, 2000; Hogendoorn and van Zoonen, 2000; van der Hoff *et al.*, 1999). It includes all the techniques that involve handling of the sample before the analysis and/or detection begin. In general, there are two basic steps implicated in most food treatments, which are extraction and clean up. However, it should be noted that nowadays it is somewhat arbitrary to separate 'extraction' from 'clean up' because many techniques carry out part or all of both simultaneously.

14.2.1 Extraction

Several sample preparation techniques, mainly solid-liquid extraction (SLE) and solid phase extraction (SPE), have been applied to extract carbamate and urea residues from food (Nunes *et al.*, 1999a; Berrada *et al.*, 2003a).

SLE is the traditional system that has been largely employed with satisfactory results in terms of recovery, precision, limits of quantification and number of analytes determined. However, the disadvantages of this technique are that it is rather laborious, time consuming and large volumes of toxic solvent are used. Table 14.1 evaluates the different methods in terms of pesticides analyzed, matrix used, recovery obtained, and determination technique applied. SLE can be carried out with solvents of different polarity, including low polarity solvents as ethyl acetate (Martínez.Galera *et al.*, 2001; Miliadis *et al.*, 1999; Blasco *et al.*, 2002a, b; Balinova, 1998; Koblizek *et al.*, 2002; Stöcklein *et al.*, 1998; Jansson *et al.*, 2004; Tsiropoulos *et al.*, 1999), cyclohexane (Goto *et al.*, 2003) or dichloromethane (Escuderos-Morenas *et al.*, 2003) and water-miscible solvents, such as acetone (Stan, 2000; Schulze *et al.*, 2002a, b; Pantiru *et al.*, 2003; Katsoudas *et al.*, 2000; Caballo-López and de Castro, 2003; Mastovska *et al.*, 2001; Nunes *et al.*, 1998b; Abad *et al.*, 2003; Del Carlo *et al.*, 2004) and methanol (Delgado *et al.*, 2001; Sawaya *et al.*, 1999; Nunes *et al.*, 1998b, c, d, 2000; Wu *et al.*, 2002; Blasco *et al.*, 2002a). Food samples are homogenized with the solvent in a Waring blender, or other type of homogenizing system including ultrasound (Caballo-López and de Castro, 2003), and then filtered to

Table 14.1 Evaluation of different solid-liquid extraction procedures

Pesticides	Matrices	Extraction	Clean up	Recovery, %	Determination	Ref.
Benzoylureas Carbamates	Plant materials	NFAS Ethyl acetate-anhydrous sodium sulphate	GPC	76.7–102.6	LC-UV LC-EM	Balinova, 1998; Koblizek *et al.*, 2002
Carbamates Ureas	Fruits and vegetables	Ethyl acetate-anhydrous sodium sulphate	—	68.9–72.4	LC-MS	Blasco *et al.*, 2002a, b; Stöcklein *et al.*, 1998; Jansson *et al.*, 2004)
Benzoylureas	Apples and pears	Ethyl acetate-anhydrous sodium sulphate	SPE silica cartridge	75–102	LC-UV	Tsiropoulos *et al.*, 1999; Miliadis *et al.*, 1999
Benzoylureas	Tomatos	Ethyl acetate-anhydrous sodium sulphate	SPE aminopropyl	78–103	LC-Fluorescence	Martínez-Galera *et al.*, 2001
Carbamates	Pears and apples	Acetone-dichloromethane-hexane	—	76.86–98.9	LC-MS	Lacassie *et al.*, 1999
Carbamates	Fruits	Cyclohexane	GPC	67–129	Flow-injection-MS	Goto *et al.*, 2003
Carbamates	Total diet Vegetable matrices	PAM I Methanol	Acetonitrile/ Petroleum ether Charcoal/celite	79–92	LC-Fluorescence LC-UV LC-MS Biosensors	Sawaya *et al.* 1999, Nunes 1998b, c, d, 1999b, 2000
Phenylureas	Total diet	PAM I Methanol	Hexane/Cl_2CH_2 Florisil	75–89	LC/photolysis/ Fluorescence	Sawaya *et al.*, 1999

Phenylurea Carbamates	Potatoes	Methanol	Petroleum ether/ Cl_2CH_2	84–101	GC-NPD GC-MS	Wu *et al.*, 2002; Blasco *et al.*, 2002a
Carbamates	Foodstuffs	DFG-S19 Acetone	Ethyl acetate/ cyclohexane GPC	79–102	GC-NPD GC-MS	Stan, 2000
Carbamates	Infant food	Acetone	Ethyl acetate/ cyclohexane	92–104	GC-MS LC-MS Biosensors	Schulze *et al.*, 2002a,b
Carbamates	Fruits and vegetables	Acetone and cyclohexane	GPC SPE silica, C_{18} or carbon	40–100	LC-UV LC-Fluorescence	Pantiru *et al.*, 2003
Carbamates Phenylureas	Fruits and vegetables	Acetone	—	—	ELISA LC-MS	Katsoudas *et al.*, 2000; Caballo-López and de Castro, 2003
Carbamates Phenylureas	Food Commodities	AOAC Acetone	Dichloromethane/ petroleum ether	70–102	GC-MS	Mastovska *et al.*, 2001
Carbamates Phenylureas	Fruits and vegetables	Acetone	C_{18} cartridge Dichloromethane Aminopropyl cartridge	64–102	LC-MS	Nunes *et al.*, 1998b
Carbamates	Cucumbers Strawberries	Acetone	Dichloromethane/ petroleum ether SPE aminopropyl	72–123	LC-fluorescence ELISA	Abad *et al.*, 2003
Carbamate	Food samples	Acetone/hexane	SPE C_{18} cartridge	89–106	GC-NPD LC-Fluorescence	Del Carlo *et al.*, 2004

recover the pesticides for subsequent steps. The tendency to thermal decomposition (to methylisocyanate and phenol, or to urea), makes most carbamate and urea pesticides difficult to extract using other conventional techniques, such as Soxhlet extraction. Long heating periods in the Soxhlet flask cause degradation of these analytes (Balinova, 1998).

The most widely employed SLE procedures are multi-residue methods that can extract a large number of pesticides and pesticide-related compounds, but are not specific for carbamate and urea residues (Hogendoorn *et al.*, 2000; van der Hoff *et al.*, 1999; Ahmed, 2001; Nunes *et al.*, 1999a). These methods include the well-known multi-residue methods described in the official literature such as the AOAC method, the German DFG S19 or that implemented by the National Food Administration of Sweden (NFAS). All of them are based on extraction with acetone and partitioning with dichloromethane, commonly known as the Luke method, or with ethyl acetate in the presence of sodium sulphate followed by solid-phase or gel permeation clean up to achieve the removal of co-extractives present in the sample extract. The technique of determination recommended for these methods is gas chromatography (GC) in combination with various selective detectors.

The US Food and Drug Administration (FDA) has also compiled special methods, which are intended for analysis of a certain groups of pesticides, in the Pesticide Analytical Manual (PAM I). The Krause's method is one of these standard methods that has been developed for carbamates determination. It involves extraction with water/methanol (depending on the moisture of products) and evaporation of methanol. Residues in aqueous extracts are transferred to acetonitrile by liquid-liquid partitioning in the presence of sodium chloride. Co-extractives are removed from acetonitrile by partitioning into petroleum ether, which is discarded. Residues are partitioned from acetonitrile into dichloromethane. Dichloromethane solution is cleaned up on a charcoal/celite column, and residues are eluted with toluene/acetonitrile. A specific method for phenylurea herbicides that involves extraction with methanol has also been reported in PAM I (Ahmed, 2001). Co-extractives are removed by adding sodium chloride to the methanol extract and partitioning with hexane, which is discarded. Residues are partitioned from methanol into dichloromethane. Concentrated dichloromethane extract is passed through a Florisil column, and residues are eluted with acetone/dichloromethane. Figure 14.1 shows a scheme of these extraction methods that points out their complexity and laboriousness.

Most analytical methods reported in the literature are modifications and variations that can improve these extraction and clean up methods by way of changes in technology to reduce the analysis time. Advances could be made by simplifying clean up, improving extraction, miniaturizing with solid phase extraction (SPE), increasing the use of liquid chromatography (LC), intensifying automation, and introducing mass spectrometry detection (MSD) (Del Carlo *et al.*, 2004; Abad *et al.*, 2003; Nunes *et al.*, 1998b; Katsoudas *et al.*, 2000; Caballo-López and de Castro, 2003; Pantiru *et al.*, 2003; Blasco *et al.*, 2002a, b;

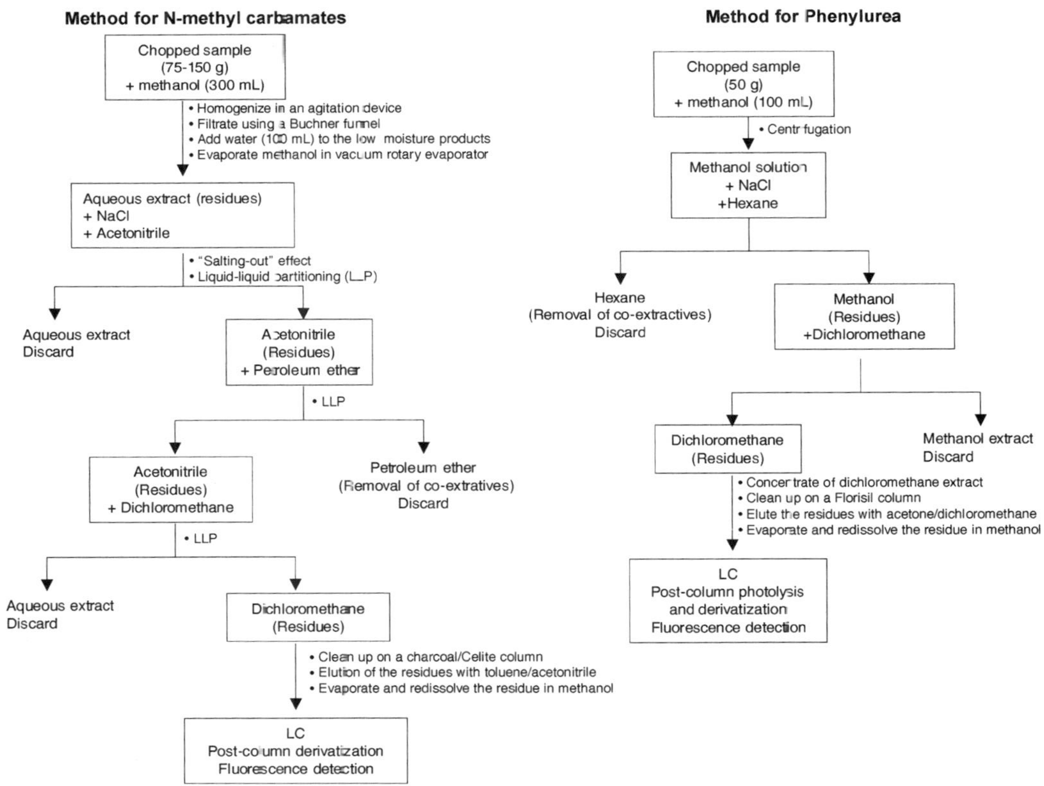

Fig. 14.1 Scheme of the extraction procedures recommended for carbamate and urea-derived pesticides by the Pesticide Analytical Manual (USA FDA).

Table 14.2 Recently developed techniques that have been used to extract carbamates and ureas from food

Extraction	Matrices	Pesticides	Clean up	Recovery, %	Determination	Ref.
ASE Acetonitrile at 100 °C under 2000 psi	Fruits and vegetables	Carbamates	Carboxylic-acid mini-column 30% acetone in hexane	70–100	LC-post-column fluorescence	Okihashi *et al.*, 1998
ASE Pressurized hot water	Fruits and vegetables	Carbamates	C_{18} column on-line	80–104	LC-post-column fluorescence	Herrera *et al.*, 2002
ASE Dichloromethane/Acetone At 40 °C under 2000 psi	Fruits and vegetables	Phenylureas	GPC	72–101	LC-MS	Bester *et al.*, 2001
MAE Acetonitrile	Food	Carbamates	C_{18} column on-line	80–102	LC-post-column fluorescence	Caballo-López and de Castro, 2003
MAE Water at 30 W for 7 min	Strawberries	Diethofencarb	SPME PDMS/DVB	22–34	LC-UV	Cao *et al.*, 2003
Ultrasound-assisted extraction (UAE) Acetonitrile	Food	Carbamates	C_{18} column on-line	85–101	LC-post-column fluorescence	Caballo-López and de Castro, 2003
SFE Celite and CO_2+DMSO (10%)	Fruits and vegetables	Carbamates	—	—	LC-post-column fluorescence	Stuart *et al.*, 1999
MSPD C_8 and dichloromethane-methanol	Fruits and vegetables	Carbamates	On-column with silica	64–106	LC-MS	Fernández *et al.*, 2000
MSPD C_8 and dichloromethane-methanol	Fruits and vegetables	Carbamates, benzoylureas and other compounds	—	85–102	LC-UV LC-MS	Valenzuela *et al.*, 1999, 2000, 2001; Blasco *et al.*, 2002b

MSPD Diatomaceous earth Ethyl acetate	Fruit juices	Carbamates	—	88–100	LC-MS	Perret *et al.*, 2002
SPE C_{18} and ethyl acetate	Wine	Carbamates Other pesticides	—	99-103	GC-MS	Soleas *et al.*, 2000
SPE C_{18} and methanol	Wine	Benzoylureas	—	69–105	LC-DAD	Miliadis *et al.*, 1999
SPE Homogenization with methanol:water C_{18} and dichloromethane-methanol	Fruits and vegetables	Urea-derived pesticides	—	42–118	CE-UV	Rodríguez *et al.*, 2001
SPME After blending and centrifuging PDMS/DVB	Strawberries	Carbamates	—	22–45	LC-UV	Wang *et al.*, 2000
SPME After diluting PDMS Carbowax TPR	Vegetables	Carbamates Phenylureas	—	8–98	GC-MS	Volante *et al.*, 2000
In tube-SPME on-line LC-EM Polypirrole coated capillary and methanol-water	Wine	Phenylureas Carbamates	—	24–35	LC-MS	Wu *et al.*, 2002
SBSE Homogenization with methanol:water PDMS stir bar and methanol	Oranges	Carbamates	—	8–13	LC-MS	Blasco *et al.*, 2002b

Stöcklein *et al.*, 1998; Jansson *et al.*, 2004; Martínez-Galera *et al.*, 2001; Lacassie *et al.*, 1999; Nunes *et al.*, 1998b, c, d, 1999b, 2000; Wu *et al.*, 2002; Schulze *et al.*, 2002a, b).

With the current trend towards miniaturization of sample preparation, several new methods have been introduced (Table 14.2). Modern techniques for extracting food based on SLE, which minimize the organic solvent used and the time required, are accelerated by using accelerated solvent extraction (ASE) and microwave-assisted solvent extraction (MASE).

ASE is a technique for extracting solid and semi-solid samples with liquid solvents at elevated temperatures and pressures, to increase the efficiency of the extraction process. Increased temperature accelerates the extraction kinetics, while elevated pressure holds the solvent below its boiling point, thus enabling safe and rapid extraction. Extractions which normally take hours, can be done in minutes. ASE offers a lower cost per sample than other techniques by reducing solvent consumption by up to 95%. ASE has been proposed for the extraction of carbamates and phenylureas from food with organic solvents or hot water (Okihashi *et al.*, 1998; Caballo-López and de Castro, 2003; Herrera *et al.*, 2002).

The hallmark of MASE is accelerated dissolution kinetics as a consequence of the rapid heating processes that occur when a microwave field is applied to a sample. The current popularity of MASE resides mainly in its applicability to a wide range of sample types. This is because selectivity can be easily manipulated by altering solvent polarities because the solvents can be heated to two to three times their atmospheric boiling points. The extraction solvent can be chosen independent of its boiling point and the amount of solvents used in routine laboratory extractions is reduced by up to 90%. Recently, MASE has given excellent results in extracting carbamates from fruit and vegetables using acetonitrile or water (Caballo-López and de Castro, 2003; Cao *et al.*, 2003).

A method for the extraction of carbamates from food based on ultrasound-assisted leaching has been proposed as an inexpensive and efficient alternative to ASE and MASE (Caballo-López and de Castro, 2003). The authors established that this is of great help in the pre-treatment of solid samples, as it facilitates and accelerates operations such as the extraction, dispersion and homogenization. However, there is only one report in the literature of the use of a flow injection manifold coupled to an ultrasound-assisted extractor for full automation of all of the steps of the analytical process.

Supercritical fluid extraction (SFE) (Stuart *et al.*, 1999) uses a supercritical fluid as the extraction solvent. Carbon dioxide (CO_2) is the most widely used one. There have been only a few studies using SFE for carbamate pesticides (Jeong *et al.*, 2003; Stuart *et al.*, 1999) and none for urea-derived pesticides. Carbamates often require the addition of small quantities of a second solvent such as methanol, dimethyl sulfoxide (DMSO), acetonitrile and/or acetone, to increase their solubility in the supercritical fluid. SFE has the advantages of increased automation, greater selectivity, reduced sample preparation time, lower operating costs and less waste generated, compared to common extraction methods. The main disadvantages of SFE, which are responsible for its infrequent application to determine carbamates and urea residues, are poor recovery because of the lack of solubility of polar and relatively polar compounds and long clean up procedure for dirty extracts.

An opportunity to reduce analysis time, solvent consumption, and overall cost might be through use of SPE, which includes different approaches such as: matrix solid-phase dispersion, solid-phase microextraction (SPME) and stir bar sorptive extraction (Ahmed, 2001; Beltrán *et al.*, 2000; Barker, 2000, 2003; Baltussen *et al.*, 2003; Hogendoorn *et al.*, 2000; van der Hoff *et al.*, 1999).

Matrix solid-phase dispersion is especially suited to extract solid samples because it simultaneously disrupts and extracts solid and semi-solid samples. The procedure involves the dispersal of the sample over a solid support such as diatomaceous earth or C_{18}. The homogenized matrix is placed in a column and analytes are eluted with a small amount of organic solvent (Barker, 2000, 2003; Ahmed, 2001). Matrix solid-phase dispersion has often been used to extract carbamates and benzoylurea pesticides from juices, fruit and vegetables because of its efficiency in reducing interfering substances (Perret *et al.*, 2002; Fernández *et al.*, 2000; Valenzuela *et al.*, 1999, 2000, 2001; Blasco *et al.*, 2002b).

The other solid-phase based techniques – solid-phase extraction, solid-phase microextraction and stir bar sorptive extraction – were initially designed to analyze water samples. They have been extended for liquid food such as milk, juices or wine (Soleas *et al.*, 2000; Miliadis *et al.*, 1999). Solid samples can also be extracted by solid-phase extraction after a separate homogenization step with a hydro-alcoholic mixture (Rodríguez *et al.*, 2001).

Solid-phase microextraction (SPME), first described by Pawliszyn and his co-workers, is a solvent-free, rapid and inexpensive technique for the extraction of organic compounds from aqueous sample matrices (Beltrán *et al.*, 2000; Ahmed, 2001). A fused silica fibre coated with a polymeric film is exposed to the extraction liquid. Extracted organic substances accumulate in the stationary phase and are desorbed thermally into a heated injector for gas chromatography or with a solvent for liquid chromatography or capillary electrophoresis. This technique comprises two separate steps, extraction (retention of the analytes on the stationary phase) and desorption, both of which must be optimized. The variables that influence the extraction step are fibre type, extraction time, ionic strength, sample pH, extraction temperature, sample agitation and matrix effect. Factors that affect desorption include temperature, desorption time and focusing oven temperature or solvent employed and its volume. Originally, polydimethylsiloxane (PDMS) and polyacrilate fibres were used, but now other coatings such as polydimethylsiloxane-divinylbencene (PDMS/DVB) or carbowax are employed. SPME of carbamates and ureas from food is becoming popular (Wang *et al.*, 2000; Volante *et al.*, 2000; Wu *et al.*, 2002; Cao *et al.*, 2003). SPME techniques can provide considerable enrichment but are not well suited to solid samples yet.

In-tube SPME can be easily coupled on-line with liquid chromatography for the analysis of less volatile and/or thermally labile compounds (Wu *et al.*, 2002). This technique, using a coated open tubular capillary, as the SPME device, allows for convenient automation of the extraction process, which not only saves analysis time but also provides better precision relative to off-line manual techniques. In-tube SPME has been applied to the analysis of carbamate and phenylurea pesticides in wine (Wu *et al.*, 2002). The authors demonstrated that the selection of a suitable coating is the key step in optimization.

Stir bar sorptive extraction (SBSE) is a new sampling technique also designed to extract organic analytes from aqueous matrices, which was developed by Sandra *et al.* (Baltussen *et al.*, 2003). Its theoretical principle is the same as that of SPME – the sorption of analytes onto polymeric film. But in SBSE the film is coated onto an iron stir bar to increase the surface area. The stir bar is immersed in the sample and extraction takes place during the stirring. The capability of SBSE to determine methiocarb in oranges has been tested using liquid chromatography-mass spectrometry (Blasco *et al.*, 2002b). However, the procedure gave a limited enrichment of this pesticide (between 8 and 13%).

SPME and SBSE are characterized by the important reduced usage of organic solvents employed. However, the time required to adsorb the analyte from the sample increases analysis time and recoveries are not always satisfactory.

Table 14.3 compares the above methods in terms of solvent used, time required, concentration factor achieved and limits of detection for the most sensitive detection systems. Several conclusions can be drawn from the information summarized in Tables 14.2 and 14.3. Microwave and accelerated-solvent extraction are particularly rapid relative to the classic SLE approaches, with extraction times of less than 30 minutes. These two techniques are becoming increasingly popular, and supplanting the use of SFE, which is becoming less used.

Matrix solid-phase dispersion (MSPD) has also attracted attention. The main advantage of MSPD is its ability to process solid samples; the main disadvantage is its limited enrichment capability. However, the reported detection limits are adequate. The use of smaller sample amounts could indicate increased sensitivity of the analytical instruments that can obtain an adequate analytical measurement with less contaminated samples.

14.2.2 Clean up

The clean up techniques most commonly employed for extracts containing residues of carbamate and/or urea pesticides are liquid-liquid partitioning (LLP), adsorption chromatography, such as column chromatography and SPE, and gel permeation chromatography (GPC). Many methods require a combination of these techniques. Simplifying a method by eliminating sample manipulation in the clean up step would shorten the analysis time, eliminating opportunities for pesticide loss and/or for extract contamination, decreased solvent and consumables usage, and reduced overall analytical cost.

As sample clean up is reduced or even removed, increasing stress is placed on the determinative step. As a result, chromatographic separation begins to suffer for the presence of large amounts of sample co-extractives. Such coextractives

Table 14.3 Comparison of different extraction procedures according to the time required, the economic cost and the detection limits

Extraction	Time	Organic solvent	DLs mg/kg	Applicability	Remarks
Conventional SLE	6–12 h	100 mL–1L	0.001–10	Carbamate and urea pesticides	Satisfactory analytical performance Adequate validation Laborious, time and time-consuming Ability to concentrate samples
ASE	20 min	< 20 mL	0.001–10	Carbamate and urea pesticides	Satisfactory analytical performance Savings in organic solvent and time Ability to concentrate samples
MASE	< 30 min	25–50 mL	0.01	Carbamates	Seems an efficient and inexpensive alternative Scarce literature
Ultrasound-assisted extraction	30 min	5 mL	0.01	Carbamates	Seems an efficient and inexpensive alternative Very scarce literature
SFE	30 to 60 min	8–50 mL	20–40	Carbamates	The technique is going out of use Low recoveries
MSPD	30 min	10–20 mL	0.001–0.1	Carbamate and urea pesticides	Useful for liquid and solid matrices Low ability to concentrate the sample Saving in organic solvent and time
SPE	30 min	10–30 mL	0.001–0.1	Carbamate and urea pesticides	Better for liquid samples Ability to concentrate sample Satisfactory analytical performance Adequate validation
SPME	2 h	0–10 mL	0.001–0.1	Carbamate and urea pesticides	Different fibres and working modes (in-tube, normal) available Low recoveries Better for liquid samples
SBSE	2–3 h	0–10 mL	0.1	Carbamates	Only one film is commercially available Scarce literature Better for liquid samples

may produce a loss of resolution of pesticides in the sample, a loss of pesticide on the chromatographic column, and a fouling of the detector. For these reasons, the chemist must weigh the need to shorten analysis time with the instrumentation 'down time' (i.e. time required to clean, repair and regenerate the instrument to its original operating specification). However, because reduction of clean up steps pays a high return in time saved for a typical analysis by reducing analytical cost and increasing sample throughput, effort should be made to explore it fully.

Several clean up procedures, which include the use of glass chromatography columns (silica gel, alumina, Florisil, silanized Celite-charcoal) and Sep-Pack cartridges, were compared for the determination of aldicarb, carbaryl, carbofuran, methomyl and propoxur in vegetable samples (potatoes and carrots) (Nunes *et al.*, 1998c). According to recoveries of the studied compounds after elution in a glass column, the most efficient systems employed 4.6% deactivated alumina and a silanized Celite-charcoal (4:1) as adsorbents, using dichloromethane-methanol (99:1) and toluene-acetonitrile (75:25) mixtures, respectively, as binary eluents. The efficiency of these procedures was also examined by analyzing other parameters such as the time required for the clean up – lower using Sep-Pack cartridges than adsorption columns; facility of operation – superior for Sep-Pack cartridges; and cost of the procedure – more expensive for SPE cartridges. This study also showed that the liquid-liquid partitioning (LLP) step is only necessary if a UV detector is used. With fluorimetric detection, recoveries of the more polar compounds are still higher if the partitioning step is omitted.

Gel permeation chromatography (GPC) has proven to be a universal clean up procedure applicable as clean up step in LC methods for carbamates and benzoylureas in fruit and vegetables (Balinova, 1998). In comparison with classical partitioning with a separating funnel, GPC is faster, formation of emulsions is avoided and the quantity of hazardous solvents is reduced. GPC clean up results in a good separation of the matrix co-extractives. The GPC column can be used for the clean up of many samples, so that less handling is required and the procedure is more cost effective. Sample extracts of apples, rape seeds, tomatoes and wheat were subjected to clean up using combinations of GPC with different SPE materials such as silica gel, graphitized carbon black (Envi-carb) and polar modified polymeric sorbents (Oasis MAX). The same sorbents were studied for the simultaneous preconcentration and group specific isolation of 15 carbamates. Highest recovery values were obtained with the MSX-sorbent by elution with ethyl/acetate cyclohexane 1:1 and acetone/buffer for the elution of carbamates. The combination of GPC and MAX cartridges also offered the cleanest UV chromatograms.

However, simple SPE clean up in disposable cartridges has become the preferred technique for clean up and concentration of selected pesticides because of its simplicity, speed and effectiveness. There are some methods reported that successfully employ these techniques for solid samples after homogenization of solid foods with water miscible solvents, such as methanol, acetonitrile, etc. SPE can discriminate between the target compounds and the matrix components to a degree that depends on the selectivity of the SPE. A new innovative concept in SPE, which can further improve the capabilities of the technique, is highly selective phases that can discriminate and isolate the target pesticide from a multitude of other contaminants.

But, selective sorbents are less useable for enrichment of many different compounds. These phases are based on immunoaffinity and molecularly imprinted polymers (MIPs). So far the most sensitive and selective phases are the immunoaffinity ones, which are constructed using biological antibodies bound to a silica or glass support. The major disadvantage of this approach is that production of antibodies is difficult and costly (Hogendoorn and van Zoonen, 2000; Nunes *et al.*, 1998d).

These problems have led to the development of MIPs, which involves the synthesis of cross-linked polymers around the template (analyte or the slightly modified analyte). Once the polymer has been formed the template is removed, leaving an 'imprint'. Both, immunosorbents and MIPs have been used for extracting carbamate and urea pesticides from water, with good clean up efficiency. Unfortunately, these selective sorbents have not yet been applied to analyze carbamates and ureas in complex matrices as food, so it is not clear how effective they would be in that context (Hogendoorn and van Zoonen, 2000; Nunes *et al.*, 1998d).

Miniaturization of the clean up step can assist in adapting robotics to multi-residue methods (MRMs). The inclusion of a mini-column packing with C_{18} in the flow injection system achieved the concentration of carbamates before chromatographic separation, derivatization and detection, thus lowering the limits of detection (Caballo-López and de Castro, 2003).

14.2.3 Derivatization

Derivatization can be performed to determine urea and carbamate residues by GC as well as by LC. For GC the objective is to transform these compounds to thermostable and volatile derivatives. This step is normally performed prior to injection in the GC. The purpose of derivatization is different in the case of the LC system, where normally, the idea is to transform the analytes to fluorescent substances because fluorescence detection is more selective and sensitive than UV. This derivatization is performed post-column, after chromatographic separation and requires additional materials such as pumps. Examples of derivatizing reagents common for carbamate and urea residues determination are presented in Table 14.4.

GC derivatization is rarely, if ever, used nowadays. The more usual derivatization reagents were heptafluorobutyric acid anhydride (HFBA), trimethylaniliniun hydroxide (TMAH) or trimethylsulfonium hydroxide (TMSH) and methyl iodine. The derivatized compounds are detected by nitrogen-phosphorus (NPD), mass spectrometry (MSD) or electron capture (ECD) detectors. However, as can be observed in Table 14.4, where there are no

Table 14.4 Derivatizating agents used for carbamate and urea residues determination

Compound	Reaction	Reagent	Determination technique	Reference
Carbamates	Post-column alkaline hydrolysis	NaOH, OPA[a]	LC-fluorimetric	Herrera *et al.*, 2002; Sawaya *et al.*, 1999; Caballo-López and de Castro, 2003; Stuart *et al.*, 1999; Okihashi *et al.*, 1998
Benzoylureas Phenylureas	Post-column photoirradiation	UV irradiation	LC-fluorimetric	Martínez.Galera *et al.*, 2001; Sawaya *et al.*, 1999
Carbamates and phenylureas	Post column photolysis	UV irradiation	LC-MS	Nunes *et al.*, 1998b

[a] o-phthaldehyde

applications of these reactions, they are not included in the recent MRMs based on GC or GC-MS because derivatization has the disadvantage of requiring more sample preparation steps and analysis time.

LC derivatization is still a very useful technique that involves, in the case of carbamates, hydrolysis with an alkaline solution (usually NaOH) to a methylamine that is subsequently derivatized in the presence of o-phthalic dicarboxyaldehyde and mercaptoethanol to create the fluorescent product (Berrada *et al.*, 2003b; Sawaya *et al.*, 1999; Caballo-López and de Castro, 2003; Stuart *et al.*, 1999; Okihashi *et al.*, 1998).

Carbamates, phenylureas and benzoylureas are also transformed to fluorescent products by photochemically-induced fluorimetry (PIF) making them photochemically reactive after UV irradiation compounds. PIF is more recent than chemical derivatization and has been much less applied to quantitative analysis (Volmer, 1998; Sawaya *et al.*, 1999).

Volmer (1998) used photolysis to enhance structural information in LC-MS spectra. After post-column irradiation and LC-MS ionization, the phototransformation products appear as apparent 'product ions' in the mass spectrum, since the unreacted precursor and the compound and the photoreaction products all co-elute. The usefulness of LC-photolysis-MS has been demonstrated for the detection and confirmation of phenylureas and carbamates in food samples.

14.3 Techniques for rapid screening of samples

The term 'screening' is used to mean a method that can analyze a large number of samples, often for one pesticide or a small group of pesticides in a relatively short period of time. This type of screening uses technologies that are less expensive and more rapid to use than conventional methods such as immunoassays or biosensors.

Enzyme-linked immunosorbent assays (ELISAs) are methods based on the interaction of an analyte with an antibody that recognizes it with high affinity and specificity. They have been found to be simple and cost-effective alternatives to instrument analysis especially when numerous samples are being analyzed. Immunoassays have been developed as commercial screening tests, while LC and GC are used to confirm the results. The applications of ELISA to food analysis are shown in Table 14.5.

Monoclonal antibody-based ELISAs have been developed for three of the most widely applied N-methyl carbamate pesticides, i.e., carbaryl, carbofuran and methiocarb. These immunoassays were applied to pesticide analysis in juices, fruits, and vegetables (Abad *et al.*, 1998, 1999, 2003; Moreno *et al.*, 2001). This immunoassay method is able to analyze the target carbamates in strawberries and cucumbers at levels of regulatory relevance with accuracy and precision comparable to those obtained by a reference method. However, the possibility of analyzing low levels of them was not tested.

Table 14.5 Immunosorbent assays (ELISA) methods developed for determining carbamate and urea pesticides in food

Analyte	Matrix	Sample treatment	Immunoassay	Sensitivity	Reference
Carbaryl	Six crops	PAM I Extraction with methanol LLP and clean up on celite-charcoal	Monoclonal antibody ELISA competitive assay format	3.9 to 5.7 μg/L	Nunes *et al.*, 1998b
Carbaryl Carbofuran Methiocarb	Cucumbers and strawberries	Extraction with acetone LLP petroleum ether/dichloromethane and clean up on aminopropyl-bonded silica	Monoclonal antibodies ELISA	10 μg/L	Abad *et al.*, 2003
Carbamates	Bananas, peaches, strawberries and tomatoes	Extraction with acetone	Monoclonal antibodies Competitive assay format ELISA	0.1–10 μmg/kg	Katsoudas *et al.*, 2000

Nunes *et al.* (1998b) applied indirect competitive ELISA for carbaryl quantification in vegetable and fruit extracts, evaluating the effect of different vegetable matrices (banana, carrot, green bean, orange, peach and potato), and the different organic solvents used for the extraction. This ELISA is free from interference from commonly found vegetable components, but a rigorous clean up procedure was carried out nevertheless. The assay compares favourably with LC determination.

The applicability of enzyme inhibition and ELISA methods to carbamate analysis in bananas, peaches strawberries and tomatoes has been addressed (Katsoudas *et al.*, 2000) showing that both methodologies provide simple and fast screening procedures to detect carbamate residues in food commodities.

The detection of phenyl urea and triazine pesticides in water, ethanol and hexane extracts by ELISA, using microtiter plates for covalent immobilization of the respective monoclonal antibodies K4E7 and B76-BF5 has been reported by Stöcklein *et al.*, 2000). Polystyrene microtiter plates are resistant against several organic solvents. Detection limits below 0.2 ng/ml were obtained for phenylurea compounds.

Despite the number of different test variations available, ELISA methods often require elaborate sample preparation and involve time consuming, and tedious protocols. In addition, specific problems may be encountered from matrix interference. As an example, Fig. 14.2 shows the matrix effect of various vegetable extracts using an ELISA for carbaryl. Regrettably, in most cases the recovery of immunoaffinity-based methods has been shown to be low.

Biosensor technology is a powerful alternative to conventional analytical techniques, by harnessing the specificity and sensitivity of biological systems in small, low cost devices (Avramescu *et al.*, 2002; Velasco-García and Mottram, 2003; Nunes *et al.*, 1998a). The principle of detection is the specific binding of the analyte of interest to the complementary recognition element immobilized on a suitable support medium. The main biological materials used in biosensor technology are: enzyme/substrate, antibody/antigen and nucleic acids/ complementary sequences.

The specific interaction results in a change in one or more physicochemical properties, (pH change, electron transfer, mass change, heat transfer, uptake or release gases or specific ions) which are detected and may be measured by the transducer. Depending on the method of signal transduction, biosensors can be divided into different groups: optical, amperometric, thermopiezoelectric or magnetic. Amperometric devices are the most commonly reported class of biosensors. Amperometric detection typically relies on an enzyme system that catalytically converts analytes into products that can be oxidized or reduced at a working electrode, maintained at a specific potential. Screen-printing is growing in popularity as a method for the fabrication of electrodes with potential use as electrochemical detectors in biosensors. This is because this technique enables mass production of biosensors at low cost (Avramescu *et al.*, 2002).

Among electrochemical sensors, enzyme-modified electrodes have gained increasing popularity in their use either directly or indirectly via inhibition of

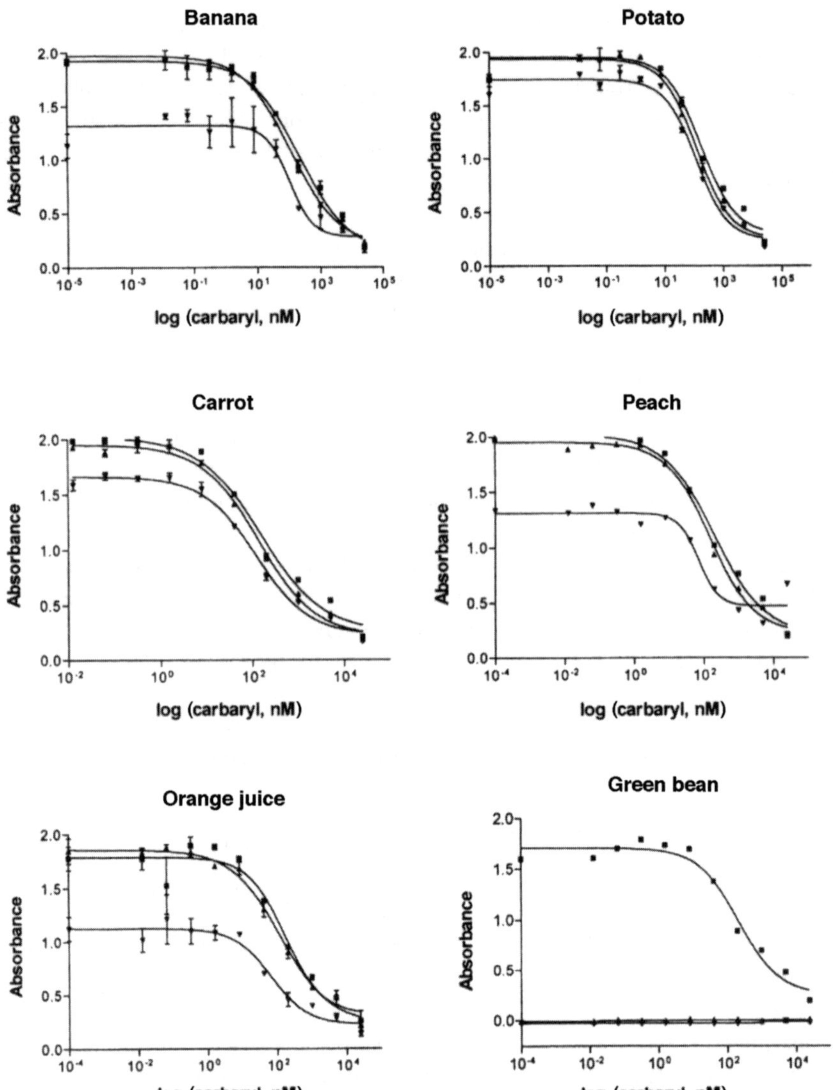

Fig. 14.2 Matrix effect of the vegetable extracts. ELISA assay performed with PBST buffer containing 10% MeOH (■) and the vegetable extract diluted 50-fold (▲) and 20-fold (▼) with PBST. Dilution of the antibody: 1/32000; concentration of the coating antigen: 0.4 μg ml^{-1} (reprinted from Nunes *et al.* (1998b) with permission from Elsevier).

enzyme activity by hazardous compounds. The development of biosensors for carbamates is based on the measurement of acetyl choline esterase (AChE) activity (Schultze *et al.*, 2002b; Xavier *et al.*, 2000; Bachmann *et al.*, 2000; Avramescu *et al.*, 2002; Nunes *et al.*, 1998a, d, 1999b; Patel, 2002; Pogacnik *et al.*, 1999):

$$\text{Acetylthiocholine} + H_2O \xrightarrow{\text{AChE}} \text{thiocholine} + CH_3COOH$$

The development of biosensors for phenylureas is based on the inhibition of the photosynthetic processes in photosystem II (PSII) (Pulido-Tofino *et al.*, 2000; Avramescu *et al.*, 2002; Patel, 2002). Phenylureas are detected by a decrease in the biosensor signal. The choice of an enzyme, as a biorecognition element, enables simultaneous detection of a wide group of related compounds, like organophosphorus and carbamate pesticides or triazine, phenylurea and phenolic herbicides. This is an advantage over other biorecognition elements, such as antibodies, where only one analyte can be detected in each analysis.

Immunosensors can be very specific for a single analyte. Fluoroimmunosensors have been developed to determine isoproturon showing negligible cross-reactivity with other phenylurea-related compounds that were tested (Stöcklein *et al.*, 1998; Pulido-Tofino *et al.*, 2000, 2001; Mallart *et al.*, 2001).

Despite the promising biosensors that have been developed in research laboratories, there are not many reports of applications in the monitoring of carbamate and urea residues in food. This is because the main limitations of this technique are complexities of sample preparation and poor stability of biological receptors (Velasco-García and Mottram, 2003). Table 14.6 shows sample pre-treatment, sensor type and basis, and sensitivity obtained in food analysis of urea and carbamate pesticides.

14.4 Separation techniques

14.4.1 Gas chromatography

Carbamates and ureas in general, and their transformation products in particular, are often described as polar and thermally labile molecules – these properties limit the use of GC (Berrada *et al.*, 2003a). With regard to this, a clear discrepancy appears in the literature. Different authors proposed methods based on GC with derivatization reactions (Berrada *et al.*, 2003a), but it seems that direct determination of carbamate and urea pesticides is possible at very low concentrations (Escuderos-Morenas *et al.*, 2003; Delgado *et al.*, 2001; Stan, 2000; Berrada *et al.*, 2003a). Other authors do not recommend this technique to determine these analytes because the compounds are thermolabile, non-volatile and/or polar (Delgado *et al.*, 2001). There are also some papers on identifying and quantifying the thermal decomposition products formed in the GC injector. However, these methods have been exclusively applied to the analysis of surface waters (Berrada *et al.*, 2001, 2003b). Selected GC applications in the analysis of carbamates and urea residues in food are presented in Table 14.7.

The first general conclusion from the data in Table 14.7 is that GC is a less popular technique for analyzing these compounds. Few workers still employ this technique because there are few carbamates and ureas that can be determined by GC, and they are normally detected by multi-residue procedures (Stan, 2000; Soleas *et al.*, 2000). There are also a few reports of sophisticated, high-cost and

Table 14.6 Biosensors developed for determining carbamate and urea pesticides in food

Analyte	Matrix	Sample treatment	Biosensor: type and basis	Sensitivity	Reference
Isoproturon	Water	Without treatment	Immunosensors Optical fluorescente	0.1 μg/l	Mallart *et al.*, 2001
Isoproturon	Water Foodstuff	Extraction with methanol	Immunosensor Optical fluorescente	μ/l level	Pulido-Tofino *et al.*, 2000, 2001)
Triazine and phenylurea herbicides	Water	Without treatment	Inhibition of the PSII Amperometric detection	10^{-9} M for diuron	Koblizek *et al.*, 2002
Carbamates	Fruit Vegetables Infant Food	Dilution with potassium phosphate buffer or isopropanol	ACh inhibition Amperometric	5 μg/kg	Schultze *et al.*, 2002a, b
Carbamates	Fruit Vegetables Water	To squeeze and to analyze directly the juice	ACh inhibition Amperometric	ppb level	Nunes *et al.*, 1999b
Carbamates	Fruits Vegetables	PAM for carbamates (see Table 14.1)	ACh inhibition Amperometric	ppb level	Nunes *et al.*, 1998d
Carbamates	Water Juices	Without treatment	ACh inhibition Photothermal detection	1–4 μg/ml	Pogacnik *et al.*, 1999
Propoxur Carbaryl	Lettuces Onions	Phosphate buffer and sonication	AChE inhibition Optical detection of pH indicator chlorophenol red	Propoxur 1 μg/kg Carbaryl 12.5 μg/kg	Xavier *et al.*, 2000
Carbamates	Egg, bovine meat, milk and honey	Extraction with acetone/hexane	ACh inhibition Amperometric	10 ng/ml	Del Carlo *et al.*, 2004

Table 14.7 GC applications to determine carbamate and urea residues in food

Analytes	Column, temperature and carrier gas	Detector	Sensitivity	Remarks	Reference
Phenylureas	HP-5, 5% diphenyl-95% dimethylpolisiloxane (30 m × 0.53 mm, 2.65 μm) Inlet temperature 220, 1 μl (splitless) injection 300 °C detector temperature Oven program from 110 °C to 250 °C	GC-NPD	6–47 ng/g	Those contained methoxy radical seem stable	Escuderos-Morenas *et al.*, 2003
Carbamates	HP-5, 5% diphenyl-95% dimethylpolisiloxane (30 m × 0.53 mm, 2.65 μm); OV-101 (10 m × 0.53 mm, 2.65 μm) Inlet temperature 220, 1 μl (splitless) injection 300 °C FID/NPD detector temperature and 220 °C mass-selective detector interface Oven program from 110 °C to 240 °C	GC-FID/NPD GC-MS	41–50 ng//g	Degradation increases when using old columns with respect to the new ones	Delgado *et al.*, 2001
Carbamates Phenylureas	HP-5, SE-54 (50 m × 0.32 mm, 0.17 m) OV-17 (25 m × 0.32 mm, 0.25 μm) HP-5, SE-54 (25 m × 0.2 mm, 0.33 m) Inlet temperature 210 °C, 1 μl (splitless) injection 300 °C ECD, 280 °C NPD and 260 °C mass selective interface Oven temperature from 100 °C to 280 °C	GC-NPD/ECD GC-MSD	< 10 ng/g	Method established for monitoring more than 400 pesticides	Stan, 2000
Carbamates	DB-5 MS (30 m × 0.25 mm, 0.25 m) Inlet temperature 270ºC, 1 μl (splitless) injection 270ºC mass-selective detector interface Oven temperature from 70ºC to 290ºC	GC-MS	2	Multiresidues method for 17 pesticides of different classes	Soleas *et al.*, 2000
Carbamates	RTX-5 Sil MS (10 m × 0.53 mm, 1 μm) He carrier gas at 20 psi (low-pressure GC) Inlet temperature 250ºC, 1 or 2 μl (splitless) injection 280ºC mass-selective detector interface Oven program from 90ºC to 290ºC	GC-MS	0.1–0.9 ng/g	Sometimes results are worse than using conventional GC	Mastovska *et al.*, 2001

undisposable modifications of GC that result in elegant methods that are not applicable to the routine analysis of real samples (Mastovska *et al.*, 2001). One of these approaches is to conduct GC at sub-ambient pressure conditions, or low-pressure gas chromatography (LP-GC). This has some advantages such as larger sample 'loadability' and lower detection limits, but it has the trade-off of poorer separation efficiency (Mastovska *et al.*, 2001).

Phenylurea herbicides are subject to decomposition in gas chromatograph inlets, and typically any peak detected corresponds to the aniline breakdown product (Balinova, 1998). However, a study on thermal stability of the phenylurea herbicides seems to confirm that the ones containing the methoxy radical, i.e. monolinuron, linuron and chlorbromuron, are stable (Escuderos-Morenas *et al.*, 2003). Thermal stability of several carbamate pesticides and metabolites has also been extensively studied showing that there is some degradation in GC (Delgado *et al.*, 2001). A way to analyze urea and carbamates pesticides by GC is to minimize thermal degradation by using short capillary columns at low temperature (Escuderos-Morenas *et al.*, 2003; Delgado *et al.*, 2001). Figures 14.3 and 14.4 show the GC-NPD chromatograms of phenylureas and carbamates in powdered potato, where the thermal degradation was minimized and/or avoided by using a thermal gradient program of weak ramps and semi-capillary columns.

14.4.2 Liquid chromatography

LC is the favoured technique for the determination of urea and carbamates, since many of these compounds lack the thermal stability required for chromatographic analysis. Most LC methods employ reversed phase chromatography with C_8 and C_{18} and aqueous mobile phases. Carbamates and ureas can be efficiently separated with two different solvent systems, methanol/water and acetonitrile/water. Table 14.8 summarizes the separation conditions and the detectors reported in representative papers on this technique.

Other recent innovations, originating from the development of new LC column packing materials, such as immunoaffinity sorbents, molecular imprinted polymers and restricted access medium columns, have not yet been used to separate carbamates or ureas (Ahmed, 2001).

14.4.3 Capillary electrophoresis

Capillary electrophoresis (CE) is a highly efficient technique for separating and quantifying a wide variety of compounds. It is more versatile than LC and GC, since there is nearly no restriction to certain classes of pesticides, and derivatization becomes unnecessary. Capillary zone electrophoresis (CZE), micellar electrokinetic capillary chromatography (MECK) and capillary electro-chromatography (CEC) are the most successful modes. The number of papers describing separation of pesticides by such techniques is increasing spectacularly (Picó *et al.*, 2003; Berrada *et al.*, 2003a; Ahmed, 2001). However, their

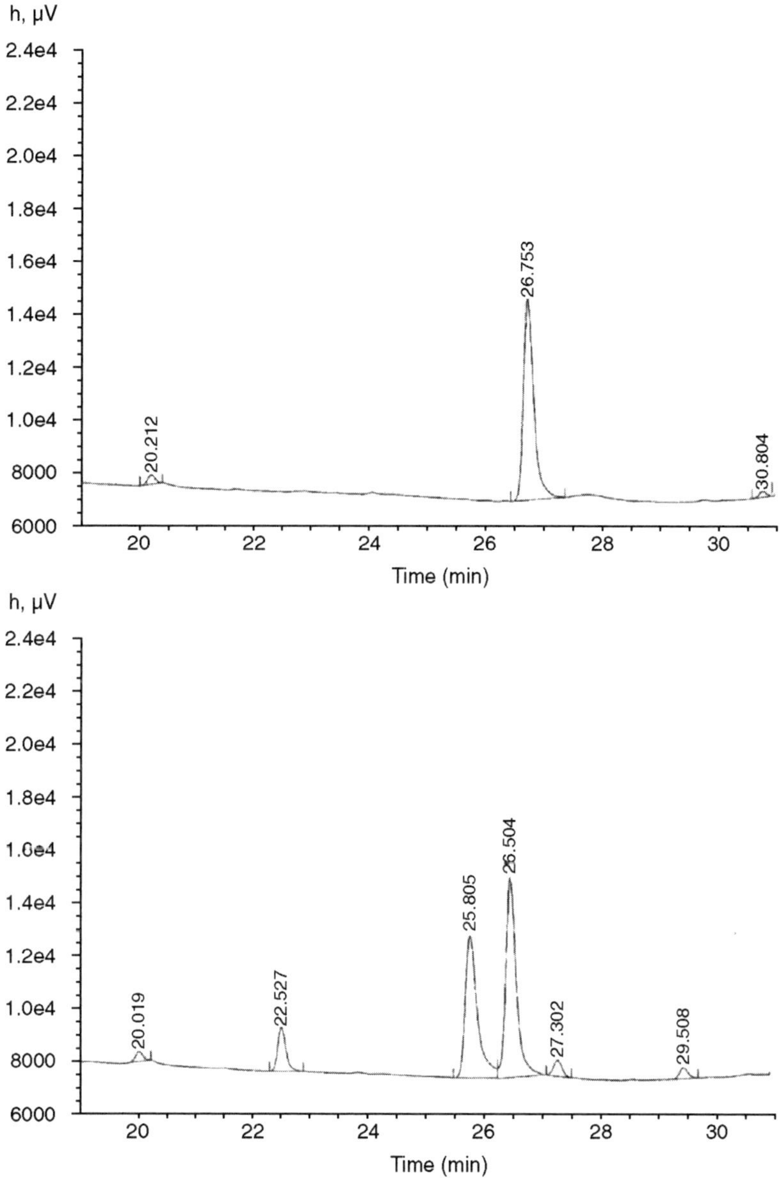

Fig. 14.3 Chromatograms of powdered potato by GC-NPD. (a) Blank, (b) 1.6 μg herbicide fortified sample. Conditions: Column HP-5 (30 m $\times$ 0.53 mm $\times$ 2.65 μm); flow rate 28.3 ml min^{-1}; injection volume, 1 μl; m_{potato}, 2.5 g; [I.S.$_{methylparathion}$], 0.5 μg ml^{-1}. Temperaure program: $T_{injector}$: 220 °C; $T_{detector}$: 300 °C; $T^{a}_{oven\ initial}$: 110 °C (2 min) Gradient 5 °C/min–140 °C (2 min); 5 °C/min–210 °C (2 min); 7 °C/min–250 °C (2 min). Elution order, fluometuron, monolinuron, monuron, I.S., linuron, chlorbromuron (reprinted from Escuderos-Morenas *et al.* (2003) with permission from Elsevier).

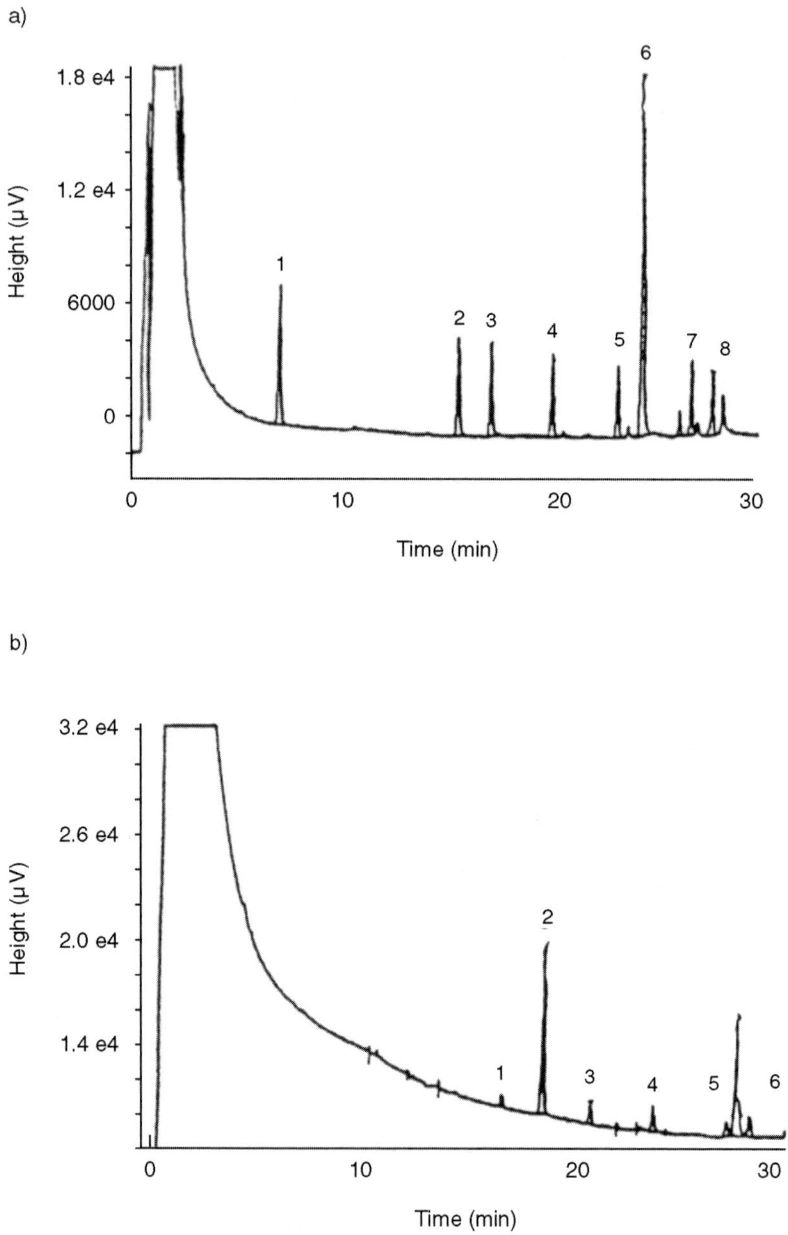

Fig. 14.4 Chromatogram obtained from a spiked powdered potato sample. HP-5 (30 m × 0.53 mm, 2.65 μm) column. (a) GCFID, [pesticide] = 10 mg kg^{-1}, injection volume, 1 μ; elution order: 1 = IPF, 2 = PHM, 3 = NAP, 4 = PRO, 5 = CBF, 6 = phenanthrene, 7 = CAR, 8 = MET. (b) GCNPD, [pesticide] = 0.5 mg kg^{-1}, injection volume, 1 μl; elution order: 1 = PHM, 2 = 4-nitrophenol, 3 = PRO, 4 = CBF, 5 = CAR, 6 = MET. (reprinted from Delgado *et al.* (2001) with permission from Elsevier).

Table 14.8 LC applications to determine carbamate and urea residues in food

Analyte	Column, mobile phase	Detector	Sensitivity	Reference
Benzoylureas	C_{18} analytical column Methanol–water (80:20) isocratic Flow-rate between 0.4 and 1 mL/min	LC-UV	0.05–2.1 mg/kg	Balinova, 1998; Martínez.Galera *et al.*, 2001
Benzoylureas Carbamates Phenylureas	C_{18} analytical column Methanol-water gradient Flow-rate between 0.3 and 1 mL/min	LC-UV LC-APCI-MS LC-Fluorescence LC-ES-MS LC-hV-MS	0.001–0.5 mg/kg	Tsiropoulos *et al.*, 1999; Miliadis *et al.*, 1999; Valenzuela *et al.*, 2000, 2001; Nunes *et al.*, 1998b; Koblizek *et al.*, 2002; Blasco *et al.*, 2002a; Okihashi *et al.*, 1998; Caballo-López and de Castro, 2003; Herrera *et al.*, 2002; Volante *et al.*, 2000
Carbamates	C_8 analytical column Methanol-water gradient Flow-rate 1 mL/min	LC-APCI-MS	0.001–0.1 mg/kg	Fernández *et al.*, 2000
Phenylureas Carbamates	C_{18} analytical column Methanol–acetic acid/ammonium acetate buffer Flow-rate 1 mL/min	LC-UV LC-ES-MS	0.5–2 μg/kg	Caballo-López and de Castro, 2003; Jansson *et al.*, 2004
Carbamates	C_{18} analytical column Acetonitrile–water (30:70) isocratic Flow-rate 1 mL/min	LC-UV	0.1 mg/kg	Nunes *et al.*, 1998c
Carbamates Phenylureas Benzoylureas	C_{18} analytical column Acetonitrile–water gradient Flow-rate between 0.5 and 1 mL/min	LC-ES-MS LC-UV	0.01–1.2 μg/L	Wu *et al.*, 2002; Valenzuela *et al.* 1999

Table 14.8 Continued

Analyte	Column, mobile phase	Detector	Sensitivity	Reference
Carbamates	C_{18} analytical column Acetonitrile–phosphate buffer (pH=6) gradient Flow-rate 1 mL/min	LC-UV	—	Pantiru *et al.*, 2003
Carbamates Other pesticides	C_{18} analytical column Acetonitrile–water (2 mM ammonium formate, pH 3–5) gradient Flow-rate between 0.04 and 0.3 mL/min	LC-ES-MS	0.02–0.05 mg/kg	Lacassie *et al.*, 1999; Perret *et al.*, 2002
Carbamates	C_{18} analytical column Acetonitrile–water (2mM ammonium formate, pH 7) gradient Flow-rate 1.0 mL/min	LC-APCI-MS	0.5–1.3 ng	Nunes *et al.*, 2000
Carbamates	C_{18} analytical column Methanol–water (2mM ammonium formate, pH 7) gradient Flow-rate 1.0 mL/min	LC-ES-MS	0.005–0.8 μg/mL	Stöcklein *et al.*, 1998
Carbamates	C_{18} analytical column Tetrahidrofuran–water gradient Flow-rate 1 mL/min	LC-Fluorescence	—	Stuart *et al.*, 1999
Carbamates	C_{18} analytical column Water–methanol–acetonitrile gradient Flow-rate 1.5 mL/min	LC-Fluorescence	0.2 and 1.3 ng	Nunes *et al.*, 2000

Table 14.9 CE applications to determine carbamate and urea residues in food

Analyte	Concentration	Injection, capillary, buffer	Detector	Sensitivity	Reference
Urea-pesticides Sulphonylurea Phenylurea Benzyolurea	Off-line concentration by SPE with C_{18} disposable column Concentration 10-fold	Fused-silica capillary of 50 m 4 mM borate (pH 9.2) containing 35 mM SDS	UV (DAD)	0.05–0.3 mg/kg	Rodríguez *et al.*, 2001
Carbamates Ureas	On-line concentration by sweeping and stacking with reverse migration micelles Concentration 3–18-fold Off-line concentration by a SLE procedure Concentration 15-fold	Fused-silica capillary of 20 mM phosphate buffer (pH 2.5) containing 25 mM SDS and 10% of methanol	UV (DAD)	2.5 μg/L	da Silva *et al.*, 2003

application to real samples analysis is still extremely scarce (da Silva *et al.*, 2003; Rodríguez *et al.*, 2001). Some typical examples are summarized in Table 14.9.

Recently, CE using MECK has been proven to have a good potential for detecting sulfonylurea, phenylurea and benzoylurea in different matrices including grain, fruit and vegetables. However, CE applications are generally limited by the high detection limits and the lack of selective detectors. One approach to improving detection limits is to employ preconcentration methods as off-column concentration by LLE or SPE and on-column preconcentration by SPE and stacking. This latter concentration strategy has been investigated for the analysis of carbamates (carbaryl and propoxur) and ureas (diuron and linuron) in drinking water and vegetables using MECK (da Silva *et al.*, 2003).

14.5 Detectors used in combination with separation techniques

Carbamate and urea pesticides can be determined using different detectors in GC, LC and CE analysis.

14.5.1 Classical detectors in GC

A characteristic of the carbamate molecule is the nitrogen atom, which forms the basis for detection; and some carbamates also contain chlorine, sulphur or other marker atom in the molecule. Prior to the development of LC-MS instruments, GC and, in particular, nitrogen-phosphorus detector (NPD) were preferred because the resolution is greater, and the detectors were more sensitive and selective than in LC.

14.5.2 Classical detectors in LC and CE

LC is widely used in carbamate and urea pesticides analysis, often with UV or diode array (DAD) detectors, probably due to its wide applicability and consequent presence in most LC systems. But these conventional techniques cannot be used for multi-residue screening, because of their insensitivity and lack of specificity, and the large amounts of co-extractives from vegetable extracts. Even though several LC-UV methods based on SLE or MSPD have been reported for carbamates and ureas, many compounds elute from the matrix and this makes identification difficult. As a typical example, Fig. 14.5 shows LC-UV chromatograms obtained by a MSPD procedure for citrus samples with and without 'spiking' with benfuracarb, diflubenzuron, flufenuxuron, hexaflumuroan and hexythiazox at levels slightly below the respective maximum residue limits (MRLs).

Fluorescence detection may seem to be an interesting alternative but, unfortunately, most urea and carbamates do not display inherent fluorescence. LC coupled to a photolysis cell in series with a fluorescence detector or post-column derivatization systems seems to be the solution. Figure 14.6 shows an

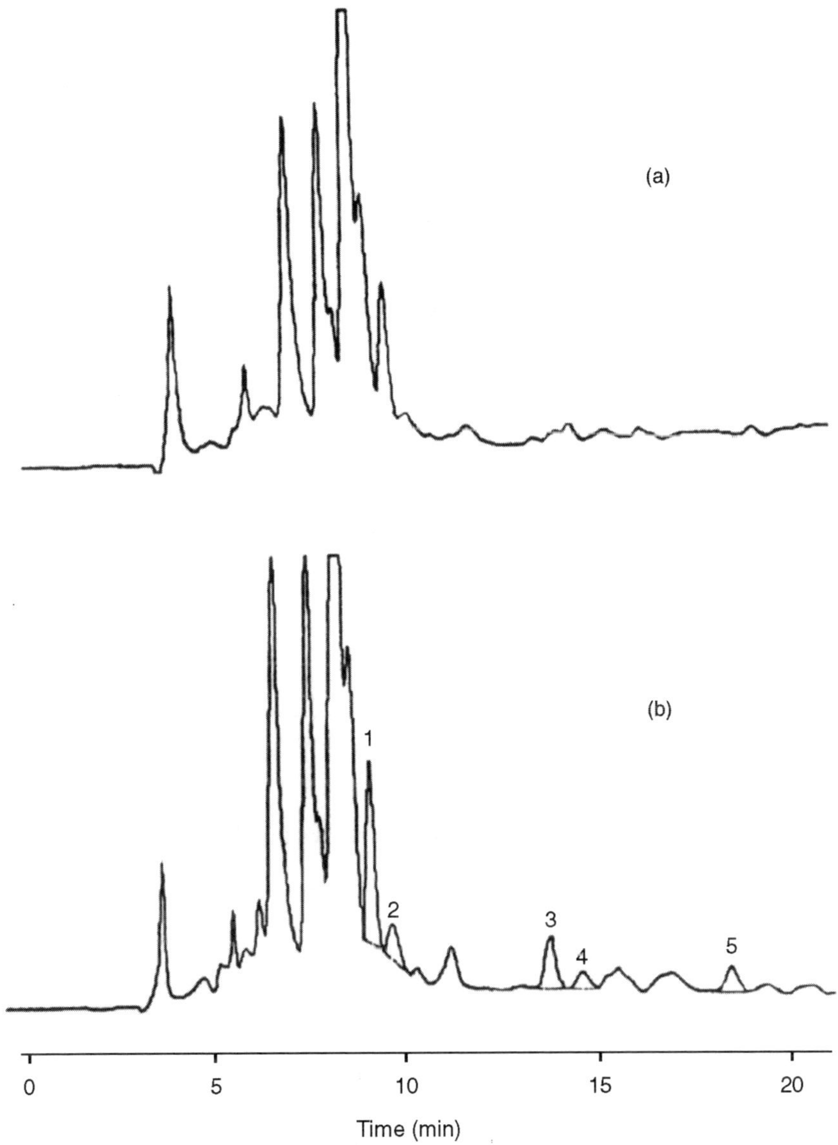

Fig. 14.5 (a) Chromatogram of a non-fortified orange sample. (b) Chromatogram showing the separation of the pesticides in a fortified orange sample (level of fortification): 1 = Diflubenzuron (0.5 μg/g), 2 = Hexaflumuron (0.3 μg/g), 3 = Benfuracarb (1 μg/g), 4 = Hexythiazox (0.2 μg/g) and 5 = Flufenoxuron (0.3 μg/g). (reprinted from Valenzuela *et al.* (1999) with permission from Elsevier).

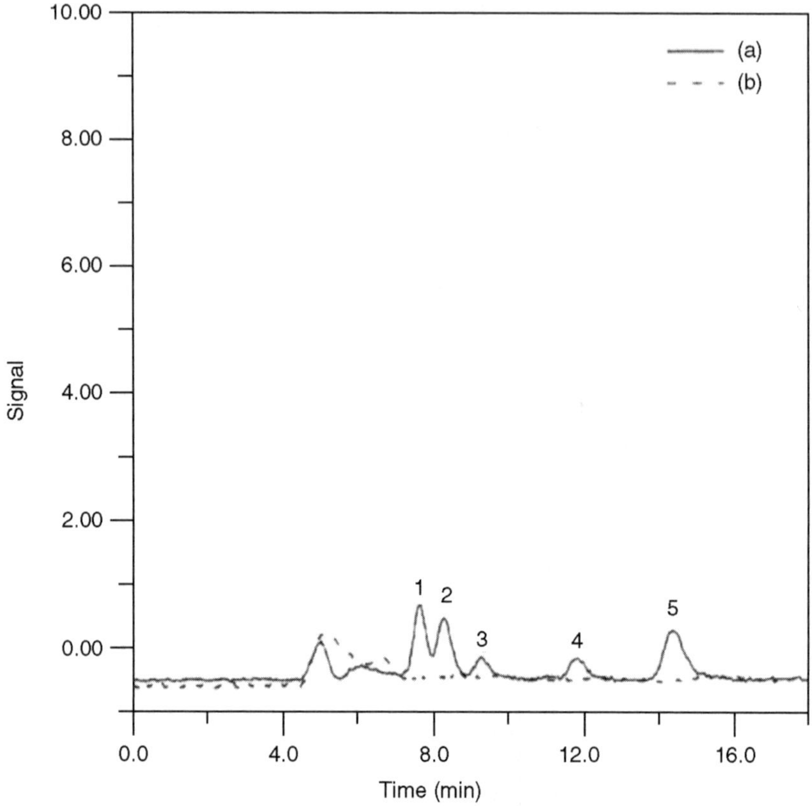

Fig. 14.6 (a) Chromatogram of a blank tomato extract. (b) Chromatogram of a tomato sample spiked with: diflubenzuron (15 ng ml^{-1}), triflumuron (14 ng ml^{-1}), hexaflumuron (18 ng ml^{-1}), lufenuron (22 ng ml^{-1}) and flufenoxuron (6 ng ml^{-1}) (reprinted from Martínez.Galera *et al.* (2001) with permission from Elsevier).

LC-fluorescence chromatogram of a tomato blank extract without interference and a tomato extract 'spiked' with four benzoylureas, detected by continuous on-line post column irradiation followed by fluorimetric detection.

Direct detection of carbamate and urea pesticides by capillary electrophoresis can be made using UV or diode array (DAD) and fluorescence detectors. These detectors have the same drawbacks as in their application to LC. As an example, Fig. 14.7 shows the MECK-DAD of some urea-derived compounds extracted from oranges by SPE. There are several peaks from the matrix that can interfere with the determination of the analytes.

14.5.3 Mass spectrometric detection

MSD can be coupled to GC, LC and CE for determining carbamate and urea pesticides. Quadrupole systems are probably the most widely used mass spectrometers because of their relatively low price and ease of operation.

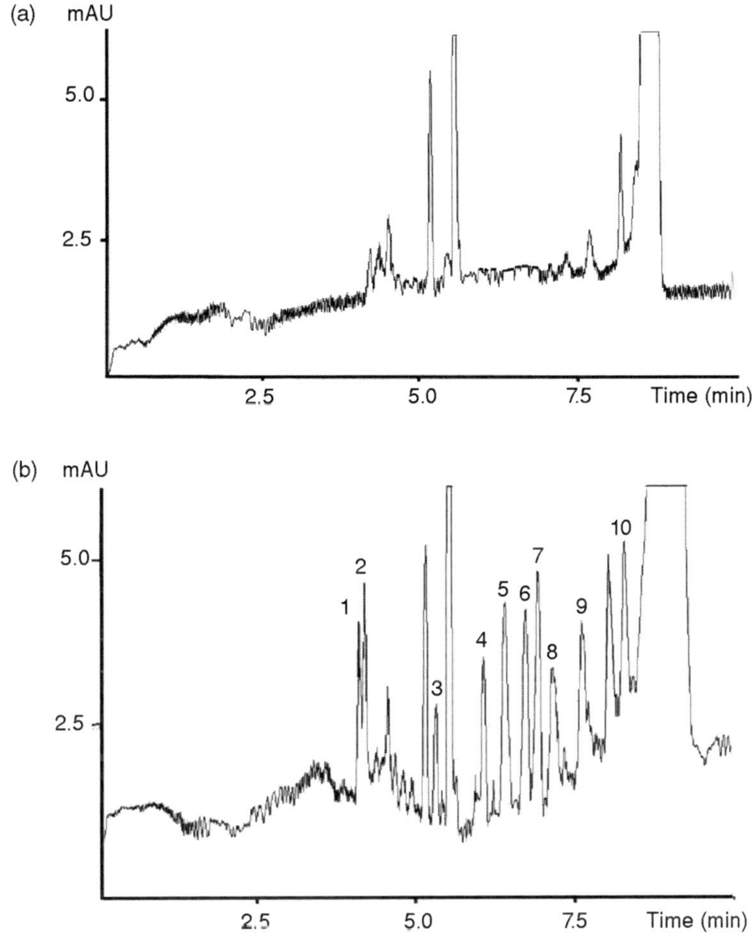

Fig. 14.7 Single wavelength (240 nm) electropherogram of (a) an extract orange blank and (b) extract of fortified orange with ten compounds at 0.5 mg kg^{-1} level. Peak identification: 1. = triasulfuron; 2. = chlorsulfuron; 3. = monuron; 4. = fluometuron; 5. = metobromuron; 6. = chlorotoluron; 7. = isoproturon; 8. = diuron; 9. = methabenzthiazuron; 10. = flufenuxuron (reprinted from Rodríguez *et al.* (2001) with permission from Wiley).

Together with the traditional single quadrupole systems, tandem mass spectrometers allow repeating the MS process a number of times and can be an ideal tool in some cases.

Tandem mass spectrometry carries out more than one stage of mass analysis, first pre-selecting an ion, and secondly analyzing the fragments obtained by collision induced dissociation (CID) with an inert gas like argon or helium. This dual analysis can be tandem in space or tandem in time. Tandem in space means that two mass spectrometers are in series and that the various steps of the process take place simultaneously but are separated in space. Many combinations have been tried: the triple quadrupole (TQ) and hybrid quadrupole-ion trap (Q-TOF) are the most successful ones. Dual analysis can also be tandem in time, as achieved in quadrupole ion traps (QIT), in which the sequence of events take place in the same space but is separated in time.

The successful combination of mass spectrometry with gas chromatography (GC-MS) can be applied to determine some carbamate and urea residues in food. Two classes of bench-top MS detector are often used in combination with capillary GC: a quadrupole MS, and an ion trap (IT). Conventional GC-MS methods are performed on a single quadrupole using electron impact ionization at 70 eV electron beam energy. Identification of unknown compounds is based on comparison of the mass spectra of the peaks in the sample with mass spectral libraries or interpretation of the fragmentation patterns. However, in full scan mode a great number of peaks are recorded and must be evaluated. This, and the lack of detection sensitivity for a few well-known active ingredients may be the reason why GC-MS is not usually applied to universal screening but more for target analysis with selected ion monitoring (SIM) (Delgado *et al.*, 2001; Stan, 2000; Soleas *et al.*, 2000; Mastovska *et al.*, 2001).

In addition to the conventional single quadrupole, a series of carbamates and phenylurea pesticides have been studied by GC-ion trap MS/MS collision-induced dissociation (CID), in the resonant excitation mode. Mass spectra of carbamates and phenylureas produced highly abundant rearrangement ions, in addition to ions produced by cleavage (Yinon and Vincze, 1997). This fact opens new perspectives to more accurate identification of the compounds. However, the problems associated with the inadequacy of GC for determining carbamates and ureas are not resolved. GC-MS and GC-MS/MS are scarcely used for the determination of these compounds in food samples (Hogendoorn and van Zoonen, 2000; van der Hoff *et al.*, 1999).

The on-line combination of liquid chromatography and mass spectrometry (LC-MS) offers significant advantages and is attracting increasing attention. This is because it meets the demands of sensitive and selective analyte detection in complex matrices, which are prerequisites in food analysis, according to recent national and international laws and regulations (Patel, 2002). Figure 14.8 illustrates the LC-MS chromatograms of the same urea herbicides and carbamates that in Fig. 14.5 were determined by LC-UV. The selectivity and sensitivity are clear.

Atmospheric pressure ionization (API) sources are the prevailing interfaces that include atmospheric pressure chemical ionization (APCI) and electrospray (ES). Thanks to the versatility of these interfaces, the detection of pesticides by mass spectrometry is now supplanting current spectrophotometric or fluorimetric detection. This is demonstrated by the many examples of applying LC-MS to analyze carbamate and urea residues that are found in recent literature (Table 14.10). Despite the methods described, there is not an exact procedure for choosing the most sensitive interface or mode of ionization (positive or negative) for carbamate and urea residues (Thurman *et al.*, 2001; Fernández *et al.*, 2000).

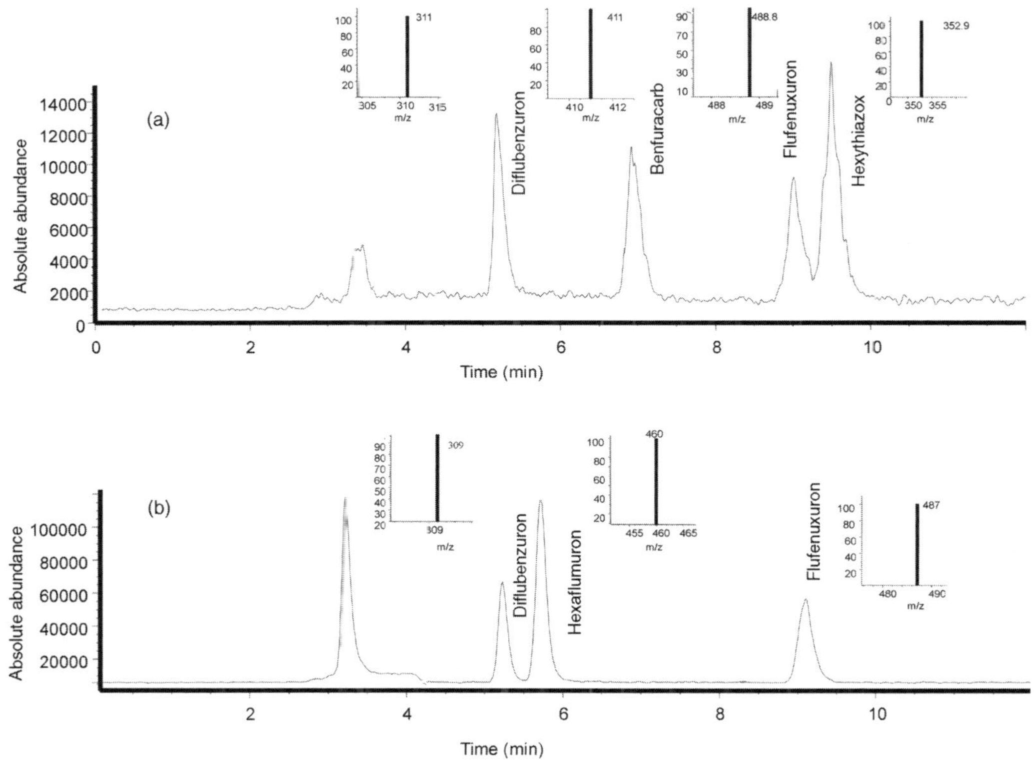

Fig. 14.8 LC-APCI-MS chromatogram of orange sample fortified with the studied pesticides at 0.5 mg kg^{-1} (a) in positive ion mode, and (b) in negative ion mode (reprinted from Valenzuela *et al.* (2001) with permission from AOAC Int).

Table 14.10 Types of LC-MS applications to determine carbamate and urea residues in food

Compounds	MS detector chracteristics	Main ions obtained	2º fragmentation (using tandem)	Reference
Carbamates	Simple quadrupole Compares APCI and ES and PI and NI modes	$[M+H]^+$ and $[M+H-CH_3NCO]^+$ (APCI, PI) $[M+H]^+$ and $[M+Na]^+$ (ES,PI) $[M-CH_3NCO]^-$, (APCI, NI)		Fernández *et al.*, 2000
Carbamates	Simple quadrupole APCI in PI mode	$[M+H]^+$ $[M+H-CH_3NCO]^+$ $[M+H-CH_3NCO_2H]^+$		Nunes *et al.*, 1998d, 2000; Blasco *et al.*, 2002a; Valenzuela *et al.*, 2001
Carbamates and phenylureas	Simple quadrupole ES in PI mode	Carbamates: $[M+H]^+$ $[M+H-CH_3NCO]^+$ Phenylureas: $[M+H]^+$, $[M+Na]^+$ $[C_3H_6NO]^+$		Wu *et al.*, 2002
Benzyolureas	Simple quadrupole APCI in NI and PI modes	NI mode: $[M-H]^-$ and $[M-H-HF]^-$ PI mode: $[M+H]^+$		Valenzuela *et al.*, 2000, 2001
Carbamates, phenylureas, and other pesticides	Triple quadrupole ES in PI mode	$[M+H]^+$ $[M+Na]^+$ $[M+NH_4]^+$ Other fragments	Carbamates: $[M+H-CH_3NCOH]^+$ $[M+H-CH_3NCO_2H]^+$ Other specific transitions Phenylureas: $[C_3H_6NO]^+$ Other specific transitions	Jansson *et al.*, 2004; Nunes *et al.*, 1998b; Hogenboom *et al.*, 2000; Bester *et al.*, 2001; Taylor *et al.*, 2002; Goto *et al.*, 2003; Perret *et al.*, 2002
Carbamates and benzoylphenylureas	Quadrupole ion trap	$[M+H]^+$	There is not multiple-stage mass spectrometry	Zrostlikova *et al.*, 2002

Despite the limited number of studies comparing best conditions and optimal sensitivity for some of the studied compounds, it is possible to draw some general conclusions. ES in any ionization mode (PI or NI) was five to ten times less sensitive than APCI for phenylurea herbicides. Benzoylureas are ionized using either APCI or ES with the same sensitivity. However, ionization in NI mode is three times more sensitive than in PI mode and some individual compounds such as hexaflumuron do not give a response in PI mode.

Carbamates are protonated both in APCI PI mode and in ES PI mode since they contain either nitrogen or oxygen atoms that have a reasonably high proton affinity (Fernández *et al.*, 2000; Nunes *et al.*, 2000). However, they are only ionized in APCI using NI mode (Fig. 14.9).

From Table 14.10 it is obvious that sodium adducts were common using an ESI interface for phenylurea and carbamates (related to the presence in the molecule of a group that donates a lone pair of electrons to form stable sodium adducts at the carbonyl group).

Although API interfaces provide 'soft' ionization that mainly produces the protonated or deprotonated molecule, ions can be fragmented, and sometimes structural information about a particular ion can be obtained. Fragmentation with a single quadrupole is performed using collision-induced dissociation (CID) by increasing the potential between the entrance capillary and the first skimmer (referred to as fragmentor or cone voltage) in the ion focusing region of the instrument.

Application of CID to carbamates commonly provides typical ions $[M\text{-}57]^+$ and $[M\text{-}75]^+$ by the loss of neutral methylisocyanate or methylcarbamic acid from the molecule. The spectra of the phenylurea pesticides give a characteristic ion at *m/z* 72. This fragment ion is characteristic to phenylurea pesticides and has been assigned to the structure $[OCN(CH_3)_2]^+$ formed by the cleavage of the N–C bond. Besides this ion, other fragments can be formed by cleavage of the lateral chains, and by migration and rearrangement of different functional groups. Benzyolureas also present some characteristic ions corresponding to $[M\text{-}20]^-$, which indicates the neutral loss of fluorhydric acid.

When single-stage mass spectrometry is used, there are still several analytical disadvantages related to the characteristics of the mass spectrum (the ionization process is 'soft' and the main ion is the protonated or deprotonated molecule). The lack of a consistent number of characteristic fragment ions could lead to erroneous results because of the presence in complex matrices of known and unknown compounds that provide isobaric interferences or negate a multiple-component spectrum. However the use of tandem mass spectrometry is extremely useful (Picó *et al.*, 2004).

The triple quadrupole (TQ) that uses three quadrupoles in series can achieve excellent sensitivity even with complex matrices, because it eliminates interference prior to measurement of ions from target compounds. The first quadrupole functions as a mass filter that passes only through ions within a small range of masses. The second quadrupole is the collision chamber, where the isolated ions are cleaved and transferred to the third quadrupole. The third

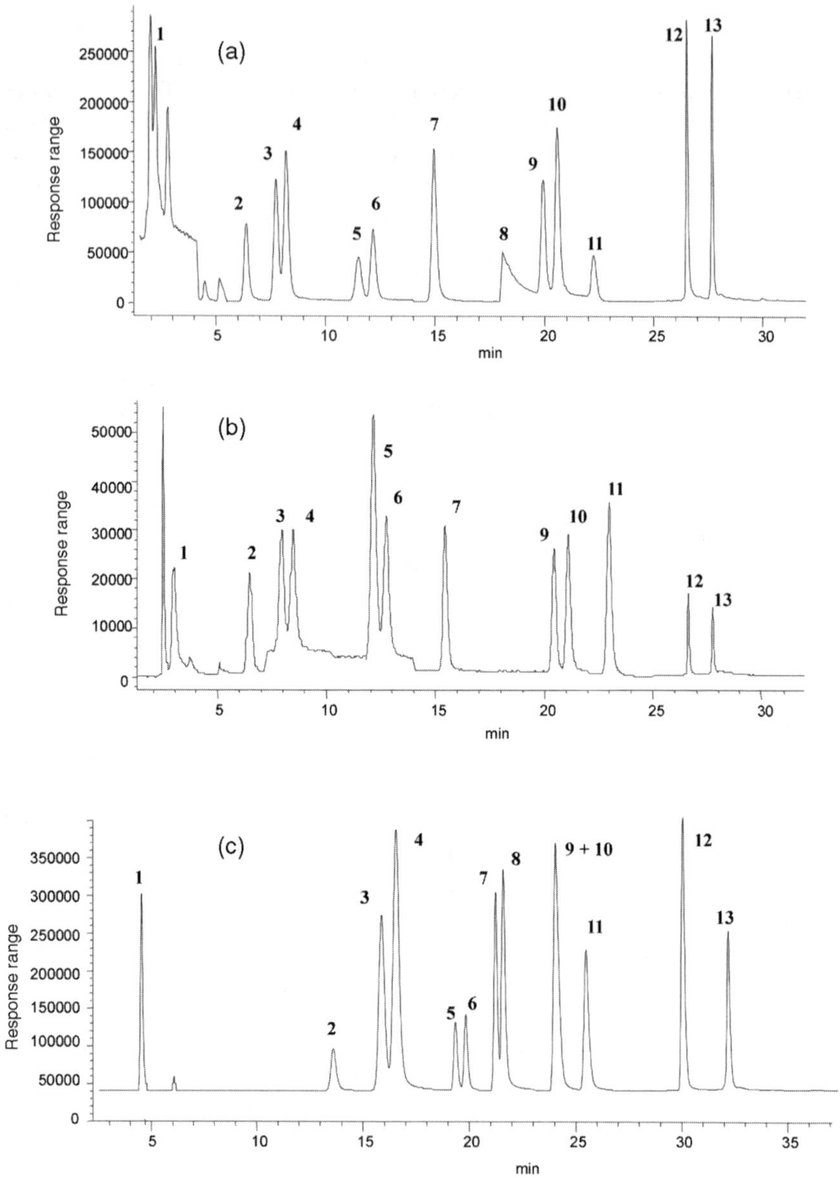

Fig. 14.9 SIM chromatograms of an orange sample spiked at $1\,mg\,kg^{-1}$ with 13 carbamates standard mixture obtained by LC-APCI-MS in positive mode (a), LC-APCI-MS in negative mode (b) and LC-ES-MS in positive mode (c). Peaks 1. Oxamyl, 2. Metholcarb, 3. Propoxur, 4. Carbofuran, 5. Carbaryl, 6. Ethiofencarb, 7. Isoprocarb, 8. Pirimicarb, 9. Fenobucarb, 10. Diethofencarb, 11. Methiocarb, 12. Fenoxycarb and 13. Thiobencarb. (reprinted from Fernández *et al.* (2000) with permission from Elsevier).

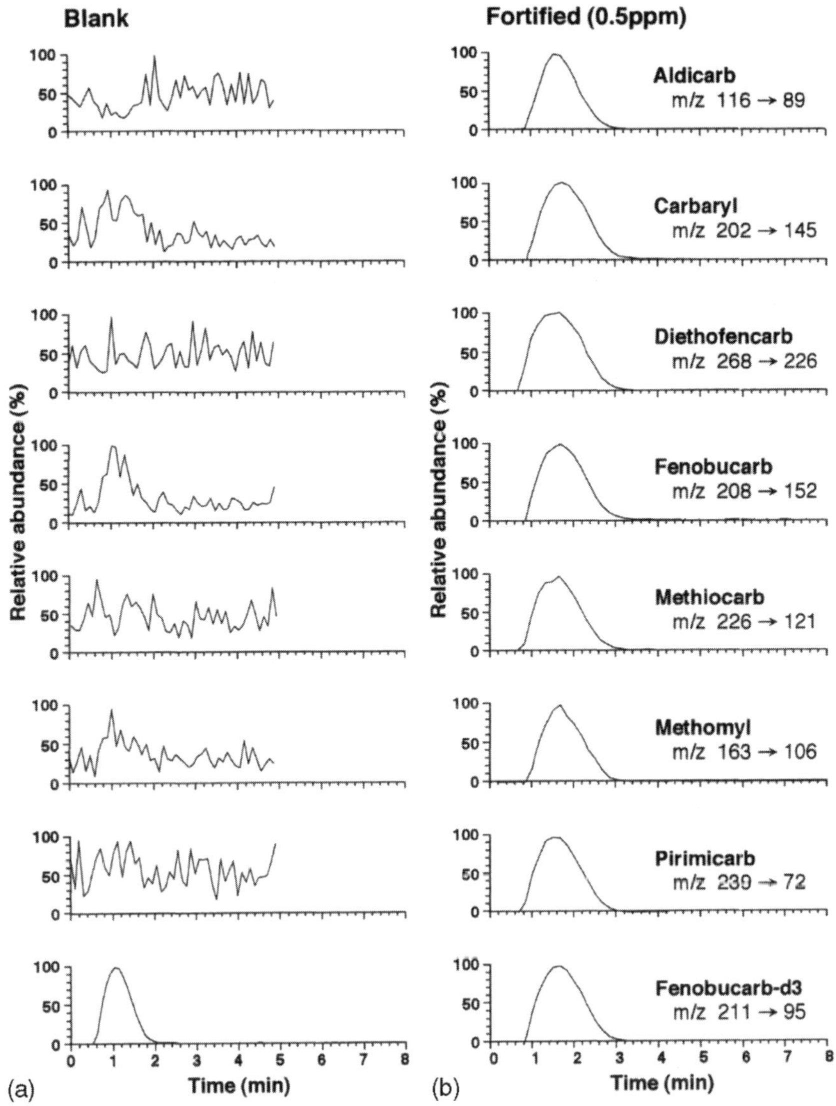

Fig. 14.10 Typical MRM profiles of the fortified and blank lemon samples (Reprinted from (Goto *et al.*, 2003) with permission from Elsevier).

quadrupole filters the results of the cleavage so they can be scanned as the product ion spectrum. Because the first quadrupole operates as a mass filter that allows through only ions within a small range of masses, an intense clean up step is not always required to prepare a sample solution (Fig. 14.10). However, co-extractives from the sample matrix influence the ion formation processes, hence the term 'matrix interferences', the central issue in this area of method development.

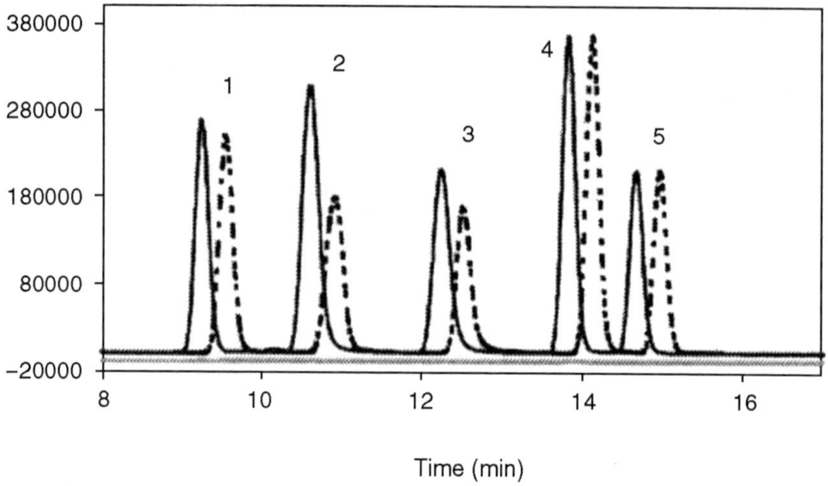

Fig. 14.11 Example of suppression of some pesticides in one injection. Injection of some pesticides at 0.05 mg kg^{-1} (0.125 $\mu g\ ml^{-1}$) in strawberry, overlaid with the same pesticides in methanol and a blank chromatogram of strawberry. Retention time of pesticides in strawberry (- - -) is manually moved 0.3 min, true retention time is identical. Only peak no. 2 and no. 3 are suppressed. ES+/MS/MS. Peak 1: ethiofencarb-sulphoxide; 2: carbendazim; 3: thiabendazole; 4: propoxur; 5: carbaryl. (Reprinted from Jansson *et al.* (2004) with permission from Elsevier).

Tandem mass spectrometry has been applied successfully to determine carbamate and urea residues in food. Matrix suppression/enhancement phenomena are effectively compensated for by using an appropriate calibration technique. Calibration often uses matrix matched standards (i.e. those with a similar matrix composition to that of the analyzed sample; Caballo-López and de Castro, 2003; Goto *et al.*, 2003). Another technique is the use of an internal standard with a retention time identical or similar to that of the analyte. Isotopically labelled internal standards are well suited for this purpose (Jansson *et al.*, 2004; Stöcklein *et al.*, 1998) (Fig. 14.11).

Quadrupole ion trap (QIT) instruments have been applied to study the spectra of phenylurea and carbamates in water using an APCI interface and ionization in PI mode. The ion fragmentation pathways were studied in detail by mass spectrometry (MS), MS^2, MS^3, and MS^4. All compounds were observed as their protonated molecules by MS and in successive fragmentations by MS^n. The structures of typical (diagnostic) product ions were tentatively identified for each class of pesticides. Phenylureas yield an ion at m/z 72 by MS2, corresponding to $[OCN(CH_3)_2]^+$. Carbamates produced $[M+H\text{-}CONCH_3]^+$ fragments by MS^2 from neutral loss of methyl isocyanate.

Applications of QIT to pesticide residues in food are scarce because of the novelty of QIT applied to LC compared with TQ. There is only one application to determine eight polar and unstable pesticides but without any fragmentation. The main disadvantage attributed to QIT is that it suffers from a limited dynamic range. It cannot handle samples in which the ion abundances vary greatly and the range of ion traps is limited (~10^6), when there are too many ions in the trap, space charge effect led to diminished performance. The use of Ion Charge Control (ICC) prevents this problem using automated scans to rapidly count the ions before they go into the trap. This can be a problem when trace elements, particularly in dirty matrices, are analyzed, because the trap fills with both matrix ions (large number) and trace sample ions (very small number). However, results so far show that QIT is a promising alternative to better established techniques.

Capillary electrophoresis coupled to MS or tandem MS/MS is also possible using an electrospray ionization interface. However, it has not been applied to determining carbamates and ureas in real matrices.

14.6 Future trends

Analysis for carbamate and urea residues is likely to improve on many different fronts, but mainly in extraction and determination. New ways should emerge of increasing the speed and efficiency of sample preparation processes, based on automated strategies. There is particular interest in carrying out selective solid-phase extraction (SPE) and clean up procedures. Future studies on sample preparation will concentrate on improving extraction techniques such as accelerated solvent extraction (ASE), microwave-assisted solvent extraction (MASE), matrix-solid-phase dispersion (MSPD), solid-phase extraction (SPE), solid-phase microextraction (SPME) and stir-bar sorptive extraction (SBSE). But one must bear in mind that sample preparation cannot be regarded as a separate step and that coupling the sample-handling techniques with selective detection modes can both simplify them and provide a more powerful analytical procedure.

Liquid chromatography methods have been developed that are suitable for automation and are thus compatible with rapid screening tests, in terms of sample throughput and turnaround time. In addition, the development of LC-MS with API interfaces has undoubtedly contributed to increasing separation efficiency and improving the sensitivities of analytical methods. Recent progress has been made on the mass spectrometry front with the development of tandem mass spectrometry. Triple quadrupole (TQ) and quadrupole ion trap (QIT) can be used for determining pesticide residues in food. However, further development of methods is required to identify unknown carbamate and urea residues. Capillary electrophoretic methods are also seen to have much potential to analyze carbamate and urea residues, but investigations are needed to extend the general applicability of these techniques and expand their use into the field of food analysis.

Although numerous methods have been developed for the direct screening of fruit and vegetables, there is little doubt that the direction being taken is that of increased utilization of biosensor-based assays. These assays are also replacing slower and less specific inhibition assays. However, there will remain a need to support biosensors by reasonably specific isolation and quantification methods that can provide rapid identification and/or degree of confirmation of the analytes. Bioanalytical techniques will be used increasingly for the trace determination of carbamates in food samples. The fact that these analytes inhibit certain class of enzymes (AChEs) must be explored for building new and simpler detectors. The development of approaches based on the coupling of chromatographic separation with biodetection systems is certainly appropriate for consideration in the near future.

New technologies in immunochemistry, chromatography, electrophoresis, and mass spectrometry are emerging rapidly. These, together with the further development in the automation of sample preparation, measurement and data handling, will provide analysts with a unique opportunity for further innovation and improvements to meet the ever-expanding requirements in the analysis of carbamate and urea residues in food products.

14.7 Sources of further information and advice

AHMED FE, 'Analysis of pesticides and their metabolites in foods and drinks' *Trends Anal Chem*, 2001, 20 (11) 649–661.

BERRADA H, MOLTÓ JC, FONT G, 'Determination of urea Pesticide residues in vegetable, soil and water samples' *Crit Rev Anal Chem*, 2003, 33 (1) 19–41.

EUROPEAN COMMISSION, 'Food Safety. Plant Health/Pesticide Safety', in The European Union on-line. http:\\europa.eu.int.

MCGARVEY BD, 'High-performance liquid chromatographic methods for the determination of N-methyl carbamate pesticides in water, soil, plants and air' *J Chromatogr A*, 1993, 640, 89–105.

NUNES GS, BARCELÓ D, 'Analysis of carbamate insecticides in foodstuffs using chromatography and immunoassay techniques' *Trends Anal Chem*, 1999, 18 (2) 99–107.

PATEL PD, '(Bio)sensors for measurement of analytes implicated in food safety: a review' *Trends Anal Chem*, 2002, 21 (2) 96–111.

PICÓ Y, MOLTÓ JC, MAÑES J, FONT G, 'Solid-phase techniques in the extraction of pesticides and related compounds from food and soils' *J Microcol Sep*, 1994, 6, 331–359.

PICÓ Y, FONT G, MOLTÓ JC, MAÑES J, 'Pesticide residue determination in fruit and vegetables by liquid chromatography-mass spectrometry' *J Chromatogr A*, 2000, 882, 153–173.

PICÓ Y, RODRÍGUEZ R, MAÑES J, 'Capillary electrophoresis for the determination of pesticide residues' *Trends Anal Chem*, 2003, 22 (3) 133–151.

PICÓ Y, BLASCO C, FONT G, 'Environmental and food application of LC-tandem mass spectrometry in pesticide residue analyis. An overview' *Mass Spectrom Rev*, 2004, 23, 45–85.

TADEO JL, SÁNCHEZ-BRUNETE C, PÉREZ RA, FERNÁNDEZ MD, 'Analysis of herbicide residues in cereals, fruits and vegetables' *J Chromatogr A*, 882 (2000) 175–191.

TORRES CM, PICÓ Y, MAÑES J, 'Determination of pesticide residues in fruit and vegetables' *J Chromatogr A*, 754 (1–2) 301–331.

14.8 References

ABAD A, MORENO MJ, MONTOYA A (1998), 'Hapten synthesis and production of monoclonal antibodies to the N-methylcarbamate pesticide methiocarb', *J Agric Food Chem*, 46, 2417–2426.

ABAD A, MORENO MJ, MONTOYA A (1999), 'Development of monoclonal antibody-based immunoassays to the N-methylcarbamate pesticide carbofuran', *J Agric Food Chem*, 47, 2475–2485.

ABAD A, MORENO MJ, PELEGRÍ R, MARTÍNEZ MI, SÁEZ A, GAMÓN M, MONTOYA A (2003), 'Determination of carbaryl, carbofuran and methiocarb in cucumbers and strawberries by monoclonal enzyme immunoassays and high-performance liquid chromatography with fluorescence detection – An analytical comparison', *J Chromatogr A*, 833, 3–12.

AHMED FE (2001), 'Analysis of pesticides and their metabolites in foods and drinks', *Tends Anal Chem*, 20, 649–661.

AVRAMESCU A, ANDREESCU S, NOGUER T, BALA C, ANDREESCU D, MARTY JL (2002), 'Biosensors designed for environmental and food quality control based on screen-printed graphite electrodes with different configurations', *Anal Bioanal Chem*, 374, 25–32.

BACHMANN TT, LECA B, VILATTE F, MARTY JL, FOURNIER D, SCHMID RD (2000), 'Improve multianalyte detection of organophosphates and carbamates with disposible multi-electrode biosensors using recombinants mutants of Drosophila acetylcholinesterase and artifical neutral networks', *Biosens. & Bioelectron.*, 15, 193–201.

BALINOVA A (1998), 'Multiresidue determination of pesticides in plants by high-performance liquid chromatography following gel permeation chromatography', *J Chromatogr A*, 823, 11–16.

BALTUSSEN E, CRAMERS CA, SANDRA PJF (2003), 'Sorptive sample preparation – a review', *Anal Bioanal Chem*, 373, 3–22.

BARKER SA (2000), 'Applications of matrix solid-phase dispersion in food analysis', *J Chromatogr A*, 880, 63–68.

BARKER SA (2003), 'Matrix solid-phase dispersion', *J Chromatogr A*, 885, 115–127.

BELTRÁN J, LÓPEZ FJ, HERNÁNDEZ F (2000), 'Solid-phase microextraction in pesticide residue analysis. Review', *J Chromatogr A*, 885, 389–404.

BERRADA H, MOLTÓ JC, FONT G (2001), 'Gas chromatography behaviour of urea herbicides', *Chromatographia*, 54, 360–364.

BERRADA H, FONT G, MOLTÓ JC (2003a), 'Determination of urea pesticide residues in vegetables, soil, and water samples', *Crit Rev Anal Chem*, 33, 19–41.

BERRADA H, MOLTÓ JC, FONT G (2003b), 'Influence of the solvent on the gas chromatographic behaviour of urea herbicides', *Chromatographia*, 54, 253–262.

BESTER K, BORDIN G, RODRÍGUEZ A, SCHIMMEL H, PAUWELS J, VANVYNCHT G (2001), 'How to overcome matrix effect in the determination of pesticides in fruit by HPLC-ESI-MS-MS', *Fresenius J Anal Chem*, 371, 550–555.

BLASCO C, FERNÁNDEZ M, PICÓ Y, FONT G, MAÑES J (2002a), 'Simultaneous determination of imidacloprid, carbendazim, methiocarb and hexythiazox in peaches and nectarines by liquid chromatography-mass spectrometry', *Anal Chim Acta*, 461, 109–116.

BLASCO C, FONT G, PICÓ Y (2002b), 'Comparison of microextraction procedures to determine pesticides in oranges by liquid-chromatography-mass spectrometry', *J Chromatogr A*, 970, 212.

CABALLO-LÓPEZ A, DE CASTRO MI (2003), 'Continuous ultrasound-assisted extraction coupled to on-line filtration-solid-phase extraction-column liquid chromatography post column derivatisation-fluorescence detection', *J Chromatogr A*, 998, 51–59.

CAO CF, WANG Z, URRUTY L, POMMIER JJ, MONTURY M (2003), 'Focused microwave assistance for extracting some pesticide residues from strawberries into water before their determination by SPME/HPLC/DAD', *J Agric Food Chem*, 49, 5092–5097.

DA SILVA CL, DE LIMA EC, TAVARES MFM (2003), 'Investigation of preconcentration strategies for the trace analysis of multi-residue pesticide in real samples by capillary electrophoresis', *J Chromatogr A*, 1014, 109–116.

DEL CARLO M, MASCINI M, PEPE A, DILETTI G, COMPAGNONE D (2004), 'Screening of food samples for carbamate and organophosphate pesticides using an electrochemical bioassay', *Food Chem*, 84, 651–656.

DELGADO MJ, BARROSO SR, FERNáNDEZ-TOSTADO GT, POLO-DíEZ LM (2001), 'Stability studies of carbamate pesticides and analysis by gas chromatography with flame ionization and nitrogen-phosphorus detection', *J Chromatogr A*, 921, 287–296.

ESCUDEROS-MORENAS ML, SANTOS-DELGADO MJ, RUBIO-BARROSO S, POLO-DíEZ LM (2003), 'Direct determination of monolinuron, linuron and chlorbromuron residues in potato samples by gas chromatography with nitrogen-phosphorus detection', *J Chromatogr A*, 1011, 143–145.

FERNÁNDEZ M, PICÓ Y, MAÑES J (2000), 'Determiantion of carbamate residues in fruit and vegetables by matrix solid-phase dispersion and liquid chromatography-mass spectrometry', *J Chromatogr A*, 871, 43–56.

GOTO T, ITO Y, OKA H, SAITO I, MATSUMOTO H, NAKAZAWA H (2003), 'Simple and rapid determination of N-methylcarbamate pesticides in citrus fruits by electrospray ionization tandem mass spectrometry', *Anal Chim Acta*, 487, 201–209.

HERRERA MC, PRADOS-ROSALES JL, LUQUE-GARCÍA JL, LUQUE DE CASTRO MD (2002), 'Static-dynamic pressurized hot water extraction coupled to on-line filtration-solid-phase extraction-high performance liquid chromatography-post-column derivatization-fluorescence detection for the analysis of N-methylcarbamates in foods', *Anal Chim Acta*, 463, 187–197.

HOGENBOOM AC, HOFMAN MP, KOK SJ, NIESSEN WMA, BRINKMAN UATH (2000), 'Determination of pesticides in vegetables using large-volume injection column liquid chromatography-electrospray tandem mass spectrometry', *J Chromatogr A*, 892, 379–390.

HOGENDOORN E, VAN ZOONEN P (2000), 'Recent and future developments of liquid chromatography in pesticide trace analysis', *J Chromatogr A*, 892, 435–453.

JANSSON C, PIHLSTRÖM T, ÖSTERDAHL BG, MARKIDES KE (2004), 'A new multiresidue method for analysis of pesticide residues in fruit and vegetables using liquid chromatography with tandem mass spectrometric detection', *J Chromatogr A*, 1023, 93–104.

JEONG ML, CHESNEY DJ (2003), 'Determination of N-methylcarbamate pesticides from spiked matrices using supercritical fluid extraction', *Anal Chim Acta*, 389, 53–57.

KATSOUDAS E, ABDELMESSEH HH (2000), 'Enzyme inhibition and enzyme-linked immunosorbent assay methods for carbamate pesticide residue analysis in fresh produce', *J Food Protec*, 63, 1758–1760.

KOBLIZEK M, MALY J, MASOJIDEK J, KOMENDA J, KUCERA T, GIARDI MT, MATTOO AK, PILLOTON R (2002), 'A biosensor for the detection of triazine and phenylurea herbicides designed using Photosystem II coupled to a screen printed electrode', *Biotechnol. & Bioeng.*, 78, 110–116.

LACASSIE E, DREYFUSS MF, DAGUET JL, VIGNAUD M, MARQUET P, LACHATRE G (1999), 'Liquid chromatography-electrospray mass spectrometry multiresidue determination of pesticides in apples and pears', *J Chromatogr A*, 830, 135–143.

MALLART E, BARCEN C, ABUKNESHA R, GAUGLITZ G, BARCELÓ D (2001), 'Part per trillion level determination of isoproturon in certified and estuarine water samples with a direct optical immunosensor', *Anal Chim Acta*, 426, 209–216.

MARTÍNEZ.GALERA M, LÓPEZ-LÓPEZ T, GIL-GARCíA-M.D., MARTÍNEZ-VIDAL JL, VÁZQUEZ PP (2001), 'Determination of benzoylureas in tomato by high-performance liquid chromatography using continuous on-line post-elution photoirradiation with fluorescence detection', *J Chromatogr A*, 918, 79–85.

MASTOVSKA K, LEHOTAY SJ, HASLOVA J (2001), 'Optimization and evaluation of low-pressure gas chromatography-mass spectrometry for the fast analysis of multiple pesticide residues in a food commodity', *J Chromatogr A*, 926, 291–308.

MILIADIS GE, TSIROPOULOS NG, APLADA-SARLIS PG (1999), 'High-performance liquid chromatographic determination of benzoylurea insecticides residues in grapes and wine using liquid and solid-phase extraction', *J Chromatogr A*, 835, 113–120.

MORENO M, ABAD A, MONTOYA A (2001), 'Production of monoclonal antibodies to the N-methylcarbamate pesticide propoxur', *J Agric Food Chem*, 49, 72–78.

NUNES GS, BARCELÓ D (1998a), 'Electrochemical biosensor for pesticide determination in food samples', *Analusis*, 26, M156–M159.

NUNES GS, MARCO MP, RIBEIRO ML, BARCELÓ D (1998b), 'Validation of an immunoassay method for the determination of traces of carbaryl in vegetable and fruit extracts by liquid chromatography with photodiode array and mass spectrometry detection', *J Chromatogr A*, 823, 109–120.

NUNES GS, RIBEIRO ML, POLESE L, BARCELÓ D (1998c), 'Comparison of different clean up procedures for the determination of N-methylcarbamate insecticides in vegetable matrice by high-performance liquid chromatography with UV detection', *J Chromatogr A*, 795, 43–51.

NUNES GS, SKLADAL P, YAMANAKA H, BARCELÓ D (1998d), 'Determination of carbamate residues in crop samples by cholinesterase-base biosensors and chromatographic techniques', *Anal Chim Acta*, 362, 59–68.

NUNES GS, BARCELÓ D (1999a), 'Analysis of carbamate insecticides in foodstuffs using chromatography and immunoassay techniques', *Tends Anal Chem*, 18, 99–107.

NUNES GS, BARCELÓ D, GRABARIC BS, DÍAZ-CRUZ MJ, RIBEIRO ML (1999b), 'Evaluation of a highly sensitive amperometric biosensor with low cholinesterase charge immobilized on a chemically modified carbon paste electrode for trace determination of carbamates in fruit, vegetable and water samples', *Anal Chim Acta*, 399, 37–49.

NUNES GS, ALONSO RM, RIBEIRO ML, BARCELÓ D (2000), 'Determination of aldicarb, aldicarb sulfoxide and aldicarb sulfone in some fruits and vegetables using high-performance liquid chromatography-atmospheric pressure chemical ionization mass spectrometry', *J Chromatogr A*, 888, 113–120.

OKIHASHI M, OBANA H, HORI S (1998), 'Determination of N-methylcarbamate pesticides in foods using accelerated solvent extraction with a mini-column cleanup', *Analyst*, 123, 714.

PANTIRU M, TSIAKATOURAS G, MARTENS D, OCHSENKÜHN M, KETTRUP A (2003), 'Development of clean up methods for determining carbamates and acidic pesticides in agricultural products', *Fresenius Environ Bull*, 12, 871–875.

PATEL PD (2002), '(Bio)sensor for measumerement of analytes implicates in food safety: a review', *Tends Anal Chem*, 21, 96–115.

PERRET D, GENTILI A, MARCHESE S, SERGI M, D'ASCENZO G (2002), 'Validation of a method for the determination of multiclass pesticide residues in fruit juices by liquid chromatography/tandem mass spectrometry after extraction by matrix solid-phase dispersion', *J AOAC Int*, 85, 724–730.

PICÓ Y, FONT G, MOLTÓ JC, MAÑES J (2000), 'Pesticide residue determination in fruit and vegetables by liquid chromatography-mass spectrometry', *J Chromatogr A*, 882, 153–173.

PICÓ Y, RODRÍGUEZ A, MAÑES J (2003), 'Capillary electrophoresis for the determination of pesticide residues', *Tends Anal Chem*, 22, 133–151.

PICÓ Y, BLASCO C, FONT G (2004), 'Environmental and food applications of LC-tandem mass spectrometry in pesticide residue analysis. An overview', *Mass Spectrom Rev*, 23, 45–85.

POGACNIK L, FRANKO M (1999), 'Determination of organophosphate and carbamate pesticides in spiked samples of tap water and fruit juices by a biosensor with photothermal detection', *Biosens. & Bioelectron.*, 14, 569–578.

PULIDO-TOFINO P, BARROSO-MORENO JM, PÉREZ-CONDE MC (2000), 'Flow-through fluoroimmunosensor for isoproturon determination in agricultural foodstuff – Evaluation of antibody immobilization on solid support', *Anal Chim Acta*, 417, 85–94.

PULIDO-TOFINO P, BARRERO-MORENO JM, PÉREZ-CONDE MC (2001), 'Sol-gel glass doped with isoproturon antibody as selective support for the development of a flow-through fluoroimmunosensor', *Anal Chim Acta*, 429, 337–345.

RODRÍGUEZ R, PICÓ Y, FONT G, MAÑES J (2001), 'Determination of urea-derived pesticides in fruits and vegetables by solid-phase preconcentration and capillary electrophoresis', *Electrophoresis*, 22, 2010–2016.

SAWAYA WN, AL-AWADI FA, SAEED T, AL-OMAIR A, AHMAD N, HUSAIN A, KHALAFAWI S, AL-OMIRAH H, DASHTI B, AL-AMIRI H, AL-SAQER J (1999), 'Kuwait's total diet study: dietary intake of organochlorine, carbamate, benzimidazole and phenylurea pesticide residues', *J AOAC Int*, 82, 1458–1465.

SCHULTZE H, SCHMID RD, BACHMANN TT (2002a), 'Rapid detection of neurotoxic insecticides in food using disposable acetylcholinesterase-biosensors and simple solvent extraction', *Anal Bioanal Chem*, 372, 268–272.

SCHULTZE H, SCHERBAUM E, ANASTASSIDES M, VORLOVA S, SCHIMD RD, BACHMAN TT (2002b), 'Development, validation, and application of an acetylcholinesterase-biosensor test for the direct detection of insecticide residues in infant food', *Biosens. & Bioelectron.*, 17, 1095–1105.

SOLEAS GJ, YAN J, NOM K, GOLDBERG DM (2000), 'Multiresidue analysis of seventeen pesticides in wine by gas chromatography with mass-selective detection', *J Chromatogr A*, 882, 205–212.

STAN HJ (2000), 'Pesticide residue analysis in foodstuffs applying capillary gas chromatography with mass spectrometry detection. State-off the art use of modified DFG-multimethod S19 and automated data evaluation', *J Chromatogr A*, 892, 347–377.

STÖCKLEIN WFM, WARSINKE A, MICHEEL B, KEMPTER G, HÖHNE W, SCHELLER FW (1998), 'Diphenylurea hapten sensing with a monoclonal antibody and its FAB fragment: Kinetic and thermodynamic investigation', *Anal Chim Acta*, 362, 101–111.

STÖCKLEIN WFM, ROHDE M, SCHARTE G, BEHRSING O, WARSINKE A, MICHEEL B, SCHELLER FW (2000), 'Sensitive detection of triazine and phenylurea pesticides in pure organic solvent by enzyme linked immunosorbent assay (ELISA): stabilities, solubilities and sensitivities', *Anal Chim Acta*, 405, 255–265.

STUART IA, ANSELL RO, MCLACHLAN J, BATHER PA (1999), 'Surface partitioning studies of N-methylcarbamate-treated post-harvest crops using SFE-HPLV-post column reaction fluorescence', *Analyst*, 124, 275–280.

TAYLOR MJ, HUNTER K, HUNTER KB, LINDSAY D, LE BOUHELLEC S (2002), 'Multi-residue method for rapid screening and confirmation of pesticides in crude extracts of fruits and vegetables using isocratic liquid chromatography with electrospray tandem mass spectrometry', *J Chromatogr A*, 982, 225–236.

THURMAN EM, FERRER I, BARCELÓ D (2001), 'Choosing between atmospheric pressure chemical ionization and electrospray ionization interfaces for the HPLC/MS analysis of pesticides', *Anal Chem*, 73, 5441–5449.

TSIROPOULOS NG, APLADA-SARLIS PG, MILIADIS GE (1999), 'Determination of benzoylurea insecticides in apples and pears by solid-phase extraction and liquid chromatography with UV detection', *J AOAC Int*, 82, 213–216.

VALENZUELA AI, LORENZINI R, REDONDO MJ, FONT G (1999), 'Matrix solid-phase dispersion microextraction and determination by high-performance liquid chromatography with UV detection of pesticide residues in citrus fruit', *J Chromatogr A*, 839, 101–107.

VALENZUELA AI, PICÓ Y, FONT G (2000), 'Liquid chromatography/atmospheric pressure chemical ionization-mass spectrometry analysis of benzoylurea insecticides in citrus fruits', *Rapid Commun Mass Spectrom*, 14, 572–577.

VALENZUELA AI, PICÓ Y, FONT G (2001), 'Determination of five pesticide residues in oranges by matrix solid-phase dispersion and liquid chromatography to estimate daily intake of consumers', *J AOAC Int*, 84, 901–909.

VAN DER HOFF GR, VAN ZOONEN P (1999), 'Trace analysis of pesticides by gas chromatography', *J Chromatogr A*, 843, 301–322.

VELASCO-GARCÍA MN, MOTTRAM T (2003), 'Biosensors technology addressing agricultural problems [Review]', *Biosyst. Eng.*, 84, 1–12.

VOLANTE M, PONTELO M, VALOTI L, CATTANEO M, BIANCHI M, COLZANI L (2000), 'Application of solid phase micro-extraction (SPME) to the analysis of pesticide residues in vegetables', *Pest Manag Sci*, 56, 618–636.

VOLMER DA (1998), 'Investigation of photochemical behaviour of pesticides in a photolysis reactor coupled on-line with liquid chromatography electrospray ionization tandem mass spectrometry system. Application to trace a confirmatory analysis in food', *J Chromatogr A*, 794, 129–146.

WANG Z, HENNION B, URRUTY L, MONTURY M (2000), 'Solid-phase microextraction coupled with high performance liquid chromatography: a complementary technique to solid-phase microextraction-gas chromatography for the analysis of pesticide residues in strawberries', *Food Add Contam*, 17, 915.

WU J, TRAGAS C, LORD H, PAWLISZYN J (2002), 'Analysis of polar pesticides in water and wine samples by automated in-tube solid-phase microextraction coupled with high-performance liquid chromatography-mass spectrometry', *J Chromatogr A*, 976, 357–367.

XAVIER MP, VALLEJO B, MARAZUELA MD, MORENO-BONDI MC, FALAI A (2000), 'Fiber optic monitoring of carbamate pesticides using porous glass with covalent bound chlorophenol red', *Biosens. & Bioelectron.*, 14, 895–905.

YINON J, VINCZE A (1997), 'Collision-induced dissociation (CID) processes in some carbamate and phenylurea pesticides', *Int J Mass Spectrom Ion Proc*, 167/168, 21–33.

ZROSTLIKOVA J, HAJSLOVA J, POUTSKA J, BEGANY P (2002), 'Alternative calibration approaches to compensate the effect of co-extracted matrix components in liquid chromatography-electrospray ionisation tandem mass spectrometry analysis of pesticide residues in plant materials', *J Chromatogr A*, 973, 13–26.

15

Detecting fungicide residues

M. M. Sheehan, H. Berney and A. Mathewson, University College Cork, Ireland

15.1 Introduction

This chapter provides the reader with an overview of fungicides, their use and their impact as contaminants in the environment and the food chain. The analytical methods that are currently in use for the detection of fungicides are described as well as the development of immunoassay methods. The new and emerging detection technologies are presented, the factors that are considered when developing a detection system for fungicide determination are highlighted, as well as predictions and comments on future trends in this sector.

15.1.1 What is a fungicide?

Fungicide is the term given to chemicals or a mixture of chemicals that are used to kill fungi (Table 15.1). They belong to the broad category of pesticides, which can be any chemical substance with biocidal properties against any organism considered a 'pest' including, insects, rodents and weeds. Apart from fungicides, other members of the pesticide family encompass herbicides, insecticides, rodenticides, germicides. Pesticides are most commonly used in accepted agricultural practices. The administering of fungicides to agricultural crops protects against or remedies infections caused by a variety of fungal diseases (Table 15.2). Failure to control such diseases may result in reduced crop yields and ultimately serious economic consequences for the producer and associated macroeconomics. However, the agrifood industry is not exclusive in its employment of fungicides. Materials such as textiles, paper, leather and wood are impregnated with fungicides which are also painted onto masonry and plaster to preserve these materials against spoilage or rot caused by fungal growth.

Table 15.1 Characteristics of some commonly used fungicides

IUPAC name	Common chemical name	Trade name	Plant type	Protects against	Manufacturer[a]	Chemical structure
4,6-dichloro-*N*-(2-chlorophenyl)-1,3,5-triazin-2-amine	Anilazine	Daconil Dyrene, Lescorene	turfgrass	dollar spot, leaf spot, brown patch, anthracnose, stem rust, grey snow mould	ISK Biotech	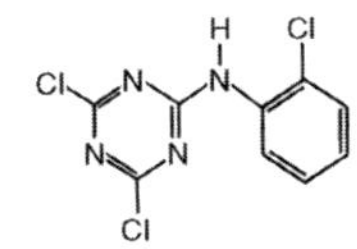
N-(trichloromethylthio) cyclohex-4-ene-1,2-dicarboximide	Captan	Captan, Orthocide50	turfgrass vegetables fruit seed	brown patch, leafspot late blight, leaf blight downy mildew decay, damping-off		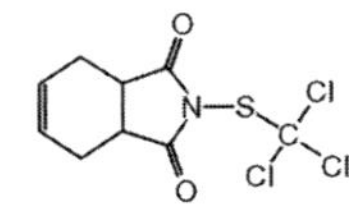
	Chlorothalonil		fruit vegetables	blossom blight, brown rot, freckle, shot hole, stone fruit rust, transit rot, bunch rot, downy mildew, leaf curl	Bayer	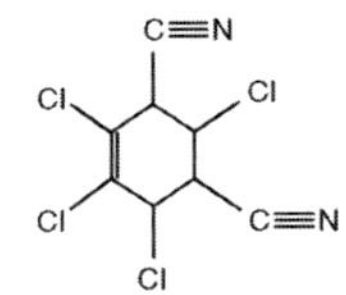
tetrachloroisophthalonitrile 1-(2-cyano-2-methoxyiminoacetyl)-3-ethylurea	cymoxanil	Curzate 60DF Sygan, and Syphal	seeds, fruit, vegetables	grey mould, leaf spot, leaf speckle, leaf blight, late blight chocolate, spot rust, anthracnose, grey mould downy mildew, leafspot phytophthora infestans, plasmopara, and peronospora	DuPont	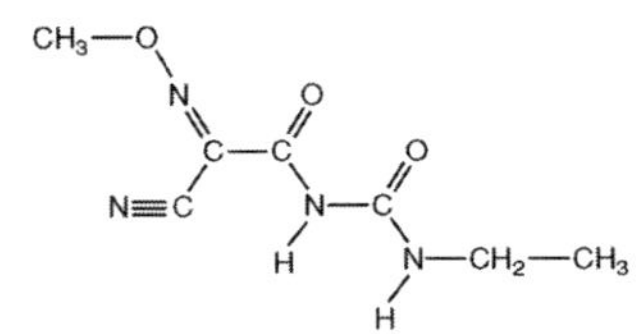

Table 15.1 Continued

IUPAC name	Common chemical name	Trade name	Plant type	Protects against	Manufacturer[a]	Chemical structure
(*RS*)-3-anilino-5-methyl-5-(4-phenoxyphenyl)-1,3-oxazolidine-2,4-dione	Famoxadone	Famoxate	vegetables fruit	late and early light blue mould, downy mildew, leaf spot	DuPont	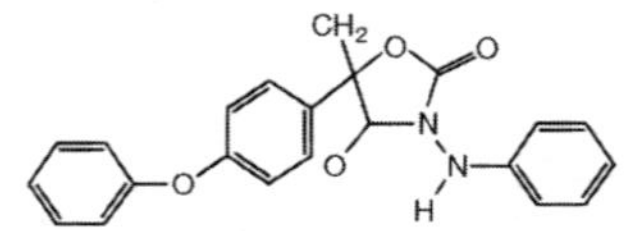
iron(III) dimethyldithiocarbamate	Ferbam	Carbomate, Ferbam Fermate	vegetables	late blight, leaf blight, downy mildew		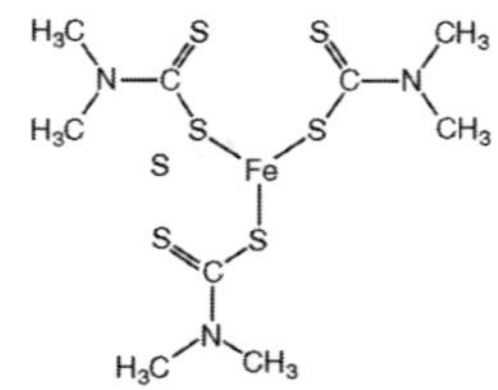
(*RS*)-1-(*β*-allyloxy-2,4-dichlorophenylethyl) imidazole	Imazalil	Bromazil, Deccozil, Fungaflor	fruit, vegetables ornamentals	powdery mildew, black spot	Janssen Pharmaceutica	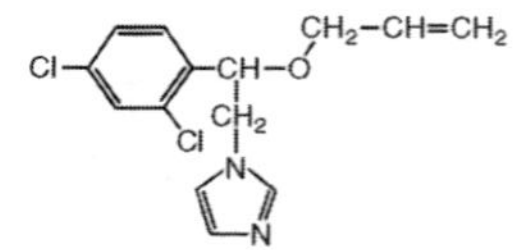
(*RS*)-2-(4-chlorophenyl)-2-(1*H*-1,2,4-triazol-1-ylmethyl)hexanenitrile)	Myclobutanil	Eagle, Mycloss	fruit ornamentals	powdery mildew black spot, mildew, rust	Dow Agrosciences, Bayer Cropscience	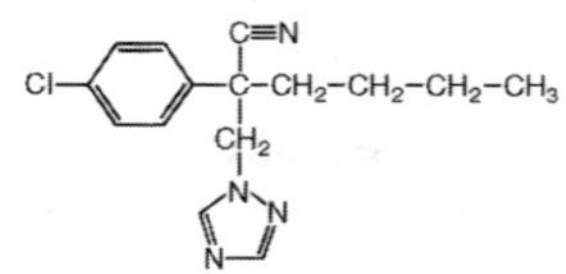

		Dowicide EC-7,	Wood	rot	Chapman Chemical	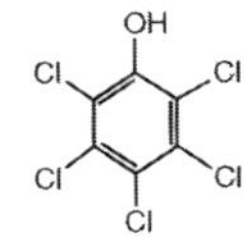
Pentachlorophenol 2-(thiazol-4-yl) benzimidazole	Thiabendazole (TBZ)	Tobaz, Apl-Luster, Arbotect, Mertect, Mycozol, TBZ, Tecto, and Thibenzole	fruit	blue mould, grey mould, brown rot, stem end rot	Merck	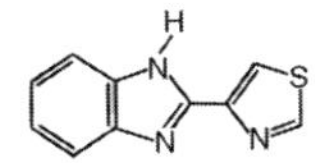
			vegetable	leaf spot, black rot, dry rot, pod and stem blight		
			ornamentals	brown spot, frog eye leaf spot, purple seed stain		
			seeds	seedling blight, seed rot		
tetramethylthiuram disulfide, TMTD	thiram	Defiant, thiram	turfgrass	Leaf spot, brown patch, damping off, dollar spot, fusarium patch.	Barmac	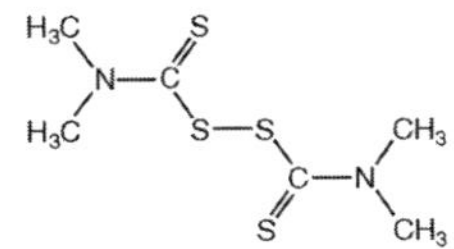
			fruit	black spot, target spot, ripe spot, brown rot, freckles, shot hole, black spot, grey mould		
			vegetables	damping off, septoria leaf spot, anthracnose		
			ornamentals	black spot, septoria spot, grey mould, fire		
			seed	decay, damping-off		

Table 15.1 Continued

IUPAC name	Common chemical name	Trade name	Plant type	Protects against	Manufacturer[a]	Chemical structure
cis-trans-1-[2-(2,4-dichlorophenyl)-4-propyl-1,3-dioxolan-2-ylmethyl]-1*H*-1,2,4-triazole	propiconazole	Banner	vegetables	dollar spot, grey leafy spot, leaf spot		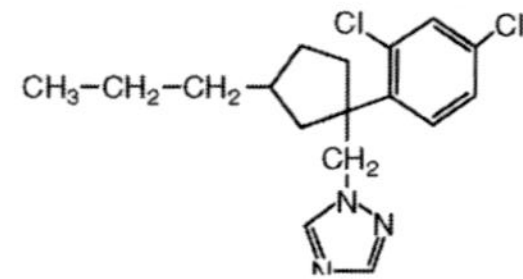
zinc ethylenebis(dithiocarbamate)	zineb	Dithane Z-78, Parzate, Zineb	turfgrass	leafspot	Barmac	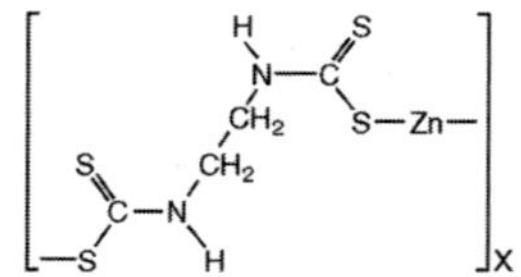

[a] *Note*: Many manufacturers produce these compounds, individual examples are given

Table 15.2 Fungal diseases and causative pathogens

Disease	Pathogen
Anthracnose	*Marssonina panattoniana*
Anthracnose, black spot	*Colletotrichum acutatum*
Basal rot, dry rot, Fusarium Patch	*Fusarium* sp.
Black spot	*Diplocarpon rosae*
Blue mould	*Penicillium* sp.
Brown patch	*Rhizoctonia solani*
Brown rot	*Monilinia fructicola*
Damping off	*Pythium* sp.
Dollar spot	*Sclerotinia homoeocarpa*
Dollar spot	*Sclerotinia* sp.
Fire	*Botrytis tulipae*
Freckles	*Venturia carpophila*
Grey leafy spot	*Pyricularia* sp.
Grey mould	*Botrytsis cinerea*
Grey snow mould	*Typhula* sp.
Leaf blight	*Alternaria dauci*
Leaf spot	*Cercospora*
Leaf spot	*Helminthosporium* sp.
Seedling blight	*Asochyta*
Septoria spot, damping off, leaf spot	*Septoria* sp.
Shot hole	*Stigimina carpophila*
Target and ripe spot	*Pezicula* sp.
Transit rot	*Rhizopus stolonifer*

The widespread use of fungicides for the variety of intended applications has meant that unintended interactions in the environment have also occurred. Traces of fungicides and evidence of fungicidal interactions have been reported in soil, water, air, food products, aquatic life, terrestrial wildlife and humans.

15.1.2 Impact of fungicides on human and animal health

Certain fungicides are known to be carcinogenic, teratogenic, mutagenic and/or goitrogenic, and it has been widely reported since the 1950s that a number of pesticides exert hormone-like effects (Colburn *et al.,* 1993). This hormone mimicry causes serious disruption to the reproductive and endocrine systems by mimicking or antagonising the effects of endogenous hormones and also by altering the synthesis or metabolism of these hormones and their receptors. Indeed, blame is being given to fungicides and other compounds that are foreign to human metabolism for the increase in incidence of breast and testicular cancers and diminishing sperm counts, conditions which are prevalent among industrialised nations (Gwereman *et al.,* 1993; Sharpe and Kekkebaek, 1993; Wolff *et al.,* 1993; Shukla *et al.,* 1996). The degradation products of the ethylene bis (dithiocarbamate) fungicides are known to be carcinogenic and teratogenic (IARC, 1987). Mercaptobenzothiazole, a mercury-containing compound used as a fungicide, is known to cause liver and kidney damage.

The toxic effects of fungicides are presented to humans and animals by exposure to contaminated food or water supplies. There is a lack of hard data in the wide area of pesticides in foods, and there are many bottlenecks in assessing toxicological effects, mainly because of a lack of sensitive methodologies.

15.1.3 Standards governing use of fungicides

Strict international standards for the use of fungicides in food production for all nations are set out by the United Nations (UN) Codex Alimentarius Commission, created jointly by the World Health Organisation (WHO) and the Food and Agriculture Organization (FAO). Codex has established Maximum Residue Limits (MRL) for over 195 active ingredients that aid in fixing standards for use of residues in food production. Fungicide use is controlled by national organisations and pesticide registration activities.

The European Union (EU) policy on fungicide use is controlled by EU Directive 91/414, which states that the safe use of pesticides must be demonstrated. Of the 840 active substances on the EU market in 1993, the European Commission (EC) decided to withdraw 348 in July 2003; a further 80 may be withdrawn thereafter. An EC proposal was submitted to the European Council and the European Parliament on 14 March 2003 to revise the existing legislation on this topic and to incorporate the expertise of the European Food Safety Authority. An EU-wide pesticide monitoring programme has been in operation since 1996 to ensure MRL legislation compliance and the monitoring of exposure levels; findings have shown that both fungicides and insecticides are the most commonly detected residues in foods (Food and Veterinary Office, EC). Information regarding food products which are found to exceed MRLs is made available to Member States through the rapid alert system.

In the United States, fungicides must be registered under the Federal Insecticide, Fungicide and Rodenticide Act (FIFRA), under which law there are 21,000 pesticide products and 860 active ingredients registered. There are three federal agencies that share responsibilities over the use and regulations of pesticides; the Environmental Protection Agency (EPA), US Department of Agriculture (USDA) and the Food and Drug Administration (FDA). The FDA conducts a monitoring program which is based on the EPA pesticide registrations. The USDA monitors and regulates imported foods, interstate food movements and all meat, poultry and egg products. The FDA Monitoring Program consists of an incidence/level monitoring and a Total Diet Study, the level of pesticides found are used in conjunction with USDA food consumption data to estimate the dietary intake of pesticide residues. Further information is provided in Chapter 12.

15.1.4 Fungicide monitoring techniques

The detection of fungicide residues and their metabolic derivatives in biological fluids from humans and animals, mainly blood and urine, gives reliable indications of exposure levels to fungicides. Analytical procedures for monitoring occupational exposure levels mostly include Gas Chromatography-Mass Spectroscopy (GC-MS) and High Performance Liquid Chromatography (HPLC). The development of a number of bioassays has also been reported. The methodologies are broad and are based mainly on monitoring the response of a biological entity (enzyme activity, cell viability) upon exposure to a suspect sample in order to elucidate any toxicological properties (mutagenic, genotoxic, etc.) of the active substance.

Cytotoxicity assays have been used to determine the effect of dithiocarbamate (DTC) fungicides on tissue cultured cells. Perocco *et al.* (1995) used BALB/c cells and found dramatic impacts of zineb on cell clonal efficiency. Soloneski *et al.* (2002) have been evaluating the effect of commercial formulations of DTC fungicides, zineb and azzurro, on cultures of CHO cells (Chinese hamster ovary) using highly sensitive *in vitro* genotoxicity studies. They report a high dose-related cytotoxicity for the fungicides, for doses greater than 50 μg/ml. Cereser *et al.* (2001) showed the cytotoxicity of thiram (tetramethylthiuram disulfide, TMTD) using human skin fibroblasts. Concentrations of 5 mg/ml were shown to cause 100% cell death. Bioassays following the effect of the fungicides maneb and mancozeb on the synthesis of bacterial enzymes β-galactosidase and α-amylase were used by Guven *et al.* (2003). As a screening method for biosynthesis, the amylase assay was sensitive to exposure levels as low as 0.1 ppm, whereas β-galactosidase synthesis was not inhibited until the cells were exposed to fungicide concentrations higher than 100 ppm. Another cell-based assay, CALUX (chemical activated luciferase expression), has proved useful for the determination of a variety of polyhalogenated chemical residues used in diverse applications. The benzimidazole group of fungicides was included in initial assay development and their detection is possible using the CALUX assay (Hoogenboom *et al.*, 1999).

The assessment of the impact of fungicidal residues on human health in particular involves the consideration of a number of complex parameters. One recent report, evaluates the impact of fungicides on human health and ecosystems (Margni *et al.*, 2002). The impact on human health is assessed by considering different routes of exposure; by inhalation, ingestion of food and of water. The estimation is based on amounts of pollutants transferred to air, soil and water and the likely amounts absorbed by the human body (e.g. from foods). Their findings suggest that the toxicological impact of the residue chlorothalonil is 30 times higher when ingested in contaminated foods than the effect induced by inhalation, and 5 times higher than that from drinking water. There is, however, consistent variation in calculating the transfer of residues to foods.

15.2 Conventional techniques and immunoassays for detecting fungicide residues

There is a range of sensitive and specific methods for the determination and quantification of chemicals, such as fungicides, from various sources, including food products. Improvements in analytical methods have impacted on the increase in reported cases of pesticide contamination in foods. Chromatography is the most widely used method for the analytical detection of active ingredients. Methods generally encompass different steps; liquid-liquid extraction followed by preconcentration and gas chromatography (GC), gas liquid chromatography (GLC) or high performance liquid chromatography (HPLC). Briefly, GLC separation is based on separation due to differences in distribution of analytes between the mobile and stationary phases and involves interaction between the gas and liquid phases. However, it is restricted to analytes that can be vaporised without degradation. HPLC offers alternative formats for separating analytes based on chemical or physical characteristics. There are three main components necessary for HPLC: a high-pressure pump, a microparticle phase column and a detector. UV detectors are the most commonly used detectors for fungicide analysis, although recently developed photoconductivity and electrochemical detectors show potential for this application. An alternative use of either GLC or HPLC permits the employment of pesticide multi-residue methods (MRM) to simultaneously determine more than one residue in one single analysis. Multi-class MRMs add functionality when a single extract is analysed with more than one chromatographic determinative step, thus providing maximum coverage of residues in different classes. This is the approach used when a sample of unknown residue composition is to be analysed.

All of these techniques are routine in suitably accredited laboratories and are well established. But they require tedious sample pre-treatment steps involving clean-up or extraction methods, expensive instruments and highly trained personnel for operation in specialised laboratories. The preparation and execution methods themselves are complicated and very labour intensive. Trends in micro-Total Analysis Systems offer a rapid alternative to existing macroscale methods. The miniaturisation of many cumbersome and expensive chemical analytical tools such as HPLC, capillary electrophoresis and gas chromatography has been reported. The manufacturing cost of these devices is significantly reduced due to the high volume fabrication processes adopted from the semiconductor industry. Often, smaller sample volumes are required thereby scaling down extraction procedures and reagents. Multifunctional integrated devices are possible using these technologies and certain less complicated sample extraction methodologies may be incorporated in an integrated device.

15.2.1 Immunoassay technology in fungicide determination

The first immunoassay systems were mainly radioimmunoassays, using radioactive ligands, which were soon followed by ELISA (enzyme linked immunosorbent assay). The first main application of immunoassays was the detection of biochemical indicators of disease (Voller *et al.,* 1976). The value of applying immunoassays for the detection of many compounds, including pesticides, has been recognised and the development of immunoassays for the detection of fungicide residues has been reported since the early 1980s (Newsome and Shields, 1981; Wie *et al.,* 1982; Wie and Hammock, 1982; Schwalbe *et al*., 1984; Huber and Hock, 1985).

The critical component for any immunoassay is the antibody which is used to 'recognise' the chemical analyte, for example a fungicide. Antibodies can be produced to recognise single chemical compounds or groups of similar compounds. Specific antibodies are generated against a foreign body or antigen by higher animals. Using this phenomenon, antibodies against any chemical compounds which have the ability to stimulate the immune system (antigenic) may be produced and extracted from serum. Polyclonal antibodies are produced by multiple cells, and are not identical to each other. They may bind different antigenic determinants or epitopes on the same molecule. Ideally for immunoassays, a supply of monoclonal antibodies which specifically recognise and bind to one site of the molecule is desired. Monoclonal antibodies are identical antibody molecules produced by a clone of cells or cell line that is derived from a single antibody-producing cell. They are generated by the fusion of a mouse B lymphocyte spleen cell (from an animal which has been challenged with the antigen of interest) with a myeloma tumour cell. The resulting cell is a hybridoma cell. A small percentage of these hybridomas will produce the desired antibody.

From the immunology perspective, there are issues concerning the immunogenicity (the ability to raise antibodies) of small molecules in raising highly specific antibodies against fungicides. Many fungicide residues are small compounds which do not stimulate the immune system sufficiently for antibody production. In these cases, a hapten is produced, where a larger molecule, often proteinaceous (bovine serum albumin, BSA, or keyhole limpet hemocyanin, KLH), is chemically conjugated to the fungicide and an immune response is raised against the conjugate (Wie *et al*., 1982; Moran *et al.,* 2002; Gueguen *et al*., 2000; Brandon *et al*., 1992, 1994). Much of the success of immunoassays for the detection of small chemical compounds such as fungicides, seems to depend on the nature of the synthetic haptens-conjugate complexes, both for multi-residue and single residue analysis with low cross-reactivity.

In order to detect antibody–antigen binding, different formats may be adopted. Immunoassays are often designed to occur on a solid substrate – in a competitive immunoassay the antibody is immobilised onto the solid substrate (e.g. plastic microtitre dish wells) and the antigen is labelled with a marker (fluorescent, radioactive or enzymatic) (Fig. 15.1). Competition is introduced by incubating the antibody with both labelled and unlabelled antigen which compete for antibody binding. Subsequently, the concentration of the antigen (analyte) is easily calculated as it is inversely related to the amount of labelled molecule.

A displacement immunoassay differs in that at the outset of the assay the antibodies are saturated with bound and labelled antigen. Upon the addition of

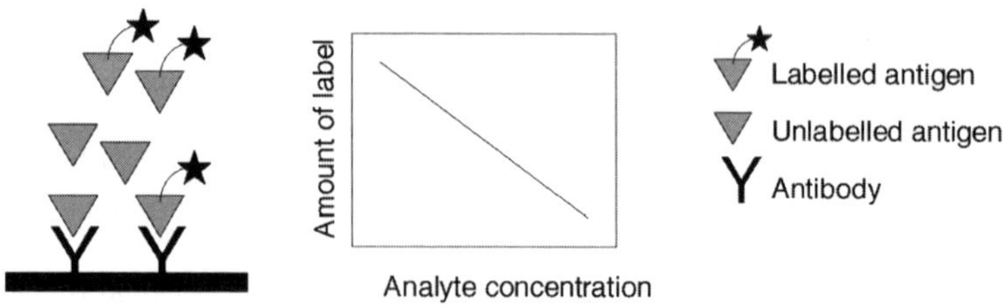

Fig. 15.1 A schematic representation of a competitive solid-phase immunoassay.

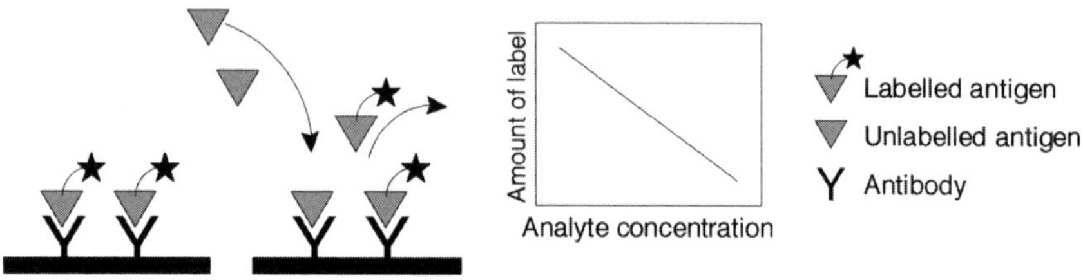

Fig. 15.2 A schematic representation of a displacement solid-phase immunoassay.

unlabelled antigen (analyte), displacement of labelled antigen occurs and again the concentration of analyte is easily calculated (Fig. 15.2).

A sandwich immunoassay format is employed only when the antigen has a high molecular weight thereby possessing more than two antigenic sites. Here, a capture antibody is attached directly or indirectly onto a solid phase and bound to the antigen. A second labelled antibody which is directed against a different epitope is added in excess and the amount of labelled antibody associated with the solid phase is directly related to the amount of analyte (Fig. 15.3).

Immunoassays may also be termed as direct or indirect. Briefly, the direct method is to label either the antibody or antigen moieties with a label and the indirect method is to employ a secondary antibody which has its antigen, and therefore binds to, the primary antibody. In this case, the secondary antibody harbours the reporter label.

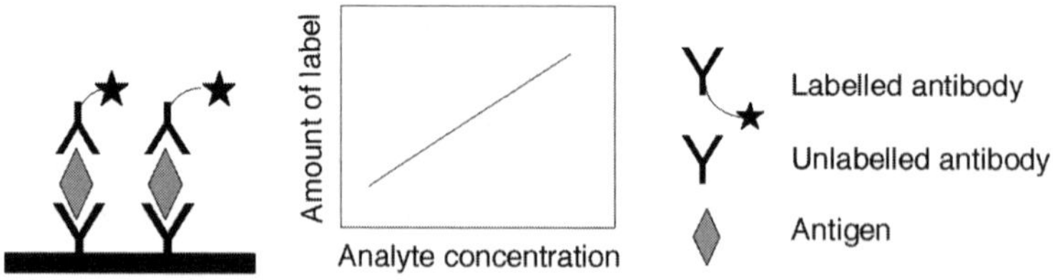

Fig. 15.3 A schematic representation of a sandwich solid-phase immunoassay.

15.2.2 Fungicide detection using immunoassays

A radioimmunoassay (RIA) was developed for the detection of benomyl and its degradation derivative, methyl 2–benzimidazolecarbamate (MBC), present on different fruits (Newsome and Shields, 1981). Results were discussed as percentage of added fungicide recovered following an extraction method and RIA. Another report for the detection of benomyl and carbendazim from a variety of matrices, describes the use of a magnetic particle-based immunoassay. Detection limits for MBC in water, fortified fruit juices and fortified soil sample were reported at 0.1 ppb, 300 ppb and 37.5 ppb, respectively (Itak *et al.,* 1993).

The fungicide fenpropimorph can be detected to limits of 13 pg/ml from of spiked soil percolation water using a competitive horse radish peroxidase (HRP) reporter immunoassay. The specificity of the antibodies developed for this assay was shown by the discrimination between *cis*- and *trans*-fenpropimorph, the sensitivity and reproducibility of this ELISA was comparable to GLC analysis (Jung *et al.,* 1989).

A commercial ELISA-based kit was used for the detection of benomyl by the determination of its byproduct methyl-2–benzimidazolecarbamate (MBC or carbendazim) from spiked wine samples. Detection limits of 5 ppb of MBC were possible (Bushway *et al.,* 1993). The same authors designed a competitive inhibition ELISA for MBC detection from bulk fruit juice concentrates. Polyclonal antibodies were employed and detection limits of 10 ppb of MBC were achieved (Bushway *et al.,* 1994).

Polyclonal antibodies were also used for the detection of the fungicide captan and its degradation product tetrahydrophthalimide (THPI), in fruits. Hapten compounds were developed and an antisera produced which is specific for captan, THPI and captafol. The detection limit reported was 1 ng/ml, where Canadian MRLs for fruits are 5.0 ppm (Newsome *et al.,* 1993).

Triazole fungicides were detected using polyclonal antibodies raised against a derivative of DTP [2–(2,4–dichlorophenyl)-3–(1*H*-1,2,4–trizol-1–yl)propanol] DTP-BSA conjugate. The polyclonals showed significant cross-reactivity with other triazole compounds; the linear ranges for all of the triazoles considered in this work was 12 to 850 ng/ml (Forlani *et al.,* 1992). Székács and Hammock (1995) described the detection of the triazole, myclobutanil, using an immunoassay, where previously, standardised methods for the specific detection of triazole fungicides in foodstuffs or environmental samples, by chromophoric or spectroscopic techniques, had not been developed. Detection limits of 0.3 μg/ml with the polyclonal-based assay were reported.

Monoclonal antibodies raised against flutolanil were employed in a competitive ELISA; detection limits of 0.3 ng/ml were achieved (Watanabe *et al.,* 1998).

Carbofuran was quantifiably detected in fruit juices using an indirect ELISA which employed monoclonal antibodies raised against a hapten-BSA conjugate. A detection limit of 0.2 ng/ml was realised, but there was some cross-reactivity observed with another methylcarbamate compound, bendiocarb. Detection was successful for spiked fruit juice samples without clean up or sample concentration steps (Abad *et al.,* 1997). Lower detection limits of 0.08 ng/ml were subsequently reported using monoclonal antibodies raised against an alternative hapten conjugate using two different ELISA methods (Abad *et al.,* 1999).

A recent immunoassay report (Queffelec *et al.,* 2001) on the quantitative detection of thiram in lettuce describes the development of two formats, a laboratory microtitre dish format and a field-based test using polystyrene tubes coated with polyclonal antibodies against an anti-serum to a thiram hapten. The authors report detection limits of 5 ng/ml for the laboratory-based method and 40 ng/ml for the field-based method. These methods are capable of detecting levels below 10 mg/kg which is below the MRL set out by Codex Alimentarius for DTC on lettuce.

The fungicide thiabendazole (TBZ) was detected down to 20 ppb in fortified liver samples by a monoclonal based immunoassay by Brandon *et al.* (1992), while US authority tolerance limits are set below 100 ppb. The complete extraction and immunoassay was performed in two hours and results were comparable to methods involving HPLC-UV analysis. Monoclonal antibodies were also produced by Abad *et al.* (2001) for the immunoassay detection of TBZ in fruit juices and for further development of multianalyte assays to determine pesticides used to protect citrus fruits, from a variety of chemical families. The authors' novel hapten approach resulted in a detection limit lower than those previously reported at 0.05 ng/ml. Multi-residue immunoassays have also been developed, for example benzimidazoles, and TBZ detection was achieved. Suitable sample preparation methods compatible with the immunoassay format were also developed here (Brandon *et al.*, 1994).

Watanabe *et al.* (2000) report an ELISA method for testing citrus fruits for the presence of the residue imazalil, otherwise detected using HPLC. The detection limit reached using monoclonal antibodies to a hapten-protein conjugate was 0.1 ng/ml where the acceptable residue level in citrus fruits in Japan is 5 ppm.

An ELISA method to determine the presence of pentachlorophenol (PCP) in water samples was demonstrated recently. Three groups of polyclonal antibodies were raised against a synthetic hapten conjugate. One antiserum in particular gave a detection limit of 0.1 ng/ml and had low cross-reactivity with halogenated and other phenolic compounds (Noguera *et al.,* 2002). An immunoassay was designed for the assessment of occupational exposure to PCP. The determination of trichlorophenols (TCP) in urine samples was adopted as an indication of PCP exposure. An indirect ELISA was developed for TCP using polyclonal antibodies against a keyhole limpet hemocyanin hapten derivative. Cross-reactivity with other chlorinated phenols was between 12 and 21%, although the level of cross-reactivity with brominated phenols was extremely high. Matrix effects for urine were overcome by a solid-phase extraction clean up step, thereby allowing a detection limit of 1 μg/ml (Galve *et al.*, 2002). The type of matrix problems common to immunosensors are those that are associated with non-specific binding of the antibody with other compounds from the sample. Changing buffers or the addition of bovine serum albumen may alleviate this.

There is a commercially available range of RaPID Assay® immunoassay kits from Strategic Diagnostics, Inc. (Newark, Delaware, USA) for the detection of a range of pesticides, including fungicides. A competitive immunoassay format is presented. The antibodies are bound to magnetic particles and a magnetic separation step is performed. The immunoassay is followed by colorimetric measurements. There are other immunoassay formats developed for the EnviroGard™ immunoassay-based kit. These do not employ magnetic particle technology. In an original article reporting the detection of procymidone a limit of detection of 20 μg/kg in samples extracted from peppers was achieved. The EU tolerance is 2 mg/kg whereas in the United States the tolerance is nil tolerance (Fernández-Alba *et al.,* 1995). An alternative manufacturer, Envirologix (Portland, Maine, USA), supplies immunoassay kits in microwell plate formats for pesticide detection assays and also for fungicides: metalaxyl with a detection limit of 0.08 ppb in water, and benomyl/carbenzadim with a detection limit 0.04 ppm in food samples.

The sensitivity and specificity of the immunoassay approach is dependent on a number of factors, including the antibody, the assay format, matrix effects and sample preparation protocols. It is clear that the immunoassay approach has to be tailored for each compound to be effective and represents a significant investment in time and money to reach a stage where a skilled operator can determine fungicide levels in a sample. There are significant benefits to be gained by using this biorecognition approach in a rapid, one-step, user-friendly format. The recognition molecules are available and redesign at a system level should permit the assay transfer from a plate reader apparatus to a biosensor format.

15.3 Detecting fungicide residues using biosensors

A biosensor is any analytical device incorporating a biological component as a sensing layer that specifically interacts with a particular analyte (Fig. 15.4). The sensing layer is coupled to a transducer. Needs for biosensor development are found in such diverse spheres as agriculture, medical monitoring and diagnosis, environment and defence. The miniature geometry of most biosensors affords portable testing and on-site analysis. Biosensors are associated with reduced running costs, short analysis times and, in some cases, greater limits of detection. The sensing layer imparts analyte specificity. Generally the analyte recognition event is based on a physical binding or hybridisation of a receptor-ligand nature, e.g. antibody–antigen binding. The transducer component measures a change in signal (current, fluorescence etc.) upon analyte binding and yields a digital signal which is proportional to the analyte concentration.

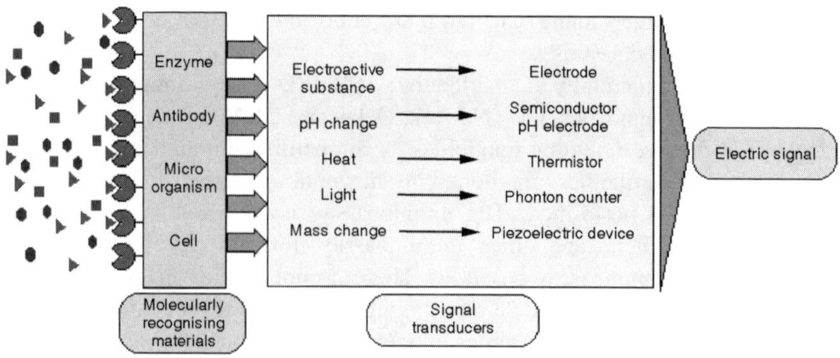

Fig. 15.4 A schematic description of biosensor formats.

15.3.1 Biosensors for fungicide detection

A number of varying biosensor formats have been reported in the literature as suitable for the detection of fungicides, the most abundant being enzyme-based sensors. However, electrochemical, optical and immunosensors have also been developed.

Immunosensors for fungicide detection

Immunosensors are detection systems that detect a biorecognition event which is measured by the sensor and the signal is interpreted as a positive binding event or a non-binding event. Immunosensor technology is based on immunoassays which use antibodies for detection, and in many cases the quantitation, of biochemical molecules. However, there is a dramatic lack of transfer of these valuable immunoassays to immunosensor formats.

A portable pollution instrument based on a multiple analyte immunosensor was developed recently which has the capacity specifically to detect a range of harmful pollutants for water monitoring. The transduction method is based on total internal reflection fluorescence and up to three analytes are detected from one sample simultaneously. This constitutes one of the few reports of multi-analyte detection capability for such an instrument (Barzen *et al.,* 2002). The instrument detects the herbicides alachor and atrazine as well as PCP in one measurement. It was capable of measuring the herbicide mixture to levels lower than the EU threshold, 0.07 μg/l alachor and 0.03 μg/l for atrazine, but the detection limits for PCP was 4.23 μg/l which is higher than the permitted level of 1 μg/l (Oubina *et al.,* 1997).

Sensors have been developed for some *N*-methyl carbamate (NTC) pesticides. This is a group of 15 active compounds that are widely applied, mainly as insecticides. Some members of this group are also used against slugs or as fungicides (Updike and Hicks, 1967). Monoclonal antibodies to carbaryl were incorporated in an immunosensor where controlled-pore glass (CPG) was used as a solid substrate for antibody immobilisation. This facilitated the development of an elaborate flow-through immunosensor format. The system detection limit for carbaryl in non-pretreated samples of drinking water is 0.029 μg/ml. One attractive feature of this format is its reusability – up to 100 immunoassays were performed using the same reactor. Also, low cross-reactivities with other methylcarbamates were reported (González-Martínez *et al.,* 1997). An alternative option for the detection of carbaryl was described more recently, where an immunoassay for the detection of its hydrolysis product, 1–naphthol, was developed in organic media (Penalva *et al.,* 2000). The success of the immunoreaction in organic media was due largely to the addition of a surfactant. However, higher amounts of antibody and antigen were necessary. Also, sensitivity and detection limits were compromised in comparison to the assay when it is performed in aqueous media. Here, however, the CPG did not possess the reusability properties that were previously reported (González-Martínez *et al.,* 1997). An additional sensor format was developed in a 'Protein A/G-based sensor' to overcome issues regarding immunoassay regeneration (Penalva *et al.,* 2000).

Fungicide residue detection using the commercially available BIAcore biosensor chip was demonstrated recently (Schlecht *et al.*, 2002). The BIAcore instrument uses surface plasmon resonance as its sensing platform. Modifications was made to the BIAcore chip for the immobilisation of carboxyl group containing haptens. This approach also allowed for repeated usage of the biochip. A detection limit of 0.1 μg/ml for 2,4–dichlorophenoxyacetic acid was achieved with monoclonal antibodies.

Enzyme-based sensors

Enzyme-based sensors involve an electrochemical method to monitor the consumption of a mediator during an enzyme-catalysed reaction and a redox reaction involving an electron-transfer mediator. The amperometric method allows for direct correlation between the concentration of the substrate and the intensity of current associated with the electrochemical transformation of the mediator. Amperometric measurements are possible when a constant potential is applied to an electrode. Charge changes occur as currents are created via electron transfer between the bioassay and the electrode. These changes in charge are monitored.

Low cost, biocompatible screen-printed carbon electrodes are an attractive electrode material for enzyme-based biosensors as the biomolecule can be incorporated at the electrode core (Gorton, 1995). Additionally, the incorporation of electronic mediators in the carbon-polymer paste prior to the printing process, improves the measurement process (Lobo *et al.,* 1997). These electrodes were demonstrated as suitable for amperometry with NAD^+-dependent dehydrogenase, tyrosinase or modified acetylcholinesterase (AChE) (Avramescu *et al.,* 2002).

Noguer and Marty (1997) reported an effective enzyme sensor for detecting the presence of DTC fungicides. Monitoring the inhibition of aldehyde dehydrogenase (ADH) activity caused by the presence of DTC fungicides was based on the oxidation of cofactor NAD^+ to NADH catalysed by ADH activity to NADH. A secondary oxidation reaction occurs in the presence of hexacyanoferrate (II) causing a subsequent reoxidation, which is monitored by the platinum electrode transducer. Amperometry is the electrochemical method employed. The authors report an improved sensitivity measurement of 1.48 ppb compared to 400 ppb achieved using spectrophotometric analysis. More recently, the same authors developed an enzyme sensor for the detection of a metabolite, MITC, of DTC fungicides. The NAD^+-dependent enzyme aldehyde dehydrogenase was immobilised on the screen-printed carbon electrode. The oxidation of NADH using Meldola's blue as the electron mediator was monitored amperometrically. Detection levels of 100 ppb were achieved with these disposable sensors (Noguer *et al.,* 2001). The determination of DTC fungicides was the focus of a bienzymic biosensor that utilised ADH immobilised onto screen-printed carbon electrodes which incorporated a surface platinum layer. Disposable sensor devices were made and the sensing process was facilitated by solubilising the fungicide analytes by a transformation methodology with EDTA. A detection limit of 8 ppb was reported and the authors highlighted that the detection limit obtained using standard spectrometry methods is 400 ppm for these compounds (Noguer *et al.,* 1999).

Schultze *et al.* (2002) developed screen-printed electrodes as biosensors for organophosphate (OP) and carbamate residues in infant foods without sample pre-treatment steps. The enzyme acetyl choline esterase was printed onto the electrode surface and immobilised by gluteraldehyde crosslinking. Interestingly, the authors eliminated matrix effects by an additional extraction step in order to incubate the sample in a solvent. The sensitivity of the biosensor compared well with standard analytical methods.

The inhibition of lactate dehydrogenase (LDH) activity by the fungicide PCP was described as a detection method for this substance in drinking water. Screen-printed carbon electrodes modified with cobalt phthalocyanine monitored the evolution of hydrogen peroxide as a result of a two enzyme system. LDH linkage to lactate oxidase and the further linkage to glucose dehydrogenase gave rise to a three enzyme system. The three-linked enzyme system enabled three- to four-fold reductions in the concentration of the non-optimal cofactor NADPH. Increased enzyme inhibition is achieved thereby, reducing the PCP detection limits of the three enzyme system to 26.6 μg/ml of PCP, which is still much higher than the 0.1 μg/ml EC maximum admissible concentration guidelines for potable water (Young *et al.,* 2001).

A warning device against the accidental pollution of waterways by pesticides has been described (Besombes *et al.*, 1995). It encompasses an amperometric biosensing tool to monitor the inhibition of the enzyme tyrosinase by a variety of pesticides including the fungicides 2,4–dichlorophenol and chloroiso-propylphenylcarbamate. The enzyme was immobilised by co-electro-polymerisation of tyrosinase and cation amphiphilic pyrrole monomer onto glassy carbon disk electrodes. Direct amperometric measurement of chlorophenols was possible as these are tyrosinase substrates; a detection limit of 0.4 μM for 2,3 dichlorophenol was achieved (Besombes *et al.,* 1995).

Biosensors for detection of many pesticides based on acetyl choline esterase (AChE) inhibition have been given considerable research attention. One report describes the detection of a number of NTC residues in a range of vegetable crop samples (Nunes *et al.*, 1998). Three sources of AChE and two of butyrylcholinesterase were examined for biosensor suitability with screen-printed platinum working electrodes which had been overlaid with an additional modified graphite layer containing CoPC. Enzyme immobilisation was realised by a crosslinking reaction with gluteralderhyde. The most promising results were reported for the detection of carbofuran in spiked potato and carrot samples which had not undergone pre-treatment steps. There was satisfactory correlation with chromatographic techniques. Conductive boron-doped diamond electrodes were demonstrated to be suitable materials for the electrochemical detection of a number of NTC residues (Rao *et al.*, 2002). The residues were first separated using liquid chromatography and purified samples were used for direct electrochemical detection. The detection limit was 5–20 ng/ml. Also, prior to injection the pesticide-containing samples underwent a phenolic derivatisation by alkaline hydrolysis and the electrochemical detection of these compounds was greatly enhanced; detection limits of 0.6–1 ng/ml were achieved.

A recombinant enzyme was developed to improve an amperometric biosensor system for the discrimination of binary mixtures of AChE-inhibiting contaminants. Three mutant enzymes of the *Drosphila melanogaster* AChE were selected that demonstrated individual sensitivity patterns towards different organophosphate and carbamate analytes. The authors adopted a novel approach by combining a range of AChE with artificial neural networks to produce a sensitive multianalyte detection system (Bachmann *et al.*, 2000). Two multisensor systems comprising 3 and 4 mutated AChE were employed in each. Simultaneous detection of pesticides was achieved and resolution errors of 0.4 mg/l for paraoxon and 0.5 mg/l for carbofuran were realised. Figure 15.5 illustrates the employment of AChE in enzyme biosensors.

An AChE-based biosensor incorporating a quartz crystal microbalance (QCM) was demonstrated as a suitable system for the detection of organophosphate and carbamate compounds (Guilbault and Ngeh-Ngwainbi, 1998; Abad *et al.*, 1998). The piezoelectric crystal resonates at a given frequency, AChE is immobilised onto a gold layer deposited on the crystal surface and a precipitate is formed as a product of the enzyme reaction. The deposition onto the crystal causes changes in the mass of the crystal which leads to measurable changes in frequency. Enzyme inhibition data is used to calculate contaminant concentrations.

Another AChE-based sensor was developed for organophosphate and carbamate residue detection, where AChE inhibition was monitored with an EnFET (enzyme field effect transistor) device. This is an ion-sensitive field-effect transistor with AChE entrapped in a membrane positioned at the gate electrode. This device is capable of detecting1.38 μg/l of paroxon and 2.21 μg/l of carbofuran from spiked tap water samples (Flores *et al.*, 2003).

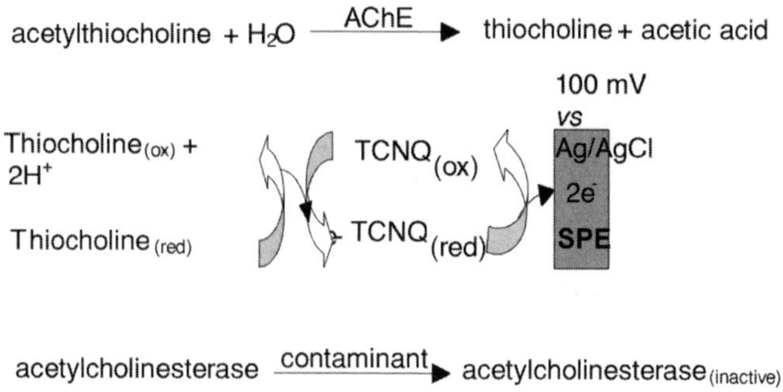

Fig. 15.5 Schematic representation of the reaction catalysed by the enzymes acetylcholinesterase (AChE).

Enzyme stability on or at the biosensing electrode is one of the most significant considerations in the development of enzyme-based sensors. Enzyme stability is affected by the immobilisation protocols or the carrier material onto which the enzyme is bound to the entrapment matrix (a porous surface such as sol-gel matrix).

The applicability of lipase enzymes in biosensors is showing promise. The main bioreaction being tested is use of a lipase to generate glycerol from a triacylglycerol. The glycerol produced is quantified by a chemical or enzymatic method. Clinical diagnostics for the quantitative determination of triacylglycerols is the main focus of lipase sensing development. However, biosensor usage can be expected to develop in the agrifood and pharmaceutical industries (Schoemaker *et al.,* 1994).

15.3.2 Optical enzyme biosensors

The inhibition of LDH activity by the fungicide PCP was described using spectrophotometric detection, and a detection limit of 1 μg/ml was reported (Young *et al*., 1999). Rogers *et al.* (1991) describe a fluorescently-labelled electric eel AChE for the detection of carbamate residues and organophosphate compounds using a fibre-optic biosensor The sensor was capable of detecting ranges of these contaminants from nanoMolar to microMolar levels.

An optical detection system was reported for the detection of organophosphate and carbamate residues in fortified fruit juices and tap water. Flow injection analysis coupled with a photothermal detector was employed to monitor the inhibition of AChE. Thermal lens spectroscopy affords sensitive measurements at low absorbance regimes. Limits of detection between 0.2 ng/ml and 4 ng/ml were achieved for the different residues (Pogačnik and Franko, 1999). More recently this biosensor system was improved by incorporating an excitation laser which increases sensitivity levels and vegetable samples were analysed without a sophisticated pre-treatment process. Contamination levels in the analysed samples were measured at concentrations below the EU regulatory limits, showing that the sensitivity of the biosensor is adequate (Pogačnik and Franko, 2003).

A dual enzyme detection system was designed for the simultaneous detection of the fungicide captan and organophosphate pesticides from water and incorporates an optical detection method (Choi *et al.,* 2003). A sol-gel film was used for the immobilisation of the enzymes glutathione-*S*-transferase and AChE. Enzyme inhibition monitoring is based on the decrease of product generation from enzyme substrates. This decrease is due to a decline in enzyme activity caused by the presence of captan and organophosphates. The concentration of hydrolysis products are measured by an optical absorbance reader. The generation of the metabolites, s-(2,4–dinitrobenzene) glutathione (yellow colour) and α-naphthol (red colour), was monitored at wavelengths of 400 and 500 nm. Concentration ranges of 0–2 ppm for both contaminants were detected successfully.

15.3.3 Biosensor development

The development of biosensors is clearly an interdisciplinary effort, from the selection of the biorecognition elements to the development of the signal processing algorithms. Expertise in many fields is essential. To outline some of the main steps in this development process; the initial work focuses on the selection of an appropriate biorecognition system specific for the target analyte of interest. Also, the transduction method and immobilisation methodologies of the biomolecules are selected. Signal processing methodologies are then exploited to develop the software and user interface. Biosensor packaging is an essential consideration from both the manufacturing and user perspectives.

In developing biosensors, immunosensors or enzyme-based sensors, for the detection of fungicide residues from either an untreated sample or from a sample that has undergone pre-treatment steps, consideration of the matrix effect is significant at the outset. The matrix effect is not to be underestimated and different matrices exert different influences on the sensing reaction. A sample to be analysed will contain an array of different molecules, apart from the analyte, that may interfere with the biosensor reaction. In the case of fruit juices, the pH is low and for an enzyme-based sensor where the optimum pH for enzyme sensing activity is near neutral, suboptimal conditions exist. This sensitivity to pH is related to the effect of ions on enzyme activity. In certain situations, dilution with an appropriate buffer is sufficient in adjusting the pH conditions to streamline the reaction constituents for optimum sensing conditions. However, it is more likely that an extraction or clean-up step is required, thus complicating the biosensor analysis. It is imperative to consider the extraction and clean-up needs of the target samples and the sensitivities of the bioassays themselves compared to the regulatory limits.

One of the overriding advantages of the development of biosensors for fungicide detection over conventional analytical methods, is the possibility of testing multiple samples simultaneously in an array format. The ability to provide screening or semi-quantitative determinations of contaminating residues on site, or at any point along the farm to fork chain would be extremely useful.

15.4 Conclusions

Despite developments in active substance testing, there is a huge and growing need to develop fast and simple biological screening tests to aid in the monitoring detection and control of fungicides, and indeed all plant protection products.

Even though there is a vast number of technologies demonstrated as effective for fungicide detection, there is a slow transfer of this technology to the marketplace. One of the major obstacles and challenges for the future of fungicide detection is designing systems that are capable of detecting more than one fungicide residue. Fungicides and their metabolites are a large group of chemically diverse compounds. Currently, there are detection systems (conventional analytical or biosensors) which, for a variety of reasons, focus on the detection of one residue or a family of closely-related compounds. The real challenge will be to develop parallel systems for the detection of multiple residues. It is easy to understand that the marketplace might resist the uptake of single sensors and systems which detect one analyte from one or a narrow range of samples. The development of suitable detection technologies must be informed by end-users and stakeholders in order to address real needs.

15.5 Sources of further information and advice

This list of information sources is not exhaustive. There is a wealth of information available from many international, governmental and non-governmental organisations on all aspects of pesticides, from their chemical structure to the regulatory information surrounding their use. They have all been referenced using their Internet sites as much of the material is available free of charge. Sources of information specific to fungicide residues are included under the term pesticide.

- Food and Agriculture Organization FAO of the United Nations *information is provided on food safety analysis and evaluation data on pesticide residues* (http://www.fao.org).
- The International Atomic Energy Agency (IAEA) and FAO: joint efforts in using nuclear techniques and related biotechnologies for developing improved strategies for sustainable food security including pesticide management
(http://www.iaea.org/programmes/nafa/dx/index.html)
- The Organisation for Economic Co-operation and Development (OECD) runs a program to help improve the efficiency and effectiveness of pesticide and biocide regulation by OECD governments – a range of publications on the subject is available
(http://www.oecd.org/).
- The European Commission Food Safety website has made available a list of active substances, information regarding Directive 91/414/EEC, a rapid alert

system for food and feed products. These weekly bulletins are reports highlighting concerns regarding food product contaminations (http://europa.eu.int/comm/food/index_en.html).

- Environmental Protection Agency, USA, *information regarding health and safety, toxicological data for pesticides is available* (http://www.epa.org).
- Food and Drug Administration (FDA): information regarding enforcement testing (http://www.fda.gov)
- National Pesticide Information Centre, USA, a service provided by EPA and Oregon State University, *this website provides information on pesticide use and management, impact on the environment and factual information on more than 600 pesticides* (http://www.npic.orst.edu).
- Pesticide Action Network UK publishes a newsletter and has fact sheets on many pesticide active ingredients, and a links page to many useful websites regarding pesticide related subjects (http://www.pan-uk.org)
- The University of Nebraska-Lincoln hosts a pesticide education resource facility with links to relevant sites including, pesticide health and safety, pesticide information databases, pesticide laws and regulations, newsletters (http://pested.unl.edu/).
- To gain an insight into the classification of pesticides and more particularly fungicides, there is a compendium of pesticide common names available which also includes an extensive list of fungicides, their chemical formulae and structures (http://www.hclrss.demon.co.uk/sitemap.html).

15.6 Acknowledgements

I would like to express my warmest appreciation and gratitude to Prof. Jean Louis Marty, Dr Alan Wood and Mr Stephen Galvin each of whom provided material for the illustrations in this chapter.

15.7 References

ABAD A, MORENO M J, MONTOYA A (1997), 'A monoclonal immunoassay for carbofuran and its application to the analysis of fruit juices', *Anal Chim Acta* 347, 103–110.

ABAD A, MORENO M J, MONTOYA A (1999), 'Development of monoclonal antibody-based enzyme immunoassays to the N-methylcarbamate pesticide carbofuran', *J Agric Food Chem* 47 (6), 2475–2485.

ABAD A, MANCLÚS J J, MORENO M J, MONTOYA A (2001), 'Determination of thiabendazole in fruit juices by a new monoclonal enzyme immunoassay', *J AOAC Int* 84, 156–161.

ABAD J M, PARIENTE F, HERNÁNDEZ L, ABRUÑA H D, LORENZO E (1998), 'Determination of organophosphorus and carbamate pesticides using a piezoelectric biosensor', *Anal Chem* 70 (14), 2848–2855.

AVRAMESCU A, ANDREESCU S, NOGUER T, CAMELIA B, ANDREESCU MARTY J-L (2002), 'Biosensors designed for environmental and food quality control based on screen-printed graphite electrodes with different configurations', *Anal Bioanal Chem* 374, 25–32.

BACHMANN T T, LECA B, VILATTE F, MARTY J-L, FOURNIER D, SCHMID R D (2000), 'Improved multianalyte detection of organophosphates and carbamates with disposable multielectrode biosensors using recombinant mutants of *Drosphila* acetylcholinesterase and artificial neural networks', *Biosens Bioelectron* 15, 193–201.

BARZEN C, BRECHT A, GAUGLITZ G (2002), 'Optical multiple-analyte immunosensor for water pollution control', *Biosens Bioelectron* 17, 289–295.

BESOMBES J-L, COSNIER S, LABBÉ P, REVERDY G (1995), 'A biosensor as warning device for the detection of cyanide, chlorophenols, atrazine and carbamate pesticides', *Anal Chim Acta* 311, 255–263.

BRANDON D L, BINDER R G, BATES A H, MONTAGUE JR WC (1992), 'Monoclonal antibody-based ELISA for thiabendazole in liver', *J Agric Food Chem* 40, 1722–1726.

BRANDON D L, BINDER R G, BATES A, H MONTAGUE JR WC (1994) 'Monoclonal Ab for multiresidues ELISA of benizimidazole anthelmintics in liver', *J Agric Food Chem* 42, 1588–1594.

BUSHWAY R J, PARADIS L R, PERKINS L B, FAN T S, YOUNG B E, WALSER P E (1993), 'Determination of methyl 2–benzimidazolecarbamate in wine by competitive inhibition enzyme immunoassay', *J AOAC Int* 76(4), 851–856.

BUSHWAY R J, YOUNG B E, PARADIS L R, PERKINS L B, MARTIN S K, BROWN M P (1994), 'Determination of methyl 2–benzimidazolecarbamate in bulk fruit juice concentrates by competitive-inhibition enzyme immunoassay', *J AOAC Int* 77(5), 1237–1243.

CERESER C, BOGET S, PARVAZ P, REVOL A (2001), 'An evaluation of thiram toxicity on cultured human skin fibroblasts', *Toxicology* 162, 89–101.

CHOI J-W, KIM Y-K, OH B-K, SONG S-Y LEE, W H (2003), 'Optical biosensor for simultaneous detection of captan and organophophorous compounds', *Biosens Bioelec* 28, 591–597.

COLBURN T, VOM SAAL F S, SOTO A M (1993), 'Developmental effects of endocrine-disrupting chemicals in wildlife and humans', *Environ Health Perspect* 101, 378–384.

FERNANDEZ-ALBA A R, VALVERDE A, AGüERA A, CONTRERAS M, RODRIGUEZ D (1995), 'Determination of procymidone in vegetables by a commercial competitive inhibition enzyme immunoassay', *Anal Chim Acta* 311, 371–376.

FLORES F, ARTIGAS J, MARTY J-L, VALDÉS F (2003), 'Development of an EnFET for the detection of organophosphorous and carbamate insecticides', *Anal Bioanal Chem* 376, 476–480.

FORLANI F, ARNOLDI A, PAGANI S (1992), 'Development of an enzyme-linked immunosorbent assay for triazole fungicides', *J Agric Food Chem* 40, 328–331.

GALVE R, NICHKOVA M, CAMPS F, SANCHEZ-BAEZA F, MARCO M P (2002), 'Development and evaluation of an immunoassay for biological monitoring chlorophenols in urine as potential indicators of occupational exposure', *Anal Chem* 74(2), 468–78.

GONZÁLEZ-MARTÍNEZ M A, MORAIS S, PUCHADES R, MAQUIERIRA A, ABAD A, MONTOYA A

(1997), 'Development of an automated controlled-pore glass flow-through immunosensor for carbaryl', *Anal Chim Acta* 347, 199–205.

GORTON L (1995), 'Carbon paste electrodes modified with enzymes, tissues and, cells', *Electroanalysis* 7 (1), 23–45.

GUEGUEN F, BOISDÉ F, QUEFFELEC A, L HAELTERS J P, THOUVENOT D, CORBEL B, NODET P (2000), 'Hapten synthesis for the development of a competitive inhibition enzyme-immunoassay for thiram', *J Agric Food Chem* 48, 4492–4499.

GUILBAULT G G, NGEH-NGWAINBI J (1988), 'Use of protein coatings on piezoelectric crystals for assay of gaseous pollutants'. In: Guilbault G G Mascini M (eds), *Analytical Uses of Immobilized Biological Compounds for Detection, Medical and Industrial Uses*, Dordrecht, The Netherlands, pp. 187–194.

GUVEN K, TOGRUL S, IYAR F, OZANT S, DE POMERAI D I (2003), 'A comparative study of bioassays based on enzyme biosynthesis in *Escherichia coli* and *Bacillus subtilis* exposed to heavy metals and organic pesticides', *Enz Microbial Technol* 32, 658–664.

GWEREMAN A, CARLSEN E, KEIDING N, SKAKKEBAEK N E (1993), 'Evidence for increasing incidence of abnormalities of the human testis: a review', *Environ Health Perspect* 101, 65–71.

HOOGENBOOM L A, HAMERS A R, BOVEE T F (1999), 'Bioassays for the detection of growth-promoting agents, veterinary drugs and environmental contaminants in food', *Analyst* 124 (1), 79–85.

HUBER S J, HOCK B A (1985), 'Solid phase enzyme immunoassay for quantitative determination of the herbicide terbutyrn', *J Plant Dis Prot* 92, 147–156.

IARC (1987) 'Genetic and related effects: an updating of selected IARC monographs from volumes 1 to 42, Monographs on the Evaluation of Carcinogenic Risks to Humans', Suppl 6, International Agency for Research on Cancer, Lyon.

ITAK J A, SELISKER M Y, JOURDAN S W, FLEEKER J R, HERZOG D P (1993), 'Determination of benomyl (as carbendazim) and carbendazim in water, soil and fruit juice by a magnetic particle-based immunoassay', *J Agric Food Chem* 41, 2329–2332.

JUNG F, METER H H D, HAMM R T (1989), 'Development of a sensitive enzyme-linked immunosorbent assay for the fungicide fenpropimorph', *J Agric Food Chem* 37,1183–1187.

LOBO M J, MIRANDA A J, TUÑÓN P (1997), 'Amperometric biosensors based on NAD(P)-dependent dehydrogenase enzymes', *Electroanalysis* 9 (3), 191 .

MARGNI M, ROSSIER D, CRETTAZ P, JOLLIET O (2002), 'Life cycle impact assessment of pesticides on human health and ecosystems', *Agriculture Ecosystems Environ* 93, 379–392.

MORAN E, O'KEEFFE M, O'CONNOR R, LARKIN A M, MURPHY P, CLYNES M (2002), 'Methods for generation of monoclonal antibodies to the very small drug hapten 5–benzimidazolecarboxylic acid', *J Immunol Meths* 271, 65–75.

NEWSOME W H, SHIELDS J B (1981), 'A radioimmunoassay for benmyl and metho 2–benzimidazolecarbamate on food crops', *J Agric Food Chem* 29, 220–222.

NEWSOME W H, YEUNG J M, COLLINS P C (1993), 'Development of enzyme immunoassay for captan and its degradation product tetrahydrophthalimide in foods', *J AOAC Int* 76, 381–386.

NOGUER T, MARTY J L (1997) 'High sensitive bienzymic sensor for the detection of dithiocarbamate fungicides', *Anal Chim Acta* 347, 63–70.

NOGUER T, GRADINARU A, CIUCU A, MARTY J L (1999), 'A new disposable biosensor for the accurate and sensitive detection of ethylenebis (dithiocarbamate) fungicides', *Anal*

Lett 32 (9), 1723–1738.

NOGUER T, BALASOIU A M, AVRAMESCU A, MARTY J L (2001), 'Development of a disposable biosensor for the detection of metam-sodium and its metabolite MITC', *Anal Lett* 34 (4), 513–528.

NOGUERA P, MAQUIERIA A, PUCHADES R, BRUNET E, CARRAMOLINO M M, RODRÍGUEZ-UBIS J C (2002), 'Development of an exzyme-linked immunosorbent assay for pentachlorophenol', *Anal Chim Acta* 460, 279–288.

NUNES G S, SKLÁDAL P, YAMANAKA H, BARCELÓ D (1998), 'Determination of carbamate residues in crop samples by cholinesterase-based biosensors and chromatographic techniques', *Anal Chim Acta* 362, 59–68.

OUBIÑA A, PUIG D, GASCÓN J, BARCELÓ D (1997), 'Determination of pentachlorophenol in certified waste waters, soil samples and industrial effluents using ELISA and liquid-solid extraction followed by liquid chromatography', *Anal Chim Acta* 346, 49–59.

PENALVA J, PUCHADES R, MAQUIERIA A, GEE S, HAMMOCK B D (2000), 'Development of immunosensors for the analysis of 1–naphthol in organic media', *Biosens Bioelectron* 15, 99–106.

PEROCCO P, COLACCI A, BONORA B, GRILLI S (1995), 'In vitro transforming effect of the fungicide metalaxyl and zineb', *Teratogen Carcinogen Mutagen* 15, 73–80.

POGAČNIK L, FRANKO M (1999), 'Determination of organophosphate and carbamate pesticides in spiked samples of tap water and fruit juices by a biosensor with photothermal detection', *Biosens Bioelec* 14, 569–578.

POGAČNIK L, FRANKO M (2003), 'Detection of organophosphate and carbamate pesticides in vegetable samples by a photothermal biosensor', *Biosens Bioelec* 18, 1–9.

QUEFFELEC A L, BOISDÉ F, LARUE J P, HAELTERS J P, CORBEL B, THOUVENOT D, NODET P (2001), 'Development of an immunoassay (ELISA) for the quantification of thiram in lettuce', *J Agric Food Chem* 49, 1675–1680.

RAO T N, LOO B H, SARADA B V, TERASHIMA C, FUJISHIMA A (2002), 'Electrochemical detection of carbamate pesticides at conductive diamond electrodes', *Anal Chem* 74 (7), 1578–1583.

ROGERS K R, CAO C J, VALDES J J, ELDEFRAWI A T, ELDFRAWI M E (1991), 'Acetylcholinesterase fiber-optic biosensor for detection of anticholinesterases', *Fundam Appl Toxicol* 16 (4), 810–820.

SCHLECHT U, NOMURA Y, BACHMANN T, KARUBE I (2002), 'Reversible surface thiol immobilization of carboxyl group containing haptens to a BIAcore biosensor chip enabling repeated usage of a single sensor surface', *Bioconjug Chem* 13 (2) 188–93.

SCHOEMAKER M, FELDBRUEGGE R, TRAU D, GRUENDIG B, SPENER F (1994), *Fat Sci Technol* 96, 420–421.

SCHULTZE H, SCHERBAUM E, ANASTASSIADES M, VORLOVÁ S, SCHMID R D, BACHMANN T T (2002), 'Development, Validation, and application of an acetylcholinesterase biosensor test for the direct detection of insecticide residues in infant food', *Biosens Bioelect* 17, 1095–1105.

SCHWALBE M, DORN E, BEYERMANN K (1984), 'Enzyme immunoassay and fluoro-immunoassay for the herbicide diclofop-methyl', *J Agric Food Chem* 32, 734–741.

SHARPE R M, KEKKEBAEK N E (1993), 'Are oestrogens involved in falling sperm count and disorders of the male reproductive tract ?', *The Lancet* 341 1392–1395.

SHUKLA Y, BAQAR S M, MEHROTRA N K (1996), 'Carcinogenic and co-carcinogenic studies of thiram on mouse skin', *Food Chem Toxicol* 34 (3), 283.

SOLONESKI S, GONZÁLEZ M, PIAGGION E, REIGOSA M A, LARRAENDY M L (2002), 'Effect of dithiocarbamate pesticide zineb and its commercial formulation, azzurro III Genotoxic evaluation on Chinese hamster ovary (CHO) cells', *Mutation Res* 514, 201–212.

SZÉKÁCS A, HAMMOCK B D (1995), 'Development of an enzyme-linked immunosorbent assay for the detection of the triazole fungicide myclobutanil', *J Agric Food Chem* 43, 2083–2091.

UPDIKE S J, HICKS G P (1967), 'The enzyme electrode', *Nature* 214 (92), 986–988.

VOLLER A, BIDWELL D E, BARTLETT A (1976), 'Enzyme immunoassay in fiagnostic medicine Theory and Practice', *Bull WHO* 53, 55–65.

WATANABE S, ITO S, OMODA N, MUNAKATA H, HAYASHI M, YUASA Y (1998), 'Development of a competitive enzyme-linked immunosorbent assay based on a monoclonal antibody for a fungicide flutolanil', *Anal Chim Acta* 376, 93–96.

WATANABE E, WATANABE S, ITO S, HAYASHI M, WATANABE T, YUASA Y, NAKAZAWA H (2000), 'Development of an enzyme-linked immunosorbent assay for the fungicide imazalil in citrus fruits', *J Agric Food Chem* 48, 5124–5130.

WIE S I, HAMMOCK B D (1982), 'Development of enzyme-linked immunosorbent assays for residue analysis of diflubenzuron and BAY SIR 8514', *J Agric Food Chem* 30, 949–947.

WIE S I, SYLWESTER A P, WING K D, HAMMOCK B D (1982), 'Synthesis of haptens and potential radioligands and development of antibodies to insect growth regulators diflubenzuron and BAY SIR 8514', *J Agric Food Chem* 30, 943–948.

WOLFF M S, TONIOLO P G, LEE E W, RIVERA M, DUBIN N (1993), 'Blood levels of organochlorine residues and risk of breast cancer', *J Natl Cancer Inst* 85, 648–652.

YOUNG S J, DOWMAN A A, COWELL D C (1999), 'The detection of pentachlorophenol by its inhibitory effectiveness on lactate dehydrogenase of rabbit muscle and bovine heart', *J Pest Biochem Physiol* 64, 1–8.

YOUNG S J, HART J P, DOWMAN A A, COWELL D C (2001), 'The non-specific inhibition of enzymes by environmental pollutants: a study of a model system towards the development of electrochemical biosensor arrays', *Biosens Bioelectron* 16, 887–894.

16

Detecting herbicide residues

J.L. Tadeo, C. Sánchez-Brunete and B. Albero, INIA, Spain

16.1 Introduction: key issues in detecting herbicide residues in food

Weeds are usually controlled in modern agriculture by treatment with herbicides to avoid the decrease in yield their presence would produce. The widespread use of these compounds has led to environmental contamination and the presence of herbicide residues in crops. These pesticides can enter the food chain through direct treatment or via environmental routes (air, water and soil). The toxicity of most of these substances makes it necessary to control their residues in food and, therefore, they are regulated by international and national legislation.[25,28]

Herbicides are a diverse group of pesticides belonging to different chemical classes. Table 16.1 shows the herbicides most often used in agriculture together with their chemical structures. The control of herbicide levels in food made necessary the development of analytical methods to determine the different types of herbicides at residue levels. Several steps are involved in the determination of herbicides in food. Sample preparation and determination are main steps in the analysis. They will be described below. Levels of herbicides in different types of food and sources of further information will also be considered.

16.2 Trends in sample preparation

Sample preparation is an important step that consists of the extraction of the analyte from the matrix and 'clean-up' of the extract, if necessary, before its detection and quantification, generally performed by using an analytical

Table 16.1 Main chemical classes of herbicides with their chemical structures

Chemical classes	Main components	Typical representative
Anilides	alachlor, butachlor, metolachlor, propachlor	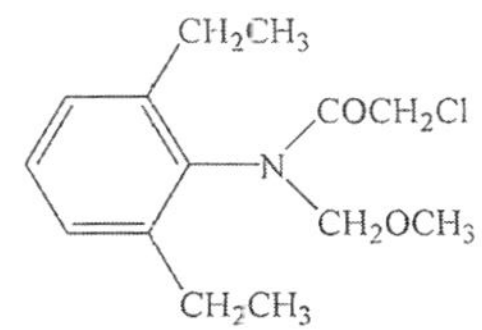 alachlor ($C_{14}H_{20}ClNO_2$)
Benzonitriles	bromoxynil, ioxynil	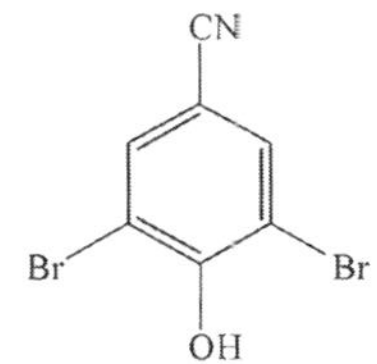 bromoxynil ($C_7H_3Br_2NO$)
Carbamates	chlorpropham, EPTC, molinate, phenmedipham, propham, thiobencarb, tri-allate	$[(CH_3)_2CH]_2NC(O)SCH_2CCl{=}CCl_2$ tri-allate ($C_{10}H_{16}Cl_3NOS$)
Dinitroanilines	benfluralin, butralin, dinitramine, ethalfluralin, pendimethalin, trifluralin,	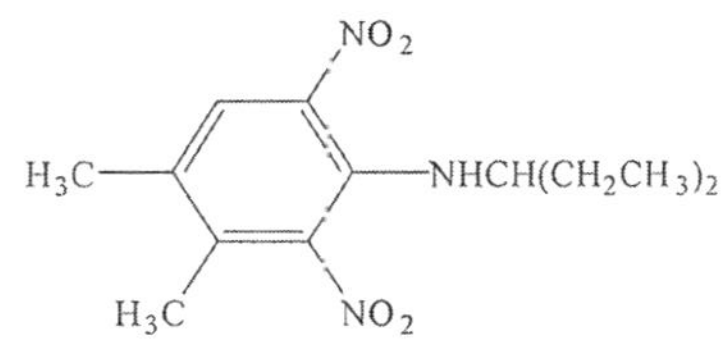 pendimethalin ($C_{13}H_{19}N_3O_4$)

Table 16.1 Continued

Chemical classes	Main components	Typical representative
Organophosphorus	glufosinate, glyphosate	$HO_2CCH_2NHCH_2P(=O)(OH)_2$ glyphosate ($C_3H_8NO_5P$)
Phenoxyacids		
Aryloxyphenoxyacids	diclofop, fenoprop, fenoxaprop, fluazifop, quizalofop	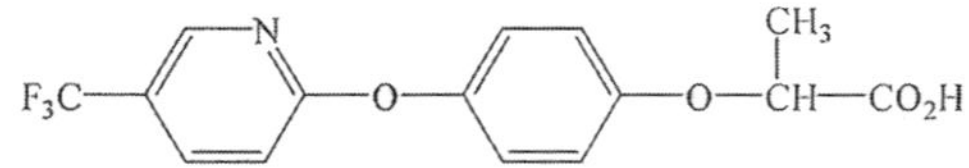 fluazifop ($C_{15}H_{12}F_3NO_4$)
Phenoxyalcanoic acids	2,4-D, dichlorprop, MCPA, MCPB, mecoprop	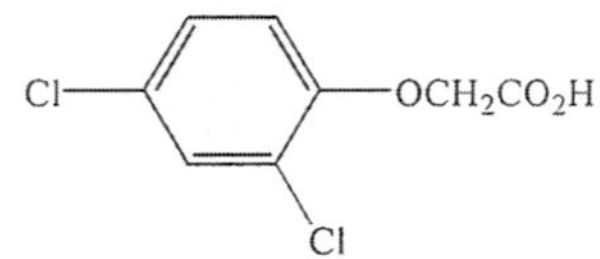 2,4-D ($C_8H_6Cl_2O_3$)
Quaternary ammonium	difenzoquat, diquat, paraquat	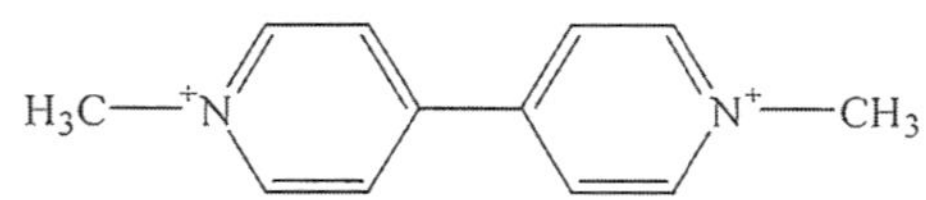 paraquat ($C_{12}H_{14}N_2$)

Triazines	atrazine, cyanazine, desmetryn, metamitron, metribuzin, prometron, prometryn, simazine, terbumeton, terbuthylazine, terbutryn, trietazine	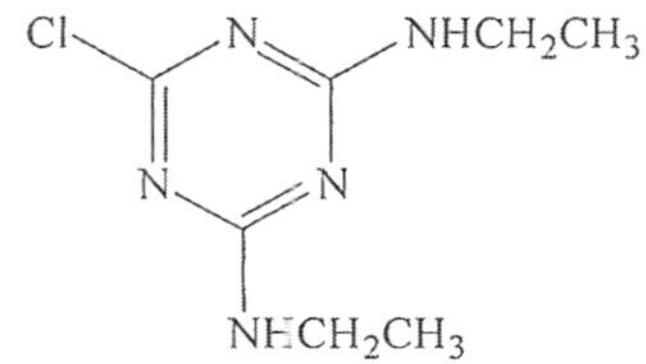 simazine ($C_7H_{12}ClN_5$)
Uracils	bromacil, lenacil, terbacil	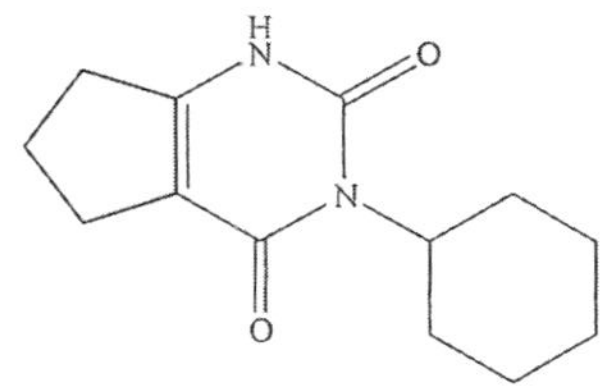 lenacil ($C_{13}H_{18}N_2O_2$)
Ureas		
Phenylureas	chlorbromuron, chlorotoluron, diuron, fenuron, isoproturon, isouron, linuron, metobenzuron, metobromuron, monolinuron, neburon, siduron, tebuthiuron	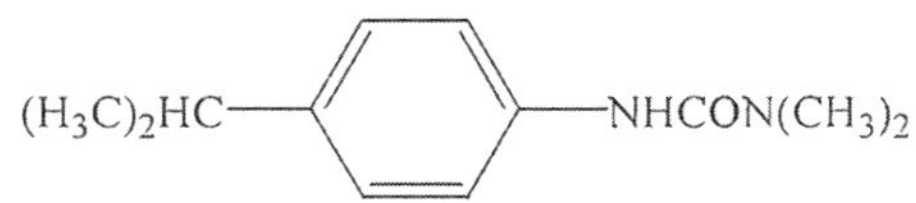 isoproturon ($C_{12}H_{18}N_2O$)

Table 16.1 Continued

Chemical classes	Main components	Typical representative
Sulfonylureas	bensulfuron, chlorsulfuron, metsulfuron, nicosulfuron, primisulfuron, pyrazosulfuron, rimsulfuron, sulfometuron, triasulfuron, tribenuron, triflusulfuron	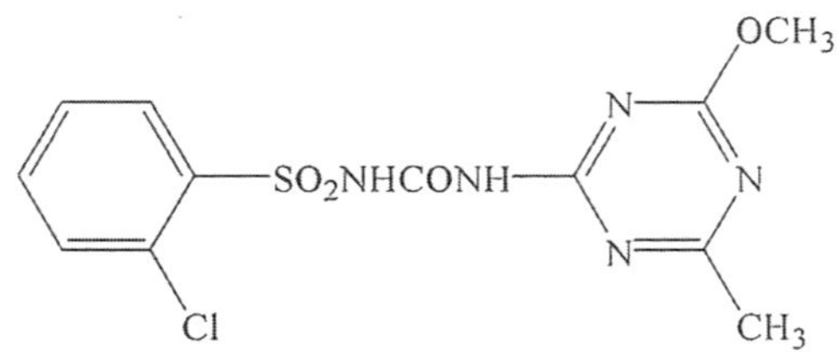 chlorsulfuron ($C_{12}H_{12}ClN_5O_4S$)

instrument. No current method is universal, allowing the extraction of all pesticides from all type of matrices. In general, multiresidue methods are used for the determination of various compounds at the same time.

16.2.1 Classical methods

Classical analytical methods are based on solvent extraction of samples, usually employing simple procedures like Soxhlet extraction. Solvent extraction is still used for herbicide analysis in food. Several solvents, for example acetone, acetonitrile, ethyl acetate and methanol, are employed in the preparation of samples, generally with a subsequent liquid–liquid partition or column clean-up.[81] The polarity of the analyte and the type of matrix are key factors in the selection of extraction methods for herbicides, Table 16.2. These methods have several drawbacks, such as the high volume of toxic organic solvents used and the amount of glassware needed, which make the procedure laborious and time consuming.

In recent years, several new technologies have been reported for sample preparation, such as solid-phase extraction (SPE), matrix solid-phase dispersion

Table 16.2 Solvent extraction of herbicides from food

Food	Herbicide	Solvent	Reference
Cereals, fruits, vegetables	Multiclass	Acetone or acetone-water	32, 46, 48, 72, 85, 96
Cereals, fruits, vegetables	Multiclass	Acetonitrile or acetonitrile-water	7, 9, 22, 24, 26, 34, 45, 53, 54, 63, 94
Cereals, fruits, vegetables, wine, crayfish	Phenoxyacids, triazines, ureas	Dichloromethane or dichloromethane-acetone	5, 29, 57, 65, 68, 87, 98
		Methanol	14, 39
Fruits, vegetables	2,4-D, simazine	Diethyl ether or diethyl ether-hexane	55, 84
Cereals, fruits, vegetables, milk	Multiclass	Ethanol or methanol	4, 11, 13, 15-18, 23, 42, 56, 64, 67, 79, 97, 99
Cereals, milk	Atrazine, tebuthiuron	Ethyl acetate or tert-buthyl ether	69, 93
Cereals	Sulfonylureas	Hexane	11
Composite dietary samples	Triazines	Hexane-acetone (Soxhlet)	66
Fruits, vegetables	Glyphosate	Water-chloroform or dichloromethane	33, 49, 73
Cereals, fruits, legumes, vegetables	Glyphosate, quaternary ammonium	Water or acidic aqueous solutions	30, 38, 74, 75, 90
Cereals, vegetables, fish	Benzonitriles, phenoxyacids	0.1 M NaOH, organic solvent extraction after acidification	12, 20, 70, 71, 77, 83

(MSPD), accelerated solvent extraction (ASE), solid-phase microextraction (SPME) and supercritical fluid extraction (SFE), with the aim of decreasing the use of organic solvents.[2,58]

16.2.2 Solid-phase extraction (SPE)

SPE is an alternative technique to liquid extraction based on the retention of the analyte on a solid sorbent by different mechanisms, like Van der Waals forces or electrostatic interactions. Several sorbents are often used in SPE, such as Florisil, alumina, various polymers and reverse-phase silica (C_{18}). In addition, anion and cation exchange resins are used for polar, ionic pesticides. The recovery of analytes from the solid phase is achieved by elution with a small volume of organic solvent. Depending on which analyte and sorbent are employed, different solvents are used, like ethyl acetate, hexane, methanol or water, or mixtures of solvents. SPE can be used as an extraction technique, which also performs a simultaneous clean up, or as a clean up procedure after extraction by other techniques, generally solvent extraction. SPE is probably one of the most frequently used techniques in sample preparation, since it is fast and robust with a low solvent consumption. Table 16.3 shows the application of this technique to sample preparation for herbicide analysis in food.

16.2.3 Matrix solid-phase dispersion (MSPD)

MSPD is a recently developed extraction method based on the dispersion of the matrix on a solid phase and the subsequent extraction of analytes by small amounts of organic solvents. Solid matrices need to be mixed with the solid phase, generally in a mortar, before being transferred to the extraction column, whereas liquid samples can be directly homogenised with the solid phase in the column.[80] Solid phases of different polarities, similar to those employed in SPE, are used and Florisil and reverse-phase silica (C_8) are those more frequently employed. Table 16.4 summarises the extraction of herbicides from food using MSPD.

16.2.4 Accelerated solvent extraction (ASE)

ASE is a new technique based on the extraction of samples using small amounts of pressurised solvent at high temperature. The efficiency of extraction increases with temperature and, as a consequence, the extraction time and volume of solvent can be reduced. The increase in pressure is necessary to keep solvents in liquid state. Moreover, analytes have to be thermally stable under the conditions employed. Table 16.5 shows the application of this technique to herbicide extraction from food.

16.2.5 Solid-phase microextraction (SPME)

SPME is a solvent-free preparation technique for extracting and concentrating herbicides from samples or their headspace. Two steps can be considered: the

Table 16.3 Use of solid-phase extraction (SPE) in sample preparation

Food	Herbicide	Sorbent	Solvent	Extraction/Clean up	Reference
Fruits, vegetables	Triazines, ureas, uracils	Alumina	Chloroform or hexane-ethyl acetate	Clean up	4, 5, 22
Fruits, vegetables	2,4-D	Aminopropyl	Acetone-hexane	Clean up	84
Cereals, fruits, vegetables	Glyphosate	Anion or cation exchange	Acidic or basic aqueous solutions	Clean up	49, 73, 75
Cereals	Sulfonylureas	Cation exchange	Basic aqueous solution	Clean up	41
Fruits, vegetables, milk	Triazines	Cation exchange	Methanolic aqueous solutions	Clean up	7, 56
Fruits, vegetables, milk	Multiclass	Carbon-celite or ionic exchange	Acetonitrile-toluene	Clean up or extraction	26, 76
Cereals, fruits, vegetables, milk	Multiclass	C_{18}	Organic solvents	Clean up	57, 63, 93, 94
Cereals, fruits, vegetables	Multiclass	Florisil	Organic solvent mixtures	Clean up	1, 12, 13, 15, 17.18 20, 23, 32, 37, 42, 72, 77, 95
Milk	Ureas	Florisil	Chloroform	Clean up	11
Beef liver	Atrazine	Molecular imprinted polymer	Acetonitrile-chloroform	Extraction	50
Cereals, fruits, vegetables	Quaternary ammonium	Silica	Acidic aqueous solutions	Clean up	38, 90
Cereals, fruits, vegetables, wine	Triazines, ureas	Silica	Organic solvent mixtures	Clean up	29, 65, 98
Cereals	Anilides	Styrene polymer	1N HCl - methanol	Clean up	53

Table 16.4 Use of matrix solid-phase dispersion (MSPD) in sample preparation

Food	Herbicide	Solid-phase	Solvent	Reference
Fruits, vegetables	Triazines, ureas, carbamates	Florisil	Ethyl acetate or dichloromethane-acetone	36
Fruits, potatoes	Propham	C_8	Dichloromethane	61
Beef kidney	Atrazine	Silica and anion exchange	Ethanol-water	21

Table 16.5 Accelerated solvent extraction (ASE) of herbicides from food

Food	Herbicide	Solvent	Reference
Fruits, vegetables	Anilides, dinitroanilines	Acetone-dichloromethane	1
Soybeans	Multiresidue	0.05 M HCl-acetonitrile	52
Oranges	Phenylureas	Dichloromethane-acetone	8
Beef kidney	Atrazine	Ethanol-water	21

extraction or retention of analytes on the solid phase, and the desorption of analytes in the injection port of a gas chromatograph or in a solvent suitable for injection in the equipment chosen. In the extraction step, the fibre is exposed to the sample, generally in an aqueous solution or suspension, or to the sample headspace. There are several factors that influence sample preparation by SPME. The type of coated fibre, the exposure time and the type of matrix are important factors in the extraction step, whereas temperature and desorption time mainly influence the desorption of analytes. There are various available commercial fibres for use in SPME that have different coating phases, such as PDMS, polypyrrole, carbowax, divinylbenzene or binary mixtures of these. SPME applications to the analysis of herbicides in food are shown in Table 16.6.

Table 16.6 Solid-phase microextraction (SPME) of herbicides from food

Food	Herbicide	Fibre[a]	Reference
Potatoes	Chlorpropham	PDMS 100 μm	88
Wine	Terbuthylazine, trifluralin	PDMS100 μ m	86
	Carbamates, ureas	Polypyrrole	35
Beef kidney	Atrazine	CW-DVB 65 μm	21

[a] PDMS: polydimethylsiloxane. CW: Carbowax. DVB: divinylbenzene

16.2.6 Supercritical fluid extraction (SFE)

SFE uses fluids under conditions where they have similar densities to liquids but higher diffusion coefficients and lower viscosities, which leads to faster extraction of solutes. Moreover, this technique can be automated with a subsequent saving of labour and time. The broad polarity range of herbicides makes necessary the use of modifiers like methanol or water. Carbon dioxide is often used as supercritical fluid, due to its low critical temperature and pressure, although additional clean up may be necessary for some matrices. Table 16.7 shows the main applications of this technique reported for herbicide analyses in food.

Table 16.7 Supercritical fluid extraction (SFE) of herbicides from food

Food	Herbicide	Fluid	Reference
Cereals, fruits, vegetables	Anilides	CO_2	95
Fruits, vegetables	Atrazine, chlorpropham	CO_2	44
	Ureas	CO_2	37
Onions	Fluzifop	CO_2	89
Eggs	Triazines	CO_2	59
Meat products	Alachlor, atrazine, 2,4-D	CO_2 modified with methanol	51

16.3 Analytical methods for particular herbicide residues

The qualitative and quantitative determination of herbicides in food will depend on their physico-chemical properties. If the herbicide is volatile and thermally stable, gas chromatography (GC) is the analytical technique most often used, due to the very sensitive and selective detectors available (nitrogen-phosphorus detector (NPD) and electron-capture detector (ECD)). Fused silica capillary columns, with low polarity stationary phases, are normally used in gas chromatographic analyses. But if the compound is not volatile or is unstable, high performance liquid chromatography (HPLC) will be the chosen technique, usually with ultraviolet (UV) detection or diode array detection (DAD). In addition, fluorescence (FL) detection is used in some cases for compounds with fluorescence emission spectra. Columns most commonly employed in HPLC are reverse-phase C_{18}.

Mass spectrometry (MS) is a very useful technique for the identification of compounds at residue level and has been widely used, in recent years, coupled to gas chromatography. Figure 16.1 shows a chromatogram of a mixture of herbicides analysed by GC-MS with selected ion monitoring (SIM). Improved robustness of HPLC-MS equipments together with a progressive decrease in cost, has led to more frequent use of this technique in residue analysis, with good sensitivity and selectivity achieved. In addition, using multiple MS analyses (MS/MS) improves sensitivity and selectivity. The use of other techniques like capillary electrophoresis (CE) and enzyme-linked immunosorbent assay (ELISA) has been reported.

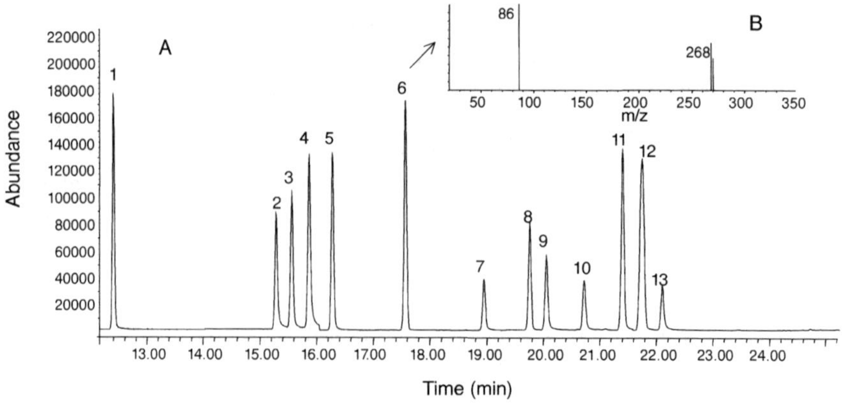

Fig. 16.1 (A) GC-MS chromatogram of a herbicide mixture. 1: propachlor, 2: simazine, 3: atrazine, 4: terbumeton, 5: terbuthylazine, 6: tri-allate, 7: metribuzin, 8: alachlor, 9: prometryn, 10: terbutryn, 11: benthiocarb, 12: metolachlor, 13: cyanazine. (B) Tri-allate identification by the mass spectrum obtained with selected ion monitoring

Herbicide residues in food need to be determined at trace levels and, therefore, the limit of detection (LOD) is an important characteristic of the method. They are normally in the parts per billion (ppb) range, ng/g. The more commonly used analytical methods for the determination of different classes of herbicides in food are described below.

16.3.1 Anilides

These herbicides have a chlorine atom in their molecule and are also named chloroacetamides. Alachlor and metolachlor are herbicides of this group more often used in agriculture. Table 16.8 summarises the analytical methods employed in their determination. The thermal stability of these compounds

Table 16.8 Analytical methods used in the analysis of anilides

Herbicide	Food	Technique	Detector	LOD (mg/kg)	Reference
Alachlor	Fruits, vegetables	GC	ECD	0.02–0.04	1, 36
			MS	0.03–0.10	26, 45, 78, 85
	Composite dietary samples	GC	MS	0.0004	66
	Meat products	ELISA		0.001–0.014	51
	Milk	ELISA		0.001	62
Metolachlor	Fruits, vegetables	GC	ECD	0.099–0.12	1
			MS	0.04–0.05	45, 78
		HPLC	MS/MS	0.5	34
Anilides	Fruits, vegetables	GC	MS	ppb range	95
			MS/MS	ppb range	76
	Milk	GC	MS/MS	ppb range	76

allows their analysis by GC and, as their molecules contain N and Cl atoms, NPD and ECD detectors can be used. In addition, MS detection has been employed with good results.

16.3.2 Benzonitriles (Table 16.9)

The main members of this group of herbicides are bromoxynil and ioxynil. They are also called hydroxybenzonitriles. The presence of several halogen atoms makes ECD a good option for their detection. These compounds are formulated as esters that hydrolyse after application. The hydroxyl group hinders GC determination, making convenient the derivatisation of these compounds to obtain a better GC response. The methyl derivative is often obtained by reaction with diazomethane or other methylation reagent. An alternative derivatisation is perfluoroacylation – the resulting derivatives can be analysed by GC-MS.

Table 16.9 Analytical methods used in the analysis of benzonitriles

Herbicide	Food	Technique	Derivatisation	Detector	LOD (mg/kg)	Reference
Bromoxynil	Onions	GC	Diazomethane	ECD	0.01	13
	Cereals	GC	Diazomethane	ECD	0.01	12
			HFBA[a]	MS	0.001	70
				ECD	0.005	42
		HPLC		UV	0.05	42
Ioxynil	Fruits, vegetables	GC		ECD	0.003	36
	Cereals	GC	HFBA	MS	0.001	70

[a] HFBA: heptafluorobutyric anhydride

16.3.3 Carbamates (Table 16.10)

Carbamates are a numerous group of pesticides derived from carbamic acid (H_2N-COOH). Most of them are insecticides and only a few compounds, such as chlorpropham, propham and tri-allate, are used as herbicides. In general, these compounds are thermolabile and may be analysed by HPLC. In some cases, their analysis by GC has been reported, after hydrolysis to the corresponding anilines, derivatisation and detection by NPD or MS.

16.3.4 Dinitroanilines (Table 16.11)

Pendimethalin and trifluralin are most often used in this group. Their thermal stability and the presence of several halogen atoms in some of them make GC-ECD the preferred analytical technique, together with GC-MS.

Table 16.10 Analytical methods used in the analysis of carbamates

Herbicide	Food	Technique	Detector	LOD (mg/kg)	Reference
Chlorpropham	Fruits, vegetables	GC	MS	0.005-0.05	44, 45, 78, 85
	Onions	GC	NPD	0.05	17
	Potatoes	GC	MS	0.01	88
	Fruits, vegetables, milk	GC	MS/MS	ppb range	76
Phenmedipham	Spinach	GC	MS		79
		HPLC	UV		79
Propham	Fruits, vegetables	HPLC	MS	0.05	61
Thiobencarb	Fruits, vegetables	GC	MS	0.05	45
Tri-allate	Fruits, vegetables	GC	MS		78, 85
Carbamates	Fruits, vegetables	GC	MS	0.03-0.05	26
			NPD	0.04-0.05	36
	Wine	HPLC	MS	0.08–0.41 ng/ml	35

16.3.5 Organophosphates: Glyphosate (Table 16.12)

Glyphosate is a herbicide widely used in agriculture. The high polarity of this compound and the need to analyse its main metabolite, aminomethylphosphonic acid (AMPA), makes determination by HPLC a preferred option. Nevertheless, as some organophosphates do not possess a good UV response, their

Table 16.11 Analytical methods used in the analysis of dinitroanilines

Herbicide	Food	Technique	Detector	LOD (mg/kg)	Reference
Ethalfluralin	Fruits, vegetables	GC	MS/MS	ppb range	76
Pendimethalin	Fruits, vegetables	GC	ECD	0.027-0.031	1
			ECD/NPD	0.004	36
			MS/MS	0.002	43, 76
	Fruits, vegetables, nuts	GC	NPD	0.022	23
	Onions	GC	ECD	0.003-0.021	63
Trifluralin	Fruits, vegetables	GC	ECD	0.026-0.11	1
			ECD/NPD	0.005	36
			MS/MS	0.002	43, 76
	Carrots	GC	ECD	0.002	48
	Grapes, wine	GC	NPD		94
	Wine	GC	MS	0.15 μg/l	86
	Composite dietary samples	GC	MS	0.0004	66
Dinitroanilines	Fruits, vegetables	GC	MS	0.02-0.05	26, 45, 78, 85
	Milk	GC	MS/MS	ppb range	76

Table 16.12 Analytical methods used in the analysis of organophosphorus herbicides

Herbicide	Food	Technique	Derivatisation[a]	Detector	LOD (mg/kg)	Reference
Glyphosate	Fruits, vegetables	HPLC, column switching	FMOC-Cl	FD	0.01	33
		HPLC	OPA-MERC	FD	0.05	49
	Kiwi, asparagus	GC	TFAA and diazomethane	FPD	0.05	73
	Cereals	HPLC		MS/MS	0.01	30
	Cereal, lentils, beans	HPLC	$NaNO_2$ and postcolumn derivatisation with KI-sulfamic acid- acetic acid- H_2SO_4	TEA	0.005–1	75

[a] FMOC-Cl: 9-fluorenylmethoxycarbonyl chloride, OPA: o-phthalaldehyde, MERC: 2-mercaptoethanol, TFAA: trifluoroacetic anhydride

determination by HPLC cannot be performed without derivatisation. Therefore, analyses of glyphosate and AMPA have been carried out by HPLC with fluorescence (FD), mass spectrometry (MS/MS) or chemiluminescence (TEA) detection and, in some cases, by GC after derivatisation with various reagents and detection using a flame photometric detector (FPD).

16.3.6 Phenoxyacids and aryloxyphenoxyacids (Table 16.13)

The oldest synthetic herbicide is the phenoxyacid 2, 4-D, synthesised after the Second World War and still in use. The acidic nature of such herbicides makes them highly polar and does not allow their direct analysis by GC. Various reagents have been used to obtain their corresponding esters. Methylation is frequently used by means of diazomethane or by other less toxic reagents like methanol-sulphuric acid or boron trifluoride-methanol. Pentafluorobenzyl esters are also obtained as they give a good GC-ECD response.

16.3.7 Quaternary ammonium herbicides (Table 16.14)

Diquat and paraquat are typical representatives of this group of herbicides. Their cationic nature favours adsorption to the matrix and makes necessary the use of strong acids for the extraction step. These compounds are not volatile and may be determined by HPLC with UV detection. Analysis by GC is only possible after hydrogenation, which can be done with sodium borohydride and nickel (II) chloride. The hydrogenated derivatives can be determined by GC-NPD or GC-MS. The analysis of these compounds in food has also been carried out by other techniques such as CE or ELISA.

Table 16.13 Analytical methods used in the analysis of phenoxyacids

Herbicide	Food	Technique	Derivatisation	Detector	LOD (mg/kg)	Reference
Diclofop	Fruits, vegetables	GC		ECD	0.052–0.14	1
Fluazifop	Fruits, vegetables	HPLC		MS/MS	0.01–0.05	9
		GC		ECD	0.01	36
	Potatoes, soybeans	GC	Diazomethane	NPD, MS	0.01	20
	Onions	GC	Diazomethane	MS	0.02	89
		HPLC		UV	0.2	89
Quizalofop	Fruits, vegetables	GC		MS	0.05	45
2,4-D	Fruits, vegetables	GC	BCl_3/ 2-chloroethanol	ECD		84
		CE		UV	0.005–0.085	52
		ELISA				64
	Lettuce	GC	PFB[a]	MS	0.5	87
	Citrus fruits	GC	BCl_3/ 2-chloroethanol	ECD	0.01	24
	Oranges	GC	BF_3/ methanol	MS		91
		ELISA				91, 92
	Wheat	GC	Diazomethane	ECD	0.05	12
		GC	BF_3/ methanol	ECD	0.20	18, 77
	Meat products	ELISA			0.001–0.014	51
	Milk	ELISA			0.001	62
MCPA	Wheat	HPLC		UV	ppb range	67
Mecoprop	Cereals	GC	BF_3/ methanol	Hall-ECD	0.001–0.002	15, 16
Phenoxy-acids	Cereals	GC	BF_3/ methanol	MS	0.04	71
	Peas	GC	Diazomethane	MS	0.0045	32
	Milk	HPLC		UV	0.5 ppb	100
	Fish	GC	Diazomethane	MS	0.1–4 ppb	83

[a] PFB: pentafluorobenzyl derivative

16.3.8 Triazines (Table 16.15)

Triazines are one of the oldest herbicide groups and comprise several compounds widely used in agriculture, such as atrazine and simazine. The wide use of atrazine and its properties make it one of the pollutants more frequently found in the environment. Triazines are thermally stable and have several nitrogen atoms. Therefore, they can be determined by GC, particularly with NPD detection, and also by GC-MS. Their determination by HPLC with UV or DAD detection is also possible, but the limit of detection (LOD) obtained is often worse. HPLC coupled with MS can also be used with a clear improvement in LOD.

Table 16.14 Analytical methods used in the analysis of quaternary ammonium

Herbicide	Food	Technique	Detector	LOD (mg/kg)	Reference
Diquat	Potatoes	CE	UV	0.01	90
		GC	NPD	0.005	31
	Cereals, vegetables	HPLC	UV	0.01	19
Paraquat	Potatoes	CE	UV	0.01	90
		GC	NPD	0.005	31
	Fruits, vegetables	ELISA		0.01	74
	Cereals, vegetables	HPLC	UV	0.01	19

Table 16.15 Analytical methods used in the analysis of triazines

Herbicide	Food	Technique	Detector	LOD (mg/kg)	Reference
Atrazine	Fruits, vegetables	GC	MS	0.004	44
			MS/MS	0.002	43
	Fruit juices	CE	UV	0.03	40
	Green beans	HPLC	DAD	0.02	57
	Oranges	GC	NPD		10
	Beef kidney	GC	MS	0.02	21
	Beef liver	HPLC	UV	0.005	50
	Meat products	ELISA		0.001–0.014	51
	Milk	ELISA		0.001	62
Cyanazine	Onions	GC	NPD	0.01	17
Metamitron	Fruits, vegetables	GC	MS		85
Prometryn	Parsley	GC	NPD	0.05	6
Simazine	Blueberries	HPLC	UV	0.08	22
	Chickpeas	GC	NPD	0.02	5
	Must	HPLC	UV	20 μg/l	55
	Wine	GC	NPD	35.7 μg/l	29
Terbuthylazine	Wine	GC	MS	0.55 μg/l	86
Triazines	Fruits, vegetables	GC	MS	0.02–0.07	26, 45, 78
			MS/MS	ppb range	76
			NPD	0.01–0.02	36, 56, 65
		HPLC	MS	1–5 ppb	54
			UV	0.01	7
	Cereals	GC	NPD	0.01–0.02	56, 65
	Composite dietary samples	GC	MS	0.002	66
	Eggs	GC	FTD[a]		59
	Milk	GC	NPD	0.02	56
			MS/MS	ppb range	76

[a] FTD: photometric detector

Table 16.16 Analytical methods used in the analysis of uracils

Herbicide	Food	Technique	Detector	LOD (mg/kg)	Reference
Bromacil	Fruits, vegetables	GC	MS	0.09–0.10	26, 45, 85
Lenacil	Fruits, vegetables	GC	MS	0.05	45, 85
	Spinach	HPLC	UV		79
		GC	MS		79
Terbacil	Fruits, vegetables	GC	NPD	0.02	36
			MS	0.04–0.05	26, 45

16.3.9 Uracils (Table 16.16)

This group of herbicides includes compounds such as bromacil, lenacil and terbacil. The presence of nitrogen atoms in their molecules, together with their stability, allows their determination by GC using NPD or MS detectors. In addition, determination by HPLC has also been reported.

16.3.10 Ureas (Table 16.17)

Ureas are an extensive group of herbicides widely used in agriculture. Phenylureas were first and diuron, linuron, chlortoluron and isoproturon are

Table 16.17 Analytical methods used in the analysis of ureas

Herbicide	Food	Technique	Detector	LOD (mg/kg)	Reference
Phenylureas					
Chlortoluron	Cereals	GC	MS	0.01	60
Diuron	Blueberries	HPLC	UV	0.17	22
	Green beans	HPLC	DAD	0.01	57
Linuron	Potatoes	GC	MS	0.1	46
Monolinuron	Fruits, vegetables	GC	MS	0.10	45
Tebuthiuron	Milk	GC	MS	0.03 μg/ml	69
Phenylureas	Fruits, vegetables	GC	NPD	0.08–0.10	36
			MS	0.03–0.21	26
			MS/MS	ppb range	76
		HPLC	UV	0.01	72, 97
			MS/MS	0.002	8, 34
	Wine	HPLC	UV	0.01–0.32 ng/ml	35
	Milk	GC	MS/MS	ppb range	76
		HPLC	UV		11
Sulfonylureas					
Bensulfuron	Rice, crayfish	HPLC	UV	0.008–0.05	98
Metsulfuron	Cereals, sugarcane	HPLC	UV	0.005	99
Sulfonylureas	Cereals	CE	UV	0.005–0.09	41, 52

typical representatives. These compounds are thermally unstable, which makes difficult their determination by GC. Nevertheless, they have been determined by this technique either directly or by analysis of their corresponding anilines obtained by hydrolysis. Direct GC determination has been achieved using low injection temperatures or by favouring the formation of isocyanate derivatives, the compounds actually determined, in the injection port of the gas chromatograph.[60]

A group of herbicides more recently developed are sulfonylureas, which have greater herbicide activity and are applied at lower doses. These compounds are also thermally unstable and may be analysed by HPLC, generally with UV detection.

16.4 Levels of herbicide residues found in food

Pesticides, and particularly herbicides, play a major role in maintaining agricultural production today. Nevertheless, their use may result in adverse effects caused by the toxicity of these chemicals. This fact, together with great public concern about food safety makes it necessary to monitor pesticide residues in food.

Pesticide monitoring programmes are operated by different countries all over the world.[27,47] In general, an important percentage of food monitored contained measurable residues. This is understandable because pesticides are widely used to produce food and the analytical detection limits for these chemicals are very low. However, the number of samples exceeding the maximum residue level (MRL), which is the maximum safe level expected following authorised pesticide application, is very low. The percentage of samples with values above MRLs in the 2001 monitoring program was 3.9% in EU and 1.1% in the United States. In the European monitoring program, the compounds most frequently found were fungicides in fruits and vegetables and insecticides in cereals, whereas in the United States monitoring program the five most often observed chemicals in total diet studies were insecticides.

Herbicide residue levels in food have not been frequently reported in the scientific literature. Table 16.18 summarises the herbicides found in those studies. The reported chemicals belong mainly to the widely used dinitroanilines, triazines and phenoxyacid groups, and the levels found are, in general, low. Some of these compounds are occasionally found in food of animal origin, particularly in milk, and the reported residue levels are also low.

16.5 Sources of further information and advice

BRAITHWAITE A and SMITH F J, 1999, *Chromatographic Methods*, Dordrecht, Kluwer Academic.

EU Plant Health/Pesticides Safety: *http://europa.eu.int/comm/food/*

Table 16.18 Herbicide residue levels found in food

Food	Herbicide	Level found (mg/kg)	Reference
Vegetable origin			
Cereals			
Corn	Atrazine	0.1	93
Rice	Benfluralin, trifluralin	0.07–0.08	96
Wheat	2,4-D	0.01–0.3	18
	Benfluralin, trifluralin	0.07	96
Fruits			
Apple	Pendimethalin	0.1-0.2	23
Fig	Pendimethalin	0.05-0.08	23
Orange	2,4-D	0.2-0.4	91, 92
Vegetables			
Asparagus	Pendimethalin	0.05	23
Carrot	Linuron	0.003	34
	Trifluralin	0.003–0.01	48
Green bean	Trifluralin	0.004	76
Lettuce	2,4-D	0.001–0.007	87
Onion	Metolachlor	0.01–0.06	82
	Pendimethalin	0.003–0.1	23, 63
Peas	MCPA	0.02	32
Potato	2,4-D	0.04	64
	Chlorpropham	0.006–0.08	88
	Metribuzin	0.008–0.04	54
Spinach	Lenacil	0.3	79
	Trifluralin	0.0002	76
Sweet potato	Trifluralin	0.0001	76
Animal origin			
Milk	2,4-D	0.02	3
	Alachlor	0.007	3
	Atrazine	0.008	3

EPA Residue Analytical Methods: *http://www.epa.gov/oppbead1/methods/ramindex.htm*

GROVER R, 1988, *Environmental Chemistry of Herbicides*, Florida, CRC Press.

HORNSBY A G, WAUCHOPE R D AND HERNER A E, 1996, *Pesticides Properties in the Environment*, New York, Springer.

HUTSON D H and ROBERTS T R, 1987, *Herbicides*, Chichester, John Wiley & Sons.

PAWLISZYN J, 1997, *Solid Phase Microextraction Theory and Practice*, Chichester, Wiley-VCH.

TOMLIN C D S, 2000, *The Pesticide Manual*, UK, British Crop Protection Council.

16.6 References

1 ADOU K, BONTOYAN W R, SWEENEY P J, 'Multiresidue method for the analysis of pesticide residues in fruits and vegetables by accelerated solvent extraction and capillary gas chromatography', *J Agric Food Chem,* 2001 **49**(9) 4153–60.

2 AHMED F E, 'Analyses of pesticides and their metabolites in foods and drinks', *Trends Anal Chem,* 2001 **20**(11) 649–61.

3 ALFERNESS P, WIEBE L, 'Determination of mesotrione residues and metabolites in crops, soil, and water by liquid chromatography with fluorescence detection', *J Agric Food Chem,* 2002 **50**(14) 3926–34.

4 ALFONSO HERNÁNDEZ M M, TRAVIESO SANTALLA A, ALVAREZ M E, 'Utilización de la cromatografía líquida en la determinación de residuos de lenacil en suelo y fre sas', *Ciencias De La Agricultura,* 1990 **39** 165–70.

5 ALLENDER W J, 'Measurement of simazine residues in chickpeas, *Cicer arietinum,* by gas-liquid chromatography', *Pestic Sci,* 1990 **29** 183–6.

6 BARDALAYE P C, WHEELER W B, 'Capillary gas chromatographic determination of prometryn and its degradation products in parsley', *J AOAC Int,* 1985 **68**(4) 750–3.

7 BATTISTA M, DI CORCIA A, MARCHETTI M, 'Extraction and isolation of triazine herbicides from water and vegetables by a double trap tandem system', *Anal Chem,* 1989 **61**(9) 935–9.

8 BESTER K, BORDIN G, RODRIGUEZ A, SCHIMMEL H, PAUWELS J, VANVYNCHT G, 'How to overcome matrix effects in the determination of pesticides in fruit by HPLC-ESI-MS-MS', *Fresenius J Anal Chem,* 2001 **371**(4) 550–5.

9 BOLYGO E, BOSELEY A, 'A liquid chromatography-tandem mass spectrometry method for Fluazifop residue analysis in crops', *Fresenius J Anal Chem,* 2000 **368**(8) 816–9.

10 BOURAID A, MARTIN ESTEBAN A, FERNÁNDEZ P, CÁMARA C, 'Microwave assisted extraction method for the determination of atrazine and four organophosphorus pesticides in oranges by gas chromatography', *Fresenius J Anal Chem,* 2000 **367**(3) 291–4.

11 BRANDSTETEROVA E, CHOVANCOVA V, MATISOVA E, HOLECKOVA J, TEKEL J, 'Application of micro-HPLC for the determination of phenylurea herbicides in milk', *J High Resolut Chromatogr,* 1991 **14**(10) 696–8.

12 CESSNA A, 'Comparison of extraction/hydrolysis procedures for the determination of acidic herbicides in plants: Residues of Mecoprop in barley following postemergence application', *J Agric Food Chem,* 1992 **40**(7) 1154–7.

13 CESSNA A, 'Gas chromatographic determination of bromoxynil in onions', *J Agric Food Chem,* 1990 **38**(9) 1844–7.

14 CESSNA A, 'HPLC determination of linuron residues in asparagus following pre- and early postemergence applications', *Can J Plant Sci,* 1990 **70**(2) 591–7.

15 CESSNA A, 'Residues of mecoprop in post-emergence- treated wheat and oat', *Pestic Sci,* 1992 **36**(1) 31–3.

16 CESSNA A, 'Simultaneous extraction and detection of residues of (2,4–dichlorophenoxy)acetic acid and bromoxynil from wheat', *J Agric Food Chem,* 1980 **28**(6) 1229–32.

17 CESSNA A, BENOIT D L, 'Weed control and herbicide residues in onion following use of chlorpropham and cyanazine', *Pestic Sci,* 1992 **35**(4) 355–62.

18 CESSNA A, HOLM F A, 'Residues of 2,4–D in wheat following application after

heading', *Can J Plant Sci,* 1993 **74**(1) 199–203.

19 CHICHILA T M, WALTERS S M, 'Liquid chromatography determination of paraquat and diquat in crops using silica column with aqueous ionic mobile phase', *J AOAC,* 1991 **74**(6) 961–7.

20 CLEGG B S, 'Gas chromatographic analysis of Fluazifop-butyl (Fusilade) in potatoes, soybeans, and soil', *J Agric Food Chem,* 1987 **35**(2) 269–73.

21 CURREN M S S, KING J W, 'Ethanol-modified subcritical water extraction combined with solid-phase microextraction for determining atrazine in beef kidney', *J Agric Food Chem,* 2001 **49**(5) 2175–80.

22 ELY C B, FRANS R E, LAVY T L, TALBERT R E, MATTICE J D, 'Determining diuron, simazine, and methiocarb residues in highbush blueberries (Vaccinium *corymbosum*)', *HORTSCIENCE,* 1993 **28**(1) 33–5.

23 ENGEBRETSON J, HALL G, HENGEL M, SHIBAMOTO T, 'Analysis of pendimethalin residues in fruit, nuts, vegetables, grass and mint by gas chromatography', *J Agric Food Chem,* 2001 **49**(5) 2198–206.

24 ERNER Y, COGGINS JR. C W, 'Free and bound residues of 2,4–D in "Marsh" grapefruit and "Washington" Navel orange fruit', *J Am Soc Hortic Sci,* 1989 **114**(5) 846–50.

25 EEC: EUROPEAN UNION COUNCIL DIRECTIVE 91/414/EEC, 1991.

26 FILLION J, HINDLE R, LACROIX M, SELWYN J, 'Multiresidue determination of pesticides in fruits and vegetables by gas chromatography mass selective detection and liquid chromatography with fluorescence detection', *J AOAC Int,* 1995 **78**(5) 1252–66.

27 FOOD AND DRUG ADMINISTRATION (FDA) PESTICIDE PROGRAM RESIDUE MONITORING 2001.

28 FQPA: FOOD QUALITY PROTECTION ACT USA, 1996.

29 GARCIA-REPETTO R, GARRIDO I, REPETTO M, 'Determination of organochlorine, organophosphorus, and triazine pesticide residues in wine by gas chromatography with electron- capture and nitrogen-phosphorus detection', *J AOAC Int,* 1996 **79**(6) 1423–7.

30 GRANBY K, VAHL M, 'Investigation of the herbicide glyphosate and the plant growth regulators chlormequat and mepiquat in cereals produced in Denmark', *Food Addit Contam,* 2001 **18**(10) 898–905.

31 HAJSLOVA J, CUHRA P, DAVIDEK T, DAVIDEK J, 'Gas chromatographic determination of diquat and paraquat in crops', *J Chromatogr,* 1989 **479**(2) 243–50.

32 HENGEL M J, MOURER C R, SHIBAMOTO T, 'Gas chromatographic/mass spectrometric method for analysis of chlorophenoxy acid herbicides MCPB and MCPA in peas', *Journal of Environmental Chemistry*, 1998 **8**(3) 429–33.

33 HERNANDEZ F, HIDALGO C, SANCHO J V, 'Determination of glyphosate residues in plants by precolumn derivatization and coupled-column liquid chromatography with fluorescence detection', *J AOAC Int,* 2000 **83**(3) 728–34.

34 HOGENBOOM A C, HOFMAN M P, KOK S J, NIESSEN W M A, BRINKMAN U A TH, 'Determination of pesticides in vegetables using large-volume injection column liquid chromatography-electrospray tandem mass spectrometry', *J Chromatogr A,* 2000 **892**(1/2) 379–90.

35 JINGCUN W, TRAGAS C, LORD H, PAWLISZYN J, 'Analysis of polar pesticides in water and wine samples by automated in-tube solid-phase microextraction coupled with high-performance liquid chromatography-mass spectrometry', *J Chromatogr A,* 2002 **976**(1/2) 357–67.

36 KADENCZKI L, ARPAD Z, GARDI I, AMBRUS A, GYORFI L, REESE G, EBING W, 'Column

extraction of residues of several pesticides from fruits and vegetables a simple multiresidue analysis method', *J AOAC Int,* 1992 **75**(1) 53–61.

37 KAIHARA A, YOSHII K, TSUMURA Y, NAKAMURA Y, ISHIMITSU S, TONOGAI Y, 'Multiresidue analysis of pesticides in fresh fruits and vegetables by supercritical fluid extraction and HPLC', *J Health Sci*, 2000 **46**(5) 336–42.

38 KESARI R, MANISH R, GUPTA V K, 'Spectrophotometric method for determination of paraquat in food and biological samples', *J AOAC Int,* 1997 **80**(2) 388–91.

39 KHAN S U, 'Electron capture gas-liquid chromatographic method for the simultaneous analysis of 2,4–D, Dicamba, and Mecoprop residues in soil, wheat and barley', *J AOAC,* 1975 **58**(5) 1027–31.

40 KHROLENKO M, DZYGIEL P, WIECZOREK P, 'Combination of supported liquid membrane and solid-phase extraction for sample pretreatment of triazine herbicides in juice prior to capillary electrophoresis determination', *J Chromatogr A,* 2002 **975**(1) 219–27.

41 KRYNITSKY A J, SWINEFORD D M, 'Determination of sulfonylurea herbicides in grains by capillary electrophoresis', *J AOAC Int,* 1995 **78**(4) 1091–6.

42 LAWRENCE J F, PANOPIO L G, MCLEOD H A, 'Comparison of liquid and gas chromatography for the determination of bromoxynil octanoate and benzoylprop ethyl in wheat products', *J Agric Food Chem,* 1980 **28**(5) 1019–22.

43 LEHOTAY S J, 'Analysis of pesticide residues in mixed fruit and vegetable extracts by direct sample introduction/ gas chromatography/tandem mass spectrometry', *J AOAC Int,* 2000 **83**(3) 680–97.

44 LEHOTAY S J, ELLER K, 'Development of a method of analysis for 46 pesticides in fruits and vegetables by supercritical fluid extraction and gas chromatography/ion trap mass spectrometry', *J AOAC Int,* 1995 **78**(3) 821–30.

45 LIAO W, JOE T, CUSICK W G, 'Multiresidue screening method for fresh fruits and vegetables with gas chromatographic / mass spectrometric detection', *J AOAC,* 1991 **74**(3) 554–65.

46 MATTERN G C, SINGER G M, 'Determination of linuron in potatoes using capillary column gas chromatography/ mass spectrometry', *J AOAC,* 1989 **72**(6) 970–4.

47 MONITORING OF PESTICIDE RESIDUES IN PRODUCTS OF PLANT ORIGIN IN THE EUROPEAN UNION, NORWAY ICELAND AND LIECHTENSTEIN 2001 REPORT, 2003.

48 MORTIMER R D, BLACK D B, DAWSON B A, 'Pesticide residue analysis on foods by NMR. III. Comparison of ^{19}F NMR and GC-ECD for analyzing trifluralin residues in field-grown carrots', *J Agric Food Chem,* 1994 **42**(8) 1713–6.

49 MOYE H A, MILES C J, SCHERER S J, 'A simplified high-performance liquid chromatographic residue procedure for the determination of glyphosate herbicide and (Aminomethyl)phosphonic acid in fruits and vegetables employing postcolumn fluorogenic labelling', *J Agric Food Chem,* 1983 **31**(1) 69–72.

50 MULDOON M T, STANKER L H, 'Molecularly imprinted solid phase extraction of atrazine from beef liver extracts', *Anal Chem,* 1997 **69**(5) 803–8.

51 NAM K S, KING J W, 'Supercritical fluid extraction and enzyme immunoassay for pesticide detection in meat products', *J Agric Food Chem,* 1994 **42**(7) 1469–74.

52 NEMOTO S, LEHOTAY S J, 'Analysis of multiple herbicides in soybeans using pressurized liquid extraction and capillary electrophoresis', *J Agric Food Chem,* 1998 **46**(6) 2190–9.

53 NORTRUP D A, 'Determination of residues of alachlor and related herbicides in crops by liquid chromatography with electrochemical detection', *J AOAC Int,* 1997 **80**(5) 1104–10.

54 OKIHASHI M, AKUTSU K, OBANA H, HORI S, 'Determination of triazine herbicides in foods with liquid chromatography mass spectrometry', *Analyst,* 2000 **125**(11) 1966–9.
55 ORTIZ-GÓMEZ M T, PÉREZ-ARRIBAS L V, LEÓN-GONZÁLEZ M E, POLO-DÍEZ L M, 'Liquid Chromatography determination of simazine and antimycin A in must', *J Agric Food Chem,* 1995 **43**(11) 2883–6.
56 PARDUE J R, 'Multiresidue method for the chromatographic determination of triazine herbicides and their metabolites in raw agricultural products', *J AOAC Int,* 1995 **78**(3) 856–62.
57 PARRILLA P, MARTINEZ VIDAL J L, 'HPLC determination of pesticides in green bean samples after SPE clean-up', *Chromatographia,* 1996 **43**(5/6) 265–70.
58 PAWLISZYN J, 'New directions in sample preparation for analysis of organic compounds', *Trends Anal Chem,* 1995 **14**(3) 113–22.
59 PENSABENE J W, FIDDLER W, DONOGHUE D J, 'Supercritical fluid extraction of atrazine and other triazine herbicides from fortified and incurred eggs', *J Agric Food Chem,* 2000 **48**(5) 1668–72.
60 PÉREZ S, MATIENZO M T, TADEO J L, 'GC-ITD analysis of chlortoluron and its metabolites in cereals', *Chromatographia,* 1993 **36** 195–200.
61 POUS X, RUIZ M J, PICO Y, FONT G, 'Determination of imidacloprid, metalaxyl, myclobutanil, propham, and thiabendazole in fruits and vegetables by liquid chromatography-atmospheric pressure chemical ionization-mass spectrometry', *Fresenius J Anal Chem,* 2001 **371**(2) 182–9.
62 PYLYPIW HM JR, HANKIN L, 'Herbicides in pooled raw milk in Connecticut', *J Food Prot,* 1991 **54**(2) 136–7.
63 RAJ M F, PATEL B K, SHAH P G, BAREDAVIA T N, 'Pendimethalin, fluchloralin and oxadiazon residue in/on onion', *Pesticide Research Journal*, 1999 **11**(1) 68–70.
64 RICHMAN S J, KARTHIKEYAN S, BENNETT D A, CHUNG A C, LEE S M, 'Low-level immunoassay screen for 2,4–Dichlorophenoxyacetic acid in apples, grapes, potatoes and oranges. Circumventing matrix effects', *J Agric Food Chem,* 1996 **44**(9) 2924–9.
65 ROSEBOOM H, HERBOLD H A, 'Determination of triazine herbicides in various crops by capillary gas chromatography with thermionic detection', *J Chromatogr* 1980 **202**(3) 431–8.
66 ROSENBLUM L, HIEBER T, MORGAN J, 'Determination of pesticides in composite dietary samples by gas chromatography/mass spectrometry in the selected ion monitoring mode by using a temperature-programmable large volume injector with preseparation column', *J AOAC Int,* 2001 **84**(3) 891–900.
67 RUCKENDORFER H, LINDNER W, 'Trace analysis of 2, 4, 5, TP and other acidic herbicides in wheat using multicolumn-HPLC', *Int J Environ Anal Chem,* 1984 **18** 87–99.
68 RUSSO C, LANZA C M, TOMASELLI F, LANZA G, ALEPPO E M DI, 'HPLC determination of 2–(2,4–Dichlorophenoxy) propionic acid used for fruit drop control of citrus', *Ital J Food* 1991 **3**(3) 231–7.
69 RUTHERFORD B S, SHACKELFORD D D, ULMER J J, 'Determination of tebuthiuron and metabolites in bovine milk by GC-MSD', *J Agric Food Chem,* 1995 **43**(8) 2110–6.
70 SÁNCHEZ-BRUNETE C, GARCÍA-VALCÁRCEL A I, TADEO J L, 'Determination of bromoxynil and ioxynil residues in cereals and soil by GC-ITD', *Chromatographia,* 1994 **38**(9/10) 624–8.
71 SÁNCHEZ-BRUNETE C, GARCÍA-VALCÁRCEL A I, TADEO J L, 'Determination of residues

of phenoxy acid herbicides in soil and cereals by gas chromatography-ion trap detection', *J Chromatogr A,* 1994 **675**(1/2) 213–8.
72 SANNINO A, 'Determination of phenylurea herbicide residues in vegetables by liquid chromatography after gel permeation chromatography and Florisil cartridge cleanup', *J AOAC Int,* 1998 **81**(5) 1048–53.
73 SEIBER J N, MCCHESNEY M M, KON R, LEAVITT R A, 'Analysis of Glyphosate residues in kiwi fruit and asparagus using high-performance liquid chromatography of derivatized glyphosate as a cleanup step', *J Agric Food Chem,* 1984 **32**(3) 678–81.
74 SELISKER M Y, HERZOG D P, ERBER R D, FLEEKER J R, ITAK J A, 'Determination of paraquat in fruits and vegetables by a magnetic particle based enzyme-linked immunosorbent assay', *J Agric Food Chem,* 1995 **43**(2) 544–7.
75 SEN N P, BADDOO P A, 'Determination of glyphosate as N-nitroso derivative by high performance liquid chromatography with chemiluminescence detection', *Int J Environ Anal Chem,* 1996 **63**(2) 107–17.
76 SHERIDAN R S, MEOLA J R, 'Analysis of pesticide residues in fruits, vegetables, and milk by gas chromatography/tandem mass spectrometry', *J AOAC Int,* 1999 **82**(4) 982–90.
77 SMITH A E, 'Gas chromatographic method for analysis of 2,4–D in wheat. Interlaboratory study', *J AOAC,* 1984 **67**(4) 794–8.
78 SOJO L E, BROCKE A, FILLION J, PRICE S M, 'Application of activated carbon membranes for on-line cleanup of vegetable and fruit extracts in the determination of pesticide multiresidues by gas chromatography with mass selective detection', *J Chromatogr A,* 1997 **788**(1/2) 141–54.
79 SORCE C, CECCARELLI N, LORENZI R, 'Residues of Lenacil and Phenmedipham in spinach leaves', *Agricultura Mediterránea*, 1994 **124** 132–41.
80 TADEO J L, SÁNCHEZ-BRUNETE C, 'Analysis of pesticide residues in fruit juices by matrix-solid phase dispersion and gas chromatographic determination', *Chromatographia,* 2003 **57**(11/12) 793–8.
81 TADEO J L, SÁNCHEZ-BRUNETE C, PÉREZ R A, FERNÁNDEZ M D, 'Analysis of herbicide residues in cereals, fruits and vegetables', *J Chromatogr A,* 2000 **882**(1/2) 175–91.
82 TAMILSELVAN C, SUNDARARAJAN R, 'Terminal residues of metolachlor in groundnut (Arachis hypogaea), soybean (Glycine max) and onion (Allium cepa)', *Indian J Agric Sci,* 1994 **64**(7) 495–7.
83 TERNES T A, BAUMANN W, NAGEL R, 'Contributions to the analysis of organic xenobiotics in fish. II. Method for the determination of chlorophenoxy herbicides in fish using GC/MS', *Fresenius J Anal Chem,* 1996 **354**(2) 237–40.
84 TING K C, KHO P K, 'Determination of trace 2,4–dicholophenoxyacetic acid in fresh produce by gas chromatography with boron trichloride/2-chloroethanol derivatization', *J AOAC Int,* 1998 **81**(1) 93–8.
85 TUINSTRA L G M T, ROOS A H, MATSER A M, TRAAG W A, RHIJN J A VAN, 'Development of a multi-residue/multi-matrix method for pesticide analysis in agricultural products', *Fresenius J Anal Chem,* 1991 **339** 384–6.
86 VITALI M, GUIDOTTI M, GIOVINAZZO R, CEDRONE O, 'Determination of pesticide residues in wine by SPME and GC/MS for consumer risk assessment', *Food Addit Contam,* 1998 **15**(3) 280–7.
87 VOGEL A, 'Methodology and determination of 2,4–D and triclopyr residues employing the GC-ITD in the analysis of lettuce plants cultivated in the Tala Valley, Republic of South Africa', *Bull Environ Contam Toxicol,* 1998 **60**(3) 371–8.
88 VOLANTE M, CATTANEO M, BIANCHI M, ZOCCOLA G, 'Some applications of solid phase

micro extraction (SPME) in the analysis of pesticide residues in food', *J Environ Sci Health, Part B,* 1998 **33**(3) 279–92.

89 WIGFIELD Y Y, LANOUETTE M, 'Supercritical fluid extraction of the fortified residues of fluazifop-P-butyl (Fusilade II) and its major metabolite, Fluazifop-P in onions', *J Agric Food Chem,* 1993 **41**(1) 84–8.

90 WIGFIELD Y Y, MCCORMACK K A, 'Simultaneous determination of residues of paraquat and diquat in potatoes using high performance capillary electrophoresis with UV detection', *J Agric Food Chem,* 1993 **41**(12) 2315–8.

91 WILLIAMS K J, JAMES R J, THORPE S A, REYNOLDS S L, 'Two analytical methods for the measurement of 2,4–D in oranges an ELISA screening procedure and a GC-MS confirmatory procedure', *Pestic Sci,* 1997 **50**(2) 135–40.

92 WILLIAMS K J, THORPE S A, REYNOLDS S L, 'The use of ELISA for the determination of pesticide residues in food', *Int J Environ Anal Chem,* 1995 **65**(1/4) 149–52.

93 WITTMANN C, HOCK B, 'Analysis of triazine residues in food by an enzyme immunoassay', *J Agric Food Chem,* 1993 **41**(9) 1421–5.

94 YING G G, WILLIAMS B, 'Herbicide residues in grapes and wines', *J Environ Sci Health, Part B,* 1999 **34**(3) 397–411.

95 YOSHII K, OKADA M, TSUMURA Y, NAKAMURA Y, ISHIMITSU S, TONOGAI Y, 'Supercritical fluid extraction of ten chloroacetanilide pesticides and pyriminobac-methyl in crops comparision with the Japanese bulletin method', *J AOAC Int,* 1999 **82**(5) 1239–45.

96 YUGANDHAN S N, REDDY S K, KUMAR R P R, JAYARAMA R S, 'Differential pulse polarographic determination of Benfluralin and Trifluralin in formulations and grains', *Int J Environ Anal Chem,* 1999 **72**(4) 247–55.

97 ZAHNOW E W, 'Analysis of the herbicide diuron in crops', *J Agric Food Chem,* 1987 **35**(3) 403–6.

98 ZHOU M, BRAMBLE F Q, DEVINE T J, NORWOOD G I, 'Determination of bensulfuron methyl in rice and crayfish by liquid chromatography with a column- and eluant-switching system and UV detection', *J AOAC Int,* 1996 **79**(3) 791–6.

99 ZHOU M, LI G Y, WHALEN S A, 'Determination of metsulfuron methyl and its two metabolites in crops by liquid chromatography with ultraviolet detection', *J AOAC Int,* 1994 **77**(6) 1654–9.

100 ZHU L, EE K H, ZHAO L, LEE H K, 'Analysis of phenoxy herbicides in bovine milk by means of liquid-liquid-liquid microextraction with a hollow-fiber membrane', *J Chromatogr A,* 2002 **963**(1/2) 335–43.

Part IV

Other chemical residues in food

17

Xenoestrogens

I. Shaw, University of Canterbury, New Zealand; B. Thomson and P. Cressey, Institute of Environmental Science & Research, New Zealand

17.1 Introduction

Guillette *et al.* (1994) reported that in Lake Apopka (Florida, USA) alligators' penises were shorter than those of alligators from neighbouring Lake Woodruff. A great deal of very elegant research linked this effect to estrogen-mimicking organochlorine pesticides (OCs) contaminating Lake Apopka which collected significant run-off from surrounding farmland. Since this important observation there have been numerous studies which have shown that a multitude of animal species are affected by a broad array of environmental estrogens. Whether humans might be among the animals affected by exposure to exogenous estrogens via their food and drinking water soon became a very real scientific question. The immediacy of this question was accentuated when effects were seen, for example a steady decline in sperm count over the past 50 years (Carlsen *et al.*, 1992), which could be attributed to estrogenic effects. There is now a great deal of interest in the exogenous estrogens and their potential effects upon people. While it is possible to show that trends exist in particular potential effects upon people (e.g. decreasing sperm count) and that the concentrations of specific xenoestrogens are increasing in our environment (including food and drinking water), so far no conclusive cause/effect links have been shown.

There are several physiological effects in humans which could be caused by estrogens. For example, the sperm count has been shown to be in decline over the past 50 years. Indeed between 1951 and 1973 there was a 2% per annum decline in sperm count in UK males (Irvine *et al.*, 1996). If this trend continues within 25 years the fertility of UK males will have declined to such an extent that the birth rate is likely to be affected. Similar observations have been made in other countries (Van Waeleghem *et al.*, 1994; Auger *et al.*, 1995). There is a great deal of controversy surrounding these data. For example, of the data used by Carlsen *et al.*, (1992):

- 48 of the 61 (79%) case studies cited were after 1970; and
- different inclusion criteria were used for these which may skew the results – in simple terms the earlier data were likely to be more representative of the general male population, whereas the later data were likely to be from men who visited infertility clinics and so were more likely to have lower sperm quality.

Despite this, scientists are agreed that there has been a decline in sperm quality; it is the magnitude of the decline that is still a matter of conjecture.

Breast cancer is related to natural estrogen in some patients. It is known that some breast cancers can be caused by particular clones of transformed breast cells possessing estrogen receptors (ER) which stimulate division when they are occupied by natural estrogen. Indeed, one of the most effective treatments for breast cancer is Tamoxifen, an ER blocker. The frequency of breast cancer is increasing (Hakulinen *et al.*, 1986), but, perhaps the most important observation is that for male breast cancer (a rare condition), the frequency of which has increased significantly (Ewertz *et al.*, 1989) over the past decade. This latter point is important in the context of potential exogenous estrogen effects because male estrogen levels are very low and so if absorbed xenoestrogens might raise the blood estrogen activity sufficiently to result in pharmacological effects, the outcome might be tumour development. This is very much less likely in females who have relatively very high natural estrogen levels and so for xenoestrogens to have an impact very high doses would be necessary (human sperm count and breast cancer will be discussed later in this chapter). Similarly, the frequency of testicular cancer in humans is also increasing and endocrine disrupters in the environment have been implicated (Adami *et al.*, 1994), but there is much less supportive data for this link.

Armed with the evidence that potentially exogenous estrogen-mediated human disease is increasing in frequency, the cause/effect relationship must be explored carefully. In light of this it is perhaps surprising that there is no concrete evidence for a cause/effect relationship between and in humans. However, despite the lack of definitive evidence for a link between exposure to xenoestrogens and human endocrine-related disorders, there is good circumstantial evidence which points firmly to the likelihood that the human effects are related, at least in part, to exposure to xenoestrogens. The main tenets of this circumstantial argument are:

- Xenoestrogens occur in the environment.
- We are exposed via food and drinking water.
- There is good evidence for animal effects (i.e. laboratory experiments linking exposure to xenoestrogens to pharmacological effects).

17.2 Mechanism of action of xenoestrogens

17.2.1 The estrogen receptor (ER)

ERs are present in the cytoplasm of many cell types. They are large protein molecules with a specific binding site which has conformational specificity for the estrogen molecule (i.e. in a natural context 17β-estradiol). When the receptor is occupied by an estrogen a signal is sent via a molecular messenger system to the cell nucleus which stimulates specific protein synthesis. The overall effect of the interaction is feminisation at a cellular and whole body level. The specificity of the ER is determined by the chemistry of the binding site (Fig. 17.1). It should be noted that the structural requirements for a ligand to bind to the ER appear to be sufficiently generic to allow binding by a wide range of natural and synthetic compounds.

Amino acid residues in the binding site interact on a conformationally specific basis with particular chemical groups on the estrogen molecule (Fig. 17.2). For example, there is a requirement for two hydrophilic groups a specific distance apart (they probably hydrogen bond to amino acid residues in the binding site) and a hydrophobic region between the hydroxyls (which is likely to interact with hydrophobic amino acids in the binding site by Van der Waals forces). 17β-Estradiol is the best fit for the ER and therefore results in a maximum response. Other molecules which have structural similarities to 17β-estradiol will also fit the site, but less well and so elicit a diminished ER-mediated response (Table 17.1). There are two ERs, α and β, which are structurally similar, but have different ligand specificities and elicit different

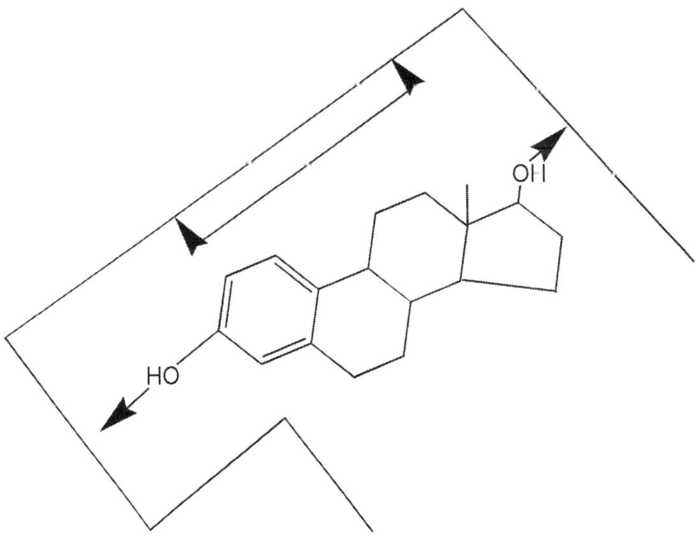

Fig. 17.1 Schematic representation of the estrogen receptor (ER) showing the requirement for specific molecular attributes of the ligand i.e., two hydrophilic groups (e.g., -OH) and a hydrophobic region (e.g., polycyclic region) (from Shaw and Chadwick, 1998).

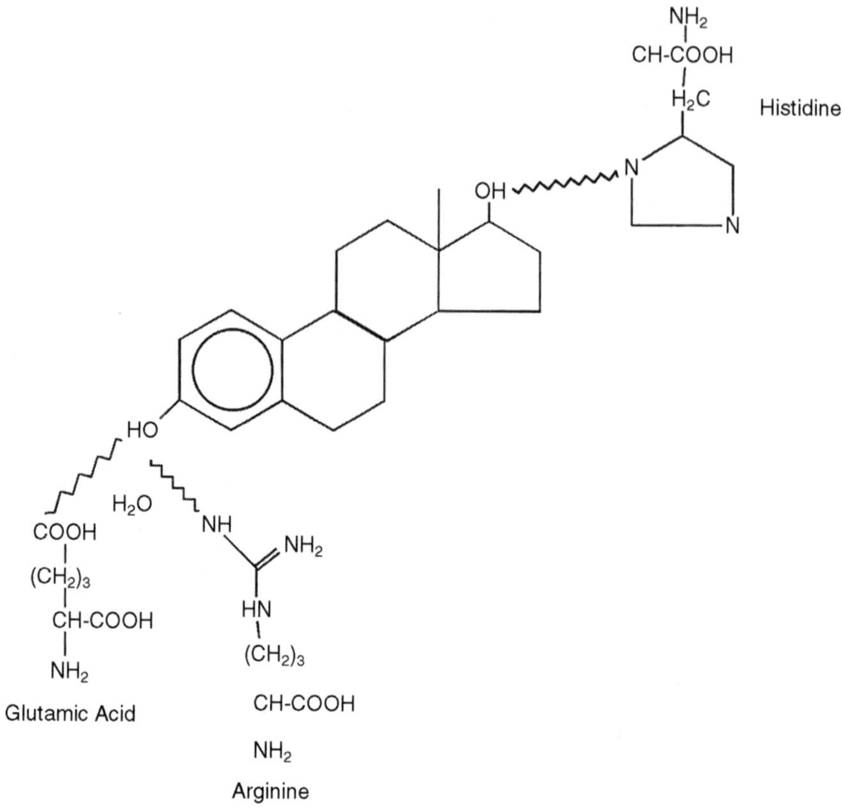

Fig. 17.2 Interaction between estrogen receptor amino acids and 17β-estradiol in the estrogen receptor active site.

Table 17.1 Relative binding affinities (the higher the number the greater the binding affinity) of different estrogens and xenoestrogens for the α- and β-estrogen receptors (Gruber *et al.*, 2002).

Estrogen/Xenoestrogen	Estrogen Receptor	
	α	β
17β-Estradiol	100	100
17α-Estradiol	58	11
Estriol	14	21
Estrone	60	37
4-Hydroxyestradiol	13	7
2-Hydroxyestrone	2	0.2
Genistein	4	87
Coumestrol	20	140
Daidzein	0.1	0.5
4-Octylphenol	0.02	0.07
Nonylphenol	0.05	0.09

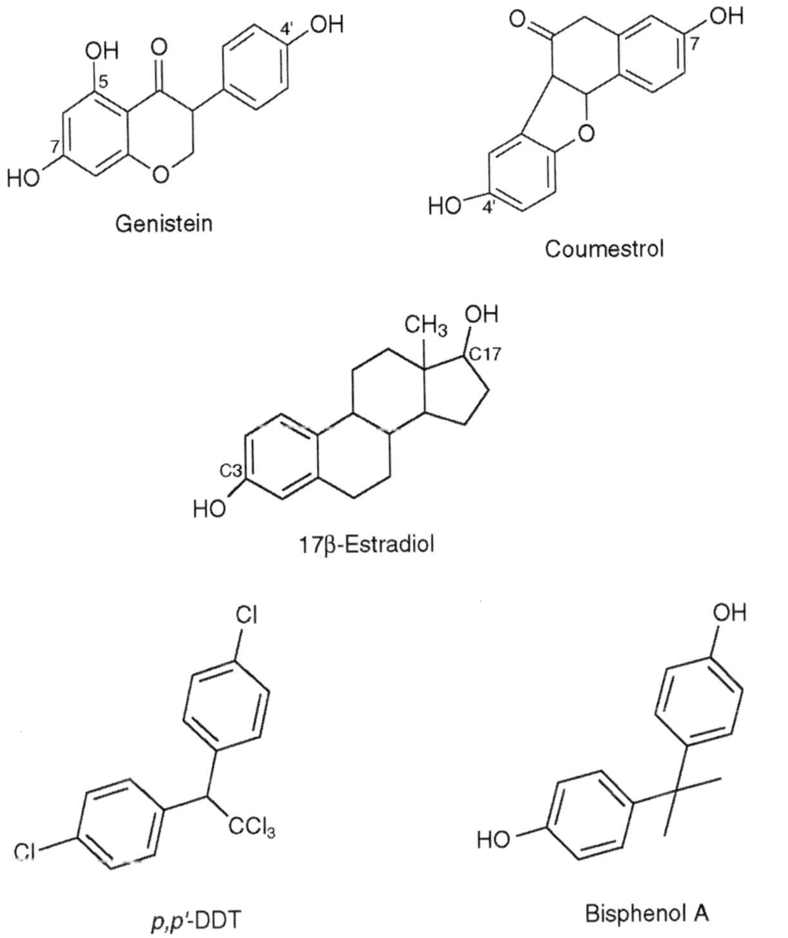

Fig. 17.3 A selection of estrogenic compounds showing their structural analogy to 17β-estradiol.

physiological responses. Structural analogy with 17 β-estradiol is a good way of predicting estrogenicity (Fig. 17.3; Shaw and McCully, 2002).

Structure activity relationships for estrogenic activity are emerging. It is now possible to make some predictions about estrogenic activity if molecular structure is known. However, there are still estrogenically active compounds that defy the emerging rules.

Structure activity relationships have been elegantly explored in detail by Fang *et al.* (2001). The basic criteria are molecular fit into the estrogen receptor, and the position of electron withdrawing groups that coincide with the key amino acids in the ER site (see Fig. 17.2). It is clear how important this fit is when xenoestrogen activity is compared with molecular dimensions, in particular separation of electron withdrawing groups (e.g. –OH) (Fig. 17.4) that are intimately involved in hydrogen bonding to the key amino acid residues.

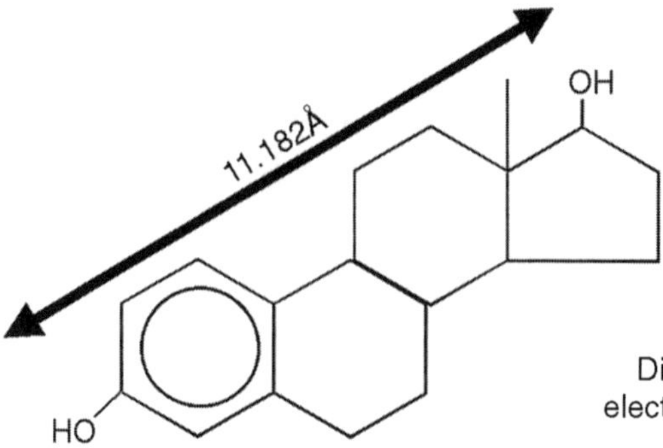

	Distance between electronegative groups (Å)	Relative estrogenicity
17β-estradiol	11.182	1
Coumestrol	11.406	2×10^{-3}
Genistein	11.773	1×10^{-4}
Dieldrin	~7.25	1×10^{-6}
DDT	9.270	3×10^{-5}

Fig. 17.4 Comparison of the separation of electronegative groups and estrogenic potency (relative to 17 β-estradiol) between selected xenoestrogens and 17β-estradiol.

17.2.2 Sexual differentiation

Sexual differentiation in humans occurs at about four weeks of gestation, at which time a gene on the Y chromosome produces an enzyme that stimulates development of the testis. In the absence of this enzyme ovaries develop. Once testes have formed they secrete a peptide (anti-Mullerian hormone), which causes regression of the potential female reproductive tract, and testosterone, which in turn stimulates development of the male reproductive tract. Estrogen does not appear to have a role in sexual differentiation at this stage. The developing fetus is protected from high levels of maternal estrogen by sex-hormone binding globulin (SHBG), which binds and inactivates estrogen.

17.2.3 The role of estrogen in males

The testis consists of a large number of seminiferous tubules lined with Sertoli cells and germ cells, with interstitial (Leydig) cells lying in the connective tissue between the tubules. During the fetal and pre-pubertal period of development, Sertoli cells are able to synthesise testosterone from estradiol. It is thought that the main function of this conversion in males is to provide a negative feedback effect on the multiplication and differentiation of Leydig cells and on their capacity to synthesise testosterone. Exposure of males to levels of estrogen found in females would have a feminising effect, resulting in breast formation, fat deposition, and reduced fertility due to suppression of gonadatrophin release.

17.2.4 The role of estrogen in females

Estrogen plays a crucial role in the maintenance and function of the female reproductive tract, including stimulating proliferation of granulosa cells within the maturing follicle and increasing oviduct motility and secretions necessary for sperm capacitation. Estrogen also stimulates proliferation of uterine endometrial cells and sensitises the myometrium to contractile influences at parturition. During puberty, estrogen stimulates breast duct growth and influences female patterns of fat deposition. In adults, estrogen is important for the maintenance of bone structure through the stimulation of calcium deposition – hence post-menopausal osteoporosis.

Exposure of adult females to abnormally high estrogenic activity may affect ovarian and oviduct function and fertility and result in proliferation of uterine and breast tissue, which may lead to carcinoma.

17.3 Assays for xenoestrogens

17.3.1 *In vitro* assays

In vitro estrogen assays fall into three groups, corresponding to steps in the estrogen receptor-dependent metabolic pathway that they assay (Fig. 17.5). The groups are:

- Receptor binding assays, which measure the strength of the interaction between the estrogen receptor and the estrogenic compound.
- Receptor-dependent gene expression assays, which measure the ability of the estrogenic compound to activate cells' biochemical responses, via the estrogen receptor and hence to produce a protein or proteins.
- Cell proliferation assays, which measure an estrogen-dependent cellular response.

17.3.2 Receptor binding assays

These assays measure the strength of the interaction between the estrogen receptor and the test xenoestrogen in a competitive binding assay with 17β estradiol. Assays utilise estrogen receptors from mouse uteri (Korach *et al.*, 1988, Krishnan *et al.*, 1993), spotted seatrout liver (Thomas and Smith, 1993), rainbow trout liver (White *et al.*, 1994), cultured MCF-7 human breast cancer cells (Nagle *et al.*, 1997) and cultured ECC-1 human endometrial carcinoma cell lines (Bergeron *et al.*, 1999).

17.3.3 Receptor-dependent gene expression assays

Receptor-dependent gene expression assays measure the ability of the estrogenic compound to cause a conformational change in the receptor leading to DNA transcription and gene expression. Examples of assays of this type include the following.

- Yeast estrogen screen (YES), created by transfecting yeast cells with the human estrogen receptor and two estrogen response elements linked to the

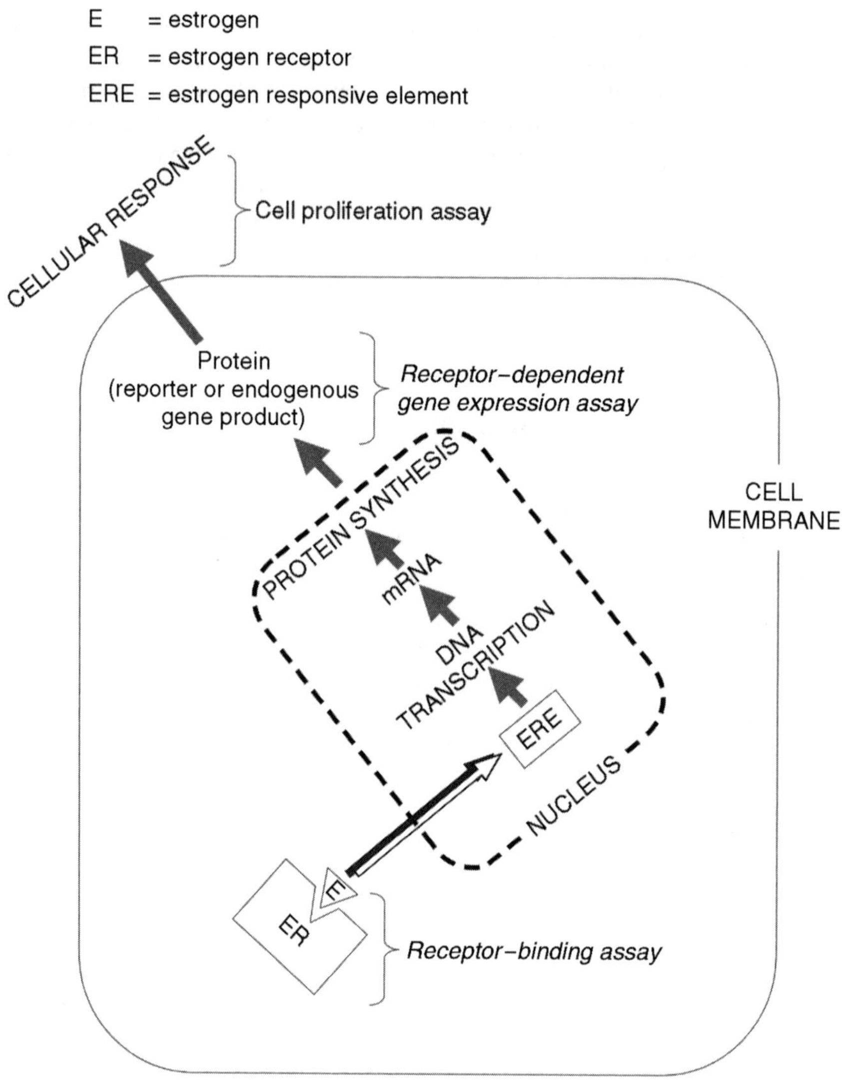

Fig. 17.5 Assays for estrogenicity showing their targets in estrogen's mechanism of action.

lacZ reporter gene, coding for β-galactosidase (Arnold *et al.*, 1996) which is upregulated and leads to the conversion of a yellow galactoside dye to red chromophore (plus galactose) that can be measured spectrophotometrically.

- HeLa cells, which do not contain an estrogen receptor, co-transfected with an estrogen responsive reporter vector (ERET81CAT) and a mouse ER vector (pRSV). Estrogenic activation results in production of chloramphenicol acetyltransferase (CAT), which is detected by ELISA (Shelby *et al.*, 1996).

- The production of cathepsin-D and pS2 from MCF-7 human breast cancer cell line can be monitored with the ELSA-CATH-D and ELSA-PS2 immunoradiometric assays following exposure to estrogenic compounds (Olea *et al.*, 1996).
- Production of complement C3, a well known estradiol-regulated protein from a cultured rat endometrial adenocarcinoma cell line (RUCA-I). Proteins are labelled with [^{35}S]-methionine and determined by autoradiography after electrophoretic separation (Hopert *et al.*, 1998).
- Production of zona radiata proteins and vitellogenin in primary hepatocytes from Atlantic salmon exposed to xenoestrogens in vitro. Protein products are determined by ELISA (Celius *et al.*, 1999).

17.3.4 Cell proliferation assays

Cell proliferation assays measure an estrogen-dependent physiological response resulting from the production of functional proteins. The ability of chemicals to induce estrogen receptor positive cell proliferation is an indicator of estrogenic activity (Soto *et al.*, 1995). Assays of this sort can be carried out *in vitro* by utilising established cell lines derived from estrogen responsive target organs, such as rat pituitary cells and human breast cancer cell lines (T47-D and MCF-7). MCF-7 is by far the most commonly used cell line for assays of estrogenicity and is the basis for the so-called E-Screen assay (Soto *et al.*, 1995).

17.3.5 *In vivo* assays

Perhaps the best assays are those that use target species response. For example, exposure of trout to xenoestrogens results in vitellogenin synthesis. These assays all rely on a measure of pharmacological response (e.g. vitellogenin production). They are applied mainly to the assessment of environmental impact.

17.3.6 Choice of assay and comparison of results from different assays

The yeast (YES) and E-Screen assays are the most widely used. Whilst the majority of assays have employed purified individual test chemicals and the response compared to a reference compound (generally 17 β-estradiol), the yeast assay has been used to study the effect of mixtures and to measure estrogenicity of foodstuffs (Silvia *et al.*, 2002). Results from the different assay methods cannot be compared directly. However it is arguable that relative estrogenicity (i.e. relative to 17 β-estradiol – estradiol equivalence factor (EQ)) can be compared between assays.

17.4 Measuring risks from different xenoestrogens

To compare exposure to xenoestrogens with endogenous levels of estrogens, xenoestrogen exposures are multiplied by 17 β-estradiol equivalence factors (EQs) for the individual xenoestrogens. EQ is the ratio of the concentration of

Table 17.2 Equivalence factors for dietary xenoestrogens showing the assays by which they were determined (Thomson *et al.*, 2003)

Xenoestrogen	Estrogenicity equivalence factor ($EQ \times 10^{-6}$)	Estrogenicity assay method and references
Genistein	260	Cell proliferation
Daidzein	110	
Enterolactone	1	Cell proliferation
Enterodiol	0.1	
Coumestrol	300	Cell proliferation
Quercetin	1	Cell proliferation
Kaempferol	70	Cell proliferation
Luteolin	59	
Apigenin	150	
Naringenin	77	
Phloretin	25	
Isoliquiritigenin	25	Assigned the same as phloretin on the basis of structural similarity, and in the absence of cell proliferation data
Zearalenone	10,000	Cell proliferation
DDT and metabolites	1	Cell proliferation
Endosulfan	1	Cell proliferation
Synthetic pyrethroids	100	Enzyme expression
Polychlorinated biphenyls (PCBs)	1	Cell proliferation
Alkyl phenols	1,000	Most conservative cell proliferation
Bisphenol A	1,000	Most conservative cell proliferation
BHA	0.6	Cell proliferation

the xenoestrogen to the concentration of 17 β-estradiol which produced the same response in an estrogenicity assay. Rudel (1997) has reviewed the use of EQs in assessing xenoestrogenic risk. He provides significant evidence that different xenoestrogens may act by different mechanisms to produce a multitude of different effects, and that the use of EQs represents a significant simplification of this complex and poorly understood system. Despite this he feels that their use is valid to provide an estimate of risk and to suggest priorities for action. A wide range of EQs have been proposed for the same xenoestrogen from a multitude of studies carried out using different assay systems (Table 17.2). Despite this, a clear indication of level of estrogenicity gives a measure of hazard to allow assessment of the risk following dietary intake.

17.4.1 Additive estrogenicity

Relative estrogenicity is important because it gives an indication of the pharmacological importance of different xenoestrogens. However, since xenoestrogens act by occupying a common receptor, additivity is important. Therefore the total estrogenicity intake determines pharmacological effect. This is important to remember when assessing impact, since it is sometimes stated that a particular xenoestrogen has low relative estrogenicity and therefore represents a low risk. This may not be the case since it adds to the estrogenicity intake of a particular consumer.

17.5 Health effects of xenoestrogens

Concern about the effects of endocrine disruptors on human health has arisen from the accumulating body of evidence of effects in wildlife. These effects vary from subtle changes in the physiology and sexual behaviour of species, to permanently altered sexual differentiation. In most cases the causal link between exposure and endocrine disruption is implied but not established – there is no clear cause/effect relationship. Examples of potential effects in wildlife include:

- *Invertebrates*: The masculinisation of female marine gastropods exposed to tributyl tin oxide (TBTO) in antifouling paints.
- *Fish*: Chemical constituents in pulp and paper mill effluents and sewage treatment effluents can affect reproductive development.
- *Amphibians*: Population declines in amphibians in both pristine and polluted habitats worldwide.
- *Reptiles*: Penis abnormalities in alligators from Lake Apopka (Florida, USA) have been attributed to high levels of organochlorine (OC) pesticide xenoestrogens.
- *Birds*: Eggshell thinning and altered gonadal development in birds of prey exposed to DDT, resulting in severe population decline.
- *Mammals*: Exposure to OC contaminants has been shown to adversely impact the reproductive and immune function in Baltic seals, resulting in population decline. Whether this is due to immune effects resulting in higher disease rates or declining reproduction is unclear.

The evidence of these adverse outcomes in wildlife combined with studies in laboratory animals substantiates our concerns about human health effects. Areas of human health concern include the following.

- *Reproductive effects*: Xenoestrogens have been implicated in declining human sperm count and quality (see Section 17.1), fertility impairment, an increase in spontaneous abortions, and a decline in the proportion of male babies. Increased frequency of abnormalities of the male reproductive tract development, namely cryptorchidism and hypospadias have been reported.
- *Precocious puberty*: Concerns have been raised about the influence of xenoestrogens (phthalate plasticisers, p,p'-DDE and *in utero* exposure to polybrominated biphenyls) on the timing of puberty.
- *Cancer*: Increasing trends of cancer in hormonally sensitive tissues such as breast, endometrial, testicular, prostate and thyroid have been attributed, in part, to widespread exposure of the general population to xenoestrogens.

17.5.1 Sperm counts and sperm quality

Reduced sperm count is controversial and to some extent the data are equivocal. However, there is evidence that sperm counts (million sperm/ml of semen) and sperm quality (motility) have decreased significantly in the last 50 years. Carlsen *et al.* (1992) analysed the results of 61 studies carried out between 1938 and 1990 and estimated an average 40% decrease in sperm counts over the period. A report covering just the period 1970–1990 showed that there had been no change during this time (Brake and Krause, 1992). More recently, Swan *et al.* (2000) looked at data from 101 studies and confirmed that there appeared to be evidence of decreasing sperm counts in Western countries, but not in non-Western countries. On balance it looks like sperm count is trending down, but at a very much lower rate than was thought originally.

17.5.2 Cryptorchidism

There is good evidence for increasing rates of cryptorchidism (undescended testes [Greek cryptos – hidden; orchid – testis]) (Chilvers *et al.*, 1984; John Radcliffe Hospital Cryptorchidism Study Group, 1986, 1992). The apparent rate of cryptorchidism in England and Wales approximately doubled between 1950 and 1980. Paulozzi (1999) reviewed data from 29 birth defect registries in 21 countries and uncovered clear increases in cryptorchidism in the United States and South America, but not in other countries' report systems included in the study. Since 1985 cryptorchidism rates appear to have declined (see Toppari *et al.*, 1995) which might indicate changes in exposure to xenoestrogens in the intervening years.

Concerns about xenoestrogenic compounds used in farming and gardening prompted a Danish register-based case-control study of rates of cryptorchidism and hypospadias (Weidner *et al.*, 1998). The study found a significantly increased rate of cryptorchidism in the sons of women working in gardening, but not in the sons of men involved in farming and gardening. The inference is that some chemicals (e.g. pesticides) used by gardeners are estrogenic.

17.5.3 Hypospadias

Hypospadia is a displacement of the urethral opening towards the scrotum. Paulozzi (1999) concluded that hypospadia increases were most marked in two American studies and in Scandinavia and Japan. According to some reports the increases appeared to level off after 1985 and were not seen at all in less affluent countries. This might again be due to reduced xenoestrogen intake in later years.

As with declining sperm count there is significant conjecture surrounding hypospadia. A Finnish study reported hypospadia rates to be essentially constant during the period 1970–1986 (Aho *et al.*, 2000). They noted that the rates observed during this period were approximately three times higher than previously reported for the same period, but ascribed this to completeness of registration. They suggested that this improved registration may be the basis for apparent increases observed in other registries. North and Golding (2000) reported an increased risk of hypospadias in sons of mothers who were vegetarian during pregnancy. While not tested by dietary questionnaires it was hypothesised that vegetarian women would be exposed to considerably higher levels of phytoestrogens than non-vegetarian women. Weidner *et al.* (1998) found no significant increase in rates of hypospadias in sons of parents involved in farming and gardening, contradicting the cryptorchidism findings by the same group.

17.5.4 Testicular cancer

Toppari *et al.* (1996) showed an increase in the incidence of testicular cancer around the world between 1960 and 1987. In addition, Bergstrom *et al.* (1996) evaluated data from six Scandinavian and Eastern European countries which indicated a general increasing trend in testicular cancer incidence from 1920 to 1996. The rate of increase varied from 2.3% per annum (Sweden) to 5.2% per annum (East Germany) which is similar to data from Canada (Weir *et al.*, 1999), the United States (McKiernan *et al.*, 1999), and New Zealand (Pearce *et al.*, 1987). Further analysis of US data has suggested that the rate may have stabilised or even decreasing during the mid-1990s (Pharris-Ciurej *et al.*, 1999). Might this be another indication of decreased exposure to xenoestrogens in recent years?

17.5.5 Breast cancer

Few studies have been reported on rates of male breast cancer, which is a rare disease. A survey of rates in four Scandinavian countries indicated an increasing trend in Denmark during the period 1955–1980, but no clear trend in any other country (Ewertz *et al.*, 1989). Female breast cancer is very much more common.

Breast cancer is, in some cases, stimulated by agonist occupancy of the estrogen receptor. There is a sub-class of the disease which is particularly estrogen-dependent. For xenoestrogens to promote female breast cancer the plasma levels would need to have a significant impact on 'normal' estrogen levels. The likelihood of xenoestrogen doses being sufficiently high to achieve this is low for pre-menopausal women, but will be more likely in post-menopausal women. However, in males the situation is different as 'normal' circulating estrogen levels are low and therefore dietary xenoestrogens are a more realistic explanation for the increased incidence of rare breast cancer in this group.

Studies in a number of countries have indicated a steady increase in the incidence of breast cancer in women through the last few decades. Breast cancer rates in the United Kingdom were reported to have increased at a rate of approximately 1% per annum during the period 1973–1987 (Department of Health, 1998). Similar trends have been reported for Scandinavia (Hakulinen *et al.*, 1986), the United States (Feuer and Wan, 1992), Singapore (Seow *et al.*,

1996), Australia (Smith *et al.*, 1998; here the trend is more complex, with a greater rise in latter years), and New Zealand (Cox, 1995).

It is very difficult to determine a cause/effect relationship for breast cancer, because of its multifactorial mechanism (genetic, hormonal, exposure to carcinogens). Therefore we will probably never fully elucidate the role, if any, of xenoestrogens. In addition, the detection rate and screening for breast cancer has improved immensely in recent years. This, of course, will have an inflationary effect on the observed incidence.

17.5.6 Positive effects

Some naturally occurring xenoestrogens (e.g. phytoestrogens) are actively promoted in functional foods, sold as dietary supplements, and as an alternative to hormone replacement therapy because of their claimed health benefits. They have been claimed to be beneficial in:

- cardiovascular disease
- hormone-dependent cancers, particularly breast cancer
- cholesterol-related disorders
- post-menopausal conditions such as osteoporosis
- stomach disorders
- cognitive functions.

A good example is a brand of bread sold in Australasia which proudly advertises its soy content (soy is rich in phytoestrogens, e.g. coumestrol) and its positive effects on women's health. Whether this and related claims are true is uncertain. Despite this, it is important to remember that xenoestrogens (i.e. phytoestrogens) in food might be beneficial in some circumstances.

17.6 Xenoestrogens in food and levels of dietary intake

Food is just one human exposure route to estrogens and xenoestrogens (Fig. 17.6). Since this book focuses on food, we will discuss only this exposure route. However, it is important to remember that the pharmacological effects of xenoestrogens are additive and the source is irrelevant.

Xenoestrogens in food can either be natural (e.g. phytoestrogens) or synthetic contaminants, which can be either direct food contaminants (e.g. some phthalates mainly from environmental contamination), or indirect contaminants via agricultural (e.g. some pesticides) or environmental contamination (e.g. polyphenolethoxylates used as surfactants in industry) (Table 17.3). There have been numerous studies that have identified xenoestrogens in particular foods, and measured their concentrations. These data (i.e. hazards) have limited value until they are set in a human intake context (i.e. risk) (Table 17.4).

Thomson *et al.* (2003) calculated exposure of New Zealand consumers to xenoestrogens in their diet (Table 17.5) with a view to estimating the potential

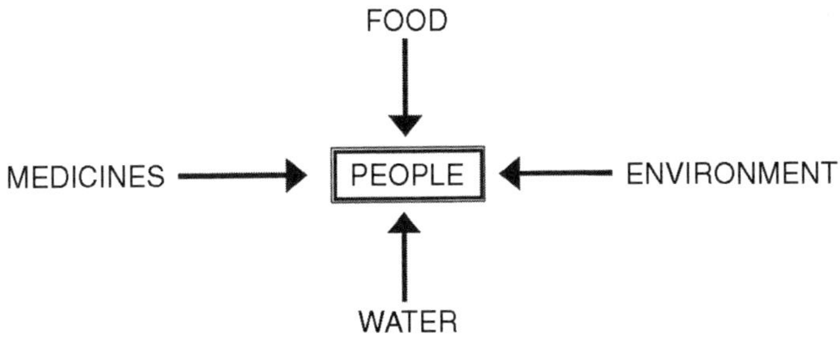

Fig. 17.6 Human exposure routes to estrogens and xenoestrogens.

Table 17.3 Natural and synthetic xenoestrogens from food

Natural compounds	Synthetic compounds
Isoflavones	DDT and its metabolites
Lignans	Dieldrin
Coumestans	Endosulfan
Flavonoids	Synthetic pyrethroid pesticides
Resorcylic lactones	PCBs
	Alkyl phenols
	Butylated hydroxyanisole (BHA)

Table 17.4 Foods contributing 5% or more to dietary exposure of xenoestrogens for a New Zealand adult male (from Thomson *et al.*, 2003)

Xenoestrogen	Food type
Genistein	Bread, soy milk, savoury pies, sausages
Daidzein	Bread, soy milk, savoury pies, sausages, cows milk
Enterolactone	Carrots, bread, potato, beans
Enterodiol	Potato, carrots, beans, bread
Coumestrol	Alfalfa
Quercetin	Tea, apples, onion
Kaempferol	Tea, broccoli
Luteolin	Celery, red pepper
Apigenin	Celery
Naringenin	Grapefruit and grapefruit juice
Phloretin	Apples and apple juice
Isoliquiritigenin	Liquorice
Zearalenone	Mixed grain bread, breakfast cereal
DDT and metabolites	Whole milk, lamb
Dieldrin and aldrin	Nil
Endosulfan	Cucumber, tomatoes
Synthetic pyrethroids	Cracker biscuits, cake, beef sausages, dry spaghetti, white bread
Polychlorinated biphenyls (PCBs)	Imported tinned fish, NZ fish, bread, potatoes
Alkyl phenols	Freshwater fish, water
Bisphenol A	Canned food (non-acid, non-oil), canned fish
BHA	Processed foods

Table 17.5 Estimated dietary intakes of xenoestrogens for three New Zealand population subgroups (Thomson *et al*, 2003)

Xenoestrogen	Estimated Dietary Exposure (mg/day)		
	Male 25 years and over	Female 25 years and over	Young male 19–24 years
Isoflavone			
Genistein	1.9	1.2	1.7
Daidzein	1.2	0.87	1.1
Lignans			
Enterolactone	0.28	0.19	0.26
Enterodiol	0.15	0.10	0.16
Coumestans			
Coumestrol	0.019	0.027	0.033
Flavonoids			
Quercetin	14	14	7.1
Kaempferol	6.9	7.0	1.8
Luteolin	0.10	0.14	0.10
Apigenin	0.31	0.54	0.31
Naringenin	2.9	1.8	2.9
Phloretin	3.7	3.2	6.8
Isoliquiritigenin	2.3	2.3	2.3
Resorcylic lactones			
Zearalenone	0.00097	0.00075	0.0012
Pesticides and industrial chemicals			
DDT and metabolites	0.0055	0.0036	0.0073
Dieldrin and aldrin	Nil	Nil	Nil
Endosulfan	0.00011	0.00013	0.00011
Synthetic pyrethroids	0.0012	0.00086	0.0014
Polychlorinated biphenyls (PCBs)	0.000084	0.000058	0.000090
Alkyl phenols	0.00018	0.00019	0.00018
Bisphenol A	0.0044	0.0041	0.0048
BHA	0.11	0.11	0.11

for pharmacological impact. This was based on the model proposed by Shaw and McCully (2002) in which plasma levels were calculated from dietary intake data based on a series of assumptions about absorption, metabolism and excretion. The studies of both Thomson *et al.* (2003) and Shaw and McCully (2002) suggest that current intakes of dietary xenoestrogens are likely to lead to pharmacological effects in some consumers because calculated xenoestrogen plasma levels exceeded 'normal' levels (Table 17.6).

It is clear from the data in Table 17.6 that there is a large discrepancy between actual and theoretical plasma levels – this probably reflects

Table 17.6 Comparison of theoretical and actual blood levels (from published data) of selected dietary xenoestrogens (Thomson *et al*, 2003). Not all dietary xenoestrogens are included here because there are no published plasma levels

Compound	Theoretical blood level* (μg/l)	Actual blood levels (μg/l) (see Thomson *et al.*, 2003 for references)	EQ (ng/l)
Genistein	265.2	83.1–110	8.1×10^{-1}
Daidzein	189.1	30.1	2.4×10^{-1}
Enterolactone	41.3	5.4–7.0	4.3×10^{-3}
Enterodiol	22.0	0.46	4.4×10^{-5}
Quercetin	2956.5	7–22	2.1×10^{-2}
Kaempferol	1521.7	ND-15	1.5×10^{-1}
Phloretin	695.7	<10	1.5×10^{-3}
DDT and metabolites	0.8	0.06–0.44	3.5×10^{-4}
Endosulfan	0.0	6.6–7.2	6.1×10^{-6}
PCBs	0.0	0.5–15.2	2.0×10^{-3}
Alkyl phenols	0.0	0.5–1.0	3.8×10^{-2}
Bisphenol A	0.9	0–1.6	8.8×10^{-1}
BHA	22.8	1.02	7.9×10^{-4}
		TOTAL	2 ng/l

*Based on estimated exposure and 100% absorption into the bloodstream
ND = not detected

bioavailabililty from food. However, comparison of the total EQ with 'normal' 17β-estradiol levels will give an indication of likelihood of pharmacological effect. The 'normal' male 17β-estradiol level in plasma is 10–50 ng/l (Greenspan and Gardner, 2001) which means that a total plasma level EQ for xenoestrogens of 2 ng/l (i.e. 4–20% of 'normal' levels) is likely to have a pharmacological impact. On the other hand, the pre-menopausal female's 17β-estradiol normal range is 20–350 ng/l (Greenspan and Gardner, 2001). At the top end of this range an additional 2 ng/l from food would be a 'drop in the ocean' of estrogens and unlikely to have any pharmacological impact whatsoever.

17.6.1 Ranking the risk of dietary xenoestrogens

It is interesting to rank the potential impact of the dietary xenoestrogens on the basis of their plasma EQ values. The most important in terms of pharmacological activity on this basis is bisphenol A (used as a monomer in epoxy coatings on food cans) with genistein (present at high levels in soy) a close second. The former is due to potentially high estrogenic activity (hazard) and low intake (exposure), whilst the latter is due to moderate estrogenicity and high intake giving comparable risk (risk = hazard $\times$ exposure). The risk associated with dietary intake of synthetic compounds and phytoestrogens (isoflavones) is comparable (Fig. 17.7).

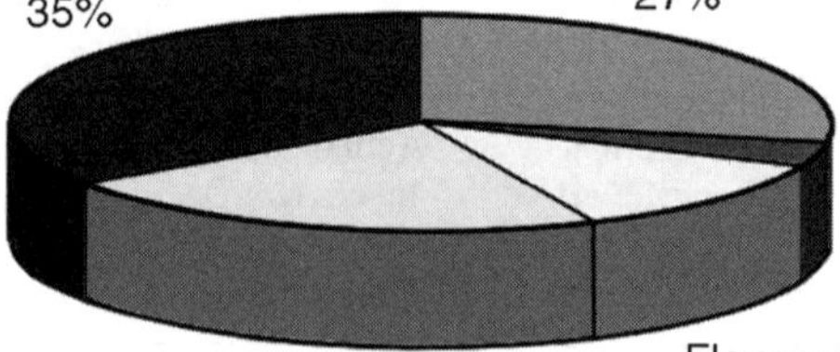

Fig. 17.7 Plasma estrogenicity (EQ) levels for the four main classes of xenoestrogen as a percentage of the total for young males – the most 'at risk' group (Thomson *et al.*, 2003).

17.7 Regulatory control of xenoestrogens

In order for regulatory authorities to introduce controls on chemicals in food, they need to be convinced that the risk to the consumer warrants legislation (usually the setting of food standards – e.g. acceptable levels in particular foods). It is clear from the evidence and discussion presented in this chapter that the effects of xenoestrogens on humans are unproven, but that there is mounting animal and *in vitro* evidence of pharmacological effects targeting the reproductive system. The point at which regulators show concern and introduce controls varies from country to country. In Europe there are controls on most of the synthetic chemicals that may have estrogenic activity, but interest in natural estrogens has led to an enormous EU-funded study under way to assess the impact of exposure to xenoestrogens on humans at a population level. We are tempted to think that if this study shows that xenoestrogens are likely to have a pharmacological effect on people that the regulators will spring into action. Regulatory committees in the UK have considered testing new chemicals for estrogenicity as a condition of approval for marketing. For example, the Advisory Committee on Pesticides (the independent committee that advises ministers via the Pesticides Safety Directorate (PSD)), discussed in the mid-1990s introducing specific tests for estrogenicity, but decided that long-term animal experiments would show estrogenic effects and that there was no need for additional tests.

Some countries (e.g. developing countries) do not see dietary exposure to xenoestrogens as important in the context of a myriad other, higher priority issues vying for government funding. The United States has taken a very different stance. They have listed xenoestrogens of concern and have appealed to industry to minimise their use, and eventually replace them with non-estrogenic alternatives. Providing reasonable timelines do accompany this approach, it is a very effective way of reducing a problem of this type. New Zealand is at an intermediate stage. Its Ministry of Health (NZMoH) funded a significant study to explore human exposure. This has been followed up by the

New Zealand Food Safety Authority (who recently took over responsibility for food safety from NZMoH) commissioning work on xenoestrogens in food. The question is will they act on the findings of the research. Or will they wait for other countries to make the first move?

In critiquing the regulatory controls it is important to remember that xenoestrogens in our diet are from many sources (see Fig. 17.6), and that they come under the jurisdiction of different government departments. Government departments often do not communicate well when cut and dried issues are placed before them, so when the issues are fuzzy and unproven it is hardly surprising that there has been little interdepartmental output worldwide. Perhaps to galvanise activity we should turn our attention away from food and focus on the environment where the effects seem to represent a significant threat to animal populations around the world.

17.8 Future trends

Taking the implications of dietary xenoestrogens seriously depends on definitive scientific proof of cause and effect. This is going to take a very long time to achieve for human exposure. In the meantime, animal and environmental impact data are all that we have to prove that exposure to xenoestrogens can cause pharmacological effects. The fact that the effects that we see in animals resemble very closely those (without a cause) that we are seeing in people should give us confidence to implicate xenoestrogens and persuade regulators to act.

Governments and their regulators are often driven by the press, because the press mirrors (or perhaps creates!), public concern. The xenoestrogen saga is difficult for the general public to appreciate and understand, and so rarely appears in the pages of the daily newspapers. This means that the public are uninformed and unaware, and so cannot bring these concerns to politicians. Having said this there have been some 'classic' newspaper articles on dietary xenoestrogens. Perhaps the best headline was in the UK's *Daily Mail* (9 May 2001): 'Gender-bending chemicals found in canned food'. The article referred to bisphenol A leaching from plastic-coated food cans.

Press interest in xenoestrogens seems to be waning. Indeed, a recent study in Japan (Kobuke *et al.*, 2002) showed peak press interest in mid-1998 with very subdued interest post-2000. We hope that the large government-funded exposure/effect studies under way worldwide (e.g. under EU Framework V) will warrant significant press interest so that the public and governments alike are kept informed about this important area with respect to the future of both people and their environment.

Delving into the vast array of data generated by research groups around the world clearly shows cause for concern. As these data are consolidated and reviewed, we have no doubt that their significance will lead regulators to introduce more controls (akin to those introduced in the United States) and that

MRLs for xenoestrogens will one day be an agenda item for Codex Alimentarius.

17.9 Sources of further information and advice

This is an area of extensive current research activity. Most of the key publications are cited in this chapter. The following government and committee reports are excellent:

Institute of Environment & Health, UK (2002), *Phytoestrogens in the human diet*
Web report W3: http://www.le.ac.uk/ieh/webpub/webpub.html

Committee on Toxicity, UK (2003), *Phytoestrogens and health*
http://www.food.gov.uk/science/ouradvisors/toxicity/COTwg/wg_phyto/

International Programme of Chemical Safety, World Health Organisation, Geneva (2002), *Global assessment of the state-of-the-science of endocrine disruptors*.

17.10 Acknowledgement

We thank Margaret Tanner for her help with the layout, figures and tables, and Anna McCarthy for her help with Fig. 17.4

17.11 References

ADAMI H-O, BERGSTROM R, MOHNER M, ZATONSKI W, STORM H, EKBOM A, TRETLI S, TREPPO L, ZEIGLER H, RAHU M, GUREVICIUS R, STENGREVICS A. (1994). Testicular cancer in nine northern European countries. *Int. J. Cancer*, 59: 33–38.

AHO M, KOIVISTO A-M, TAMMELA TLJ, AUVINEN A. (2000). Is the incidence of hypospadias increasing? Analysis of Finnish hospital discharge data 1970–1994. *Environ Health Perspect.*, 108(5): 463–5.

ARNOLD SF, KLOTZ DM, COLLINS BM, VONIER PM, GUILLETTE LJ JR, MCLACHLAN JA. (1996). Synergistic activation of estrogen receptor with combinations of environmental chemicals. *Science*, 272: 1489–94.

AUGER J, KUNSTMANN JM, CZGLIK F, JOUANNET P. (1995). Decline in semen quality among fertile men in Paris during the past 20 years. *New Engl. J. Med.*, 332: 281–5.

BERGERON RM, THOMPSON TB, LEONARD LS, PLUTA L, GAIDO KW. (1999). Estrogenicity of bisphenol A in a human endometrial carcinoma cell line. *Molecular and Cellular Endocrinology*, 150: 179–187.

BERGSTROM R, ADAMI HO, MOHNER M, ZATONSKI W, STORM H, EKBOM A, TRETLI S, TEPPO L, AKRE O, HAKULINEN T. (1996). Increase in testicular cancer incidence in six European countries: a birth cohort phenomenon. *Journal of the National Cancer Institute*, 88: 727–733.

BRAKE A, KRAUSE W. (1992). Decreasing quality of semen. *BMJ*, 305: 1498.

CARLSEN E, GIWERCMAN A, KEIDING N, SKAKKEBAEK NE. (1992). Evidence for decreasing quality of semen during the past 50 years. *BMJ*, 305: 609–13.

CELIUS T, HAUGEN TB, GROTMOL T, WALTHER BT. (1999). A sensitive zonagenetic assay for rapid in vitro assessment of estrogenic potency of xenobiotics and mycotoxins. *Environ .Health Perspec.*, 107(1): 63–68.

CHILVERS C, PIKE MC, FORMAN D, FOGELMAN K, WADSWORTH MEJ. (1984) Apparent doubling of frequency of undescended testis in England and Wales. *Lancet*, i: 330–3.

COX B. (1995). Projections of the cancer burden in New Zealand. Analysis and Monitoring Report 5. Wellington: Public Health Commission.

DEPARTMENT OF HEALTH. (1998). Nutritional aspects of the development of cancer. Report on Health and Social Subjects No. 48. Norwich: The Stationery Office.

EWERTZ M, HOLMBERG L, KARJALAINEN S, TRETLI S, ADAMI H. (1989). Incidence of male breast cancer in Scandinavia, 1943–1982. Int. J. Cancer, 43: 27–31.

FANG H, TONG W, SHI LM, BLAIR R, PERKINS R, BRANHAM W, HASS BS, XIE Q, DIAL SL, MOLAND CL, SHEEHAN DM. (2001). Structure-activity relationships for a large diverse set of natural, synthetic, and environmental estrogens. Chem. Res. Toxicol., 14: 280–94.

FEUER EJ, WAN L-P. (1992). How much of the recent rise in breast cancer incidence can be explained by increases in mammography utilisation? *American Journal of Epidemiology*, 136: 1423–36.

GREENSPAN FS, GARDNER DG (eds). (2001). *Basic and Clinical Endocrinology*, 6th edn. New York: Lange Medical Books, McGraw-Hill.

GRUBER CJ, TSCHUGGUEL W, SCHNEEBERGER C, HUBER JC. (2002). Production and action of estrogens *New Eng. J. Med*, 346: 340–352

GUILLETTE LJ JR, GROSS TS, MASSON GR, MATTER JM, PERCIVAL HJ, WOODWARD AR. (1994) Developmental abnormalities of the gonad and abnormal sex hormone concentrations in juvenile alligators from contaminated and control lakes in Florida. *Environ. Health Perspect.*, 102: 680–8.

HAKULINEN T, ANDERSEN AA, MALKER B, RIKKALA E, SHOU G, TULINIUS H. (1986). Trends in cancer incidence in the Nordic countries. A collaborative study of the five Nordic Cancer Registries. *Acta Pathologica Microbiologica Immunologica Scandinavia*, 94 (Section A), Supplement 288: 1–151.

HOPERT A-C, BEYER A, FRANK K, STRUNCK E, WÜNSCHE W, VOLLMER G. (1998). Characterization of estrogenicity of phytoestrogens in an endometrial-derived experimental model. *Environmental Health Perspectives*, 106 (9): 581–6.

IRVINE S, CAWOOD E, RICHARDSON D, MACDONALD E, AITKEN J. (1996). Evidence of deteriorating semen quality in the United Kingdom: birth cohort study in 577 men in Scotland over 11 years. *BMJ*, 312: 467–71.

JOHN RADCLIFFE HOSPITAL CRYPTORCHIDISM STUDY GROUP. (1986). Cryptorchidism: an apparent substantial increase since 1960. *BMJ*, 293: 1401–4.

JOHN RADCLIFFE HOSPITAL CRYPTORCHIDISM STUDY GROUP. (1992). Cryptorchidism: a prospective study of 7,500 consecutive male births, 1984–8. *Archives of Disease in Childhood*, 67: 892–9.

KOBUKE Y, TANAKA H, MAGARA Y. (2002). Research in Japan: Nationwide and regional river monitoring studies as well as bioassays and treatment of EDs in waterworks. IWA World Water Congress, Melbourne, Australia, Workshop Endocrine Disruptors Proceedings (eds Schafer AI and Jacobsen BN), p. 53.

KORACH KS, SARVER P, CHAE L, MCLACHLAN JA, MCKINNEY JD. (1988). Estrogen receptor-binding activity of polychlorinated hydrobiphenyls: Conformationally restricted structural probes. *Molecular Pharmacology*, 33: 120–6.

KRISHNAN AV, STATHIS P, PERMUTH SF, TOKES L, FELDMAN D. (1993). Bisphenol-A: an estrogenic substance is released from polycarbonate flasks during autoclaving. *Endocrinology*, 132: 2279–86.

MCKIERNAN JM, GOLUBOFF ET, LIBERSON GL, GOLDEN R, FISCH H. (1999). Rising risk of testicular cancer by birth cohort in the United States from 1973 to 1995. *J. Urol*, 162 (2): 361–3.

NAGLE SC, VOM SAAL FS, THAYER CA, DHAR MG, BOECHLER M, WELSHONS WV. (1997). Relative binding affinity-serum modified access (RBA-SMA) assay predicts the relative *In vivo* bioactivity of the xenoestrogens Bisphenol A and octylphenol. *Environ. Health Perspect.*, 105 (1): 70–76.

NORTH K, GOLDING J. (2000). A maternal vegetarian diet in pregnancy is associated with hypospadias. *British Journal of Urology*, 85(1): 107–13.

OLEA N, PULGAR R, PÉREZ P, OLEA-SERRANO F, RIVAS A, NOVILLO-FERTRELL, PEDRAZA V, SOTO AM, SONNENSCHEIN C. (1996). Estrogenicity of resin-based composites and sealants used in dentistry. *Environ. Health Perspect.*, 104 (3): 298–305.

PAULOZZI LJ. (1999). International trends in rates of hypospadias and cryptorchidism. *Environ. Health Perspect.*, 107 (4): 297–302.

PEARCE N, SHEPPARD RA, HOWARD JK, FRASER J, LILLEY BM. (1987). Time trends and occupational differences in cancer of the testis in New Zealand. *Cancer*, 59 (9): 1677–82.

PHARRIS-CIUREJ ND, COOK LS, WEISS NS. (1999). Incidence of testicular cancer in the United States: Has the epidemic begun to debate. *American Journal of Epidemiology*, 150 (1): 45–46.

RUDEL R. (1997), Predicting health effects of exposures to compounds with estrogenic activity: methodological issues. *Environ. Health Perspect.*, 105 Suppl 3, 655–63.

SEOW A, DUFFY SW, MCGEE MA, LEE J, LEE HP. (1996). Breast cancer in Singapore: trends in incidence 1968–1992. *International Journal of Epidemiology*, 25: 40–45.

SHAW IC, CHADWICK J. (1998). *Principles of Environmental Toxicology*, Taylor & Francis, London.

SHAW IC, MCCULLY S. (2002) The potential impact of dietary endocrine disrupters on the consumer. *Int. J. Food Sci. Technol.* 37, 471–476.

SHELBY MD, NEWBOLD RR, TULLY DB, CHAE K, DAVIS VL. (1996). Assessing environmental chemicals for estrogenicity using a combination of In vitro and In vivo assays. *Environ. Health Perspect.*, 104 (12): 1296–1300.

SILVIA E, RAJAPAKSE N, KORTENKAMP A. (2002). Something from 'Nothing' – Eight weak estrogenic chemicals combined at concentrations below NOECs produce significant mixture effects. *Environ. Sci. Technol.*, 36: 1751–6.

SMITH CL, CRICKER A, ARMSTRONG BK. (1998). Breast cancer mortality trends in Australia: 1921 to 1994. *Medical Journal of Australia*, 168: 11–14.

SOTO AM, SONNENSCHEIN C, CHUNG KL, FERNANDEZ MF, OLEA N, OLEA-SERRANO F. (1995). The E-SCREEN assay as a tool to identify estrogens: an update on estrogenic environmental pollutants. *Environ. Health Perspect.*, 103 (Supplement 7): 113–22.

SWAN SH, ELKIN EP, FENSTER L. (2000). The question of declining sperm density revisited; An analysis of 101 studies published 1934-1996. *Environ. Health Perspect.*, 108 (10): 961–6.

THOMAS P, SMITH J. (1993). Binding of xenobiotics to the oestrogen receptor of the spotted seatrout: a screening assay for potential oestrogenic effects. *Marine Environmental Research*, 35: 147–51.

THOMSON BM, CRESSEY PJ, SHAW IC. (2003). Dietary exposure to xenoestrogens in New

Zealand. *J. Environ. Monit.*, 5: 229–35

TOPPARI J, LARSEN JC, CHRISTIANSEN P, GIWERCMAN A, GRANDJEAN P, GUILLETTE LJ, JÉGOU B, JENSEN TK, JOUANNET P, KEIDING N, LEFFERS H, MCLACHLAN JA, MEYER O, MÜLLER J, RAJPERT-DE MEYTS E, SCHEIKE T, SHARPE R, SUMPTER J, SKAKKEBÆK NE. (1995). Male reproductive health and environmental estrogens. *Environ. Health Perspect.*, 104 (Supplement 4): 741–803.

VAN WAELEGHEM K, DE CLERCQ N, VERMEULEN L, SCHOONJANS F, COMHAIRE F. (1994). Deterioration of sperm quality in young healthy Belgian men. *Hum. Reprod.*, 11: 325–9.

WEIDNER IS, MØLLER H, JENSEN TK, SKAKKEBÆK NE. (1998). Cryptorchidism and hypospadias in sons of gardeners and farmers. *Environ. Health Perspect.*, 106 (12): 793–6.

WEIR HK, MARRETT LD, MORAVAN V. (1999). Trends in the incidence of testicular germ cell cancer in Ontario by histologic subgroup, 1964-1996. *CMAJ*, 160 (2): 201–5.

WHITE R, JOBLING S, HOARE SA, SUMPTER JP, PARKER MG. (1994). Environmentally persistent alkylphenolic compounds are estrogenic. *Endocrinology*, 135: 175–82.

18

Dietary estrogens

S. Hendrich, Iowa State University, USA

18.1 Introduction: defining dietary estrogens

Dietary estrogens are substances found in the diet that act like estrogens that are produced endogenously in higher organisms. 17-β-Estradiol is considered to be most representative of a complete estrogen in that it binds to estrogen receptors and triggers numerous changes in gene expression that lead to sexual maturation in female mammals, including increased expression of estrogen receptors. Operationally, estrogenic potency is defined as relative ability to displace 17-β-estradiol from binding to presumptive estrogen receptors in crude preparations of cytosol from organs rich in estrogen receptors, especially estrogen receptor-α (ER-α, e.g., uterus) (Mueller 2002). The ability to cause significant uterine enlargement in sexually immature mice (typically ~21 days old), i.e., the mouse uterine growth assay, is arguably the most well accepted standard for determination of estrogenicity (Diel *et al.* 2002). Estrogenicity may be defined in several other ways:

- ability to stimulate aromatase activity, the key enzyme in estrogen synthesis
- ability to bind to sex hormone binding globulin in place of endogenous estrogens
- ability to function as a selective estrogen receptor modulator (SERM) that induces some estrogen-like changes in gene expression in certain tissues.

With the relatively recent discovery of another estrogen receptor, ER-β (Kuiper *et al.* 1996), which has different patterns of tissue expression and relative binding affinity of various estrogens compared with ER-α, defining estrogenicity has become more complex. Other novel estrogen receptors or estrogen-binding proteins may remain to be discovered. This review will focus on dietary substances that are capable of causing uterine enlargement and modulating gene expression as mediated by known estrogen receptors α and/or β.

The definition of what types of SERM activities are beneficial and what are detrimental constitutes a major current controversy in health sciences. For example, the antiestrogen, tamoxifen, is a potent antineoplastic agent against human mammary cancer, but it also increases the risk of hepatic cancer (Law and Tandan 1999). Estrogenic activity stimulates some types of cancer (e.g., mammary cancer (Safe 1998)) but early exposure to estrogens stimulates mammary maturation and creates resistance against later exposure to mammary carcinogens; early exposure to the phytoestrogen genistein also suppressed prostate carcinogenesis in two animal models (Lamartiniere *et al.* 2002). Protection against hot flushes and other menopausal symptoms by hormone replacement therapies is accompanied by increased risk of mammary cancer (Beral 2003, Burger 2003), and is of uncertain effect on some aspects of cardiovascular disease (Burger 2003). Sorting out all of these effects to the point of being able to offer clear strategies for health optimization will require new knowledge of estrogen-regulated gene expression, environmental and host factors, including individual genetic composition, that affect this expression in tissue-specific detail. Hopefully, this review can provide some guidance as to which avenues of exploration are most likely to facilitate this knowledge quest.

18.2 The range of dietary estrogens

There are several classes of dietary components that may be estrogenic. Animal products, such as cheeses, meats, organ meats, or milk, may contain endogenous estrogens or synthetic or microbial estrogens used to improve food production efficiency. For example, derivatives of zearalenone, an estrogen derived from *Fusarium* spp. fungi, and its derivatives, are used in some parts of the world as feed additives to enhance feed efficiency and muscle deposition in livestock (Welshons *et al.* 1990). These compounds will not be discussed further in this chapter as feed additives.

Environmental estrogens are discussed in Chapter 17. These compounds include a broad range of substances that are not naturally occurring, but that enter the food supply as contaminants from industrial pollution, agricultural applications, automobile exhaust and other combustion reactions, that have at least partial estrogenicity as defined above (Section 18.1). Such compounds as dioxins, polychlorinated biphenyls, and various chlorinated hydrocarbon pesticides such as dieldrin, aldrin, and DDT, are under investigation for their potential to disrupt normal endocrine function due to their ability to act as SERMs or in other ways to modify functions of estrogens and androgens in higher organisms.

Some authors include in the broad category of environmental estrogens the phytoestrogens, or plant-derived estrogens. Of course, these are found in the environment as components of the typical diets of many humans and animal species, but this review draws the distinction that the phytoestrogens are naturally produced, and not environmental contaminants. This chapter will focus on naturally occurring dietary estrogens, which include

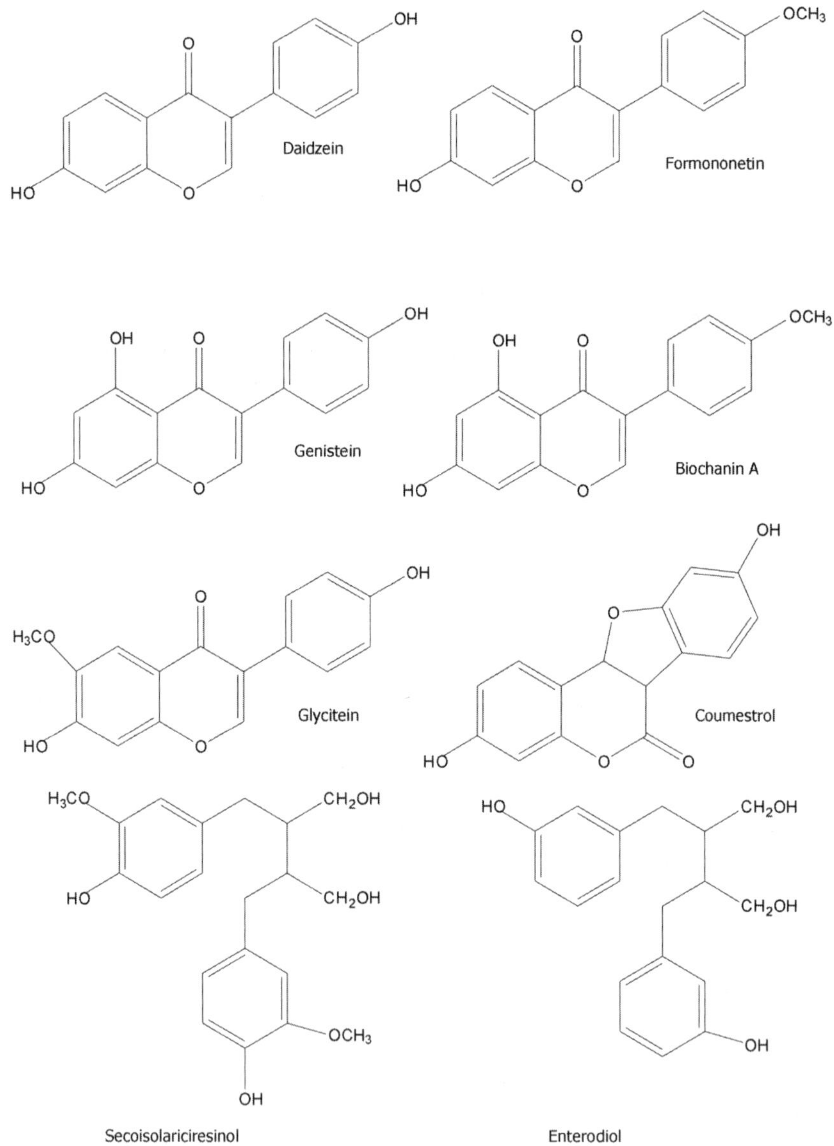

Fig. 18.1 Phytoestrogens in the human diet.

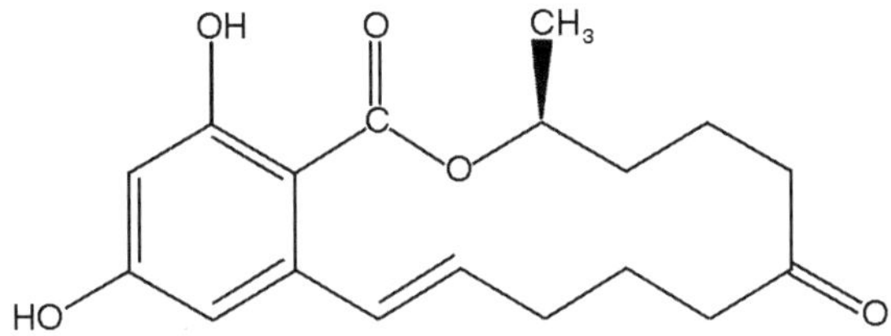

Fig. 18.2 Zearalenone, a Fusarium fungal estrogen in the food supply.

phytoestrogens (Fig. 18.1) and the microbial estrogen, zearalenone (Fig. 18.2), a *Fusarium* fungal toxin commonly contaminating grains. There are three major classes of phytoestrogens, using a strict definition (see Section 18.1): coumestrol, lignan derivatives and isoflavones (Fig. 18.1). Among the three classes, coumestrol is found in the most limited range of foods: alfalfa sprouts and a few other foods are their sources.

Lignans are associated with dietary fibers, and found most generally in whole grains. The main estrogenic lignan derivatives, enterodiol and enterolactone, are produced by bacterial action on lignan precursors in the gut. Isoflavones are predominantly found in soybeans. Genistein and daidzein are present in the greatest amounts in most soybean foods. Glycitein is a minor isoflavone, but present in amounts similar to the predominant daidzein in soygerm, which may be used as a food ingredient. Biochanin A is another minor isoflavone, apparently found mostly in clover sprouts. The isoflavone equol is a gut bacterial fermentation product of daidzein formed in about one-third of humans studied. Equol may be the most potent of the isoflavones in estrogenicity, at least by some criteria.

Several recent reviews have described present knowledge regarding phytoestrogen effects in humans and animals, including their toxicity, relative potency, modes of action, and major health effects (Potter and Steinmetz 1996, Kurzer and Xu 1997, Tham *et al.* 1998, Adlercreutz 1998, Anderson *et al.* 1999, Wiseman 2000, Hendrich and Murphy 2001, Murphy and Hendrich 2002, Fitzpatrick 2003, Wuttke *et al.* 2003). This chapter will focus on summarizing more recent literature than included in these previous reviews. This review will include *in vitro* and *in vivo* studies of human responses to dietary estrogens, as well as discussion of *in vitro* and *in vivo* animal model studies. The primary focus will be to examine estrogenicity and toxicity of these compounds, with more abbreviated discussion of the range of other largely beneficial health effects associated with dietary estrogens, because other reviews (see above) have described these beneficial effects in detail.

18.3 Assessing the estrogenicity of dietary estrogens

Estrogenicity involves interactions of ligands such as the dietary estrogens with estrogen receptors (ER-α and -β) and what effects these ER interactions have on gene expression in various tissues. Sex hormone binding globulin (SHBG) interactions also determine the effects of dietary estrogens to act as estrogens, in their ability to either displace or augment endogenous estrogen action. The extent of free estrogens in circulation is a major determinant of estrogenicity *in vivo* and the extent of SHBG binding by estrogens conversely limits estrogenicity. The expression of SHBG as well binding to SHBG may be influenced by dietary estrogens. Modulation of estrogen metabolizing enzymes by dietary estrogens may also determine estrogenicity. *In vivo* effects may not always be predicted by *in vitro* binding of ERs, SHBG or estrogen-metabolizing enzyme inhibition or potentiation, and so studies of effects of dietary estrogens *in vivo* will be compared with the *in vitro* effects, taking into account both animal models and human studies.

18.3.1 *In vitro* studies

Estrogen receptor binding studies and ER-mediated gene expression in cell cultures

The binding of genistein, formononetin, biochanin A and coumestrol to purified human ER-α and -β in competition with 17β-estradiol showed that genistein was ~100–1000-fold less able to bind ER$-alpha$ than was estradiol, formononetin was ~1000-fold less able to bind than estradiol, and coumestrol was about tenfold less potent than estradiol, whereas biochanin A was not an effective competitor with estradiol for ER-α. With respect to ER-β, genistein was only about tenfold less potent a binder than was estradiol, formononetin was ~100–1000-fold less potent than estradiol and biochanin A was ~1000-fold less potent than estradiol; coumestrol was equally able to bind ER-β compared with estradiol (Morito *et al.* 2002). In a rabbit reticulocyte lysate system containing human ER-α or rat ER-β translated from their respective cDNAs, coumestrol showing relative binding affinity similar to 17β-estradiol for ER-α and approximately twofold greater for ER-β; β-zearalenol (a zearalenone metabolite) showed about sixfold less affinity than estradiol and threefold greater affinity for ER-α than did genistein, and genistein showed threefold less affinity than estradiol and threefold greater affinity for ER-β than did β-zearalenol (Kuiper *et al.* 1997). In a subsequent study comparing human ER-α and -β binding affinities using receptor proteins from *in vitro* ER cDNA translational systems, coumestrol showed fivefold less affinity than did estradiol for ER-α but about 40% greater affinity than estradiol for ER-β. Zearalenone had similar affinities for ER-α and -β, both twentyfold less than estradiol. Whereas genistein had 25-fold less affinity for ER-α than did estradiol, genistein had ER-β binding ability nearly equal to estradiol. Daidzein had 1000-fold less affinity for ER-α than did estradiol and 200-fold less affinity than estradiol for

ER-β, with formononetin and biochanin A at least an order of magnitude less potent than daidzein for both ERs (Kuiper *et al.* 1998). In another study of relative binding affinity, coumestrol had 25-fold greater affinity than did genistein for ER-α but only twofold greater affinity for ER-β than did genistein (Mueller *et al.* 2003).

In 188R1 yeast reporter system containing ER-α, the relative potency of various dietary estrogens to induce transactivation was as follows (in molar concentrations): coumestrol 10^{-8} > zearalenone 10^{-8} > genistein 10^{-6} = biochanin A 10^{-6} > formononetin 10^{-6} > daidzein 10^{-5} (Jungbauer and Beck 2002). In a yeast reporter model (*Saccharomyces cerevisiae* Y190) carrying ER-α or ER-β genes that when induced also induce β-galactosidase (β-gal), the relative concentration of phytoestrogen needed to induce this enzyme compared with 17β-estradiol was 10,000-fold for genistein and 1,000-fold for coumestrol for ER-α; biochanin A and formononetin were ineffective. For ER-β, 100 fold more genistein, 1000–10,000-fold more biochanin A, 100,000-fold more formononetin and 100-fold more coumestrol were needed than estradiol to induce β-gal. When the phytoestrogens were added with estradiol to the yeast ER-α reporter system, micromolar concentrations of coumestrol and genistein potentiated estradiol's efficacy to induce β-gal, although genistein was somewhat less effective, and biochanin A and formononetin in micromolar concentrations moderately antagonized estradiol's efficacy. Coumestrol also potentiated estradiol in an ER-β yeast reporter system but genistein neither activated nor inhibited estradiol's effect; biochanin A and formononetin had similar effects as when added to the ER-α reporter system.

In a 293 human embryonal kidney cell model transfected with ER-α or -β using a luciferase reporter system, coumestrol, zearalenone and daidzein (1 μM) had similar abilities to induce ER-α-mediated gene expression but genistein was approximately twofold more potent, formononetin 20-fold less potent, and biochanin A one-third as potent. With respect to ER-β transactivation, activities at 1 μM concentrations were relatively as follow: genistein (1.8), coumestrol (1.0), daidzein (0.8), biochanin A (0.5), and zearalenone (0.25) (Kuiper *et al.* 1998). In Ishikawa (human endometrial) cells transfected with ER-α or ER-β and luciferase reporter, genistein and coumestrol had similar efficacy and required about three- or four-fold lesser concentrations for ER-β transactivation than for ER-α transactivation (Mueller *et al.* 2003). In MCF-7 cells transfected with ERs from various species and a luciferase reporter, α- or β-zearalenol, coumestrol, and genistein showed similar effects on human or mouse ER-α, with relative transactivation potencies compared with 17β-estradiol of 10-fold less for α-zearalenol, 100-fold less for β-zearalenol, and 10,000-fold less for coumestrol or genistein. Coumestrol and genistein were only 100-fold less potent than estradiol in transactivation of mouse ER-β, but the zearalenols had roughly the same potency for ER-β as they did for ER-α (Matthews *et al.* 2002). In a more specific cell model, GT1-7 neurones, coumesterol was 100-fold less potent than estradiol in stimulating gonadotropin-releasing hormone mRNA expression and this action of coumestrol was blocked by an ER-β antagonist,

R,R′-diethyl tetrahydrochyrsene, that did not block estradiol's action, suggesting that coumestrol's effect was largely mediated by ER-β (Bowe *et al.* 2003). Ishikawa human endometrial carcinoma cells showed increased alkaline phosphatase activity, another potential biomarker of estrogenicity. Effective concentrations of dietary estrogens for this endpoint were 1 nM for zearalenone, 10 nM for coumestrol (estradiol was similarly potent), 100 nM for genistein and 1 μM for daidzein (Wober *et al.* 2003); thus this assay showed high sensitivity to dietary estrogens, equal to or greater than the yeast reporter system (Jungbauer and Beck 2002).

Altogether, these studies indicate that zearalenone and related compounds were more potent binders and activators of ER-α than were the phytoestrogens, and for the most part zearalenone and related compounds were similar in effects on ER-α and -β. Coumestrol was somewhat more potent an activator of ER-α than was genistein, but genistein and coumestrol were generally similarly potent as activators of ER-β and similar to zearalenone or even more potent as effectors of ER-β. Daidzein was generally more than an order of magnitude less potent than genistein in ER binding and activation, and biochanin A and formononetin were even less effective; when biochanin A may have been more effective, it was possibly due to its partial conversion to genistein (Kuiper *et al.* 1998) whereas formononetin might be partially converted to daidzein, a much less potent estrogen than genistein.

Sex hormone binding globulin modulation studies

Modulation of sex hormone binding globulin (SHBG) is another mechanism of action of dietary estrogens. The extent of SHBG binding is thought to be inversely related to the effective estrogenicity of a compound *in vivo*. In an *in vitro* model system measuring access of radiolabeled estradiol to MCF-7 human mammary tumor cells, the effective free fraction of estradiol in serum from adult men was approximately 4%, whereas coumestrol, genistein and the gut microbial metabolite of daidzein, equol, had effective free fractions of approximately 46–50% and biochanin A an effective free fraction of approximately 2% (Nagel *et al.* 1998). Thus, the relative estrogenicity of several, but not all, phytoestrogens in humans may be considerably greater than that predicted by cell culture assays or ER binding. But this model system may be questioned as to its relevance to conditions *in vivo*. *In vitro*, displacement of radiolabeled estradiol from adult human female serum was 54–59% by coumestrol, genistein, or daidzein, but daidzein was an order of magnitude less effective in human pregnancy serum stripped of endogenous sex steroid hormones (Jury *et al.* 2000). When specific binding to human SHBG was measured *in vitro*, genistein had 1000-fold less affinity than did estradiol (Dechaud *et al.* 1999). Binding of human pregnancy plasma sex hormone binding proteins showed that daidzein, coumestrol and genistein had virtually no ability to displace 5α-dihydrotestosterone (DHT) (Milligan *et al.* 1998). Lignans were also examined for their interactions with human SHBG. The concentration required for enterolactone to inhibit binding of DHT to human pregnancy serum proteins by 50% was 620 μM (Schöttner and Spiteller 1998), a several hundredfold greater concentration of this major lignan metabolite than observed typically in human plasma. Thus, in general the dietary estrogens would be much more likely to be found circulating freely than would be the endogenous sex steroids, and studies of such compounds in cell cultures might be able to approximate the *in vivo* efficacy of dietary estrogens.

Modulation of sex steroid-metabolizing enzymes
Human 17β-hydroxysteroid dehydrogenase type 5 is a multifunctional enzyme located in many tissues of relevance for endogenous sex steroid production. This enzyme catalyzes testosterone synthesis and degrades DHT to androstanediol and androsterone in prostate. Concentrations of dietary estrogens that inhibited activities of this enzyme 50% were > 20 μmol/L for daidzein and genistein, 8–14 μmol/L for biochanin A, 5–11 μmol/L for coumestrol and 2–4 μmol/L for zearalenone (Krazeisen *et al.* 2002). It is possible that these effects of the dietary estrogens might reduce sex drive by decreasing testosterone levels or potentiate prostate cancer by preventing DHT degradation, but this remains to be verified *in vivo*.

18.3.2 Animal models

Animal models of *in vivo* estrogenicity of dietary estrogens have shown a variety of effects of these compounds. Mouse uterine enlargement required ~0.04 mmol coumestrol/kg body weight, ~1 mmol/kg of genistein or daidzein, ~3 mmol/kg of biochanin A and ~5 mmol/kg for formononetin (Verdeal and Ryan 1979). Song *et al.* (1999) showed that glycitein (~1 mmol/kg per day for 4 days) was somewhat more effective than an equivalent dose of genistein in stimulating mouse uterine growth, although glycitein was a less potent binder of mouse uterine cytosolic estrogen receptors than was genistein. Jefferson *et al.* (2002) showed that in groups of 10 female CD-1 mice injected subcutaneously (SC) from day 17 for 3 days with dietary estrogens, coumestrol and zearalenone at 0.04 mmol/kg and genistein at 0.4 mmol/kg caused significant uterine enlargement. In a Tier I estrogenicity screening battery in Sprague-Dawley rats, 7-week-old females dosed intraperitoneally (IP) with 0.01–0.05 mmol coumestrol/kg (for 4 days) had increased uterine weight, and 0.002–0.05 mmol/kg increased uterine stromal cell proliferation. 0.02–0.05 mmol coumestrol/kg also increased follicle stimulating hormone levels significantly (O'Connor *et al.* 2000).

Genistein at ~0.005–0.05 mmol/kg body weight fed from conception to 70 days postnatal increased plasma testosterone and decreased androgen receptor and ER-α expression in dorsolateral prostate significantly. 0.05 mmol genistein/kg also decreased ER-β expression significantly. Feeding of 0.05 mmol genistein/kg from day 56–70 postnatal had similar effects. This down-regulation might limit growth responsiveness of prostate to endogenous sex hormones, possibly a mechanism for decreasing prostate cancer risk in soy-consuming populations (Fritz *et al.* 2002a). In male 10-week-old Sprague-Dawley rats dosed IP with coumestrol for 15 days, 0.002–0.05 mmol/kg per day had no effect on prostate weight, but 0.02–0.05 mmol/kg per day significantly decreased serum DHT and thyroid hormone (T_4) and 0.05 mmol/kg per day increased prolactin (O'Connor *et al.* 2000). Sprague-Dawley rats exposed in utero from day 14 to birth to 0.004–0.4 mmol coumestrol or 0.0004–0.04 mmol genistein/kg per day had increased expression of platelet derived growth factor receptors (PDFR) α and β in testes (gonocytes) at 3 days of age. This effect was similar to effects of other exogenous estrogens and is significant in that PDFRs seem to be crucial to testicular germ cell growth and development (Thuillier *et al.* 2003). This study suggests that dietary estrogens might impair processes related to spermatogenesis and fertility, but much more work needs to be done.

Applicability to humans is open to question due to potential differences between rat and human spermatogenesis and variation in effects from oral exposure, compared with SC exposure in this study in rats. Exposure of Sprague-Dawley rats from 0–5 days of age to 0.08 mmol coumestrol/kg did not affect testes or prostate weight or FSH, testosterone or luteinizing hormone (LH) levels in these rats at 9 weeks of age (Awoniyi *et al.* 1998). Wistar rats dosed subcutaneously with 0.016 mmol genistein/kg from day 2–18 of age showed greater testes weight, decreased plasma FSH, decreased spermatocytes and seminiferous tubule formation. Later mating of genistein-treated animals was somewhat impaired. Rats fed soy-containing standard lab chow-type diet had significantly lower testes weight and increased plasma FSH compared with rats fed a soy-free diet from 0–90 days of age. Thus, perhaps longer-term exposure to dietary estrogen may adversely affect reproductive potential, but route of exposure may complicate applicability to human dietary exposure (Atanassova *et al.* 2000). Adult male Crj:CD(SD) rats dosed intraperitoneally (IP) with genistein or daidzein for 5 days at 0.04 mmol/kg showed no effect on the male-specific protein, α_{2u}-globulin, although more potent estrogens did affect the levels of this protein (Nagahori *et al.* 2001). While some studies of coumestrol, genistein and soy suggest reproductive impairments in male animals, other studies indicate no effects. Route of exposure should be carefully considered in applicability to humans, but these studies on the whole provide some reason for concern regarding male reproductive toxicity of dietary estrogens.

18.3.3 Human studies

In humans, early exposure to soy and therefore isoflavonoid dietary estrogens was studied in a retrospective cohort of approximately 250 adults aged 20–34 years fed soy as infants. The study indicated no effect of early soy exposure on pubertal maturation in males or females; women fed soy as infants had slightly longer menstrual bleeding and more discomfort. This study suggests no obvious adverse effects on reproductive function in adults fed soy as infants (Strom *et al.* 2001).

An analysis of several studies of effects of soy feeding on sex hormones and menstrual cycle in women indicated that 0.0006–0.012 mmol isoflavones/kg fed for 1–3 months tended to increase cycle length and decreased serum estradiol (Kurzer 2002). Overall ten women fed 0.009 mmol isoflavones/kg for one menstrual cycle showed decreased serum estradiol and progesterone but no effect on FSH, LH or cycle length (Lu *et al.* 2000). These changes suggest potential protection from mammary cancer due to effects of soy isoflavones on hormonal status. Forty young women fed 0.0015–0.003 mmol isoflavones/kg for one month caused no significant effects on sex hormones or menstrual cycle (Watanabe *et al.* 2000). Several studies of effects of soy isoflavone feeding (0.002–0.006 mmol/kg, 6–24 weeks) on menopausal symptoms showed that the isoflavones alleviated symptoms to some extent; efficacy was significantly correlated with initial hot flush frequency (Messina and Hughes 2003). Studies so far, at best show only modest effects of isoflavones on female hormonal status.

When several studies were reviewed, men fed 0.002–0.004 mmol isoflavones/kg for 1–2 months showed minimal to no effects on serum sex hormones (Kurzer 2002). Six men, 40–53 years of age, were fed Trinovin, a red clover isoflavone supplement containing biochanin A, formononetin, daidzein and genistein, at a total estimated isoflavone dose ~0.002 mmol/kg per day for 3 weeks. Plasma DHT was increased significantly over baseline at the end of treatment; other sex hormones were not affected. The health significance of modest increase in DHT is uncertain and potentially adverse (Lewis *et al.* 2002). An epidemiological study of soy intake and hormonal status in 69 Japanese men of mean age 60 years with mean overall soy isoflavone intake estimated at 0.0015 mmol/kg showed a significant inverse correlation between isoflavone intake and serum estradiol (Nagata *et al.* 2000), but the health significance of a modest decrease in estradiol is uncertain. Fifteen healthy men, 18–35 years of age, were fed a soy extract supplement containing ~0.002 mmol isoflavones/kg per day for 2 months and monitored for 4 months after supplementation. No changes were observed in serum sex hormones or sperm quality during or after supplementation (Mitchell *et al.* 2001).

Table 18.1 Relative estrogenicity of dietary estrogens in 3–4 day mouse uterine growth assays

Compound	Estimated estrogenic dose (mmol/kg d)	Reference
Zearalenone	0.04	Jefferson *et al.* 2002
Coumestrol	0.04	Jefferson *et al.* 2002
		Verdeal and Ryan 1979
Genistein	0.4	Jefferson *et al.* 2002
	1.0	Song *et al.* 1999
Daidzein	1.0	Verdeal and Ryan 1979
Glycitein	1.0	Song *et al.* 1999
Biochanin A	3.0	Verdeal and Ryan 1979
Formononetin	5.0	Verdeal and Ryan 1979
Lignans (enterodiol, enterolactone)	No data	

18.3.4 Summary

Dietary estrogens vary in their potency to some extent as evident in the comparison of rodent uterine growth data (Table 18.1), but they are generally relatively weak estrogens and typical human dietary intakes or modest supplementation with such compounds seems to have a modest to no effect on sex hormonal status or reproductive health. Larger-scale and longer-term epidemiological studies in humans, probably requiring the use of markers of induction of ER-responsive gene expression and examination of key health endpoints such as mammary and prostate cancer risk are needed. This may be the case especially for zearalenone, because it is a relatively potent estrogenic fungal contaminant of commonly consumed staple foods.

18.4 Assessing the toxicity of dietary estrogens

High dose exposure to dietary estrogens, the equivalent of grams per person, could cause infertility and other disruptions of reproductive function, based on extrapolation from animal models, but such exposures would be highly unlikely. More subtle potentially toxic effects from typical dietary exposures or from supplement overdosing may be due to weakly estrogenic effects or to other effects of these compounds.

18.4.1 *In vitro* studies

Exposure to dietary estrogens in unlikely to pose a significant risk of genotoxicity. Syrian hamster embryo (SHE) cells were used to study the genotoxic potential of dietary estrogens. These cells may be transformed by carcinogens into neoplastic cells and do not contain ER-α; thus making them useful for studying ER-α independent effects. The extent of SHE cell transformation was significantly increased by 50 μM daidzein, 12.5 μM genistein or coumestrol, or 100 μM biochanin A. Chromosomal aberrations were induced by 50 μM genistein or coumestrol, and aneuploidy was induced by 12.5 μM genistein and 50 μM biochanin A (Tsutsui *et al.* 2003). In human peripheral blood leukocytes from three subjects, chromosomal aberrations were induced tenfold by 25 μM genistein or fourfold by 50 μM coumestrol compared with 100 μM daidzein or DMSO vehicle (Kulling *et al.* 1999) but no statistical analysis was performed. In Chinese hamster V79 fibroblasts, induction of micronuclei and genetic mutations at the hypoxanthine-guanine phosphoribosyl transferase locus was assessed for 100 μM enterodiol or enterolactone. Neither lignan showed any clastogenic or mutagenic activity in this model (Kulling *et al.* 1998). Even though genotoxic effects were observed for some isoflavones and coumestrol, the concentrations needed for such effects were well above levels achievable by dietary exposure (e.g., Xu *et al.* 1995).

Cytotoxicity including inhibition of proliferation and apoptosis toward various tumor cell lines has been demonstrated for some dietary estrogens (for a recent review, see Birt *et al.* 2001). Three mouse testicular cell lines were studied for cytotoxicity by measuring lactate dehydrogenase (LDH) leakage; 80–200 μM genistein showed a dose-dependent increase in cytotoxicity but no statistical analysis was performed to compare doses. 40–200 μM genistein induced apoptosis in the three cell lines as well, by fluorescent microscopic analysis (Kumi-Diaka *et al.* 1999). Primary cortical neurons from rat pups showed significant cytotoxicity (LDH leakage) from 50 μM genistein, associated with apoptosis, whereas daidzein did not have this effect. The apoptotic effect of genistein seemed to be partly dependent on p42/44 and p38 mitogen-activated protein kinases (Linford *et al.* 2001). Again, given the high concentrations needed for these cytotoxic effects *in vitro*, dietary estrogens are unlikely to cause such effects in humans as a result of dietary exposure.

Alterations in hormonal function were seen in Male Wistar rat adipocytes treated with daidzein, coumestrol and zearalenone (Szkudelska *et al.* 2002). All three compounds significantly inhibited conversion of glucose to total cellular lipids (0.01–1 mmol/L for daidzein and zearalenone; 0.001–0.1 mmol/L for coumestrol). But with insulin stimulation, only daidzein (0.01–1 mol/L) and zearalenone (0.01–1 mmol/L) inhibited this conversion. Zearalenone (1 mmol/L) alone inhibited *de novo* lipogenesis, and 1 mmol/L daidzein and 0.01–0.1 mmol/L zearalenone inhibited insulin-stimulated lipogenesis. But 1 mmol zearalenone/L stimulated insulin-induced lipogenesis. Lipolysis was enhanced by daidzein and zearalenone but epinephrine-induced lipolysis was enhanced only by coumestrol and inhibited by daidzein and zearalenone. These results are of uncertain physiological significance due to the high doses of the compounds generally needed for the observed effects, but suggest that alterations in hormonal response not related to estrogenicity of the compounds should not be overlooked.

18.4.2 Animal models

A limited number of studies in animal models suggest potential anti-thyroid and anti-insulin effects, and immune and neurological toxicities from some dietary estrogens. Genistein and daidzein inhibited thyroid peroxidase and related enzymes from several species (Doerge and Chang 2002). Thyroid peroxidase is the key enzyme in thyroid hormone synthesis. The inhibition binding constant for this enzyme for genistein was 50 nmol/L and for daidzein was ~150 nmol/L. Such concentrations are theoretically achievable from exposure to these compounds in a diet rich in soy foods. Rats fed genistein at doses of 5, 100 and 500 mg/kg diet from 4 weeks before mating through weaning of pups at 3 weeks of age; pups were fed to 20 weeks after birth. All genistein doses (~0.002–0.2 mmol/kg body weight for adult rats) caused significantly decreased thyroid peroxidase activity (Doerge and Chang 2002, Doerge and Sheehan 2002), but serum thyroid hormone status remained normal in genistein-fed animals. This suggests that although thyroid peroxidase activity was decreased by genistein, thyroid hormone synthesis was still adequate. Only with concomitant iodine deficiency did soy feeding cause hypothyroidism in rats (Ikeda *et al.* 2000). It should be noted that in a study by Ikeda *et al.* (2000), soy protein feeding was only compared with feeding wheat gluten rather than a standard control diet, so whether the soy diet without iodine deficiency caused any thyroid abnormality could not be determined.

Altogether, the following, limited studies support effects of isoflavones on thyroid hormone synthesis but no functional impairment likely from dietary exposures. Red clover silage containing 0.007 mmol total isoflavones/kg diet (0.0003 mmol/kg body weight), predominantly formononetin, was fed to eight ovariectomized ewes for 14 days after 6 days acclimatation to the red clover diet; 5 months later four of the same ewes were fed the red clover again as above, compared with the other four ewes fed non-estrogenic hay. After both periods of feeding estrogens, plasma triiodothyronine (T_3) levels were significantly greater than after feeding non-estrogenic hay, but tetraiodothyronine (T_4): T_3 was only decreased significantly after the first time period of estrogen feeding. This effect on T_3 seemed to be associated with increased expression of ER-α (Madej *et al.* 2002). This effect of dietary estrogens would probably not be of functional significance because T_4, the more active thyroid hormone, was not decreased.

The following results suggest anti-insulin effects of coumestrol especially, and also show heterogeneity in effects of dietary estrogens. Genistein, coumestrol and zearalenone were compared for effects on insulin function in 130–140 g ovariectomized female Wistar rats injected with the compounds at ~0.004 mmol/kg per day for 3 days (Nogowski *et al.* 2002). Coumestrol and zearalenone but not genistein increased uterine weight, indicating frank estrogenic effects. Coumestrol increased blood glucose significantly compared with the other dietary estrogens and a control group. All three dietary estrogens increased blood concentrations of free fatty acids compared with the controls. Coumestrol and genistein decreased liver glycogen and insulin binding to both high and low affinity receptors in liver membranes.

The effect of genistein on prostate tissue and function is also of interest, due to potential impact on prostate cancer risk. Male Sprague-Dawley rats were fed 0, ~0.1 or ~0.4 mmol genistein/kg from age 21–35 days. The higher genistein dose decreased lateral prostate bud formation significantly but testosterone and dihydrotestosterone levels, and dorsolateral prostate weight were similar in genistein-fed rats compared with controls fed AIN-76A diet (Fritz *et al.* 2002b). This suggests an absence of prostate functional impairment in individuals consuming isoflavones in amounts similar to, or somewhat greater than those found in soy-containing human diets.

Immune system effects were observed in mice fed genistein (Yellayi *et al.* 2002). To attempt to mimic human infants, 70-day-old male C57Bl/6 mice were castrated and injected SC with 0.8 mmol genistein/kg for 21 days. This treatment decreased thymus weight compared with controls injected with DMSO, 100 day-old ovariectomized female C57Bl/6 mice were injected SC with 0.008–0.8 mmol genistein/kg for 7 or 21 days. 0.03 mmol genistein/kg or more significantly decreased thymus weight in females, altered T lymphocyte populations and stimulated T cell apoptosis in both males and females. In 32–34-day-old ovariectomized C57Bl/6 mice fed ~0.8–1.2 mmol genistein/kg body weight for 12 days, thymus weight was significantly decreased compared with control animals fed AIN-93G diet. The serum genistein found in these animals was similar to levels of genistein found after soy formula feeding, suggesting the possibility of impaired T cell mediated immunity in such infants, but the dose of genistein needed to achieve these serum levels was greater in mice than the dietary dose likely in human infants fed soy formula (~0.04 mmol/kg based on the USDA/Iowa State University isoflavone database indicating content of ~0.16 mmol total isoflavones/1000 mL formula, an intake of 1000 mL formula per day and a body weight of 4 kg). Due to a tenfold greater body surface area of mice than in man, the mouse's intake of 0.8 mmol/kg would be the human equivalent of 0.08 mmol/kg, only twice the estimated intake of soy-fed human infants. But ovariectomized or castrated adult mice may not be an appropriate model for human infancy, although mice in general are frequently used models for human immune functional testing. This work suggests the need for further studies of immune function and infection sensitivity of soy-fed infants. It also should be clarifed whether this effect is genistein-specific, isoflavone-specific, or generalizable to all or most dietary estrogens.

The following findings support further study of potential immunotoxic effects of isoflavones, and perhaps other dietary estrogens. Guo *et al.* (2002) fed Sprague-Dawley mothers 0.08–0.21 mmol genistein/kg housed with their pups from the pups' birth to 22 days of age. Spleen and thymus weights were unaffected by genistein in the pups although thymocyte population changes were noted with both genistein doses, but mothers fed 800 mg genistein/kg had suppressed thymus weight. Male pups had increased splenic NK activity, but female pups had decreased NK activity when fed genistein in comparsion with controls. This effect had been previously noted *in vitro* with human female peripheral blood NK cells (Zhang *et al.* 1999), but inhibition of NK activity was only noted at concentrations of genistein of $> 5\ \mu$mol/L; lower concentrations activated NK cells. Mice showed gender differences in isoflavone bioavailability with males experiencing greater levels than females (Adams *et al.* 2002). If such differences occurred in rats, males would be expected to experience suppression rather than activation of NK cells because higher isoflavone doses would cause greater toxicity.

Potentially neurotoxic effects of dietary estrogens have also been reported recently. Female Sprague-Dawley rats exposed to 0.4 mmol coumestrol/kg in the diet of their dams from birth to 21 days of age seemingly were not able to ovulate, as reflected in a lack of luteining hormone surge after being primed with estradiol and progesterone. Male Sprague-Dawley rats exposed in the same way to coumestrol from birth to 10 days of age showed significantly lessened mounting behavior and fewer ejaculations. Ovariectomized Long-Evans rats were fed 0.18 mmol isoflavones (mixture of daidzein and genistein)/kg diet showed increased ER-β expression in the paraventricular nucleus of the hypothalamus but no change in sexual behavior (Whitten et al 2002). This effect of isoflavones was the opposite of the effect of estradiol. These studies altogether support potentially adverse effects of some dietary estrogens, although mild antiestrogenic effects might protect against adverse effects of endogenous estradiol such as the stimulation of estrogen-dependent neoplasms.

Several studies support the potential for alterations in sexual behavior, sexually dimorphic functions of the nervous system, emotional status, and learning as a result of exposure to some dietary estrogens. But several dietary estrogens have not been studied in this regard, and extrapolation from rodents to humans is uncertain, although the doses studied are arguably relevant to possible human exposures. Male Long-Evans rats exposed to 1.7 mmol isoflavones/kg diet, the amount of isoflavones commonly found in standard laboratory chow diets, from conception to 120 days of age, showed greater volume of the sexually dimorphic nucleus in the pre-optic area of the brain than in females. An isoflavone-free diet did not cause this sex difference. Sexual dimorphism in visual/spatial memory was observed in Long-Evans rats after the same exposure to dietary isoflavones: females showed enhanced memory whereas males showed less memory after isoflavone feeding. A similar exposure to dietary isoflavones also significantly suppressed anxiety response in male and female Long-Evans rats in a maze test involving exploration of more and less open environments (Lephart *et al.* 2002). Eight-week-old male Lister rats fed 0.6 mmol isoflavones/kg diet for 14 days showed less social interaction and greater anxiety as reflected in fewer entries into open maze spaces (Hartley *et al.* 2003). It is difficult to resolve the disparity in results regarding anxiety from the longer-term study (Lephart *et al.* 2002) to the short-term study (Hartley *et al.* 2003). Strain differences might be the most likely explanation, although it is possible that the length of dosing period or hormonal adaptation to isoflavone exposure could be factors as well. Male Sprague-Dawley rats exposed from conception to adulthood to 0.16 mmol genistein/kg showed increased dopamine release from the striatum, a region of the nervous system controlling movement. Females did not show as strong a response to genistein, and a dose of 0.03 mmol/kg did not cause this effect (Ferguson *et al.* 2002). Further studies are warranted.

18.4.3 Human studies

Few human studies have explored the toxicity of dietary estrogens. A recent review of literature on effects of isoflavone-containing soy milk formulas on infant health indicated that six studies showed no adverse effects of soy milk feeding on growth or nutritional status in infants 0–1 year of age, except for the possibility of lower calcium bioavailability – suggested by increased 1,25-dihydroxy-vitamin D in soy-fed infants compared with infants fed human milk supplemented with vitamin D. Asthma and allergic symptoms seemed to be somewhat more common later in life for infants fed soy milk compared with human milk or some types of cow's milk formulas, but that is probably not associated with dietary estrogens from soy. Visual acuity and cognitive development seemed unaffected by soy milk, and supplementation of soy milk formulas with iodide since the 1960s has apparently prevented the hypothyroidism associated with soy milk feeding (Mendez *et al.* 2002). Limited data regarding effects of dietary estrogens on infant health support the need for additional studies given the potential for these compounds to alter development, for benefit or harm.

The relationship between intake of dietary estrogens (not including zearalenone) and thyroid cancer in women (mean age ~43 years) was studied in 608 patients and 558 case controls. Dietary intake during the year before diagnosis or interview was assessed by a food frequency questionnaire and nutrient database. Significantly reduced risk of thyroid cancer was noted for the highest quintile of intake of genistein, daidzein, formononetin, total isoflavones, secoisolariciresinol (lignan precursor), total lignans and total phytoestrogens, compared with the lowest quintile of intake when data were adjusted for age, ethnicity and energy intake. But, when data were adjusted additionally for a set of risk factors for thyroid cancer, only the highest quintile of intake of secoisolariciresinol was significantly associated with reduced thyroid cancer risk compared with the lowest quintile of intake for this phytoestrogen (Horn-Ross *et al.* 2002). These data suggest that thyroid cancer risk, thought to be estrogen dependent, may be ameliorated by at least some dietary estrogens probably acting as antiestrogens in pre-menopausal women. This study also suggests a beneficial effect of dietary estrogens on some aspects of thyroid function, rather than thyroid toxicity, at least with thyroid cancer as the endpoint.

To begin to address isoflavone toxicity, post-menopausal women (ages 46–68, n = 6/treatment) were fed a single dose of isoflavone aglucones (predominantly genistein) of ~0.01, 0.02, 0.04 or 0.08 mmol/kg. Mild toxic events related to isoflavone dose (trace pedal edema and breast tenderness) were noted in three subjects. Although a few changes in clinical chemistry were noted after isoflavone treatment, such as a transient decrease in neutrophil count, neither the standard panel of clinical blood chemistry measured at screening, day 1, 3, 6, 14 and 30 post-dosing nor clinical examination revealed any adverse effects of a single dose of as much as 1 g/day of soy isoflavones composed predominantly of genistein (Bloedon *et al.* 2002). This does not suggest that longer-term doses of such magnitude would be beneficial or without adverse effects. More studies are required.

18.4.4 Summary

Toxicity data on dietary estrogens is quite limited, but immunotoxic and neurotoxic effects are suggested by some intriguing data in recent studies in which animals were fed dietary estrogens in doses arguably relevant to human dietary exposures (e.g., Yellayi *et al.* 2002, Lephart *et al.* 2002). Human epidemiology is needed to clarify the picture of risk from these compounds. The immuno- and neuro-toxicology of zearalenone seems to be unknown. This should be a priority given the relatively strong estrogenic potency and potential for human exposure to this common fungal contaminant of grains. Toxicology of the lignans is also lacking and deserves attention. Soy isoflavones also deserve further focus, especially because they are becoming more popular as supplements and food ingredients, with less attention to coumestrol needed due to its limited occurrence in human diets.

18.5 The benefits of dietary estrogens: cancer prevention

There have been several recent reports of varied beneficial effects of dietary estrogen intake including effects on cognitive function in women. Twenty-seven women, 55–74 years of age, fed a soy isoflavone supplement providing ~0.07 mmol total isoflavones/kg daily for 6 months showed enhanced verbal memory in a category fluency test, compared with 26 similar women given a placebo during this time period (Kritz-Silverstein *et al.* 2003). These results deserve further study. Recent reviews have discussed potentially beneficial effects of dietary estrogens to prevent cancer (Persky and Van Horn 1995, Stephens 1999, Peeters *et al.* 2003), atherosclerosis (Clarkson 2002) and osteoporosis (Messina *et al.* 2001). More recent studies in each of these aspects of chronic disease prevention will be reviewed in this chapter.

Isoflavones and lignans are receiving significant attention as potential cancer-preventive dietary components. *In vitro* studies of potential mechanisms, animal models and human epidemiology have added to recent knowledge in this field.

18.5.1 *In vitro* studies

The following studies have bearing on recommendations for dietary estrogen intake for women who have estrogen-dependent neoplastic disease. In MCF-7 mammary tumor cells, genistein and coumestrol at 0.01–10 μmol/L and enterolactone at 10 μmol/L enhanced estradiol-stimulated DNA synthesis, only 50 μmol genistein/L and 100 μmol coumestrol/L suppressed estradiol's effect on DNA synthesis. Given likely plasma concentrations of these compounds from dietary exposure, genistein, coumestrol and enterolactone might actually stimulate estrogen-dependent mammary neoplastic cell growth; only pharmacological concentrations of genistein and coumestrol exerted anti-neoplastic effects (Wang and Kurzer 1998). Further studies of potentially adverse effects of dietary estrogens during cancer treatment are warranted.

Together, the following results suggest that pharmacological doses of dietary estrogens may have potential for cancer treatment against a variety of neoplasms, but *in vivo* studies assessing efficacy and safety are needed. A study of mechanisms of inhibition of MCF-7 cell proliferation showed that 25–50 mmol genistein/L induced $p21^{WAF1}$, a cyclin-dependent kinase inhibition, partly responsible for cell cycle arrest (Chinni *et al.* 2003). Human hepatoma cell lines (HepG2, Hep3B, Huh 7, PLC, HA22T) were studied for ability of genistein, biochanin A, and daidzein to inhibit proliferation and induce apoptosis. The concentration of each compound needed to inhibit growth by 50% (IC_{50}) was ~44 μmol genistein/L, ~80 μmol biochanin A/L and ~200 μmol daidzein/L. Cell cycle arrest at G2/M phase was noted especially for genistein – the effect was accompanied by inhibition of Cdc2 kinase. The isoflavones activated caspase-3 and suppressed expression of Bcl-2 and Bcl-X_l as they caused apoptosis (Su *et al.* 2003). Growth of PC-3 prostate cancer cells was inhibited significantly by 100 μmol/L of genistein, daidzein or coumestrol or 0.1–100 μmol equol/L after 6 days. LNCaP cells were growth-inhibited after 6 days by 1–100 μmol/L genistein or coumestrol, or 10–100 μmol/L daidzein or equol. Comet assay for DNA damage showed an effect of genistein at 10 μmol/L and equol at 500 μmol/L in PC-3 and LNCaP cells, with coumestrol at 100 μmol/L causing DNA damage only in PC-3 cells (Mitchell *et al.* 2000). Colo205 colon cancer cells were tested for ability of dietary estrogens to alter growth and expression of NADPH:quinone reductase (QR), an enzyme involved in detoxification of some carcinogens. Biochanin A and especially enterolactone at 1–10 μmol/L inhibited cell growth; genistein did so at 10 μmol/L. Daidzein, coumestrol and formononetin had no such effects, but biochanin A and coumestrol induced QR at 1–10 μmol/L; enterolactone and genistein induced QR at 0.1–10 μmol/L (Wang *et al.* 1998). To the extent that colon cancer cells may resemble normal colonocytes in QR induction, this effect of some dietary estrogens may be potentially anti-neoplastic in amounts obtainable from the diet. In colon cancer cell lines LS174T, Caco-2, HCT-15 and T84, enterodiol and to a greater extent enterolactone at 100 μmol/L inhibited cell proliferation after 8–10 days (Sung *et al.* 1998).

18.5.2 Animal models

Studies by Lamartiniere *et al.* (2002) showed protection from cancer by moderate dietary exposure to genistein, although daidzein exposure at 1 mmol/kg diet from conception through adulthood did not protect Sprague-Dawley female rats from DMBA-induced mammary carcinogenesis (Lamartiniere *et al.* 2002). Female Sprague-Dawley rats exposed to 1 mmol genistein/kg diet from birth to 230 days of age (genistein dose in adult rats of ~0.05 mmol/kg body weight) developed significantly fewer mammary tumors from dimethylbenz[a]anthracene (DMBA) given at 50 days of age, compared with DMBA dosed controls. TRAMP mice, transgenically altered to rapidly develop prostate cancer resembling the disease in humans, fed 1 mmol genistein/kg diet showed significantly less prostate tumor development than did controls fed AIN-76A lacking genistein. Male Lobund-Wister rats exposed to 1 mmol genistein/kg diet from conception to 48 weeks of age showed less prostate tumor incidence compared with controls exposed to the same cancer treatment regimen (chemical castration by flutamide, testosterone injections and implant, methylnitrosourea cancer-initiating agent).

Transgenic mice having the mouse mammary tumor virus (MMTV)-neu/ErbB-2 genes develop mammary tumors spontaneously. Such mice were fed genistein or daidzein (~0.2 mmol/kg body weight) from 7 to 33 weeks of age. Both isoflavones significantly lengthened tumor latency period (Jin and MacDonald 2002). GR mice carrying the MMTV gene fed biochanin A developed less mammary cancer than similar mice fed a control diet or daidzein-containing diet (Mizunuma *et al.* 2002). Both isoflavones were fed at ~0.16 mmol/kg body weight from 1 to 15 months of age. In similar mice made germfree, biochanin A was not anticarcinogenic, supporting the need for gut microbial metabolism of this compound to genistein to be effective against mammary cancer. DMBA-initiated mice were assessed for prevention of skin carcinogenesis by genistein during O-tetradecanoylphorbol-13-acetate-induced tumor promotion. Genistein at 1 or 5 μmol per mouse given twice a week for 17 weeks significantly suppressed the numbers of skin tumors per mouse (Wei *et al.* 1995).

Female C57Bl/6 mice implanted SC with MB49 bladder tumor cell were injected IP with 0.2 mmol genistein/kg for 3 weeks before and 3 weeks after tumor implantation, or fed ~0.2 mmol or 0.9 mmol total isoflavones/kg from soy isoflavone extracts. All of these treatments significantly suppressed tumor volumes compared with controls not fed the isoflavones, by decreasing angiogenesis and increasing apoptosis (Zhou *et al.* 1998). In female B6C3F1 mice challenged with B16F10 melanoma tumor cells intravenously, daily oral genistein of 0.024 or 0.08 mmol/kg for 28 days significantly suppressed lung tumor nodules and increased cytotoxic T-cell activity. Natural killer cell activity stimulated by IL-2 was also increased by 0.08 mmol genistein/kg (Guo *et al.* 2001).

Not only do studies on isoflavones show anticarcinogenic effects, but several studies have shown that lignans also exert anticancer effects. Fifty-day-old female Sprague-Dawley rats treated with 5 mg DMBA/rat were fed 0.006–0.013 mmol secoisolariciresinol diglucoside (SDG)/kg for 20 weeks beginning 1 week after DMBA (SDG dose decreased with increasing body weight over time). Number of tumors/rat and per group was significantly decreased by SDG feeding compared with controls (Thompson *et al.* 1996a). In a similar DMBA model, rats gavaged with similar amounts of SDG for 7 weeks beginning 13 weeks after carcinogen dosing showed decreased mammary tumors (Thompson *et al.* 1996b). Female Sprague-Dawley rats given 12 mg DMBA at 50 days of age and 0.004 or 0.04 mmol enterolactone/kg for 50 days starting 9 weeks after DMBA showed regressed mammary tumors at the end of treatment, and the higher dose of enterolactone significantly suppressed growth of all tumors (new and ones appearing before lignan treatment) (Saarinen *et al.* 2002).

Using methylnitrosourea, female Sprague-Dawley rats were initiated at 50 days of age, then 2 days later, fed two doses of flaxseed (2.5 or 5% of diet) or gavaged with SDG (~0.004 or 0.008 mmol/kg per day) for 22 weeks. Tumor multiplicity was significantly less only with the high dose of SDG compared with basal diet treatment. Tumor incidence and overall tumor weight did not differ among treatments (Rickard *et al.* 1999). Male Sprague-Dawley rats, 40 days of age, were dosed with azoxymethane, and one week later dosed with

~0.007 mmol SDG/kg per day by gavage for 100 days. Aberrant crypt foci (preneoplasia) in the distal colon and number of aberrant crypts/focus were significantly fewer after SDG treatment than in controls (Jenab and Thompson 1996). In male C57Bl/6 mice injected intravenously with B16BL6 melanoma cells and fed 0.015, 0.029 or 0.059 mmol SDG/kg for 2 weeks before and after cancer cell treatment, number of mice per treatment group with > 50 lung tumors was significantly less in mice fed the higher two doses of SDG than in controls. The highest dose of SDG caused lower median number of tumors/mouse than in controls (Li *et al.* 1999).

In summary, the above-cited studies showed that in cancer cell cultures and *in vivo*, tumor transplantation models, genistein and SDG suppressed neoplasia, for the most part. A few studies indicate the potential for genistein to stimulate tumor cell growth (Wang and Kurzer 1998). Hsieh *et al.* (1998) showed that ovariectomized athymic mice implanted SC with MCF-7 tumor cells and fed ~0.6 mmol genistein/kg showed greater tumor growth compared with controls. MCF-7 cells are estrogen-dependent tumor cells, so these results reasonably raise a note of caution for the use of dietary estrogens in cancer prevention and treatment. But similarly high doses of genistein in other transplanted tumor models showed benefits (e.g. Zhou *et al.* 1998). Prevention of cancer, especially during the phase of promotion, but also due to lifelong exposure, has been generally observed for genistein and SDG consumed in doses relevant to human diets. Other dietary estrogens deserve further study regarding their effects during carcinogenesis.

18.5.3 Human studies

A number of case control, prospective and other human studies have examined the roles of soy isoflavones and lignans in cancer risk. Among ~25,000 women in the Japan Public Health Center-Based Prospective Study on Cancer and Cardiovascular Diseases, when grouped into quartiles according to estimated isoflavone intake based on a food frequency questionnaire, there was a significant trend for greatest breast cancer incidence in the lowest quartile of isoflavone intake. Intake of miso soup, a soy food source of significaint isoflavone content was similarly associated with breast cancer incidence (Yamamoto *et al.* 2003). Wu *et al.* (1998) summarized evidence from four case control studies of soy intake and breast cancer risk. Two such studies (Yuan *et al.* 1995, Hirose *et al.* 1995) showed no effect of soy intake on breast cancer risk. Lee *et al.* (1991) showed a significant trend for reduced risk according to increased soy intake for pre-menopausal women only. Wu *et al.* (1996) showed a significant trend for decreased breast cancer risk with increasing soy intake for non-US born Asian women but not for US-born Asian women. In the Shanghai Breast Cancer Study, 60 breast cancer case control pairs were assessed for urinary isoflavone excretion – total isoflavone and glycitein excretion differed significantly between cases and controls (Zheng *et al.* 1999), suggesting an association between greater isoflavone intake and reduced risk of breast cancer.

Comparing 18 Australian female breast cancer patients with 20 matched controls showed fourteen-fold greater mean 24 h urinary excretion of daidzein by controls than cases. Genistein excretion showed a similar trend (Murkies *et al.* 2000), again suggesting a protective role for isoflavones in breast cancer risk.

Lignans were also studied with respect to breast cancer risk. Enterolactone was present in significantly greater amounts (by tenfold) in fluid from type I than in type II breast cysts, among 191 patients studied. Enterolactone was significantly but weakly correlated with cyst fluid epidermal growth factor (EGF), a potent cell proliferative risk factor for breast cancer, although among cyst patients who later developed breast cancer, greater breast cyst fluid EGF but not enterolactone was significantly associated with breast cancer risk (Boccardo *et al.* 2003). In women in Northern Sweden, 248 breast cancer cases and 492 controls were compared for plasma enterolactone. Both plasma enterolactone levels below the 12.5th percentile and above the 87.5th percentile were associated with greater breast cancer risk. Somewhat more pre-menopausal women were in the group with high enterolactone levels and increased breast cancer risk (Hulten *et al.* 2002). Another study of 207 breast cancer cases and 188 controls analyzed lignan intake by food frequency questionnaire. For pre- but not post-menopausal women, the highest tertile of daily lignan intake (0.04–0.2 μmol/kg) was associated with significantly decreased breast cancer risk compared with the lowest tertile of intake (0.004–0.03 μmol/kg). Pre-menopausal women having the A2 allele for cytochrome P450c17α, a key steroid hormone metabolizing enzyme showed especially reduced breast cancer risk associated with the highest tertile of lignan intake (McCann *et al.* 2002).

Effects of isoflavones and lignans has also been assessed with respect to prostate cancer risk in a limited number of studies. Messina (2003) reviewed 12 human epidemiologic studies relating soy food intake to prostate cancer risk. In two of these studies, isoflavone intake was estimated, but in both studies, the range of isoflavone intake was limited or total intake of isoflavones nearly negligible. Neither study showed cancer risk reduction with greater isoflavone intake. Of the other ten studies, only one showed a significant linear trend for reduced prostate cancer risk with greater soy milk intake, suggesting a benefit of soy isoflavones. Men with elevated prostate serum antigen (PSA $> 4\ \mu$g/L) (n = 34) showed no change after consuming soy protein with isoflavones (0.003 mmol/kg per day) or without them, each treatment for 6 weeks in a randomized, double-blind crossover design (Urban *et al.* 2001). Tissue content of dietary estrogens was examined in 15 men with benign prostate hyperplasia and 10 controls. Genistein, but not daidzein, equol, enterodiol or enterolactone, was significantly less in hyperplastic prostate than in normal prostate, suggesting a role for this dietary estrogen in preventing preneoplastic prostate growth (Hong *et al.* 2002). In a case control study of 794 prostate cancer cases and 2550 controls among Norwegian, Swedish and Finnish men, serum enterolactone divided into quartiles did not differ across the overall cohort or within each nationality between cases and controls (Stattin *et al.* 2002). A case control study of 159 cases compared with 139 controls examined intake of dietary estrogens by questionnaire, and showed no relationship between intake of coumestrol, isoflavones or lignans and testicular cancer risk (Walcott *et al.* 2002). At present there is little basis from human studies to support prostate or other reproductive cancer protective effects in men from dietary estrogens.

18.5.4 Summary

Isoflavones and lignans have shown promise in preventing, and to some extent treating, mammary cancer development. Human epidemiology provides modest support for these effects as well. But the possibility for adverse effects of some dietary estrogens on estrogen-dependent cancers has been demonstrated in a few animal and human epidemiological studies. Evidence is nearly nil that isoflavones or lignans prevent prostate cancer in humans, although some animal studies are encouraging. Clearly, this field deserves additional exploration. Zearalenone is completely unstudied, and approaches other than epidemiological case control are needed to test preventive effects of dietary estrogens.

18.6 The benefits of dietary estrogens: preventing osteoporosis and atherosclerosis

18.6.1 Osteoporosis prevention

Animal models

Several rodent studies in ovariectomized animals have shown that isoflavones or isoflavone-containing foods prevent bone mineral loss (e.g. Arjmandi *et al.* 1996). Twelve-week-old ovariectomized (OVX) Sprague-Dawley rats were gavaged with 0.18 mmol genistein/kg per day for 12 weeks. Distal femur density was significantly greater in genistein-treated rats than in OVX controls. Both interleukin (IL)-1β and tumor necrosis factor (TNF)α were decreased significantly by genistein treatment, indicating prevention of bone resorption. These effects were similar to effects of estradiol treatment, but estradiol also suppressed osteocalcin in OVX rats, compared with OVX controls. Genistein also increased uterine weight compared with OVX rats, and suppressed body weight gain due to ovariectomy (Li and Yu 2003). Thus, genistein may have anti-osteoporotic effects, suppressing bone resorption as a SERM, targeting sites of action similar in part to effects of estradiol.

Human studies

Pre-menopausal women were fed ~0.005 mmol isoflavones/kg for 24 weeks in soy protein (n = 24), compared with groups fed soy protein without isoflavones (n = 24), or whey protein (n = 21). Lumbar spine bone mineral content was significantly greater in women fed isoflavones than in women fed whey protein (Alekel *et al.* 2000). Post-menopausal women, mean age 60 years, were fed a soy isoflavone supplement of 0.004 mmol/kg for 3 months (n = 38), compared with a placebo-dosed control group (n = 40). Although the isoflavone treatment lowered plasma LDL cholesterol compared with the placebo-treated group, urinary pyridinoline and deoxypyridinoline, two markers of bone resorption, did not differ between the treatments (Dalais *et al.* 2003). This study may have been of insufficient duration to see effects of isoflavones on indices of osteoporosis.

Epidemiological studies of effects of dietary estrogens on osteoporosis also suggest potential benefits of the compounds. In 357 post-menopausal Chinese women (mean age 63 years), dietary estrogen intake was assessed by food frequency questionnaire and food compositional database (Mei *et al.* 2001). Lumbar spine bone mineral density was significantly greater in women in the highest tertile of isoflavone intake compared with the lowest tertile of isoflavone intake (~0.002 mmol isoflavone/kg v. ~0.0002 mmol isoflavone/kg). Post-menopausal Korean women (mean age 57 years) without bone disease (n = 25) were compared with subjects with osteopenia (n = 29) or osteoporosis (n = 21). Urinary excretion of enterolactone was significantly positively associated with bone density in lumbar spine, femoral neck and Ward's triangle femoral bone, but excretion of other dietary estrogens (enterodiol, daidzein, genistein, equol) showed no such significant relationships (Kim *et al.* 2002). Epidemiological studies provide modest support for anti-osteoporotic effects of some dietary estrogens, but more studies are needed.

Summary

A few studies in animal models and in humans, both intervention trials and epidemiology, suggest that isoflavones and lignans may be anti-osteoporotic. More well-controlled and long-term studies are under way, but additional attention to dietary estrogens beyond isoflavones may be warranted.

18.6.2 Atherosclerosis risk reduction

Animal models

Dietary daidzein fed to provide 0.07 mmol/kg to 8–10-week-old male and female Syrian Golden hamsters for 10 weeks significantly lowered total and non-HDL cholesterol compared with a control group fed casein (Song *et al.* 2003). There was lowering of total and non-HDL cholesterol similar to that after daidzein feeding of hamsters (they were fed isolated soy protein providing a similar total molar amount of isoflavones or fed isolated soy protein containing less than 1% the amount of isoflavones of intact isolated soy protein). This study not only supports a health-beneficial role of the dietary estrogen, daidzein, but also shows a plateau of cholesterol-lowering efficacy. Studies comparing soy protein with isoflavone-extracted soy protein that show no difference between the two in cholesterol-lowering may erroneously conclude a lack of involvement of isoflavones in this effect. More studies with purified isoflavones ought to be performed, especially dose/response studies to determine the range of effective doses.

Twelve-week-old New Zealand white rabbits were fed 1% cholesterol diets with and without isoflavone extracts (~1.1 mmol or 3.0 mmol/kg) for 8 weeks.

Isoflavone feeding did not lower serum cholesterol or LDL cholesterol compared with controls fed cholesterol alone. Oxidized LDL cholesterol measured as cholesterol hydroperoxide after *in vitro* addition of copper (0.5 mmol/L) was significantly lessened by isoflavone feeding compared with cholesterol-fed controls, and aortic atherosclerotic lesion area was also significantly reduced by isoflavone feeding (Yamakoshi *et al.* 2000). A note of caution in extrapolating such results: these levels of dietary isoflavones were quite high in comparison to typical or likely human dietary exposures.

In contrast to studies in hamsters and rabbits, ovariectomized cynomolgous monkeys fed a casein-based atherogenic diet and 0.04 mmol total soy isoflavones/kg per day for 20 weeks showed HDL cholesterol and total cholesterol: HDL cholesterol ratios intermediate between positive controls fed casein and monkeys fed soy protein containing isoflavones (Greaves *et al.* 2000). Thus, the isoflavones in soy protein could not totally account for effects of soy protein to improve plasma lipids in these monkeys.

Cynomolgous monkeys fed an atherogenic diet (45% of energy as fat, 0.28 mg cholesterol/Cal) for 26 months were ovariectomized and fed a control diet (soy protein without isoflavones), or soy protein with isoflavones (~0.03 mmol/kg) for 36 months. Addition of isoflavones to the monkeys' diets decreased plasma total cholesterol and LDL cholesterol, and increased plasma HDL cholesterol and apo A-1 contents significantly (Clarkson *et al.* 2001). Isoflavones decreased carotid atherosclerosis significantly and showed a trend toward decreasing coronary artery atherosclerosis. These effects suggest that a high intake of isoflavones in soy protein may prevent atherosclerosis to some extent.

New Zealand white rabbits, ages 6–8 weeks, 1.3–1.8 kg, were fed the lignan precursor, SDG at 0.02 mmol/kg body weight, in a 1% cholesterol diet for 8 weeks. SDG in the cholesterol-containing diet significantly lowered total serum cholesterol and LDL cholesterol compared with feeding a diet containing only cholesterol, and significantly increased HDL cholesterol. Aortic fatty streaks were also significantly lessened by adding SDG to the high cholesterol diet (Prasad 1999). The extent of formation of lignans from SDG was not measured or discussed, so it is not clear from this study whether these dietary estrogens were directly involved in this effect of SDG. The dietary cholesterol content in this study was supraphysiologic, as was the SDG content. Flaxseed contains ~0.02 mmol SDG/kg, so human exposure to SDG even on a high flaxseed diet would be unlikely to exceed 30 μmol/kg body weight. The lowest effective dose of SDG for anti-atherogenesis remains to be defined. The roles of enterodiol and enterolactone in this effect also deserve further study.

Human studies

A randomized double-blind placebo human trial of the effect of ~0.003 mmol isoflavones/kg per day fed for 8 weeks showed no effect of isoflavones on serum lipids or lipoproteins. Forty-six men and 13 post-menopausal women not taking hormone replacement therapy, 35–69 years of age and all normocholesterolemic participated (Hodgson *et al.* 1998). Thirteen normocholesterolemic, pre-menopausal women were fed 0.0006, 0.004 and 0.008 mmol total isoflavones/kg per day in soy protein for three menstrual cycles of each treatment in a randomized cross-over design. The diet with highest isoflavone content lowered LDL cholesterol in midfollicular and periovulatory phases of the menstrual cycle compared with the other diets (Merz-Demlow *et al.* 2000). These mixed results are not surprising in that soy protein and its components are known to benefit cholesterol status to a much greater extent in hypercholesterolemic than in normocholesterolemic subjects (Anderson *et al.* 1995, Crouse *et al.* 1999). But Sirtori *et al.* (2002) showed no effect on lipoprotein cholesterol status of feeding soy milk providing ~0.01 mmol total isoflavones/kg to 20 Type II hypercholesterolemic subjects (16 women, 4 men, ages 38–76 years) for 4 weeks in a randomized cross-over design with cow's milk as the control treatment. The isoflavone source was much higher in glycitein and lower in genistein compared with previous soy protein feeding studies that had shown cholesterol-lowering from soy feeding. Thus, recent human studies have largely failed to show a benefit of isoflavones on cholesterol status, but controlling such studies and having sufficient power to detect modest benefits are problems that need to be addressed further.

Cholesterol status is not the only determinant of atherosclerotic risk. A few studies have described effects of isoflavones on arterial function as well. A randomized, cross-over, double-blind placebo study in 80 subjects (mean age 54 years, 43% women) consuming ~0.005 mmol biochanin A or formononetin/kg per day for 6 weeks showed improved arterial compliance, pulse wave volume and total peripheral resistance after formononetin treatment, compared with placebo (Teede *et al.* 2003). Twenty-eight post-menopausal women (mean age 54 years) were fed milk protein, soy protein without isoflavones or soy protein providing ~0.007 mmol total isoflavones/kg for 6 weeks each in a randomized cross-over design, with 4 week washout periods between treatments. Peak flow velocity in the brachial artery was significantly less after treatment with isoflavone-containing soy than after milk protein treatment. Subjects were normocholesterolemic and experienced no effect of soy protein or isoflavones on plasma lipoproteins (Steinberg *et al.* 2003). These studies suggest effects of some isoflavones on arterial function that might prevent atherosclerosis-related ailments.

Isoflavones and lignans may be of benefit in reducing atherosclerosis risk. Offspring of the Framingham Heart Study participants, 939 post-menopausal women, were assessed for atherosclerosis risk factors according to estimated intake of isoflavones and lignans by a food frequency questionnaire. Subjects in the highest quartile of lignan intake had significantly lower waist/hip ratio and plasma triglycerides than subjects in the lowest quartile of lignan intake. Subjects in the highest quartiles of both isoflavone and lignan intakes had significantly lower metabolic syndrome scores than subjects in the lowest quartile of intake of these dietary estrogens (de Kleijn *et al.* 2002). Metabolic syndrome score was based on blood pressure, triglycerides, HDL cholesterol, waist/hip ratio and body mass index (higher score = greater cardiovascular disease risk). This study suggests potential atherosclerosis risk reduction from greater intake of some dietary estrogens.

Summary
Although a recent study with a purified isoflavone, daidzein, showed lowering of blood cholesterol in hamsters, human studies have shown mixed results from isoflavone feeding with respect to cholesterol status. A few such studies have compared isoflavone-rich soy with soy sources from which isoflavones have been removed. Even when isoflavone supplements have been used, there may be other components in such products that might also account for cholesterol-lowering, such as soyasaponins. Lignans as well as isoflavones may have some beneficial effects with respect to atherosclerosis risk, but probably not from effects on cholesterol status. Improved arterial function is also suggested for some isoflavones from human studies. Other dietary estrogens may deserve further study for similar benefits. Mechanisms of action of anti-atherosclerotic effects of dietary estrogens are seemingly quite varied, although they are understudied.

18.6.3 The overall benefits of dietary estrogens

A range of dietary estrogen intakes may have beneficial effects for preventing some chronic diseases of partial hormonal origins (Table 18.2), but results of a number of studies related to cancer, osteoporosis and atherosclerosis have also shown no benefit from a range of doses similar to those showing health

Table 18.2 Intakes of dietary estrogens associated with health benefits in recent human studies

Disease/type of study	Dietary estrogen	Intake (estimated mmol/kg body weight per d)	Reference
Cancer/case control	Lignans	0.00004–0.0002	McCann *et al.* 2002
Osteoporosis/observational	Isoflavones	~0.002	Mei *et al.* 2001
Osteoporosis/6 months intervention	Isoflavones	0.005	Alekel *et al.* 2000
Atherosclerosis/6 weeks intervention, arterial function	Formononetin	~0.005	Teede *et al.* 2003
Atherosclerosis/6 weeks intervention, arterial function	Isoflavones	~0.007	Steinberg *et al.* 2003
Atherosclerosis/3 menstrual cycle intervention, cholesterol status	Isoflavones	0.008	Merz-Demlow *et al.* 2000
Atherosclerosis/9 weeks intervention, cholesterol status	Isoflavones	0.002	Crouse *et al.* 1999

protective effects. Control of such studies is quite challenging. Developing a better understanding of specific subpopulations that may experience benefit or harm from dietary estrogens ought to be a priority (e.g. McCann *et al.* 2002). Coumestrol and zearalenone are almost unstudied in the context of disease prevention, but a significant body of knowledge exists at least indirectly examining isoflavones and lignans. Mechanisms of action of these compounds with respect to disease prevention remain to be determined. Some dietary estrogens may be of health benefit in amounts obtainable from traditional foods. The advent of engineering of functional foods with enhanced dietary estrogen contents poses a challenge to assure safety and efficacy of these unproven and potentially potent actors.

18.7 Dietary intakes of estrogens

Limited data exist on dietary estrogen contents in the human food supply. The mean daily intake of dietary estrogens in 17,357 Dutch women based on food frequency questionnaire and literature search for food analysis data showed mean daily intakes of ~8 nmol/kg for daidzein and genistein, ~4 nmol/kg for formononetin, negligible amounts of biochanin A and coumesterol and ~20 nmol/kg for SDG (Boker *et al.* 2002). Southern Chinese women (n = 650) assessed in a similar way were estimated to have daily intakes of 2000 nmol isoflavones/kg, 5 nmol coumesterol/kg, and 70 nmol lignans/kg (Mei *et al.* 2001). Conceivably, a diet containing 30 g flaxseed per day (2 tablespoons) would provide 63 nmol lignans/kg (based on Thompson *et al.* 1996a). The main source of coumestrol, biochanin A and formononetin in the human diet is alfalfa, soy and clover sprouts, with coumestrol content ranging from 1.12–18.6 mmol/kg, biochanin A content from 0–118 mmol/kg, and formononetin from 10–71 mmol/kg. The greatest amounts of these three dietary estrogens come from mixed clover and alfalfa sprouts (USDA-Iowa State University Database on Isoflavone Contents of Foods, 2002). For example, eating one half cup serving of such sprouts per day, ~35 g, could provide 0.01 mmol coumestrol, 0.064 mmol biochanin A, and 0.04 mmol formononetin/kg body weight. Based on one report of zearalenone contents of grain foods, 26% of samples tested contained a mean of 76 nmol/kg (Abouzied *et al.* 1991). From the Continuing Survey of Food Intake of Individuals data from 1994–1996, people surveyed in the United States consumed an average of 6.7 Food Guide Pyramid servings/d of grain foods (Cleveland *et al.* 2000). From USDA food composition databases (USDA Food Composition Data Release 16), serving sizes of grain food range from ~25–100 g, roughly averaging 50 g, so total daily grain intake is ~300 g/d with an estimated zearalenone intake of ~6 nmol per person per d or ~0.1 nmol/kg body weight for an average adult, if ~25% of that grain is zearalenone contaminated.

There are no regulatory action levels set for any of the dietary estrogens in the human food supply, but voluntary surveillance is commonly practiced by grain

Table 18.3 Estimated human daily intake of dietary estrogens compared with estimated toxic doses

Dietary estrogen	Estimated human daily intake (nmol/kg body weight)[1]	Estimated toxic dose (nmol/kg body weight)
Genistein	8–2000[#]	80,000 (extrapolated from mice, Yellayi *et al.* 2002)
Daidzein	8–2000[#]	?
Biochanin A	0–64,000*	?
Formononetin	4–40,000*	300 (extrapolated from ewes, Medej *et al.* 2002)
Coumestrol	5–10,000*	~600 (extrapolated from rats, Nogowski *et al.* 2002)
Lignans	20–70	?
Zearalenone	0.1	~600 (extrapolated from rats, Nogowski *et al.* 2002)

[#] High intake from diet containing soy foods.
* High intake from daily serving of 0.5 cup alfalfa/clover sprouts.
[1] Data from Boker *et al.* 2002, Mei *et al.* 2001

millers. When estimated daily intake levels are compared with estimated toxic doses as extrapolated from animals with correction for animal/human body surface area differences (7-fold for rats, 10-fold for mice) (Table 18.3), human intakes are likely to be vanishingly small in comparison with toxic exposures. Routinely high intakes of some types of legume sprouts are probably unwise, but these foods are usually used as a salad topping, with exposure to much less than a half cup serving and then, only occasionally. Continuing surveillance of the food supply for trends in consumption of foods rich in dietary estrogens, or in zearalenone contamination is warranted, but these compounds generally seem to pose minimal health risk, and some may be of health benefit, although this remains uncertain.

18.8 Future trends and sources of further information and advice

Research on health benefits of dietary estrogens is expanding (see reviews cited at the beginning of this chapter), with an emphasis on well-controlled intervention studies. Feeding specific dietary estrogens may require investigational new drug permits in the United States for human studies, and the process of obtaining appropriate data to receive the permit may be costly. Some such permits have been obtained, but for some of the dietary estrogens, this is not feasible due to established toxicity concerns for compounds such as zearalenone. Some discussion of action levels for zearalenone is ongoing. A recent outbreak in the eastern United States of heavy contamination of wheat with deoxynivalenol (DON), one of the most common mycotoxins in human foods, may raise some concerns about zearalenone, which usually occurs along with *Fusarium* trichothecenes such as DON (Herrman 2002).

Effects of mixtures of the dietary estrogens would be a potentially important realm for further investigation, because many people may want to consume flaxseed, whole grains, and soy together on a daily basis due to purported health benefits. Such a combination of foods would provide isoflavones, lignans, and potentially zearalenone. It would be of some interest to determine whether additive, synergistic or mutually antagonistic effects of such combinations occur.

Developing clearer biomarkers and disease-related endpoints for effects of dietary estrogens is a crucial need for progress in this field. Advances are being made in understanding key gene products regulated by ERs and influenced by dietary estrogens (e.g., Wober *et al.* 2003). Each dietary estrogen seems to be a unique SERM, so multiple endpoints will be needed, in order to do meaningful comparisons. Studies in human tissues should be emphasized, with assessment of exposure being done consistently in quantifying dietary contents and body burdens (from plasma and/or urinary excretion) of the compounds, although appropriate animal models will be essential for long-term disease endpoints to be effectively assessed. Progress in transgenic manipulation to create models more effectively resembling humans is ongoing, and will probably be crucial.

Availability of dietary estrogen supplements is increasing markedly, and quality control of such products is seemingly improving, with sophistication of consumers and availability of appropriate analytic methods. Such supplements are of no proven benefit, so it would probably be wiser to avoid them at this time. Consumption of dietary estrogen-rich foods in forms relatively close to their naturally-occurring state may be of some health benefit, and is most probably of negligible risk to health. Dietary estrogens pose a complex and exciting challenge to nutrition, toxicology, food and hormonal research communities, as well as to regulatory and public health agencies, and food and pharmaceutical industries. Increasingly multidisciplinary collaborations keeping public health as the central concern ought to be of highest priority in future work with these compounds.

18.9 References

ABOUZIED MM, AZCONA JI, BRASELTON WE, PESTKA JJ (1991) Immunochemical assessment of mycotoxins in 1989 grain foods: evidence for deoxynivalenol (vomitoxin) contamination. *Appl Environ Microbiol* 57: 672–677.

ADAMS MR, GOLDEN DL, ANTHONY MS, REGISTER TC, WILLIAMS JK (2002) The inhibitory effect of soy protein isolate on atherosclerosis in mice does not require the presence of LDL receptors or alteration of plasma lipoproteins. *J Nutr* 132: 43–49.

ADLERCREUTZ H (1998) Epidemiology of phytoestrogens. *Bailliere's Clin Endocrinol Metab* 12: 605–623.

ALEKEL DL, ST. GERMAIN A, PETERSON CT, HANSON KB, STEWART JW, TODA T (2000)

Isoflavone-rich soy protien isolate attenuates bone loss in the lumbar spine of perimenopausal women. *Am J Clin Nutr* 72: 844–852.

ANDERSON JJB, ANTHONY M, MESSINA M, GARNER SC (1999) Effects of phyto-oestrogens on tissues. *Nutr Res Rev* 12: 75–116.

ANDERSON JW, JOHNSTONE BM, COOK-NEWELL ME (1995) Meta-analysis of the effects of soy protein intake on serum lipids. *New Engl J Med* 333: 276–282.

ARJMANDI BH, ALEKEL L, HOLLIS BW, AMIN D, STACEWICZ-SAPUNTZAKIS M, GUO P, KUKREJA SC (1996) Dietary soybean protein prevents bone loss in an ovariectomized rat model of osteoporosis. *J Nutr* 126: 161–167.

ATANASSOVA N, MCKINNELL C, TURNER KJ, WALKER M, FISHER JS, MORLEY M, MILLAR MR, GROOME NP, SHARPE RM (2000) Comparative effects of neonatal exposure of male rats to potent and weak (environmental) estrogens on spermatogenesis at puberty and the relationship to adult testis size and fertility: evidence for stimulatory effects of low estrogen levels. *Endocrinol* 141: 3898–3907.

AWONIYI CA, ROBERTS D, CHANDRAKESHAR V, VEERAMACHANENI DNR, HURST BS, TUCKER KE, SCHLAFF WD (1998) Neonatal exposure to coumestrol, a phytoestrogens, does not alter spermatogenic potential in rats. *Endocrine* 7: 337–341.

BERAL V (2003) Breast cancer and hormone-replacement therapy in the Million Women Study. *Lancet* 362: 419–427.

BIRT DF, HENDRICH S, WANG W (2001) Dietary agents in cancer prevention: flavonoids and isoflavonoids. *Pharmacol Therap* 90: 157–177.

BLOEDON LT, JEFFCOAT AR, LOPACZYNSKI W, SCHELL MJ, BLACK TM, DIX KJ, THOMAS BF, ALBRIGHT C, BUDBY MG, CROWELL JA, ZEISEL SH (2002) Safety and pharmacokinetics of purified soy isoflavones: single-dose administration to postmenopausal women. *Am J Clin Nutr* 76: 1126–1137.

BOCCARDO F, LUNARDI GL, PETTI AR, RUBAGOTTI A (2003) Enterolactone in breast cyst fluid: correlation with EGF and breast cancer risk. *Breast Cancer Res Treat* 79: 17–23.

BOKER LK, VAN DER SCHOUW YT, DE KLEIJN MJ, JACQUES PF, GROBBEE DE, PEETERS PHM (2002) Intake of dietary phytoestrogens by Dutch women. *J Nutr* 132: 1319–1328.

BOWE J, LI XF, SUGDEN D, KATZENELLENBOGEN JA, KATZENELLENBOGEN BS, O'BYRNE KT (2003) The effects of the phytoestrogen, coumestrol, on gonadotropin-releasing hormone (GnRH) mRNA expression in GT1-7 GnRH neurones. *J Neuroendocrinol* 15: 105–108.

BURGER H (2003) Hormone replacement therapy in the post-Women's Health Initiative era. *Climacteric* 6 (Suppl 1): 11–36.

CHINNI SR, ALHASAN SA, MULTANI AS, PATHAK S, SARKAR FH (2003) Pleotropic effects of genistein on MCF-7 breast cancer cells. *Int J Mol Med* 12: 29–34.

CLARKSON TB (2002) Soy, soy phytoestrogens and cardiovascular disease. *J Nutr* 132: 566S–569S.

CLARKSON TB, ANTHONY MS, MORGAN TM (2001) Inhibition of postmenopausal atherosclerosis progression: a comparison of the effects of conjugated equine estrogens and soy phytoestrogens. *J Endocrinol Clin Metab* 86: 41–47.

CLEVELAND LE, MOSHFEGH AJ, ALBERTSON AM, GOLDBERG JD (2000) Dietary intake of whole grains. *J Am Coll Nutr* 19: 331S–338S.

CROUSE JR III, MORGAN T, TERRY JG, ELLIS J, VITOLINS M, BURKE GL (1999) A randomized trial comparing the effect of casein with that of soy protein containing varying amounts of isoflavones on plasma concentrations of lipids and lipoproteins. *Arch Intern Med* 159: 2070–2076.

DALAIS FS, EBELING PR, KOTSOPOULOS D, MCGRATH BP, TEEDE HJ (2003) The effects of soy protein containing isoflavones on lipids and indices of bone resorption in postmenopausal women. *Clin Endocrinol* 58: 704–709.

DECHAUD H, RAVARD C, CLAUSTRAT F, BRAC DE LA PERRIERE A, PUGEAT M (1999) Xenoestrogen interaction with human sex hormone-binding globulin. *Steroids* 64: 328–334.

DE KLEIJN MJ, VAN DER SCHOUW YT, WILSON PWF, GROBBEE DE, JACQUES PF (2002) Dietary intake of phytoestrogens is associated with a favorable metabolic cardiovascular risk profile in postmenopausal U.S. women: the Framingham study. *J Nutr* 132: 276–282.

DIEL P, SCHMIDT S, VOLLMER G (2002) *In vivo* test sytems fo the quantitative and qualitative analysis of the biological activity of phytoestrogens. *J Chromatog B* 777: 191–202.

DOERGE DR, CHANG HC (2002) Inactivation of thyroid peroxidase by soy isoflaovnes, *in vitro* and *in vivo*. *J Chromatog B* 777: 269–279.

DOERGE DR, SHEEHAN DM (2002) Goitrogenic and estrogenic activity of soy isoflavones. *Environ Health Perspect* 110 (suppl 3): 349–353.

FERGUSON SA, FLYNN KM, DELCLOS KB, NEWBOLD RR, GOUGH BJ (2002) Effects of lifelong dietary exposure to genistein or nonylphenol on amphetamine-stimulated striatal dopamine release in male and female rats. *Neurotoxicol Teratol* 24: 37–45.

FITZPATRICK LA (2003) Soy isoflavones: hope or hype? *Maturitas* 44: S21–S29.

FRITZ WA, WANG J, ELTOUM IE, LAMARTINIERE CA (2002a). Dietary genistein down-regulates androgen and estrogen receptor expression in the rat prostate. *Mol Cell Endocrinol* 186: 89–99.

FRITZ WA, ELTOUM I-E, COTRONEO MS, LAMARTINIERE CA (2002b) Genistein alters growth but is not toxic to the rat prostate. *J Nutr* 132: 3007–3011.

GREAVES KA, WILSON MD, RUDEL LL, WILLIAMS JK, WAGNER JD (2000) Consumption of soy protein reduces cholesterol absorption compared to casein protein alone or supplemented wth an isoflavone extract or conjugated equine estrogen in ovariectomized cynomolgous monkeys. *J Nutr* 130: 820–826.

GUO TL, MCCAY JA, ZHANG LX, BROWN RD, YOU L, KARROW NA, GERMOLEC DR, WHITE KL JR (2001) Genistein modulates immune responses and increases host resistance to B16F10 tumor in adult female B6C3F1 mice. *J Nutr* 131: 3251–3258.

GUO TL, ZHANG XL, BARTOLUCCI E, MCCAY JA, WHITE KL JR, YOU L (2002) Genistein and methoxychlor modulate the activity of natural killer cells and the expression of phenotypic markers by thymocytes and splenocytes in F_0 and F_1 generations of Sprague-Dawley rats. *Toxicol* 172: 205–215.

HARTLEY DE, EDWARDS JE, SPILLER CE, ALOM N, TUCCI S, SETH P, FORSLING ML, FILE SE (2003) The soya isoflavone content of rat diet can increase anxiety and stress hormone release in the male rat. *Psychopharmacol* 167: 46–53.

HENDRICH S, MURPHY P (2001) Isoflavones: Source and Metabolism. In: Wildman REC, ed., *Handbook of Nutraceuticals and Functional Foods*, CRC Press LLC, Boca Raton, FL, pp. 55–75.

HERRMAN T (2002) Mycotoxins in feed grains and ingredients. Kansas State University Extension Publication MF-2061 (http://www.oznet.ksu.edu/agronomy-block2/aflatoxin.pdf).

HIROSE K, TAJIMA K, HAMAJIMA N, INOUE M, TAKEZAKI T, KUROISHI T, YOSHIDA M, TOKUDOME S (1995) A large-scale, hospital-based case-control study of risk factors of breast cancer according to menopausal status. *Jpn J Cancer Res* 86: 146–154.

HODGSON JM, PUDDEY IB, BEILIN LJ, MORI TA, CROFT KD (1998) Supplemetation with isoflavonoid phytoestrogens does not alter serum lipid concentrations: a randomized coltrnoled trial in humans. *J Nutr* 128: 728–732.

HONG SJ, KIM SI, KWON SM, LEE JR, CHUNG BC (2002) Comparative study of concentration of isoflavones and lignans in plasma and prostatic tissues of normal control and benign prostatic hyperplasia. *Yonsei Med J* 43: 236–241.

HORN-ROSS PL, HOGGATT KJ, LEE MM (2002) Phytoestrogens and thyroid cancer risk: the San Francisco Bay Area thyroid cancer study. *Cancer Epidemiol Biomarkers Prev* 11: 43–49.

HSIEH CY, SANTELL RC, HASLAM SZ, HELFERICH WG (1998) Estrogenic effects of genistein on the growth of estrogen receptor-positive human breast cancer (MCF-7) cells *in vitro* and *in vivo*. *Cancer Res.* 58: 3833–3838.

HULTÉN K, WINKVIST A, LENNER P, JOHANNSON R, ADLERCREUTZ H, HALLMANS G (2002) An incident case-referent study on plasma enterolactone and breast cancer risk. *Eur J Nutr* 41: 168–176.

IKEDA T, NISHIKAWA A, IMAZAWA T, KIMURA S, HIROSE M (2000) Dramatic synergism between excess soybean intake and iodine deficiency on the development of rat thyroid hyperplasia. *Carcinogenesis* 21: 707–713.

JEFFERSON WN, PADILLA-BANKS E, CLARK G, NEWBOLD RR (2002) Assessing estrogenic activity of phytochemicals using transcriptional activation and immature mouse uterotrophic responses. *J Chromatogr B* 777: 179–189.

JENAB M, THOMPSON LU (1996) Influence of flaxseed and lignans on colon carcinogenesis and glucuronidase activity. *Carcinogenesis* 17: 1343–1348.

JIN Z, MACDONALD R (2002) Soy isoflavones increase latency of spontaneous mammary tumors in mice. *J Nutr* 132: 3186–3190.

JUNGBAUER A, BECK V (2002) Yeast reporter system for rapid determination of estrogenic activity. *J Chromatogr B* 777: 167–178.

JURY HH, ZACAHREWSKI TR, HAMMOND GL (2000) Interactions between human plasma sex hormone binding globulin and xenobiotic ligands. *J Steroid Biochem Molec Biol* 75: 167–176.

KIM MK, CHUNG BC, YU VY, NAM JH, LEE HC, HUH KB, LIM SK (2002) Relationships of urinary phyto-oestrogen excretion to BMD in postmenopausal women. *Clin Endocrinol* 56: 321–328.

KRAZEISEN A, BREITLING R, MöLLER G, ADAMSKI J (2002) Human 17 beta-hydroxysteroid dehydrogenase type 5 is inhibited by dietary flavonoids. *Adv Exp Med Biol* 505: 151–161.

KRITZ-SILVERSTEIN D, VON MüHLEN D, BARRETT-CONNOR E, BRESSEL MAB (2003) Isoflavones and cognitive function in older women: the Soy and Postmenopausal Health In Aging (SOPHIA) Study. *Menopause* 10: 196–202.

KUIPER GGJM, ENMARK E, PELTO-HUIKKO M, NILSSON S, GUSTAFSSON J-Å (1996) Cloning of a novel estrogen receptor expressed in rat prostate and ovary. *Proc Natl Acad Sci* USA 93: 5925–5930.

KUIPER GGJM, CARLSON B, GRANDIEN K, ENMARK E, HäGGBLAD J, NILSSON S, GUSTAFSSON J-Å (1997) Comparison of the ligand binding specificity and transcript tissue distribution of estrogen receptors α and β. *Endocrinol.* 138: 863–870.

KUIPER GGJM, LEMMEN JG, CARLSSON B, CORTON JC, SAFE S, VAN DER SAAG PT, VAN DER BURG B, GUSTAFSSON J-Å (1998) Interaction of estrogenic chemicals and phytoestrogens with estrogen receptor β. *Endocrinol* 139: 4252–4263.

KULLING SE, JACOBS E, PFEIFFER E, METZLER M (1998) Studies on the genotoxicity of the mammalina lignans enterodiol and enterolactone and their metabolic precursors at various endpoints *in vitro*. *Mutat Res* 416: 115–124.

KULLING SE, ROSENBERG B, JACOBS E, METZLER M (1999) The phytoestrogens coumestrol and genistein induce structural chromosomal aberrations in cultured human peripheral blood lymphocytes. *Arch Toxicol* 73: 50–54.

KUMI-DIAKA J, NGUYEN V, BUTLER A (1999) Cytotoxic potential of the phytochemical genistein isoflavone (4',5',7-trihydroxyisoflavone) and certain environmental chemical compounds on testicular cells. *Biol. Cell* 91: 515–523.

KURZER MS (2002) Hormonal effects of soy in premenopausal women and men. *J Nutr* 132: 570s–573s.

KURZER MS, XU X (1997) Dietary phytoestrogens. *Annu Rev Nutr* 17: 353–381.

LAMARTINIERE CA, COTRONEO MS, FRITZ WA, WANG J, MENTOR-MARCEL R, ELGAVISH A (2002) Genistein chemoprevention: timing and mechanisms of action in murine mammary and prostate. *J Nutr* 132: 552S–558S.

LAW CH, TANDAN VR (1999) The association between tamoxifen and the development of hepatocellular carcinoma: case report and literature review. *Can J Surg* 42: 211–214.

LEE HP, GOURLEY L, DUFFY SW, ESTEVE J, LEE J, DAY NE (1991) Dietary effects on breast-cancer risk in Singapore. *Lancet* 331: 1197–1200.

LEPHART ED, WEST TW, WEBER KS *et al.* (2002) Neurobehavioral effects of dietary soy phytoestrogens. *Neurotoxicol Teratol* 24: 5–16.

LEWIS JG, MORRIS JC, CLARK BM, ELDER PA (2002) The effect of isoflavone extract ingestion, as Trinovin, on plasma steroids in normal men. *Steroids* 67: 25–29.

LI B, YU S (2003) Genistein prevents bone resorption diseases by inhibiting bone resorption and stimulating bone formation. *Biol Pharm Bull* 26: 780–786.

LI D, YEE JA, THOMPSON LU, YAN L (1999) Dietary supplementation with secoisolariciresinol diglucoside (SDG) reduces experimental metastasis of melanoma cells in mice. *Cancer Lett* 142: 91–96.

LINFORD NJ, YANG Y, COOK DG, DORSA DM (2001) Neuronal apoptosis resulting from high doses of the isoflavone genistein: role for calcium and p42/44 mitogen-activated protein kinase. *J Pharmacol Exp Therap* 299: 67–75.

LU L-JW, ANDERSON KE, GRADY JJ, KOHEN F, NAGAMANI M (2000) Decreased ovarian hormones during a soya diet: implications for breast cancer prevention. *Cancer Res* 60: 4112–4121.

MADEJ A, PERSSON E, LUNDH T, RIDDERSTRåLE Y (2002) Thyroid gland function in ovariectomized ewes exposed to phytoestrogens. *J Chromatog B* 777: 281–287.

MATTHEWS JB, FERTUCK KC, CELIUS T, HUANG Y-W, FONG CJ, ZACHAREWSKI TR (2002). Ability of structurally diverse natural products and synthetic chemicals to induce gene expression mediated by estrogen receptors from various species. *J Steroid Biochem Mol Biol* 82: 181–194.

MCCANN SE, MOYSICH KB, FREUDENHEIM JL, AMBROSONE CB, SHIELDS PG (2002) The risk of breast cancer associated with dietary lignans differs by CYP17 genotype in women. *J Nutr* 132: 3036–3041.

MEI J, YEUNG SSC, KUNG AWC (2001) High dietary phytoestrogen intake is associated with higher bone mineral density in postmenopausal but not premenopausal women. *J Clin Endocrinol Metab* 86: 5217–5221.

MENDEZ M, ANTHONY MS, ARAB L (2002) Soy-based formulae and infant growth and development: a review. *J Nutr* 132: 2127–2130.

MERZ-DEMLOW BE, DUNCAN AM, WANGEN KE, XU X, CARR TP, PHIPPS WR, KURZER MS (2000) Soy isoflavones improve plasma lipids in normocholesterolemic, premenopausal women. *Am J Clin Nutr* 71: 1462–1469.

MESSINA M, HUGHES C (2003) Efficacy of soyfoods and soybean isoflavone supplements for alleviating menopausal symptoms is positively related to initial hot flush frequency. *J Med Food* 6: 1–11.

MESSINA M (2003) Emerging evidence on the role of soy in reducing prostate cancer risk. *Nutr Rev* 61: 117–131.

MESSINA M, GUGGER ET, ALEKEL DL (2001) Soy protein, soybean isoflavones and bone health: a review of the animal and human data. In: Wildman REC, ed., *Handbook of Nutraceuticals and Functional Foods*, CRC Press LLC, Boca Raton, FL, pp. 77–98.

MILLIGAN SR, KHAN O, NASH M (1998) Competitive binding of xenobiotic oestrogens to rat alpha-fetoprotein and to sex steroid binding proteins in human and rainbow trout (Oncorhyncus mykiss) plasma. *Gen Comp Endocrinol* 112: 89–95.

MITCHELL JH, CAWOOD E, KINNIBURGH D, PROVAN A, COLLINS AR, IRVINE DS (2001) Effect of a phytoestrogen food supplement on reproductive health in normal males. *Clin Sci* 100: 613–618.

MITCHELL JH, DUTHIE SJ, COLLINS AR (2000) Effects of phytoestrogens on growth and DNA integrity in human prostate tumor cell lines: PC-3 and LNCaP. *Nutr Cancer* 38: 223–228.

MIZUNUMA H, KANAZAWA K, OGURA S, OTSUKA S, NAGAI H (2002) Anticarcinogenic effects of isoflavones may be mediated by genistein in mouse mammary tumor virus-induced breast cancer. *Oncology* 62: 78–84.

MORITO K, AOMORI T, HIROSE T *et al.* (2002) Interaction of phytoestrogens with estrogen receptors alpha and beta (II). *Biol Pharm* Bull 25: 48–52.

MUELLER SO (2002) Overview of *in vitro* tools to assess the estrogenic and antiestrogenic activity of phytoestrogens. *J Chromatog B* 777: 155–165.

MUELLER SO, KLING M, ARIFIN FIRZANI P, MECKY A, DURANTI E, SHIELDS-BOTELLA J, DELANSORNE R, BROSCHARD T, KRAMER P-J (2003) Activation of estrogen receptor alpha and ERbeta by 4-methylbenzylidene-camphor in human and rat cells: comparison with phyto- and xenoestrogens. *Toxicol Lett* 142: 89–101.

MURKIES A, DALAIS FS, BRIGANTI EM, BURGER HG, HEALY DL, WAHLQVIST ML, DAVIS SR (2000) Phytoestrogens and breast cancer in postmenopausal women: a case control study. *Menopause* 7: 289–296.

MURPHY P, HENDRICH S (2002) Phytoestrogens in foods. *Adv Food Nutr Res* 44: 195–246.

NAGAHORI H, KOMAI K, TOMIGAHARA Y, SAITO K, ISOBE N, KANEKO H (2001) Initial induction and subsequent reduction of α_{2u}-globulin in urine and serum of mature male rats after repeated intraperitoneal injections of (anti)estrogen. *Toxicol* 162: 73–80.

NAGATA C, INABA S, KAWAKAMI N, KAKIZOE T, SHIMIZU H (2000) Inverse association of soy product intake with serum androgen and estrogen concentrations in Japanese men. *Nutr Cancer* 36: 14–18.

NAGEL SC, VOM SALL FS, WELSHONS WV (1998) The effective free fraction of estradiol and xenoestrogens in human serum measured by whole cell uptake assays: physiology of delivery modifies estrogenic activity. *Proc Soc Exp Biol Med* 217: 300–309.

NOGOWSKI L, NOWAK KW, KACZMAREK P, MACKOWIAK P (2002) The influence of coumestrol, zearalenone, and genistein administration on insulin receptors and insulin secretion in ovariectomized rats. *J Recept Signal Transduct Res* 22: 449–457.

O'CONNOR JC, DAVIS LG, FRAME SR, COOK JC (2000) Evaluation of a Tier I screening battery for detecting endocrine-active compounds (EACs) using the positive controls testosterone, coumestrol, progesterone, and RU486. *Toxicol Sci* 54: 338–354.

PEETERS PH, KEINAN-BOKER L, VAN DER SCHOUW YT, GROBBEE DE (2003) Phytoestrogens and breast cancer risk. Review of the epidemiological evidence. *Breast Cancer Res Treat* 77: 171–183.

PERSKY V, VAN HORN L (1995) Epidemiology of soy and cancer: perspectives and directions. *J Nutr* 125: 709S–712S.

POTTER JD, STEINMETZ K (1996) Vegetables, fruits and phytoestrogens as preventive agents. In: Stewart BW, McGregor D, Kleihues P, eds, *Principles of Chemoprevention*, IARC Scientific Publication No. 139, International Agency for Research on Cancer, Lyon, France, pp. 61–90.

PRASAD K (1999) Reduction of serum cholesterol and hypercholesterolemic atherosclerosis in rabbits by secoisolariciresionol diglucoside isolated from flaxseed. *Circulation* 99: 1355–1362.

RICKARD SE, YUAN YV, CHEN J, THOMPSON LU (1999) Dose effects of flaxseed and its lignan on N-methyl-N-nitrosourea-induced mammary tumorigenesis in rats. *Nutr Cancer* 35: 50–57.

SAARINEN NM, HUOVINEN R, WÄRRI A, MÄKELÄ SI, VALENTIN-BLASINI L, SJÖHOLM R, ÄMMÄLÄ J, LEHTILÄ R, ECKERMAN C, COLLAN YU, SANTTI RS (2002) Enterolactone inhibits the growth of 7, 12-dimethylbenz(a)anthracene-induced mammary carcinomas in the rat. *Mol Cancer Ther* 1: 869–876.

SAFE SH (1998) Interactions between hormones and chemicals in breast cancer. *Ann Rev Pharmacol Toxicol* 38: 121–58.

SCHÖTTNER M, SPITELLER G (1998) Lignans interfering with 5α-dihydroxytestosterone binding to human sex hormone binding globulin. *J Nat Prod* 61: 119–121.

SIRTORI CR, BOSISIIO R, PAZZUCCONI F, BONDIOLI A, LOVATI MR, MURPHY P (2002) Soy milk with a high glycittein content does not reduce low-density lipoprotein cholesterolemia in Type II hypercholesterolemia patients. *Ann Nutr Metab* 46: 88–92.

SONG TT, HENDRICH S, MURPHY PA (1999) Estrogenic activity of glycitein, a soybean isoflavone. *J Agric Food Chem*. 47: 1607–1610.

SONG TT, LEE SO, MURPHY PA, HENDRICH S (2003) Soy protein with or without isoflavones, soy germ and soy germ extract, and daidzein lessen plasma cholesterol levels in Golden Syrian hamsters. *Exp Biol Med* 228: 1063–1068.

STATTIN P, ADLERCREUTZ H, TENKANEN L, JELLUM E, LUMME S, HALLMANS G, HARVEI S, TEPPO L, STUMPF K, LUOSTARINEN T, LEHTINEN M, DILLNER J, HAKAMA M (2002) Circulating enterolactone and prostate cancer risk: a Nordic nested case-control study. *Int J Cancer* 99: 124–129.

STEINBERG FM; GUTHRIE NL; VILLABLANCA AC, KUMAR K, MURRARY MJ (2003) Soy protein with isoflavones has favorable effects on endothelial function that are independent of lipid and antioxidant effects in healthy postmenopausal women. *Am J Clin Nutr* 78: 123–130.

STEPHENS FO (1999) The rising incidence of breast cancer in women and prostate cancer in men. Dietary influences: a possible preventive role for nature's sex hormone modifiers – the phytoestrogens (Review). *Oncol Reports* 6: 865–870.

STROM BL, SCHINNAR R, ZIEGLER EE, BARNHART KT, SAMMEL MD, MACONES GA, STALLINGS VA, DRULIS JM, NELSON SE, HANSON SA (2001) Exposure to soy-based formula in infancy and endocrinological and reproductive outcomes in young adulthood. *J Am Med Assoc* 286: 807–814.

SU SJ, CHOW NH, KUNG ML, HUNG T-C, CHANG K-L (2003) Effects of soy isoflavones on apoptosis induction and G2-M arrest in human hepatoma cells involvement of caspase-3 activation, Bcl-2 and Bcl-XL downregulation, and Cdc2 kinase activity. *Nutr Cancer* 45: 113–123.

SUNG M-K, LAUTENS M, THOMPSON LU (1998) Mammalian lignans inhibit the growth of estrogen-independent human colon tumor cells. *Anticancer Res* 18: 1405–1408.

SZKUDELSKA K, SZKUDELSKI T, NOGOWSKI L (2002) Daidzein, coumestrol and zearalenone affect lipogenesis and lipolysis in rat adipocytes. *Phytomedicine* 9: 338–345.

TEEDE HJ, MCGRATH BP, DESILVA L, CEHUN M, FASSOULAKIS A, NESTEL PJ (2003) Isoflavones reduce arterial stiffness: a placebo-controlled study in men and postmenopausal women. *Arterioscler Thromb Vasc Biol* 23: 1066–1071.

THAM DM, GARDNER CD, HASKELL WL (1998) Potential health benefits of dietary phytoestrogens: a review of the clinical, epidemiological and mechanistic evidence. *J Clin Endocrinol Metab* 83: 2223–2235.

THOMPSON LU, SEIDL MM, RICKARD SE, ORCHESON LJ, FONG HHS (1996a) Antitumorigenic effect of a mammalian lignan precursor from flaxseed. *Nutr Cancer* 26: 159–165.

THOMPSON LU, RICKARD SE, ORCHESON LJ, SEIDL MM (1996b) Flaxseed and its lignan and oil components reduce mammary tumor growth at a late stage of carcinogenesis. *Carcinogenesis* 17: 1373–1376.

THUILLIER R, WANG Y, CULTY M (2003) Prenatal exposure to estrogenic compounds alters the expression pattern of platelet-derived growth factor receptors α and β in neonatal rat testis: identification of gonocytes as targets of estrogen exposure. *Biol Reprod* 68: 867–880.

TSUTSUI T, TAMURA Y, YAGI E, *ET AL.* (2003) Cell-transforming activity and mutagenicity of 5 phytoestrogens in cultured mammalian cells. *Int J Cancer* 105: 312–320.

URBAN D, IRWIN W, KIRK M, MARKIEWICZ MA, MYERS R, SMITH M, WEISS H, GRIZZLE WE, BARNES S (2001) The effect of isolated soy protein on plasma biomarkers in elderly men with elevated serum prostate specific antigen. *J Urol* 165: 294–300.

USDA FOOD COMPOSITION DATA RELEASE 16, http://www.nal.usda.gov/fnic/foodcomp/Data/

USDA-IOWA STATE UNIVERSITY DATABASE ON THE ISOFLAVONE CONTENT OF FOODS, RELEASE 1.3, 2002 http://www.nal.usda.gov/fnic/foodcomp/Data/isoflav/isoflav.html

VERDEAL K, RYAN DS (1979) Naturally-occurring estrogens in plant foodstuffs – a review. *Food Protection* 42: 577–583.

WALCOTT FL, HAUPTMANN M, DUPHORNE CM, PILLOW PC, STROM SS, SIGURDSON AJ (2002) A case-control study of dietary phytoestrogens and testicular cancer risk. *Nutr Cancer* 44: 44–51.

WANG W, KURZER MS (1998) Effects of phytoestrogens on DNA synthesis in MCF-7 cells in the presence of estradiol or growth factors. *Nutr Cancer* 31: 90–100.

WANG W, LIU LC, HIGUSHI CM, CHEN H (1998) Induction of NADPH:quinone reductase by dietary phytoestrogens in coloinc Colo205 cells. *Biochem Pharmacol* 56: 189–195.

WATANABE S, TERASHIMA K, SATO Y, ARAI S, EBOSHIDA A (2000) Effects of isoflavone supplement on healthy women. *BioFactors* 12: 233–241.

WEI H, BOWEN R, CAI Q, BARNES S, WANG Y (1995) Antioxidant and antipromotional effects of the soybean isoflavone genistein. *Proc Soc Exp Biol Med* 208: 124–130.

WELSHONS WV, ROTTINGHAUS GE, NONNEMAN DJ, DOLAN-TIMPE M, ROSS PF (1990) A sensitive bioassay for detection of dietary estrogens in animal feeds. *J Vet Diagn Invest* 2: 268–273.

WHITTEN PL, PATISAUL HB, YOUNG LJ (2002) Neurobehavioral actions of coumestrol and related isoflavonoids in rodents. *Neurotoxicol Teratol* 24: 47–54.

WISEMAN H (2000) The therapeutic potential of phytoestrogens. *Exp Opin Invest Drugs* 9:

1829–1840.

WOBER J, WEIßWANGE I, VOLLMER G (2003) Stimulation of alkaline phosphatase activity in Ishikawa cells induced by various phytoestrogens and synthetic estrogens. *J Steroid Biochem Mol Biol* 83: 227–233.

WU AH, ZIEGLER RG, HORN-ROSS PL, NOMURA AM, WEST DW, KOLONEL LN, ROSENTHAL JF, HOOVER RN, PIKE MC (1996) Tofu and risk of breast cancer in Asian Americans. *Cancer Epidemiol Biomarkers Prev* 5: 901–906.

WU AH, ZIEGLER RG, NOMURA AMY, WEST DW, KOLONEL LN, HORN-ROSS PL, HOOVER RN, PIKE MC (1998) Soy intake and risk of breast cancer in Asians and Asian Americans. *Am J Clin Nutr* 68: 1437S–1443S.

WUTTKE W, JARRY H, BECKER T, SCHULTENS A, CHRISTOFFEL V, GORKOW C, SEIDLOVA-WUTTKE D (2003) Phytoestrogens: endocrine disrupters or replacement for hormone replacement therapy. *Maturitas* 44: S9–S20.

XU X, HARRIS K,WANG H.-J, MURPHY P, HENDRICH S (1995) Bioavailability of soybean isoflavones depends upon gut microflora in women. *J. Nutr.* 125: 2307–2315.

YAMAKOSHI J, PISKULA MK, IZUMI T, TOBE K, SAITO M, KATAOKA S, OBATA A, KIKUCHI M (2000) Isoflavone aglycone-rich extract without soy protein attenuates athersclerosis development in cholesterol-fed rabbits. *J Nutr* 130: 1887–1893.

YAMAMOTO S, SOBUE T, KOBAYASHI M, SASAKI S, TSUGANE S (2003) Soy, isoflavones, and breast cancer risk in Japan. *J Natl Cancer Inst* 95: 906–913.

YELLAYI S, NAAZ A, SZEWCZYKOWSKI MA, SATO T, WOODS JA, CHANG J, SEGRE M, ALLRED CD, HELFERICH WG, COOKE PS (2002) The phytoestrogen genistein induces thymic and immune changes: a human health concern? *Proc Nat Acad Sci* 99: 7616–7621.

YUAN JM, WANG QS, ROSS RK, HENDERSON BE, YU MC (1995) Diet and breast cancer in Shanghai and Tianjin, China. *Br J Cancer* 71: 1353–1358.

ZHANG Y, SONG TT, CUNNICK JE, MURPHY PA, HENDRICH S (1999) Daidzein and genistein glucuronides *in vitro* are weakly estrogenic and activate human natural killer cells in nutritionally relevant concentrations. *J. Nutr.* 129: 399–405.

ZHENG W, DAI Q, CUSTER LJ, SHU X-O, WEN W-Q, JIN F, FRANKE AA (1999) Urinary excretion of isoflavonoids and the risk of breast cancer. *Cancer Epidemiol Biomarkers Prev* 8: 35–40.

ZHOU J-R, MUKHERJEE P, GUGGER ET, TANAKA T, BLACKBURN GL, CLINTON SK (1998) Inhibiton of murine bladder tumorigenesis by soy isoflavones via alteratinos in the cell cycle, apoptosis, and angiogenesis. *Cancer Res* 58: 5231–5238.

19

Polycyclic aromatic hydrocarbons (PAHs)

K. Tamakawa, Sendai City Institute of Public Health, Japan

19.1 Introduction

Polycyclic aromatic hydrocarbons (PAHs) are a group of organic compounds containing two or more fused aromatic rings. These compounds are generally formed by the incomplete combustion of organic materials through natural and anthropogenic processes, such as forest fires, residential heating (oil, coal and wood), vehicle traffic, incinerators, the production of coke, coal tar and asphalt, industrial power generation, cooking, smoking and so on. Because of such widespread sources, PAHs have been detected in air (Tamakawa *et al.*, 1988; Arey *et al.*, 1991; Atkinson *et al.*, 1994; Davis *et al.*, 1987; Gordon *et al.*, 1973; Pfeffer, 1994), water (Lewis, 1975; Davis *et al.*, 1942; Herbes, 1981; Basu *et al.*, 1978), soil (Tamakawa *et al.*, 1985; Tamakawa *et al.*, 1987; Bieri *et al.*, 1986; Jones *et al.*, 1989; Maliszewska-Kordybach, 1996, 2000; Maliszewska-Kordybach and Smreczak, 1988), indoor air (Alfeim and Ramdahl 1984; Daisey *et al.*, 1989; Mukerjee *et al.*, 1997), daily diet and almost everywhere in the environment. Many of these compounds are of concern to public health because of their known and suspected carcinogenicity and/or mutagenicity. PAHs generally occur as complex mixtures of hundreds of isomers, the composition of which varies according to the conditions of their formation.

Most PAHs have no commercial use other than in research. However, some PAHs are used as intermediates during production. Naphthalene (Naph), Anthracene (An) and Phenanthrene (Phe) are important raw materials used in the manufacture of dyes, celluloid, lubricants, fibers, plastics and insecticides. PAHs detected in the environment are, nevertheless, considered as mainly resulting from incomplete combustion rather than from commercial use, because the amounts used for production are small.

Among several routes for human exposure to PAHs, food is estimated to be one of the major pathways. According to Menzie *et al.* (1992), the daily dietary intake of carcinogenic PAHs is estimated to be nearly 3 μg/day. This amount is calculated to be about twenty times more than the exposure level by inhalation (0.13 μg/day) and 500 times more than the dose from drinking water (0.006 μg/day). Butler *et al.* (1993) considered lifetime cancer risks from multimedia exposure to Benzo[*a*]pyrene(B[*a*]P), which is one of the typical carcinogenic PAHs. Potential carcinogenic risks of B[*a*]P were estimated to be 4×10^{-7} in inhalation and 1×10^{-5} in dietary intake. This means that the health risk by daily dietary intake is about 25 times higher than exposure by inhalation.

In the 1970s, Doll (1977) and Wynder and Gori (1977) showed that most human cancer might be attributable to daily diet, and 40 per cent of the cancers in men and 60 per cent in women are potentially preventable. So far, a variety of carcinogens has been detected in foods. Among them, PAHs in the daily diet might be one of the major chemical factors contributing to human cancer, although their level in the environment is quite low. Therefore, it is very important to develop a simple and accurate analytical procedure, and to monitor these PAHs isomers for carcinogenic risk assessment to humans.

In this chapter, physicochemical properties and health effects of PAHs, analytical methods for PAH determination in foods and their occurrence in foods are summarized. In addition, promising analytical methods for PAHs are also critically reviewed.

19.2 Physical and chemical properties of PAHs

The term 'polycyclic aromatic hydrocarbons (PAHs)' is generally used for compounds containing only carbon and hydrogen atoms (i.e. the unsubstituted parent PAH and its alkyl-substituted derivatives). The more general term 'polycyclic aromatic compounds' commonly refers to the PAHs derivatives (e.g. nitro-PAHs (nitroarens) and hydroxy-PAH) and the heterocyclic analogues (aza-, oxa-, and thia-arenes).

PAHs have two or more aromatic rings and two adjacent benzene rings that share two carbon atoms in their chemical structures. Consequently, they have many structural isomers. In the US National Institute of Standards and Technology (NIST) Special Publication 922 'Polycyclic Aromatic Hydrocarbon Structure Index', 660 common (and not so common) PAHs are presented (Sander and Wise, 1997). This electronic version of the Structure Index allows searching via display name(s), chemical structures, Chemical Abstract Service (CAS) Registry numbers, molecular weights, and molecular descriptors.

Thus far, approximately 500 PAHs and their related compounds have been found in the environment. Among these PAHs, comparatively low molecular weight compounds, containing 24 or fewer ring carbons, have been chosen for environmental monitoring owing to their biological effects. In the United States the Environmental Protection Agency has chosen sixteen PAHs as target compounds for environmental monitoring. These PAHs include: Naph, Acenaphthene (Ace), Acenaphtylene (Acn), Fluorene (Fl), Phenanthrene (Phe), An, Fluoranthene (Flu), Pyrene (Py), Benz[a]anthracene (B[*a*]A), Chrysene (Chry), Benzo[*b*]fluoranthene (B[*b*]F), Benzo [k] fluoranthene (B[*k*]F), B[*a*]P, Dibenz[*ah*]anthracene (DB[*ah*]A), Benzo[*ghi*]perylene (B[*ghi*]P), Indeno [1,2,3-*cd*] pyrene (In[*cd*]P). The structural formulae of selected PAHs are shown in Fig. 19.1 including these sixteen PAHs. It is obvious that PAHs generally have planar structures. The chemical and physical properties of selected PAHs are also summarized in Table 19.1. These compounds were selected for inclusion in this chapter because they are suspected to be more harmful than some others and there is a greater possibility that people will be exposed to these compounds than to the others.

At ambient temperature, most PAHs are generally solids. Some have a faint, aromatic odour. As pure chemicals, PAHs exist as a pale or greenish yellow, white or colorless crystal. PAHs generally have high melting and boiling points and low vapor pressures. As PAHs are nonpolar and highly hydrophobic most of them are very soluble in organic solvents, and show low water solubility. These physical properties tend to decrease with the increase of their molecular size, and affect the distribution of PAHs in the environment. For example, in the atmospheric environment, PAHs having comparatively low molecular weight, such as An and Phe, are found almost exclusively in the gas phase. On the other hand, the heavier PAHs having four or more aromatic rings, such as B[*a*]P and B[*ghi*]P, are found almost exclusively in airborne particulates.

PAHs are primarily rather inert. However, in the presence of sunlight, they are easily decomposed to oxygenated PAHs and/or react with nitrogen oxides and nitric acid easily to form nitro-substituted PAHs (nitroarenes). Among them, nitroarenes are noteworthy compounds. Although they are usually present in much smaller quantities than the parent PAHs, most of the nitroarenes are clearly more potent mutagens than PAHs. There are three nitroarenes (1,3-, 1,6-, and 1,8-dinitropyrene) that show exceptionally strong mutagenic activity (over 100,000 revertants/n mol) (Rosenkranz and Howard, 1986; Tokiwa, 1992; Tokiwa and Ohnishi, 1986). These nitroarenes in the environment originate from direct emissions from an incomplete combustion source, especially diesel exhaust, and nitration of PAHs in the atmosphere (Rosenkranz and Howard, 1986: Tokiwa, 1992: Tokiwa and Ohnishi, 1986).

As for foods, Schlemitz *et al.* (1996) found seven nitroarenes in the daily diet, i.e. vegetables, smoked and grilled foods, oils, tea, coffee, and spices. Dafflon *et al.* (2000) detected three nitroarenes (2-nitrofluorene, 1-nitropyrene and 1- and 2-nitronaphthalene) in smoked foods from the market, such as fish and meat products. Ohnishi *et al.* (1986) found 1-nitropyrene in grilled corn, mackerel and (in considerable amounts: up to 43 ng/g) in pork and 'yakitori' (Japanese chicken) grilled with sauce.

Table 19.1 Physical and chemical properties of polycyclic aromatic hydrocarbons*

IUPAC name (abbreviation used)	CAS no.	Chemical formula, Mol.wt.	m.p. (°C)	b.p. (°C)	Water solubility (mg/l)	Octanol–water (Log P)	Vapor pressure (mm Hg)
Acenaphthene (Ace)	83-32-9	$C_{12}H_{10}$ 154.21	93.4	279	3.9 (25°C)	3.92	0.0025 (25°C)
Acenaphtylene (Acn)	208-96-8	$C_{12}H_8$ 152.2	92.5	280	16.1 (25°C)	3.94	0.000912 (25°C)
Anthracene (An)	120-12-7	$C_{14}H_{10}$ 178.24	215	339.9	0.0434 (24°C)	4.45	2.67E-006 (25°C)
Benz[*a*]anthracene (B[*a*]A)	56-55-3	$C_{18}H_{12}$ 228.3	84	437.6	0.0094 (25°C)	5.76	1.9E-006 (25°C)
Benzo[*b*]fluoranthene (B[*b*]F)	205-99-2	$C_{20}H_{12}$ 252.32	168	no data	0.0015	5.78	5E-007 (25°C)
Benzo[*j*]fluoranthene (B[*j*]F)	205-82-3	$C_{20}H_{12}$ 252.32	166	no data	0.0025	6.11	2.62E-008 (25°C)
Benzo[*k*]fluoranthene (B[*k*]F)	207-08-9	$C_{20}H_{12}$ 252.32	217	480	0.0008	6.11	9.65E-010 (25°C)
Benzo[*a*]naphthacene (B[*a*]naph)	226-88-0	$C_{22}H_{14}$ 278.36	no data	no data	0.00194 (25°C)	6.81	3.73E-009 (25°C)
Benzo[*ghi*]perylene (B[*ghi*]P)	191-24-2	$C_{22}H_{12}$ 276.34	278	>500	0.00026	6.63	1E-010 (25°C)
Benzo[*c*]phenanthrene (B[*c*]Phe)	195-19-7	$C_{18}H_{12}$ 228.3	68	no data	0.00345 (25°C)	5.25	6.66E-007 (25°C)
Benzo[*a*]pyrene (B[*a*]P)	50-32-8	$C_{22}H_{12}$ 252.32	176.5	311 (at 1E+01mmHg)	0.00162 (25°C)	6.13	5.49E-009 (25°C)

Benzo[*e*]pyrene (B[*e*]P)	192-97-2	$C_{22}H_{12}$ 252.32	177.5	310-312 (at 1E+01mmHg)	0.0063 (25°C)	6.44	5.7E-009 (25°C)
Chrysene (Chry)	218-01-9	$C_{18}H_{12}$ 228.3	258.2	448	0.002	5.81	6.23E-009 (25°C)
Coronene (Cor)	191-07-1	$C_{24}H_{12}$ 300.36	437.3	525	0.00014 (25°C)	7.64	2.17E-012 (25°C)
Dibenz[*ah*]anthracene (DB[*ah*]A)	53-70-3	$C_{22}H_{14}$ 278.36	269.5	524	0.00249	6.75	1E-010(20°C)
Dibenzo[*ah*]pyrene (DB[*ah*]P) 302.38	189-64-0	$C_{24}H_{12}$	317	no data	3.5E-005 (25°C)	7.28	6.41E-012 (25°C)
Dibenzo[*ai*]pyrene (DB[*ai*]P)	189-55-9	$C_{24}H_{12}$ 300.38	302.38	275 (at 5.00E-02mmHg)	0.000554	7.28	1.78E-011 (25°C)
Fluoranthene (Flu)	206-44-0	$C_{16}H_{10}$ 202.26	107.8	384	0.26 (25°C)	5.16	9.22E-006 (25°C)
Fluorene (Fl)	86-73-7	$C_{13}H_{10}$ 166.22	114.8	295	1.89 (25°C)	4.18	0.00842 (25°C)
Indeno[1,2,3-*cd*]pyrene (In[*cd*]P)	193-39-5	$C_{22}H_{12}$ 276.34	163.6	536	0.0019 (25°C)	6.7	1.25E-010 (25°C)
Naphthalene (Naph)	91-20-3	$C_{10}H_8$ 128.18	80.2	217.9	31 (25°C)	3.3	0.085 (25°C)
Perylene (Per)	198-55-0	$C_{20}H_{12}$ 252.32	252.32	274	0.0004 (25°C)	6.25	5.25E-009 (25°C)
Phenanthrene (Phe)	85-01-8	$C_{14}H_{10}$ 178.24	99.2	340	1.15 (25°C)	4.46	0.000112 (25°C)
Pyrene (Py)	129-00-0	$C_{16}H_{10}$ 202.26	151.2	404	0.135 (25°C)	4.88	4.5E-006 (25°C)

*Interactive PhysProp Database Demo, http://esc.syrres.com/interkow/physdemo.htm

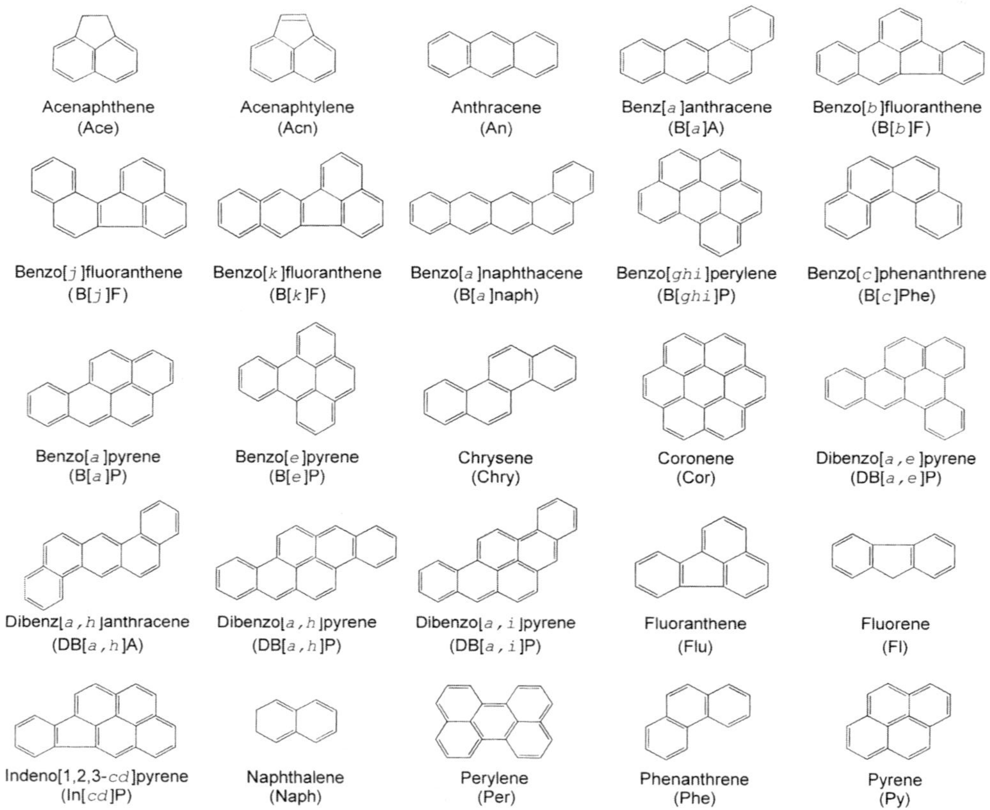

Fig. 19.1 Structural formulae of polycyclic aromatic hydrocarbons.

19.3 Health effects of PAHs

19.3.1 Effects in experimental animals and *in vitro* bioassay

Biological characteristics of the majority of PAHs have not been clarified yet. Among them, B[*a*]P has been most widely studied as a model compound for toxicological effects of the other PAHs.

Concerning acute toxicity, PAHs generally show moderate response. Available data on the acute toxicity of PAHs are few. The values of oral LD_{50} reported are: B[*a*]P over 1600 mg/kg body weight in mice (Awogi and Sato, 1989); Phe, 700,100 mg/kg in mice (Montizaan *et al.*, 1989); Naph, 490–9430 mg/kg in rats (Montizaan *et al.*,1989: US EPA, 1978). Adverse effects such as myelotoxicity, haemolymphatic changes and anemia were observed in the short-term studies of these compounds (Legraverend *et al.*, 1983). A systemic effect caused by long-term testing is substantial carcinogenicity.

Many PAHs are known to be capable of producing tumours in experimental animals. Among these PAHs, B[*a*]P, B[*a*]A and DB[*ah*] have been studied as potent carcinogens in a variety of bioassays for the estimation of carcinogenicity. These carcinogenic compounds generally cause hyperkeratosis in studies of adverse effects after dermal application, while non- or weakly-carcinogenic PAHs, such as An, Py, and Benzo[*e*]pyrene (B[*e*]P), are inactive. After oral administration to rodents by B[*a*]P and several PAHs, tumors are observed in the forestomach, liver, lungs, and mammary glands (IARC, 1983). Although primary tumors may be induced at the site of administration, final target organs seems to be the proliferating tissues, for example in the intestinal epithelia and bone marrow, in which the active metabolite of B[a]P may react in the S-phase of the mitotic cycle.

As concerns transplacental carcinogenicity, B[*a*]P can cross the placenta in mice and rats, inducing pulmonary adenomas and skin papillomas in the progeny (Shendrikova *et al.*, 1974: Takahashi, 1974; Bulay, 1970). Transplacental carcinogenesis has also been reported by Beniashvili (1978). Newborn mice seem to be susceptible to the carcinogenic effects of PAHs (IARC, 1972, 1983; Platt *et al.*, 1990: Busby *et al.*, 1988). Carcinogenic PAHs such as B[*a*]P, B[*a*]A and DB[*ah*]A also show embryotoxic effects in rodents.

As the testes and ovaries contain proliferating cells, their organs might be susceptible to PAH exposure. In pregnant rats, significant increases in the number of resorptions and fetal wastage were observed after B[*a*]P exposure. In these animals, decreases in uterine weights may be due to an antiestrogenic effect of B[*a*]P (Bui *et al.*, 1986). According to Legraverend *et al.* (1984), intraperitoneal administration of B[*a*]P to pregnant mice induced stillbirths, resorptions and malformations.

As PAHs are generally lipophilic, these compounds tend to be stored in fatty tissues, including mammary fat and bone marrow. In the detoxification pathway of PAHs, they are initially oxidized to several arene oxides and phenols by the mixed-function oxidase system, which converts non-polar PAHs into polar hydroxy and epoxy derivatives. These metabolizing systems are widely distributed in animal tissues. Among them, liver is the most active in metabolizing capacity, followed by lung, intestinal mucosa, kidneys and so on. It is noteworthy that B[*a*]P as well as the other PAHs are potent inducers of mixed-function oxidases and potentiate their own toxicity. The induction of isozymes is reported to be mediated by binding to a cytosolic receptor protein, the Ah receptor (Nebert *et al.*, 1993).

B[*a*]P is initially converted to several epoxides such as 7,8-epoxide, and then hydrolyzed to the corresponding stereoisomeric dihydrodiols. These intermediates are further converted to diolepoxides such as 7,8-dihydrodiol-9,10-epoxide. These metabolic intermediates are then conjugated with glutathione, sulphates and mercapturic or glucuronic acids. These conjugates are much more water-soluble than the other hydroxylated intermediates, which enable excretion to occur via the kidney. Formation of conjugates is regarded as a true detoxification reaction.

Microbial mutation tests have been widely used for the estimation of the genotoxicity of chemicals. Among them, the Ames test is a well-known bacterial mutagenicity test (Ames *et al.*, 1975). According to Weisburger, the Ames test has been shown to be over 90% accurate in predicting genotoxicity (Weisburger, 2001). The bacterium used in the Ames test is a strain of *Salmonella typhimurium* that has a mutation in the *his* operon. Test strains of the Ames test can regain their functions by back mutation ($His^- \rightarrow His^+$) after exposure to mutagens. Consequently, revertants in this assay can grow in the absence of exogenous histidine. Moreover, these histidine-requiring strains also have other mutations, such as the *rfa*, *uvbr*, and *R-factor* that increase mutagenic sensitivity. In the Ames test, several strains of bacteria are available. The typical test strains commonly used and their detectable mutation type are as follows: *S. typhimurium* TA98, TA1537 (frame-shift), and *S. typhimurium* TA100, TA1535, and TA102 (base-pair substitution). Mutagenicity of PAHs to *S. typhimurium* TA98 and TA100 with metabolic activation are summarized in Table 19.2. In order to examine the genotoxic profiles of PAHs, a bibliographic database, TOXNET (Toxicology Data Network), by the Environmental Mutagen Information Center (EMIC) is available. It covers environmental mutation literature from 1950. Users can search by subject terms, title words, chemical names, Chemical Abstracts Service Registry Numbers (CAS No.), and authors (EMIC).

PAHs such as B[*a*]P generally show mutagenic response after metabolic activation with S9 mix. The diol-epoxide metabolites of B[*a*]P, including trans-9, 10- epoxy-7,8-dihydrodiol B[*a*]P, are considerably more mutagenic than the parent compounds. These vicinal or so-called 'bay-region' (e.g., stereo-chemically hindered, cup-shaped area between carbons 10 and 11 of benzo[a]pyrene, or 1 and 12 of benz[a]anthracene) diol-epoxides are considered to be the ultimate mutagenic and/or carcinogenic species of alternant PAHs (ATSDR, 1995). In addition to base pair substitutions by these ultimate mutagens, it is thought that bulky adducts of PAH to DNA bases also induce frameshift mutations, deletions, strand breakage, and a variety of chromosomal

Table 19.2 Mutagenicity of polycyclic aromatic hydrocarbons in the Ames test

	TA98/+S9mix	Reference	TA100/+S9mix	Reference
Acenaphthene	—	1	—	1
Acenaphtylene	—	1	—	1
Anthracene	—	2, 3	—	2, 3
Benz[*a*]anthracene	+	2, 4	+	2, 4
Benzo[*b*]fluoranthene	+	4	+	5
Benzo[*j*]fluoranthene	No data	No data	+	5
Benzo[*k*]fluoranthene	+	4	+	5
Benzo[*a*]naphthacene	No data	No data	No data	No data
Benzo[*ghi*]perylene	+	6	+	7, 8
Benzo[*c*]phenanthrene	+	9	+8, 9	
Benzo[*a*]pyrene	+	2, 10	+	2, 10
Benzo[*e*]pyrene	±	234	±	2, 11
Chrysene	+	1, 2	+	2, 4
Coronene	+	1	No data	No data
Dibenz[*ah*]anthracene	+	4	+	2
Dibenzo[*ah*]pyrene	+	12	+	12
Dibenzo[*ai*]pyrene	+	4	+	2
Fluoranthene	+	6, 13	+	13
Fluorene	+	2	+	2
Indeno[1,2,3-*cd*]pyrene	+	14	+	15
Naphthalene	No data	No data	No data	No data
Perylene	+	4, 16	+	16
Phenanthrene	—	1, 2	—	1, 2
Pyrene	—	1, 2	—	1, 2

Reference
1 Florin I, Rutberg L, Curvall M and Enzell C R (1980)
2 McCann J, Choi E, Yamasaki E and Ames B N (1975)
3 Purchase I F H, Longstaff E, Ashby J, Styles J A, Anderson D, Lefevre P A and Westwood F R (1976)
4 Hermann M (1981)
5 Hecht S S, LaVoie E, Amin S, Bedenko V and Hoffmann D (1980)
6 Tokiwa H, Morita K, Takeyoshi H, Takahashi K and Ohnishi Y (1977)
7 Katz M, Heddle J A and Salamone M F (1981)
8 Carver J H, Machado M L and MacGregor J A (1986)
9 Wood A L, Bouchard D C, Brusseau M L and Rao P S C (1990)
10 Simmon V F, Rosenkranz H S, Zeiger E and Poirier L A (1979)
11 Dunkel V C, Zeiger E, Brusick D, McCoy E, McGregor D, Mortelmans K, Rosenkranz H S and Simmon V F (1984)
12 Wood A W, Chang R L, Levin W, Ryan D E, Thomas P E, Lehr R E, Kumar S, Sardella D J, Boger E, Yagi H, Sayer J M, Jerina D M and Conney A H (1981)
13 Bos R P, Theuws J L G, Jongeneelen F J and Henderson P T (1988)
14 Hermann M, Durand J P, Charpentier J M, Chaude O, Hofnung M, Petroff N, Vandecasteele J P and Weill N (1980)
15 Rice J E, Coleman D T, Hosted T J, LaVoie E J, McCaustland D J and Wiley J C (1985)
16 Lofroth G, Toftgard R, Nilsson L, Agurell E and Gustafsson J A (1984)

alterations. Furthermore, B[*a*]P induces forward mutations in cultured mammalian cells (Oberly *et al.*, 1984). Sister chromatid exchange is also induced in Chinese hamster cells after intraperitoneal administration of B[*a*]P (Tong *et al.*, 1983).

As mentioned above, some nitroarenes show exceptionally strong mutagenicity in the Ames test. These compounds are generally 'direct-acting-mutagens', i.e. being mutagenic without S9 mix. The mononitro-PAHs undergo reductive metabolism in bacterial test strains at the nitro group to their corresponding *N*-hydroxylamines, which are generally reactive to DNA molecules.

An overview of the genotoxicity of selected PAHs considered by the International Programme on Chemical Safety (IPCS) is summarized in Table 19.3. Short-term tests used for the evaluation of genotoxicity are as follows:

- reverse mutation test in *Salmonella typhimurimum* (Ames test)
- forward mutation test in *S. typhimurimum* strain TM677
- bacterial tests for DNA damage *in vitro*
- tests for mutagenicity in yeasts and *Drosophila melanogaster,* including host-mediated assays
- various assays carried out on mammalian cells *in vitro*, and various tests *in vivo*.

Among the selected PAHs in the EHC Monograph, only three PAHs, anthracene, fluorene, and naphthalene, were inactive in all short-term tests and sixteen PAHs showed mutagenic responses. The other PAHs could not be clearly classified as mutagenic.

Overall evaluations on the carcinogenicity of selected PAHs are also cited from the IPCS in Table 19.4 (EHC, 1998). This synopsis shows the classification of selected PAHs as carcinogenic, non-carcinogenic, or questionably carcinogenic. The PAHs found to be carcinogenic were as follows: Anthanthrene (Anth), B[*a*]A, B[*b*]F, B[*j*]F, B[*k*]F, B[*a*]P, Chry, cyclopenta[*cd*]pyren (cyclopenta[*cd*]P), DB[*ah*]A, Dibebzo[*ae*]pyrene (D[*ae*]P), Dibebzo[*ah*]pyrene (DB[*ah*]P), Dibebzo[*ai*]pyrene (DB[*ai*]P), Dibebzo[*al*]pyrene (DB[*al*]P), In[*cd*]P, 5-Methylchrysene (5MeChry). In addition, B[*c*]Phe and Flu were suspected of being carcinogenic. Non-carcinogenic PAHs were An, B[*ghi*]P, Fl, Naph, Ace, Acn, Phe, Py, Benzo*[ghi]*fluoranthene (B[*ghi*]Flu), 1-Methylphenanthrene (1-MePhe), Per, and Triphenylene (Triphen). Carcinogenicity of the remaining PAHs was considered questionable.

19.3.2 Effects on humans

The fact that cancer could be due to environmental causes was described for the first time by Sir Percival Pott in 1775 (Pott, 1775). He attributed the scrotal cancers of his patients to their professional exposure (chimney sweeping) to soot and tar. Later, Yamagiwa and Ichikawa succeeded in inducing neoplastic changes experimentally on the ears of rabbits by the long-term application of

Table 19.3 Overview of genotoxicity of polycyclic aromatic hydrocarbons

Compound	Results
Acenaphthene	Inconsistent, limited database
Acenaphthylene	Inconsistent, limited database
Anthanthrene	Positive, limited database
Anthracene	Negative, with a few exceptions
Benz[*a*]anthracene	Positive
Benzo[*b*]fluoranthene	Positive
Benzo[*k*]fluoranthene	Positive
Benzo[*k*]fluoranthene	Positive
Benzo[*ghi*]fluoranthene	Positive, limited database
Benzo[*a*]fluorene	Inconsistent, limited database
Benzo[*b*]fluorene	Inconsistent, limited database
Benzo[*ghi*]perylene	Positive
Benzo[*c*]phenanthrene	Positive, limited database
Benzo[*a*]pyrene	Positive
Benzo[*e*]pyrene	Positive
Chrysene	Positive
Coronene	Positive, limited database
Cyclopenta[*cd*]pyrene	Positive
Dibenz[*ah*]anthracene	Positive
Dibenzo[*ae*]pyrene	Positive
Dibenzo[*ah*]pyrene	Positive, limited database
Dibenzo[*ai*]pyrene	Positive
Dibenzo[*al*]pyrene	Positive, limited database
Fluoranthene	Positive
Fluorene	Negative, with a few exceptions
Indeno[1,2,3-*cd*]pyrene	Positive
5-Methylchrysene	Positive
1-Methylphenanthrene	Positive
Naphthalene	Negative
Perylene	Positive
Phenanthrene	Inconsistent
Pyrene	Inconsistent
Triphenylene	Positive

*Cited from EHC (1998), 'Selected non-heterocyclic aromatic hydrocarbons', *Environmental Health Criteria (EHC) Monographs 202*, WHO, Geneva.

coal tar (Yamagiwa and Ichikawa, 1918). The fact that a pure chemical compound (DB[*ah*]A) might induce cancer in mammals was demonstrated by Kennaway in 1930 (Kennaway, 1930) – in seeking to identify the carcinogenic substance in high-boiling fractions of coal tar distillates. A few years later, Cook and co-workers identified B[*a*]P in the fluorescent fraction of coal tar. In this study, two tons of medium soft pitch were used as a starting material (Cook *et al.*, 1977).

Most of the studies on the effects of PAHs, to human health, concern occupational exposure via inhalation or the skin. Epidemiological studies reported high incidences of tumours of workers exposed to coke oven emissions

Table 19.4 Overview of carcinogenicity of polycyclic aromatic hydrocarbons

Compound	Carcinogenicity (weight of evidence)	Species	Route of administration No. of studies with positive, negative, and questionable results																	
			Oral			Dermal			s.c./i.m.			i.p./i.v.			inh./tr.			Other		
			+	−	±	+	−	±	+	−	±	+	−	±	+	−	±	+	−	±
Acenaphthene	Questionable	Mouse					1	1												
Acenaphthylene			No studies																	
Anthanthrene	Positive	Mouse				2	6			1					1				1	
Anthracene	Negative	Mouse					6	1		1			1							
		Rat	2						1	2				1		1				
		Rabbit																	1	
Benz[*a*]anthracene	Positive	Mouse	2		1	7	4		4	2			2					1		
		Rat		1			1			2			1						1	
		Hamster					2											1		
Benzo[*b*]fluoranthene	Positive	Mouse				7			1			1								
		Rat													1					
		Hamster														1				
Benzo[*j*]fluoranthene	Positive	Mouse				3		1				1								
		Rat													1					
Benzo[*ghi*]fluoranthene	(Negative)	Mouse					2													
Benzo[*k*]fluoranthene	Positive	Mouse				1	2	1	1					1						
		Rat													1					
Benzo[*a*]fluorene	(Questionable)	Mouse					1	1		1										
Benzo[*a*]fluorene	(Questionable)	Mouse						1												
Benzo[*ghi*]perylene	Negative	Mouse					8			2										
		Rat														1				
Benzo[*c*]phenanthrene	(Positive)	Mouse				2		2		1	1									
		Rat									1									

Benzo[*a*]pyrene	Positive	Mouse	5		26			6			3			1			2	
		Rat	2					1			1			9			3	
		Hamster	1		1	1	1							11	1	1		
		Dog															1	
		Cattle							1									
		Pig							2									
		Monkey						1	1	1				1				
Benzo[*e*]pyrene	Questionable	Mouse			2	1	5						1					
		Rat													1			1
Chrysene	Positive	Mouse			11	9	1	3	3	1	1	2	1					
		Rat						1	2					1				
Coronene	(Questionable)	Mouse				1	1											
Cyclopenta[*cd*]pyrene	Positive	Mouse			4		1				1							
		Rat																1
Dibenz[*ah*]anthracene	Positive	Mouse	1	1	6			8			1							
		Rat						2		1				1				1
		Hamster				1								1		1		
		Monkey																1
Dibenzo[*ae*]pyrene	Positive	Mouse			3			2										
		Rat																1
Dibenzo[*ah*]pyrene	Positive	Mouse			6			2			1							
		Rat															1	
Dibenzo[*ai*]pyrene	Positive	Mouse			7			4			1							
		Rat															1	
		Hamster						2						2				
		Monkey																1
Dibenzo[*al*]pyrene	Positive	Mouse			7			1										
		Rat																2

Table 19.4 Continued

Compound	Carcinogenicity (weight of evidence)	Species	Route of administration No. of studies with positive, negative, and questionable results Oral			Dermal			s.c./i.m.			i.p./i.v.			inh./tr.			Other		
			+	−	±	+	−	±	+	−	±	+	−	±	+	−	±	+	−	±
Fluoranthene	(Positive)	Mouse					6			2		3								
Fluorene	Negative	Mouse					3			1			1							
		Rat		2																
Indeno[1,2,3-*cd*]pyrene	Positive	Mouse				2	1	2	1				1							
		Rat													1					
5-Methylchrysene	Positive	Mouse				13			1		1	1	1							
		Rat																	1	
1-Methylphenanthrene	(Negative)	Mouse					1													
Naphthalene	(Questionable)	Mouse					1	2									2		1	
		Rat	1							1	1		1							
Perylene	(Negative)	Mouse					2													
Phenanthrene	(Questionable)	Mouse				1	3	3		3			1							
		Rat														1				
Pyrene	(Questionable)	Mouse				1	7	3		1			1							
		Hamster														1				
Triphenylene	(Negative)	Mouse					2													

+, positive; -, negative; questionable; parentheses, limited number of studies
s.c., subcutaneous; i.m., intramuscular; i.p., intraperitoneal; i.v., intravenous;
inh., inhalation; tr., intratracheal
Other: e.g. intramammary injection, bladder implant, bronchial implant
* Cited from EHC (1998), 'Selected non-heterocyclic aromatic hydrocarbons', *Environmental Health Criteria (EHC) Monographs 202*, WHO, Geneva.

(Lloyd, 1971; Mazumdar *et al.*, 1975), roofing-tar emissions (Hammond *et al.*, 1976), and cigarette smoke (Wynder and Hoffmann, 1967; Maclure and MacMahon, 1980). Coke-oven workers were found to have the highest carcinogenic risk and to have a decreased immune function. In aluminum plants, health effects such as bladder cancer, asthma-like symptoms and chronic bronchitis have been observed.

There is a little information on the influences of oral exposure to PAHs in humans. Thorsteinsson (1967) linked the presence of a comparatively high level of PAHs in Icelandic smoked fish and roast meat with a high prevalence of stomach cancer in Iceland. In a similar study, Emerole reported that some smoked foods, which are contaminated by PAHs, might be a causative factor in the high incidence of stomach cancer in some Nigerian communities (Emerole, 1980). Recently, Lopez-Abente *et al.* have reported the relationship between the oral exposure of PAHs and its human health effects in a rural area in Spain. In this area, wine has traditionally been stored in tar impregnated leather bottles, which may contain PAHs (Lopez-Abente *et al.*, 2001). In the analysis of the multi-centre study, the odds ratio was reported to be increased but the population was too small to allow the observation of statistically significant changes.

Overall evaluations of the carcinogenicity of selected PAHs by IARC and the U.S. Environmental Protection Agency (USEPA) are listed in Table 19.5. The International Agency for Research on Cancer (IARC) classified PAHs into categories according to the evidence of their carcinogenicity. Group 1 is classified as 'confirmed human carcinogen for substances, for which there is sufficient evidence for a causal relationship with cancer in humans'. Potent animal carcinogens, B[*a*]P, B[*a*]A and DB[*ah*]A, are classified as 'Group 2A: probably carcinogenic to humans'. This is for substances for which there is less evidence in humans but sufficient evidence in animal studies. B[*b*]F, B[*k*]F, B[*j*]F and DB[*ah*]A are classified as 'Group 2B: possible human carcinogen'. This is for substances for which there is sufficient evidence in animal tests, or degrees of evidence considered appropriate to this category (Table 19.5) (IARC, 1983, 1987).

In order to assess the carcinogenic potency of complex mixtures, the concept of toxic equivalence has been proposed. This concept is based on an assumption of summed risk for individual PAHs. In the process of calculation, concentrations of carcinogenic PAHs in the mixture are measured as B[*a*]P relative equivalent values. Toxic equivalents (TEQs) are defined as follows:

$$\mathrm{TEQs} = \sum (\mathrm{C_i} \times \mathrm{TEF_i})$$

where C_i: concentration of individual PAHs identified in a complex mixture and TEF_i = relative potencies of PAH_i in comparison with that of B[*a*]P. The toxicity equivalence factors (TEFs) reported are listed in Table 19.5.

The concept of TEFs was initially developed to estimate the potential toxicity of complex mixtures of polychlorinated dibenzo-*p*-dioxins (PCDDs) and dibenzofurans (PCDFs). For PAHs, several attempts have been made to

Table 19.5 Evaluations of carcinogenicity of selected polycyclic aromatic hydrocarbons

IUPAC name	Toxicity equivalency factors (TEFs)					Evaluation of carcinogenicity	
	Nisbet *et al.*	Malcolm *et al.*	Larsen *et al.*	US EPA	McClure *et al.*	IARC[a]	US EPA[b]
Acenaphthene	0.001	0.001		0			
Acenaphtylene	0.001	0.001					D
Anthracene	0.01	0.01	0.0005			3	D
Benz[*a*]anthracene	0.1	0.1	0.005	0.1	0.1	2A	B2
Benzo[*b*]fluoranthene	0.1	0.1	0.1	0.1	0.1	2B	B2
Benzo[*j*]fluoranthene			0.05		0.1	2B	
Benzo[*k*]fluoranthene	0.1	0.1	0.05	0.01	0.1	2B	B2
Benzo[*ghi*]perylene	0.01	0.01				3	D
Benzo[*c*]phenanthrene						3	
Benzo[*a*]pyrene	1.0	1.0	1.0	1.0	1.0	2A	B2
Benzo[*e*]pyrene		0.01				3	
Chrysene	0.01	0.01	0.03	0.001	0.01	3	B2
Coronene		0.001				3	
Dibenz[*ah*]anthracene	5	1.0		1.0	1.0	2A	B2
Dibenzo[*ah*]pyrene					1.0	2B	
Dibenzo[*ai*]pyrene					0.1	2B	
Fluoranthene	0.001	0.001	0.05			3	D
Fluorene	0.001	0.001	0.0005			2B	D
Indeno[1,2,3-cd]pyrene	0.1	0.1		0.1	0.1	2B	B2
Naphthalene	0.001	0.001					
Perylene		0.001				3	
Phenanthrene	0.001	0.001	0.0005			3	D
Pyrene	0.001	0.001	0.001			3	D
Reference	1	2	3	4	5	6, 7	8

Table 19.5 Continued

Reference
1 Nisbet I C T and LaGoy P K (1992)
2 Malcolm H M, Dobson S (1994)
3 Larsen J C, and Larsen P B (1998)
4 USEPA (1993)
5 McClure P and Schoeny R (1995)
6 IARC (1987)
7 IARC (1983)
8 US EPA (1999)

Notes
[a] IARC; International Agency for Research on Cancer, Evaluation: Group 1; carcinogenic to humans. Group 2A; probably carcinogenic to humans, Group 2B; possibly carcinogenic to humans, Group 3; not classifiable as to its carcinogenicity to humans, Group 4; probably not carcinogenic to humans
[b] US EPA; United States, Environmental Protection Agency, Evaluation: Group A; human carcinogen. Group B1; probable human carcinogen – based on limited evidence of carcinogenicity in humans and sufficient evidence of carcinogenicity in animals. Group B2; probable human carcinogen – based on sufficient evidence of carcinogenicity in animals. Group C; possible human carcinogen. Group D; not classifiable as to human carcinogenicity. Group E; evidence of noncarcinogenicity for humans.

estimate the total carcinogenicity from TEFs of individual PAHs (Nisbet and La Goy, 1992; Malcolm and Dobson, 1994; US EPA, 1993; McClure and Schoeny, 1995; Larsen and Larsen, 1998). In the case of oral administration, however, there is a lack of adequate data on the carcinogenic effects of PAHs. Therefore, the oral toxicity of PAHs has been speculated from studies by other routes: skin application, pulmonary instillation, intraperitoneal injection, and so on.

There is another problem in using the TEFs approach in the carcinogenic risk assessment of PAHs. This approach relies on the theory that there is no interaction (synergistic and/or antagonistic) between the components of a complex mixture. However interacting effects have been reported among PAHs. PAHs such as B[*e*]P, B[*ghi*]P, Flu and Py show synergistic effects to B[*a*]P-induced tumor incidence. B[*e*]P, Flu and Py have a weak tumor promoting activity followed by B[*a*]P (ATSDR, 1995). Interactions between some PAHs are also reported to reduce the carcinogenic activity of B[*a*]P in animal experiments (ATSDR, 1995). Schneider *et al.* (2002) indicated that the TEFs approach may underestimate the carcinogenic potencies of PAHs mixtures in most cases.

19.4 Analytical methods for PAHs

As food samples generally contain lipids, it is critical to eliminate interference from these for the determination of PAHs in the first step of the analysis. The concentrations of PAHs in foods are extremely low (ppb, μg/kg) PAH analysis is therefore problematic and requires sophisticated procedures for the purification of samples from the food matrices.

As mentioned in Section 19.2, some PAHs are labile to photo-irradiation. Consequently, it is important to pay attention at all stages to the instability of

PAHs to avoid the photodecomposition of PAHs. Tamakawa *et al.* (1992) showed the decomposition of some PAHs in acetonitrile by photo-irradiation under usual experimental conditions. In the analysis of PAHs, therefore, it is recommended that samples be handled under UV-protected fluorescent lamps at all stages to achieve an accurate analysis (US EPA, 1990).

Comparatively low molecular weight PAHs, containing three or fewer aromatic rings (e.g., An, Flu, and Py), are easily sublimated during the drying-up processes in the preparation of PAHs (Tamakawa *et al.*, 1992). It is also critical to concentrate the extracting solvent carefully so as not to dry it completely. It is recommended that internal standards (surrogates) are added to the samples prior to extraction for quantification by instrumental analysis such as GC-MS (DouAbul *et al.*, 1997; Guillen *et al.*, 2000a, b, c). Dunn and Armour (1980) reported high performance liquid chromatographic (HPLC) determination using tritium-labeled B[*a*]P as an internal standard, to correct the losses of B[*a*]P during the purification procedure. In the recent United Kingdom (UK) Total Diet Study (UK, 2002), the food samples were fortified with ^{13}C-labeled PAHs as internal standards. Contamination should be considered carefully and noted, e.g. smoke from tobacco during and throughout all stages of the experiments.

Many procedures for the multi-residue analysis of PAHs have been developed. Typical methods include gas chromatography (GC) coupled with flame ionization detection (FID) or mass spectrometry (MS), and high performance liquid chromatography coupled with a ultra-violet (UV) detection or fluorescence detection. Recent typical analytical procedures for PAHs in foods are composed of alkaline saponification for extraction, chromatographic clean up and HPLC with fluorescence detection or GC-MS for determination.

19.4.1 Extraction

In this section, the existing analytical methods and procedures for extraction, preparation and clean up of PAHs, and their instrumental determination, are critically examined.

As most food samples contain only small amounts of PAHs, sophisticated procedures are generally required for their quantification. In the first step, the most efficient extraction procedures are usually adopted, so that the samples are as free as possible from analytical interference. Many extraction methods have been proposed and validated. Typical methods for PAH extraction are liquid-liquid extraction, alkaline saponification/solvent extraction and Soxhlet extraction.

Liquid-liquid extraction is applicable to food samples, which contain comparatively low fat content. In the case of analysis of the samples containing a high fat content, e.g. fats, vegetable and mineral oils, it is necessary to eliminate lipids using a further purification process such as liquid-liquid partition, column chromatography and size exclusion chromatography. The characteristics of these preparation and clean up methods for PAHs analysis will be mentioned in Section 19.4.2. Liquid-liquid extraction is useful for simultaneously analyzing both PAHs and the other environmental contaminants such as pesticide residues, polychlorinated dibenzo-*p*-dioxine (PCDDs) and polychlorinated dibenzofurans (PCDFs), which are unstable under other extraction procedures, e.g. alkaline saponification.

Alkaline saponification/solvent extraction is most commonly used for analyzing PAHs in foods. This method is applied to eliminate fat, pigments, and other organic contaminants (Grimmer and Boehnke, 1975; Tatatsuki *et al.*, 1985), which may interfere in subsequent analysis. Alkaline digestion is adopted as an official method in the United States Food and Drug Administration (Joe, 1984) and by the Pharmaceutical Society of Japan (Pharm Soc Jap, 2000).

Tatatsuki *et al.* (1985) reported that direct extraction with acetonitrile was not sufficient for the accurate quantitative extraction of PAHs, because the saponification of the residue from acetonitrile extraction yielded a greater PAH content. In order to extract PAHs from foods quantitatively, alkaline digestion prior to solvent extraction is absolutely necessary (Grimmer and Boehnke, 1975; Tatatsuki *et al.*, 1985).

Some PAHs might be labile under harsh saponification conditions (Tatatsuki *et al.*, 1985; Griest *et al.*, 1983; Potthast, 1977; Potthast and Eigner 1975). B[*a*]P was easily decomposed in the presence of light, oxygen and oxidant, especially under alkaline conditions, by peroxide in aged ethyl ether; and by oxygen when absorbed on silica gel (Dunn and Armour, 1980). To avoid decomposition and to gain good recovery, Tatatsuki *et al.* used Na_2S as an antioxidant during the alkaline digestion (Tatatsuki *et al.*, 1985). The recoveries of PAHs in the digestion mixture with sodium sulphide were comparatively greater (92.8–106.0%) than those without sodium sulphide (86.1–97.2%). The addition of sodium sulphide to alkaline digestion mixture is recommended to ensure quantitative determination of PAHs.

Soxhlet extraction (Winkler *et al.*, 1977; Birkholtz *et al.*, 1988; Voutsa and Samara, 1998; Jarvenpaa *et al.*, 1996) has been commonly used for PAH extraction from environmental samples such as soil, sewage sludge, and airborne particulates. Concerning food analysis, this method has an advantage of enabling the preparation of the extract without emulsification. This method, however, requires from six to twenty-four hours to perform and is too time-consuming. Ultrasonic extraction has much faster extraction time but it is less efficient than Soxhlet extraction.

Caffeine complexation, another extraction procedure, uses a caffeine-PAH complex. Food samples are dissolved into cyclohexane, and mixed with a caffeine-formic acid solution. After the caffeine-PAH complex is destroyed, with sodium chloride solution, PAHs are back-extracted with cyclohexane. Moret *et al.* reported that the caffeine complexation method has advantages in terms of the reduced time of extraction, but the recovery of PAHs was comparatively low (Moret *et al.*, 1996a).

Coates and Elzerman (1986) compared four procedures for extraction of PAHs: sonication, shaking, Soxhlet extraction, and continuous liquid extraction, looking at recovery efficiencies and convenience for routine analysis for plant tissue. Among these methods, sonication was the most reliable.

19.4.2 Preparation and clean up

Clean up of extracts is needed to separate target compounds from interferants, on analysis. Several clean up methods for PAH analysis, such as liquid-liquid partition, thin layer chromatography, column chromatography and a solid-phase extraction (SPE) clean up, have been studied.

Liquid-liquid partition is the most effective way of cleaning up samples with high lipid content, e.g. fats and vegetable oils (Grimmer and Boehnke., 1975; Coates and Elzerman, 1986; Menichini *et al.*, 1991a; Speer *et al.*, 1990). Oil samples are first dissolved into a non-polar solvent, such as cyclohexane or n-hexane. Subsequently, target PAHs are extracted with a polar solvent such as dimethylsulphoxide (DMSO) or a mixture of DMSO/water, while most of the interfering lipids in the samples remain in the organic phase. After the addition of water to change the partition balance between the two solvent phases, PAHs are back-extracted into non-polar solvent. Menichini *et al.* (1991b) performed the liquid-liquid partition of the oil sample dissolved into pentane using dimethyl sulphoxide, followed by preparative silica gel thin layer chromatography (TLC). Speer *et al.* (1990) purified the PAH extracts using silica gel column chromatography followed by a size exclusion chromatography.

For the clean up of PAHs, gel permeation chromatography (GPC) is also applicable. The purification of PAHs from biogenic interferences by GPC were carried out with Sephadex and μStyragel by Grimmer and Boehnke (1975), Winkler *et al.* (1977) and Hanus *et al.* (1979). GPC is ideal for estimating the extent of PAH contamination in tested samples. The application of GPC to highly contaminated marine samples (25–18,000 ng/g) was recommended by Musial and Uthe (1986). Column chromatography has also been commonly applied to further purification of crude extracts. Alumina and silica gel have been commonly used as adsorbents. Silica gel column chromatography is often followed by size exclusion chromatography using Sephadex (Grimmer, 1983; Jacob and Grimmer, 1979). As column chromatography requires a column packing process and large quantities of organic solvent as an eluant, this procedure is generally too time-consuming. Moreover, dealing with a large amount of organic solvent is also a burden in the extraction and evaporation process. As an alternative to column chromatography, a solid-phase extraction (SPE) clean up is quicker.

For routine screening purposes, conventional chromatographic columns have been substituted by commercial SPE cartridges (France *et al.*, 1991; Tamakawa *et al.*, 1986). SPE cartridges have been commonly used for the analysis of PAHs in environmental samples such as water (Cavelier, 1980; Robinson *et al.*, 1987; Mochizuki *et al.*, 1987; Landrum *et al.*, 1987; Xia *et al.*, 1988) and airborne particulates (Obuchi *et al.*, 1984: May and Wise, 1984; Tomkins *et al.*, 1985; Wise *et al.*, 1986; Benner *et al.*, 1989). Tsuji *et al.* (1985) reported a simplified analysis for PAHs in sediment and shellfish using Sep-Pak silica cartridges (Waters Assoc. Ltd.) for purification. They reported that the recoveries of 10 PAHs, i.e., An, Flu, Py, B[*a*]A, Benzo[e]pyrene (B[*e*]P), Per, B[*k*]F, B[*a*]P, DB[*ah*] A, B[*ghi*]P, ranged from 92.3 to 99.6

percent. Tamakawa *et al.* (1986) developed a simplified method for the daily diet using a Sep-Pak silica cartridge. The procedure involves alkaline digestion with is sodium sulphide as an antioxidant, extraction with n-hexane, purification by Sep-Pak silica cartridge, and HPLC quantification with fluorescence detection. Recoveries and coefficients of variation (CV) were respectively: from 90.2% for An and to 102.6% for Py; and from 2.97% for B[*a*]A to 7.56% for B[*a*]P, respectively.

19.4.3 Analytical determination

A variety of methods has been reported for PAH determination. These include:

- a thin layer chromatography (TLC) (IUPAC,1987),
- GC (Coates and Elzerman, 1986; Menichini *et al.*, 1991a, b: Lebo *et al.*, 1991) coupled with the mass spectrometry (DouAbul *et al.*, 1997; Guillen *et al.*, 2000a, b: Coates and Elzerman, 1986; Nakano and Fukushima, 1994; Husain *et al.*, 1997; Nemoto *et al.*, 1998; Naf *et al.*, 1992; Broman *et al.*, 1990; Korenaga *et al.*, 1999), and
- HPLC (Jarvenpaa *et al.*, 1996; Musial and Uthe, 1986) with a fluorescence detector (Cook *et al.*, 1977; Tatatsuki *et al.*, 1985; Perfetti *et al.*, 1992; Kayali-Sayadi *et al.*, 1998; van Stijin *et al.*, 1996; Tamakawa *et al.*, 1987a, b; Nakagawa *et al.*, 1991; Sanders, 1995; Falcon *et al.*, 1999; Moret *et al.*, 1996a; Moret and Conte 1998; Moret *et al.* 1999, 2000, 2001; Simko and Bruncova, 1993; Chiu *et al.*, 1997).

As TLC is an inexpensive and quick analytical technique, this method was commonly used for the analysis of PAHs in the past. However, its separation efficiency is not large enough to carry out the simultaneous determination of many PAHs. Borneff and Kunte (1979) improved this by using two-dimensional TLC.

GC or HPLC have been commonly used for the routine screening of PAHs in foods. HPLC is superior to conventional column chromatography and TLC because of its separation efficiency and reproducibility of analysis. HPLC is generally carried out at ambient temperature and is suitable for the analysis of labile compounds, especially high molecular weight PAHs that may decompose thermally during analysis by GC.

High-resolution GC with capillary column is commonly used for PAH analysis. Typically this is with a flame ionization detector (FID), or photo-ionization detector (PID) or by quadrupole mass spectrometry (QUAD). FID has broad linearity, and is non-selective to chemicals. Therefore, samples for GC/FID should be highly purified. For PAH analysis, GC-MS using electron impact (EI) is commonly used in selected ion monitoring (SIM) mode (Nemoto *et al.*, 1998). As the stationary phases of the separation column, methylpolysiloxanes (SE-52; 5% phenyl-substituted, SE-54; 5% phenyl-, 1% vinyl-substituted) and OV-17 (50% phenyl-substituted), have been widely used for PAH analysis. Fused silica capillary columns, which can separate more than 100 PAHs in complex mixtures, have an excellent resolution (~3000 plates per meter).

As most PAHs have strong fluorescence, HPLC coupled with fluorescence spectrometry is a powerful method for the routine analysis of PAHs, because of its sensitivity and selectivity. The linearity of calibration curves is also satisfactory, ranging from nanograms to the order of micrograms. A wavelength-programmed fluorescence detection system, which changes the excitation and emission wavelength to the optimal values automatically in the time preset during a chromatographic run, has been recently used (van Stijin *et al.*, 1996; Moret *et al.*, 1999; Chiu *et al.*, 1997). A variety of separation columns for HPLC is commercially available. Among them, the octadesyl-bonded column is most frequently used, because of its high-resolution efficiency for the target compounds.

19.5 The occurrence of PAHs in foods

Examples of individual PAHs in foods are summarized in Tables 19.6–19.11. A variety of PAHs is found in substantial quantities in many kinds of food. Among them, B[*a*]P has been most commonly determined in foods. This substance has been used as an indicator for the presence of PAHs since Sandi (Lo and Sandi, 1978) cited it as such in 1954. The occurrence of PAHs in food is influenced by their physical and chemical characteristics. PAHs are lipophilic and have a relatively low aqueous solubility. Therefore, PAHs are not generally accumulated into a plant with high water content. As mentioned above, PAHs with three or fewer aromatic rings are present in the vapor phase, while PAHs with four or more rings are predominantly detected in particulate matter. PAH concentration is generally influenced by the fallout of airborne particulates and is greater on a plant surface than in its internal tissue. In the neighborhood of industrial areas or close to an emission source such as a road, high concentrations of PAHs are detected in soil and plant surfaces. Very high level contamination of PAHs was detected in lettuce grown close to a road in Sweden (Larsson and Sahberg, 1982).

Spinach and lettuce, which are vegetables with large and rough leaf surfaces, are often highly contaminated by PAHs, perhaps due to deposition from the ambient air (Crössmann and Wüstemann, 1992). Differences in contamination levels of PAHs in vegetables may be attributed to variation in the growing season and location. Examples of individual PAHs in vegetables, fruits and cereals are shown in Table 19.6. Vaessen *et al.* studied PAH concentrations in vegetables, cereals and kale in the Netherlands, and found a sample highly contaminated with Flu (117 νg/kg), Py (70 νg/kg), Chry (62 νg /kg), and B[*a*]P (15 νg/kg) (Vaessen *et al.*, 1984). Tateno examined PAHs produced in grilled vegetables, i.e. small sweet pepper, green pepper, pumpkin, eggplant, Welsh onion, onion, corn, sweet potato, potato, *shiitake* mushroom, *shimeji* mushrooms and *matsutake* mushroom (Tateno, 1990) (Table 19.6). Higher amounts of carcinogenic PAHs were detected after grilling than in raw vegetables (Tateno, 1990).

Table 19.6 Polycyclic aromatic hydrocarbon concentrations in foods: vegetables and fruit ($\mu g/kg$)

	Lettuce	Lettuce	Lettuce	Kale	Potatoes	Vegetable (average)	Grilled vegetable (average)	Fresh fruit
	Sweden 1982	Greece 1998	Germany 1994	Netherlands 1984	Netherlands 1990	Japan 1990	Japan 1990	Netherlands 1990
Acenaphthene						0.10	1.4	
Acenaphthylene								
Anthracene	<0.1–0.3					0.11	0.1	
Benz[*a*]anthracene	0.7–4.6			15	0.4	0.05	0.2	0.5
Benzo[*b*]fluoranthene	0.5–7.3		6.1		0.2			0.1
Benzo[*k*]fluoranthene			3.7		0.1	0.02	0.1	0.1
Benzo[*ghi*]perylene	0.5–10.8		10.0	7.7	0.1			0.9
Benzo[*a*]pyrene	0.3–6.2	0.08–0.75	5.6	4.2		0.09	0.3	
Chrysene				62	0.8			0.5
Dibenz[*ah*]anthracene				1		nd	nr	
Fluoranthene	2.8–9.1		28.0	117		1.26	1.1	3.6
Fluorene						nd	nd	
Indeno[1,2,3-*cd*]pyrene	0.3-8.3		2.4	7.9				
Naphthalene								
Phenanthrene	1.8–7.5					2.22	4.5	7.8
Pyrene	3.4–10.4			70		0.28	1.0	
Reference[1]	1	2	3	4	5	6	6	5

Notes:
nd: not detected; nr: not reported
[1] For list of references, see page 501.

Table 19.7 Polycyclic aromatic hydrocarbon concentrations in foods: cereals (μg/kg)

	Wheat Canada 1984	Whole grain oats Canada 1984	Barley malt Canada 1984	Oats Finland 1988	White flour United Kingdom 1996	Breakfast cereal United Kingdom 1996	Bread United Kingdom 1990	High bran and granary bread United Kingdom 1987
Acenaphthene				0.7	nr	nr		
Acenaphthylene								
Anthracene				1.3	nr	nr	<0.3	nr
Benz[*a*]anthracene	0.3–0.8	0.4	0.1–4.2	<0.1/0.2	0.04–0.19	0.06–0.15	0.2	0.11–0.21
Benzo[*b*]fluoranthene	0.1/0.2		0.1–0.5		0.02–0.06	0.02–0.05	0/2	0.07–0.09
Benzo[*k*]fluoranthene					0.03–0.08	0.02–0.07	0.1	0.1–0.14
Benzo[*ghi*]perylene					0.06–0.19	0.06–0.08	<0.7	0.13–0.20
Benzo[*a*]pyrene	0.1		nd–0.3	0.3/0.4	0.02–0.09	0.03–0.05	0.1	0.10–0.12
Chrysene					nr	nr	<0.4	
Dibenz[*ah*]anthracene	3.0		nd–1.2		<0.01–0.01	<0.01		0.01–0.02
Fluoranthene	1.5–7.4	2.9	0.8–26	1.5/13	0.07–0.40	0.22–0.60	1.0	0.58–0.69
Fluorene				2.3/2.7	nr	nr		nr
Indeno[1,2,3-*cd*]pyrene	3.0		nd–0.4		0.06–0.24	0.08–0.15		0.24–0.33
Naphthalene								nr
Phenanthrene						nr	<2.0	
Pyrene	2.6–8.5	2.8	1.1–48	1.6/5.4	0.04–0.88	0.26–1.18		0.38–0.62
Reference[1]	7	7	7	8	9	9	10	11

Notes:
nd: not detected; nr: not reported
[1] For list of references, see page 501.

Table 19.8 Polycyclic aromatic hydrocarbon concentrations in foods: fish and marine products ($\mu g/kg$)

	Fish	Fish	Fish	Fish (smoked)	Fish (unsmoked)	Fish (smoked)	Sea mussels (canned)	Oysters (fresh and canned)
	Netherlands	United Kingdom	Yemen	United Kingdom	United Kingdom	Germany	Germany	Germany
	1997	1983	1997	1982	1982	1996	1990	1990
Acenaphthene			1.1, 1.2					
Acenaphthylene			1.0, 1.0					
Anthracene	0.9		0.7, 0.8			21.0	nd–1.9	nd–0.6
Benz[*a*]anthracene	1.3	0.14	0.3, 0.4	nd–86	tr–0.09	2.5	0.8–5.7	0.8–3.0
Benzo[*b*]fluoranthene	2	0.13	0.3, 0.5			1.2		
Benzo[*k*]fluoranthene	0.7	0.04	0.3, 0.5			0.5		
Benzo[*ghi*]perylene	0.9	0.12	0.2, 0.5	nd–25	tr–0.39	0.7	0.3–1.5	0.3–0.8
Benzo[*a*]pyrene	1.4	0.13	0.7, 0.9	nd–18	tr–0.35	1.2	0.3–1.7	0.2–1.0
Chrysene	2.9	0.65	1.6, 1.9			2.5		
Dibenz[*ah*]anthracene		0.03	0.1, 0.1			<0.1		
Fluoranthene	1.8	0.1	1.5, 1.5			26.0	4.5–13.5	5.1–17.5
Fluorene			5.0, 5.5					
Indeno[1,2,3-*cd*]pyrene	1.6		0.1, 0.1	nd–37	nd–0.33	1.1	0.2–1.2	0.3–0.6
Naphthalene			19.6, 20.4					
Phenanthrene	3.5		13.0, 14.0			65.3	1.9–19.6	2.1–5.1
Pyrene		0.79	1.7, 1.8			20.5	3.2–11.2	2.6–12.4
Reference[1]	12	9	13	14	14	15	16	16

Notes:
nd: not detected; tr: trace
[1] For list of references, see page 501.

Table 19.9 Polycyclic aromatic hydrocarbon concentrations in foods: meat and dairy products (μg/kg)

	Smoked sausage United States 1984	Smoked beef Netherlands 1990	Meat and meat product Netherlands 1990	Chichen liver Kuwait 1997	Milk (raw) Japan 1999	Milk (long-life) Japan 1999	Sheep milk Kuwait 1997	Chicken egg Kuwait 1997
Acenaphthene								
Acenaphthylene								
Anthracene			0.9	100	0.01	0.0	nd	29.73
Benz[*a*]anthracene	–0.5	0.02–0.64	0.5	3.63		0.0	3.0	4.46
Benzo[*b*]fluoranthene	0.1–0.2		1	6			2.1	3.49
Benzo[*k*]fluoranthene			0.2	2			nd	4.53
Benzo[*ghi*]perylene		0.03–0.31	0.6	nd			nd	1.25
Benzo[*a*]pyrene	–0.1	0.02–0.45	0.6	3.25	0.01	0.0	1.6	7.49
Chrysene			0.6	6.36			21.5	5.57
Dibenz[*ah*]anthracene				nd			nd	4.75
Fluoranthene	0.2–0.7		1.1	10.5	0.15	0.2	14.2	1.19
Fluorene					0.07	0.0		
Indeno[1,2,3-*cd*]pyrene		0.04–0.38	0.7	nd			nd	8.73
Naphthalene								
Phenanthrene	–1.7			47.43	0.06	0.3	10.0	18.53
Pyrene	0.3–0.9			14.5	0.37	0.1	139.3	5.55
Reference[1]	17	18	18	12	19	19	12	12

nd: not detected
[1] For list of references, see page 501.

Table 19.10 Polycyclic aromatic hydrocarbon concentrations in foods: vegetable oils ($\mu g/kg$)

	Vegetable oils (olive, safflower, wheat germ, etc.) Germany 1990	Virgin olive oils Italy 1991	Olive oils Italy 1991	Extra virgin olive oil (ppb) Italy 1997	Olive oil (refined + virgin) (ppb) Italy 1997	Margarine United Kingdom 1991	Chocolate United Kingdom 1991	Sunflower Germany 1988
Acenaphthene								
Acenaphthylene								
Anthracene	nd–4.8	5–8	nd–4	tr–3.01	<0.01–0.46			0.3
Benz[*a*]anthracene	nd–6.1			tr–10.30	0.355–0.565	0.22–3.98	0.28–0.70	0.9
Benzo[*b*]fluoranthene				tr–1.330	0.618–1.398	0.16–3.0	0.11–0.22	
Benzo[*k*]fluoranthene				tr–0.476	0.229–0.458	0.20–3.40	0.10–0.25	
Benzo[*ghi*]perylene	nd–4.2			tr–0.735	0.648–1.853	0.38–5.21	0.23–1.32	0.5
Benzo[*a*]pyrene	nd–4.1			tr–1.210	0.460–1.335	0.19–6.0	0.13–0.32	0.7
Chrysene				tr–9.35	0.66–1.47	0.26–7.36	0.39-1.55	
Dibenz[*ah*]anthracene				tr–0.258	<0.01–0.104	0.05–1.02	<0.01–0.03	
Fluoranthene	0.2–16.1	7–12	3–15	tr–52.70	<0.01–4.38	0.09–4.50	2.18–3.02	3.1
Fluorene		3–7	nd	0.56–4.57	<0.01–0.57			
Indeno[1,2,3-*cd*]pyrene	nd–4.3			tr–0.63	0.288–1.960	0.49–9.14	0.18–0.45	0.4
Naphthalene				tr–22.4	<0.01–6.4			
Phenanthrene	nd–69.4	25–42	4–41	1.7–35.0	0.4–6.7			3.8
Pyrene	0.1–13.6	7–11	2–14	0.4–27.9	<0.01–4.2	0.29–6.03	2.20–4.98	2.6
Reference[1]	16	20	20	21	21	22	22	23

Notes:
nd: not detected; tr: trace
[1] For list of references, see page 501.

Table 19.11 Polycyclic aromatic hydrocarbon concentrations in foods: others (μg/kg)

	Smoke flavoring	Smoke flavoring	Smoke flavoring	Whisky	Soup	Seasoning (soybean paste)	Tea infusion (μg/l)	Soy sauce (ppb)
	Spain	Spain	Spain	United Kingdom	Netherlands	Japan	Spain	Japan
	2000	2000	2000	1991	1990	2000	1998	2000
Acenaphthene						nd–2.22		nd
Acenaphthylene								
Anthracene	0.41–1.75	113.7	8.81–118.36			nd–0.08		nd–0.10
Benz[*a*]anthracene	0.05–0.24	4.1	0.07–4.41	0.01–0.02		nd–0.06	0.0028–0.0434	nd–0.03
Benzo[*b*]fluoranthene	0.07	1.6	0.60–1.48	<0.01	0.05			
Benzo[*k*]fluoranthene	0.05–0.07	1.7	0.78–1.72	<0.01–0.01	0.08	nd–0.04		nd–0.01
Benzo[*ghi*]perylene	0.02–0.08	1.9	0.63–1.94	<0.01–0.02			0.0056–0.0273	
Benzo[*a*]pyrene	0.04–0.06	2.8	0.27–0.62	<0.01		0.01–0.08	0.0021–0.0238	nd–0.68
Chrysene		3.3		0.02–0.03	0.4			
Dibenz[*ah*]anthracene				<0.01–0.01			0.0023–0.0237	nd–0.03
Fluoranthene	0.15–0.60	43.4	0.20–43.26	0.03–0.19		0.06–0.44	0.0042–0.0301	nd–2.09
Fluorene	0.72–15.07	336.9	0.62–380.45			nd		nd–0.49
Indeno[1,2,3-*cd*]pyrene		1.6	0.38–1.57	<0.08				
Naphthalene	5.21–172.77	678.8	9.74–677.55					
Phenanthrene	0.58–6.07	627	0.94–664.92			nd–0.98	0.119–0.658	nd-3.79
Pyrene	0.17–0.62	33.5	0.16–33.50	0.02–0.24		nd–3.32	0.0184-0.168	nd-0.28
Reference[1]	26	25	24	27	5	28	29	28

Notes:
nd: not detected
[1] For list of references, see page 501.

References to Tables 19.6–19.11
1 Larsson B and Sahberg G (1982)
2 Voutsa D and Samara C (1998)
3 Germany, Ministry of Environment (1994)
4 Vaessen H A M G, Schuller P L, Jekel A A and Wilbers A A M M (1984)
5 de Vos R H, van Dokkum W, Schouten A and de Jong-Berkhout P (1990)
6 Tateno T (1990)
7 Lawrence J F and Weber D F (1984)
8 Tuominen J P, Pyysao H S and Sauri M (1988)
9 Dennis M J, Massey R C, McWeeny D J, Knowles M E and Whatson D (1983)
10 de Vos R H, van Dokkum W, Scouten A and de Jong-Berkhout P (1990)
11 FAO/WHO (1987)
12 Husain A, Naeemi E, Dashti B, Ai-Omirah H and Al-Zenki S (1997)
13 DouAbul Ali A-Z, Heba Hassan M A and Fareed K H (1997)
14 McGill A S, Mackie P R, Parsons E, Bruce C and Hardy R (1982)
15 Karl, H., and Leinemann M (1996)
16 Speer K, Steeg E, Horstmann P, Kuhn Th and Montag A (1990)
17 Joe F L Jr, Salemme J and Fazio T (1984)
18 de Vos R H, van Dokkum W, Schouten A and de Jong-Berkhout P (1990)
19 Tateno T and Kageyama Y (1999)
20 Menichini E, Bocca A, Merli F, Ianni D and Monfredini F (1991a)
21 Moret S, Piani B and Bortolomeazzi R (1997)
22 Dennis MJ, Massey RC, Cripps G, Venn I, Howarth N and Lee G (1991)
23 Speer K and Montag A (1988)
24 Guillen M D, Sopelana P and Partearroyo M A (2000a)
25 Guillen M D, Sopelana P and Partearroyo M A (2000b)
26 Guillen M D, Sopelana P and Partearroyo M A (2000c)
27 Dennis MJ, Massey RC, Cripps G, Venn I, Howarth N and Lee G (1991)
28 Tateno T (2000)
29 Kayali-Sayadi M N, Rubio-Barroso S, Cuesta-Jimenez M Pand Polo-Diez L M (1998)

Data on individual PAHs in fish, meat and dairy products are also shown in Table 19.6. A high concentration was observed in sheep milk studied in Kuwait (Husain *et al.*,1997). Comparatively high-level contamination of PAHs was detected in smoked cheese (Lintas *et al.*,1979; McGill *et al.*, 1982). According to Lintas *et al.*, B[*a*]P was detected at 1.3 μg/kg in a smoked Italian Provola cheese (Lintas *et al.*, 1979).

Cooking (such as grilling, roasting and frying) and processing (such as smoking and drying) are major sources of PAH contamination in foods. Doremire *et al.* (1979) detected the highest concentration of B[*a*]P (130 νg /kg) in cooked fatty beef. The greatest amounts of carcinogenic PAH were observed after the smoking of duck breast samples (53 νg/kg) (Chen and Liu, 1997). Concerning charcoal grilling, PAH formation was dependent on the fat content of the meat, the time of cooking and the temperature. For example, Mottier *et al.* showed high concentrations of carcinogenic PAHs (14 νg/kg) in heavily barbecued lamb sausage (Mottier *et al.*, 2000).

Vegetable oils and fats are another major source of PAHs in the diet. The levels of PAHs found in vegetable oils are listed in Table 19.6. Moret *et al.* reported the levels of 14 PAHs in 51 olive oil samples (Moret *et al.*, 1997a, b). Data show that the amount of B[*a*]P and total PAHs in olive oils ranges from trace to 1.210 μg/kg and from 2.946 μg/kg to 143.124 μg/kg, respectively. They are usually used as seasoning and margarine for cooking such as in biscuits and cakes (Dennis *et al.*, 1991). As vegetable oils are reported to be naturally free of

PAHs, their contamination of vegetable oils is mainly attributed to the drying processes of oilseeds by using combustion gases (Speer *et al.*, 1990). The refining process reduces the amount of these contaminants. High molecular PAHs are mainly removed by charcoal treatment, while 'light' PAHs (up to four aromatic rings) are generally reduced by the deodorization process (Larsson *et al.*, 1987).

Some smoke flavorings showed extremely high levels of PAHs (see Table 19.6). Guillen *et al.* (2000a, b, c) detected 34 PAHs in commercial liquid flavorings, used in the European food industry. Concerning the generation of liquid smoke flavorings, Guillen *et al.* showed that poplar wood generated a large amount of PAHs rather than oak, cherry tree and beech samples (Guillen *et al.*, 2000a).

As regards the main source of B[*a*]P in dietary intake, Dennis *et al.* estimated that 80% of B[*a*]P came from either cereal (30%) or oils and fats (50%) in the United Kingdom (Dennis *et al.*, 1983, 1991). Although cereals did not contain a high concentration of PAHs, they made a significant contribution to the dietary intake of PAHs by weight according to the total diet. They also showed that margarine was the major dietary source of PAHs in the oils and fats total diet group (Dennis *et al.*, 1991). These statistics were substantially confirmed by De Vos *et al.* in a Dutch survey (de Vos *et al.*, 1990). The major contributors to the daily intake of B[*a*]P were as follows: 'oils and fats' (47%), 'cereal products' (36%), 'sugar and sweets'(14%). In Sweden, the major contributors of PAHs to the total dietary intake seemed to be cereals (about 34%), followed by vegetables (about 18%) and oils and fats (about 16%) (Larsson *et al.*, 1987). Although smoked meat and fish had a high level of contamination of PAHs, they made very small contributions to the total dietary intakes, because they are minor components of the usual Swedish diet (Larsson *et al.*, 1987). Recently, the United Kingdom Food Standard Agency reported 'PAHs in the UK diet: 2000 Total Diet Study Samples (FSIS No. 31/02)'. Daily intakes of B[*a*]P and B[*a*]A were estimated to be two to five-fold lower in 2000 compared with 1979 for average and high-level intakes (UK, 2002). Average and high-level daily dietary intakes of B[*a*]P had fallen to 1.6 and 2.7 ng/kg bodyweight/day, respectively.

In order to assess the carcinogenic risk of PAHs to humans, it is necessary to estimate their daily dietary intake. Table 19.12 shows a comparison of daily intakes of PAHs from different studies. Tamakawa *et al.* reported that daily dietary intake of B[*a*]P for 117 meal samples was 0.0017–1.6 μg/day [geometric mean: 0.032 μg/day] by the duplicate portion method (Tamakawa *et al.*, 1992). Using the same method, Shiraishi and Shiratori estimated the daily intake of B[*a*]P in dormitory students (Shiraishi and Shiratori, 1981). The mean value was estimated to be 0.06 μg/day, ranging from 0.025 to 0.131 μg/day. Obana *et al.* reported similar data for the daily intake of B[*a*]P (0.05 μg/day) via the market basket method (Obana *et al.*, 1984). Dennis *et al.* reported that the total dietary intake of Py, which was the most abundant of PAHs investigated, was estimated to be 1.1 μg/day, followed by 0.99 μg/day for Flu, 0.50 μg/day for Chry, 0.25 μg/day for B[*a*]P, 0.22 μg/day for B[*a*]A, 0.21 μg/day for B[*ghi*]P, 0.18 μg/day for

Table 19.12 Daily dietary intake of polycyclic aromatic hydrocarbons (μg/day)

	Daily dietary intakes Austria 1991	Daily dietary intakes[b] Netherlands 1990	Daily dietary intakes[a] Netherlands 1988	Daily dietary intakes[b] United Kingdom 1983	Daily dietary intakes[a] Japan 1991	Daily dietary intakes[a] Japan 1987	Daily dietary intakes[a] Japan 1992	Daily dietary intakes[b] Japan 1984
Acenaphthylene								
Acenaphthene								
Anthracene	<0.03–5.6					0.23	0.34	0.148
Benz[*a*]anthracene	<0.02–0.14	0.20–0.36[c]	0.16	0.21				0.061
Benzo[*b*]fluoranthene	<0.05–1.02	0.31–0.36[c]		0.18		0.23	0.17	0.103
Benzo[*k*]fluoranthene	<0.02–0.30	0.10–0.14[c]		0.06	0.029–0.085	0.041	0.065	0.039
Benzo[*ghi*]perylene	<0.01–7.6	0.20–0.36[c]	0.16	0.21	0.039–0.108	0.088	0.100	0.070
Benzo[*a*]pyrene	<0.01–0.36	0.12–0.29[c]	0.08	0.25	0.045–0.109	0.084	0.064	0.050
Chrysene	<0.03–0.90	0.86–1.53[c]	1.2	0.50				
Dibenz[*ah*]anthracene	<0.01–0.10			0.03				
Fluoranthene	<0.04–4.30	0.99–1.66[c]	2.7	0.99				
Fluorene								
Indeno[1,2,3-*cd*]pyrene	<0.02–0.31	0.08–0.46[c]	0.16					
Naphthalene								
Phenanthrene	<0.33–2.0							
Pyrene	<0.02–3.97		1.1			0.98	1.00	0.620
Reference	1	2	3	4	5	6	7	8

[a] Duplicate portion method; [b] Market basket method; [c] Lower- and upper-bound values.

References

1 Pfannhauser W (1991)
2 de Vos R H, van Dokkum W, Schouten A and de Jong-Berkhout P (1990)
3 Vaessen H A M G, Jekel A A and Wilbers A A M M (1983)
4 Dennis M J, Massey R C, McWeeny D J, Knowles M E and Whatson D (1983)
5 Nakagawa T, Seshimo A, Yamamoto C, Sato Y and Kawamura T (1991)
6 Tamakawa K, Katoh Y, Ohgane Y, Mishima Y, Seki T and Tsunoda A (1987)
7 Tamakawa K, Seki T and Tsunoda A (1992)
8 Obana H, Hori S, Tanaka R and Kashimoto T (1984)

B[*b*]F, 0.17 μg/day for B[*e*]P, 0.06 μg/day for B[*k*]F, and 0.03 μg/day for DB[*a,h*]A (Dennis *et al.*, 1983). De Vos *et al.* showed that PAH intake was 0.12–0.29 μg/day by testing 221 different food items in a market basket survey of PAHs in the Netherlands (de Vos *et al.*, 1990). In a US survey, the mean level of PAH intakes was estimated to be 1.6–16.0 μg/day with the intake of carcinogenic PAHs 1–5 μg/day (Santodonato *et al.*, 1981). As shown in Table 19.7, the values of daily intake for B[*a*]P range from ~0.01-0.29 μg/day. Despite the differences in protocols for surveys and in dietary habits, it can be seen that the PAH intake estimates are remarkably similar.

19.6 Future trends

A variety of promising methods has recently been developed for PAH analysis in foods. Supercritical fluid extraction (SFE) has gained attention as a rapid alternative to conventional methods in offering shorter extraction times with higher efficiency and lower consumption of organic solvents. Liquid carbon dioxide is commonly used for extraction, because of its mild physical properties which make it suitable as an extraction fluid in SFE. France *et al.* used this method for the determination of pesticides in animal tissues (France *et al.*, 1991). Moreover, Jarvenpaa *et al.* applied SFE for the extraction of PAHs from smoked and broiled fish (Jarvenpaa *et al.*, 1996). In this case, the overall extraction procedure was reported to be completed in 20 minutes.

Accelerated solvent extraction (ASE) is another promising method for extracting from solid samples. ASE is carried out by using a conventional organic solvent at elevated temperatures and pressures to enhance extraction efficiency under closed conditions. Wang *et al.* compared the recoveries of sixteen PAHs between ASE and Soxhlet extraction (Wang *et al.*, 1999). They showed the advantages of the ASE method in the extraction of PAHs from fish and smoked meat samples in terms of reducing the amount of solvent consumed (20–30 mL/aliquot) and the time for extraction (10–20 min).

Application of semi-permeable membranes to the extraction of PAHs from lipid samples was demonstrated by Strandberg *et al.* (1998). Depending on the species and the amount of lipid, 90 percent of lipids can be reduced.

Capillary electrophoresis (CE) is also promising for the quantification of environmental pollutants (Takeda, 2001), because of its high sensitivity and selectivity. Two modes have been proposed in the CE method. One is the capillary zone electrophoresis (CZE), and the other is electrokinetic chromatography (EKC). As EKC is generally superior to CZE in the separation efficiency of electrically neutral analytes, EKC has more advantages for the analysis of environmental pollutants.

As mentioned above, purification procedures have been greatly simplified by using SPE cartridges instead of packed columns. This preparation, however, is still time-consuming. For routine screening purposes, an on-line purification system is promising. Grob (1991), Vreuls *et al.* (1991) and Moret *et al.* (1996b, c,

1997a, b, 2001) developed an on-line LC-GC and LC-LC-GC analytical system for PAHs in fats and oils. The system is composed of coupled normal phase-reversed phase HPLC. The main difficulty in this system is an exchange of the mobile phase between different solvent systems, which are not miscible. Moret *et al.* developed an exclusive interface with two additional 10-port valves. Good recoveries (above 80 percent), repeatability (CV%: 2.4–5.7 percent) and linearity characteristics were obtained (Moret *et al.*, 2001). According to the author, a complete analysis can be performed in less than 30 minutes using this system. So-called hyphenated techniques such as LC-LC and LC-LC-GC seem to be ideal for the routine screening purpose (Moret *et al.*, 2001). Moreover, these on-line systems may open new possibilities as automated analytical systems.

For sensitive detection, LC/MS is a promising technique. Galceran *et al.* (1996) and Stavric *et al.* (1997) applied this method to the analysis of mutagenic heterocyclic aromatic amines in beef and processed food flavor samples, respectively.

Gas chromatography time-of-flight mass spectrometry (GC-TOF-MS) is also reported to be a very powerful method with the limits of detection in the low picogram range for PAHs (0.3–6 pg). This is another promising technique for the sensitive determination of organic micro-contaminants in the environment (Rene *et al.*, 1999).

19.7 Sources of further information and advice

Further information on PAHs is available at the websites of the US National Institute of Standards and Technology (NIST), the International Programme on Chemical Safety (IPCS) and the US Agency for Toxic Substances and Disease Registry (ATSDR). Their addresses and the outlines of each file are as follows.

- Lane C. Sander and Stephen A. Wise. NIST Special Publication 922, Polycyclic Aromatic Hydrocarbon Structure Index. http://ois.nist.gov/pah/

NIST Special Publication 922 'Polycyclic Aromatic Hydrocarbon Structure Index' is presented by the NIST as an aid in the identification of the chemical structures and nomenclature of 660 PAHs. This file allows you to display name(s), chemical structures, CAS numbers, molecular weights, and so on.

- Environmental Health Criteria (EHC) Monographs 202: Selected non-heterocyclic aromatic hydrocarbons, WHO, Geneva, 1998, available at http://www.inchem.org/documents/ehc/ehc/ehc202.htm

Environmental Health Criteria (EHC) series are issued by the IPCS. These series are based on a comprehensive search of available original publications, scientific literature and reviews. Each monograph generally includes physical and chemical properties and analytical methods, sources of human exposure and environmental exposure, kinetics and metabolism in laboratory animals and humans, effects on humans and an evaluation of risks for human health, effects on the environment and so on. The EHC series are published by the World Health Organization (WHO) and hard copies can be obtained from the Office of Distribution and Sales, WHO, 1211 Geneva 27, Switzerland.

- ATSDR Toxicological Profile Information:
  Toxicological Profile for Polycyclic Aromatic Hydrocarbons (PAHs), available at http://www.atsdr.cdc.gov/toxprofiles/tp69.html

The ATSDR toxicological profile information is presented by the Agency for Toxic Substances and Disease Registry (US ATSDR) to provide public health information to prevent harmful exposures and disease related to toxic substances. This file succinctly characterizes the toxicological and adverse health effects information for the hazardous substance described.

- Polycyclic Aromatic Hydrocarbons: Occurrence in foods, dietary exposure and health effects, European Commission, 2002, available at
  http://europa.eu.int/comm/food/fs/sc/scf/index_en.html

This report gives background information on PAHs with an emphasis on the occurrence in foods, dietary exposure and health effects prepared by the Scientific Committee of Food Task Force on PAH, European Commission.

- Irwin R J, VanMouwerik M, Stevens L, Seese M D and W. Basham. *Environmental Contaminants Encyclopedia,* US National Park Service, Water Resources Division, Fort Collins, Colorado, 1998 (242).

This file is available at the website of the US Park Service Home Page (*http://www.nps.gov/*). This product differs from the other existing databases in that it deals with environmental toxicology rather than human health effects. 118 document files on chemical substances are available.

19.8 Acknowledgements

The author is grateful to the editor and reviewers for their valuable comments and suggestions, and would like to express his appreciation to Ms Ajet Blondy for the English language amendments.

19.9 References

ALFEIM I and RAMDAHL T (1984), 'Contribution wood combustion to indoor air pollution as measured by mutagenicity in Salmonella and polycyclic aromatic hydrocarbon concentration', *Environ Mutagen*, 6 121–130.

AMES B N, MCCANN J and YAMASAKI E (1975), 'Methods for detecting carcinogens and mutagens with Salmonella/mammalian-microsome mutagenicity test', *Mutation Res*, 31 347–364.

AREY J, ZIELINSKA B, ATKINSON R and WINTER A M (1991), 'Analysis of PAH and their nitroderivatives in ambient air', in Cooke M, Loening K, Merritt J (eds), *Polynuclear aromatic hydrocarbons: measurement, means, and metabolism,* Columbus, OH, Battelle Press, 51–67.

ATKINSON R and AREY J (1994), 'Atmospheric chemistry of gas-phase polycyclic aromatic hydrocarbons: Formation of atmospheric mutagens', *Environ Health Perspectives,* 102 (Suppl 4) 117–126.

ATSDR (1995), 'Polycyclic Aromatic Hydrocarbons (PAHs)', *ATSDR Toxicological Profiles*, US Department of Health and Human Services, Public Health Service, Agency for Toxic Substances and Disease Registry. CRC Press LLC, available at http://www.atsdr.cdc.gov/toxprofiles/tp69.html

AWOGI T and SATO T (1989), 'Micronucleus test with benzo*[a]*pyrene using a single peroral administration and intraperitoneal injection in males of the MS/Ae and CDl-1 mouse strains', *Mutat Res*, 223 353–356.

BASU D K and SAXENA J (1978), 'Polynuclear aromatic hydrocarbons in selected US drinking water and their raw water sources', *Environ Sci Technol*, 12 795–798.

BENIASHVILI D S H (1978), A comparative study on the action of some carcinogens inducing transplacental blastomogenesis in rabbits', *Vopr Onkol*, 24 77–83.

BENNER B A, GORDON G E and WISE S A (1989), 'Mobile sources of atmospheric polycyclic aromatic hydrocarbons: a roadway tunnel study', *Environ Sci Technol*, 23(10) 1269–1278.

BIERI R H, HEIN C, HUGGETT R J, SHOU P, SLONE H, SMITH C and SU C (1986), 'Polycyclic aromatic hydrocarbons in surfacee sediments from the Elizabeth River subsetuary', *Int J Env Anal Chem,* 26 97–113.

BIRKHOLTZ D A, COUT R T and HRUDEY S E (1988), 'Determination of polycyclic aromatic compounds in fish tissue', *J Chromatogr*, 449 251–260.

BORNEFF J and KUNTE H (1979), 'Method 1. Analysis of polycyclic aromatic hydrocarbons in water using thin layer chromatography and spectrofluorometry', in Egan H, Castegnaro M, Bogovski P, Kunte H and Walker EA (eds), *Environmental carcinogens: Selected methods of analysis. Volume 3: Analysis of polycyclic aromatic hydrocarbons in environmental samples*, Lyon, International Agency for Research on Cancer (IARC Scientific Publications No. 29), 129–139.

BOS R P, THEUWS J L G, JONGENEELEN F J and HENDERSON P T (1988), 'Mutagenicity of bi-, tri- and tetra-cyclic aromatic hydrocarbons in the 'taped-plate assay' and in the conventional *Salmonella* mutagenicity assay', *Mutat Res*, 204 203–206.

BROMAN D, NAF C, LUNDBERGH I and ZEBUHR Y (1990), 'An in situ study on the distribution, biotransformation and flux of polycyclic aromatic hydrocarbons (PAHs) in an aquatic food chain (seston-*Mytilus edulis* L.-*Somateria mollissima* L.) from the Baltic: an ecotoxicological perspective', *Environ Toxicol Chem,* 9 429–442.

BUI Q Q TRAN M B and WEST W L (1986), 'A comparative study of the reproductive effects of methadone and benzo[a]pyrene in the pregnant and pseudopregnant rat. *Toxicology,* 42 195–204.

BULAY O M (1970), The study of development of lung and skin tumors in mice exposed in utero to polycyclic hydrocarbons, *Acta Med Turk*, 7 3–38.

BUSBY W F JR, STEVENS E K, KELLENBACH E R, CORNELISSE J and LUGTENBURG J (1988), 'Dose–response relationships of the tumorigenicity of cyclopenta[cd]pyrene, benzo[a]pyrene and 6-nitrochrysene in a newborn mouse lung adenoma bioassay',

Carcinogenesis, 9 741–746.

BUTLER J P, POST G B, JOY P L and WALDMAN J M (1993), 'Assessment of carcinogenic risk from personal exposure to benzo(a)pyrene in the total human environmental exposure study (THEES)', *J Air Waste Manage Assoc*, 43 970–977.

CARVER J H, MACHADO M L and MacGREGOR J A (1986), 'Application of modified *Salmonella*/microsome prescreen to petroleum-derived complex mixtures and polynuclear aromatic hydrocarbons (PAH)', *Mutat Res*, 174 247–253.

CAVELIER C (1980), 'Analysis of polynuclear aromatic hydrocarbons by HPLC with fluorimetric detection', *Analysis*, 8(2) 46–48.

CHEN B H and LIN Y S (1997), 'Formation of Polycyclic Aromatic Hydrocarbons during processing of duck meat', *J Agric Food Chem*, 45 1394–1403.

CHIU C P, LIN Y S and CHEN B H (1997), 'Comparison of GC-MS and HPLC for overcoming matrix interferences in the analysis of PAHs in smoked food', *Chromatographia*, 44(9/10) 497–504.

COATES J T and ELZERMAN A W (1986), 'Extraction and determination of selected polycyclic aromatic hydrocarbons in plant tissues', *J Assoc Off Anal Chem*, 69(1) 110–114.

COOK J W, HEWETT C L and HIEGER I (1977), 'The isolation of a cancer-producing hydrocarbon from coal tar. Part I, II, III', *J Chem Soc*, 1933 29 395–405.

CRÖSSMANN G and WÜSTEMANN M (1992) [Loadings in domestic gardens and allotments by anorganic and organic substances with damaging potential: Actual documentation. Part I: Soils and garden wastes and Part II: Vegetables and fruits.] Berlin, Ministry of Environment, pp. 40–42, 108–124.

DAFFLON O, SCHEURER L, KOCH H and BOSSET J O (2000), 'Quantitation of nitrated polycyclic aromatic hydrocarbons in fish, meat products and cheese using liquid chromatography', *Mitt Geb Lebensmittelunters Hyg*, 91(2) 158–171.

DAISEY J M, SPENGLER J D and KAARAKKA P (1989), 'A comparison of the organic chemical composition of indoor aerosols during wood burning and non-woodburning periods', *Environ Int*, 15 435–442.

DAVIS C S, FELLIN P and OTSON R (1987), 'A review of sampling methods for polyaromatic hydrocarbons in air', *J Am Pollut Control Assoc,* 37 1397–1408.

DAVIS W W, KRAHL M E and CLOWES G H A (1942), 'Solubility of carcinogenic and related hydrocarbons in water', *J Am Chem Soc*, 64 108–110.

DENNIS M J, MASSEY R C, MCWEENY D J, KNOWLES M E and WHATSON D (1983), 'Analysis of polycyclic aromatic hydrocarbons in UK total diets', *Food Chem Toxicol*, 21 569–574.

DENNIS MJ, MASSEY RC, CRIPPS G, VENN I, HOWARTH N and LEE G (1991), 'Factors affecting the polycyclic aromatic hydrocarbons content of cereals, fats and other food products', *Food Addit Contam*, 8 517–530.

DE VOS R H, VAN DOKKUM W, SCHOUTEN A and DE JONG-BERKHOUT P (1990), 'Polycyclic aromatic hydrocarbons in Dutch total diet samples (1984–1986)', *Food Chem Toxic*, 28 263–268.

DOLL R (1977), 'Strategy for detection of cancer hazards to man', *Nature*, 265 589–596.

DOREMIRE M E, HARMON G E and PRATT D E (1979), '3,4-Benzopyrene in charcoal grilled meats', *J Food Sci*, 44 622–623.

DOUABUL ALI A-Z, HEBA HASSAN M A and FAREED K H (1997), 'Polynuclear aromatic hydrocarbons (PAHs) in fish from the Red sea coast of Yemen', *Hydrobiologia*, 352 251–262.

DUNKEL V C, ZEIGER E, BRUSICK D, MCCOY E, MCGREGOR D, MORTELMANS K, ROSENKRANZ H S and SIMMON V F (1984), 'Reproducibility of microbial mutagenicity assays: 1. Tests with *Salmonella typhimurium* and *Escherichia coli* using a standardized protocol', *Environ Mutag*, 6 (Suppl 2) 1–39.

DUNN B P and ARMOUR R J (1980), 'Sample extraction and purification for determination of polycyclic aromatic hydrocarbons by reverse-phase chromatography', *Anal Chem*, 52 2027–2031.

EHC (1998), 'Selected non-heterocyclic aromatic hydrocarbons', *Environmental Health Criteria (EHC) Monographs 202,* WHO, Geneva, 47–96.

EMEROLE G O (1980), 'Carcinogenic polycyclic aromatic hydrocarbons in some Nigerian foods', *Bull Environm Contam Toxicol*, 24 641–646.

FALCON M S G, AMIGO S G, YUSTY M A L and LOZANO J S (1999), 'Determination of benzo[a]pyrene in some Spanish commercial smoked products by HPLC-FL', *Food Addit Contam*, 16(1) 9–14.

FAO/WHO (1987), *31st Report of the Joint Committee on Food Additives*, WHO: Geneva, Switzerland, 759p.

FLORIN I, RUTBERG L, CURVALL M and ENZELL C R (1980), 'Screening of tobacco smoke constituents for mutagenicity using the Ames' test', *Toxicology,* 18 219–232.

FRANCE J E, KING J W and SNYDER J M (1991), 'Supercritical fluid-based cleanup technique for the separation of organochlorine pesticides from fats', *J Agric Food Chem*, 39 1871–1874.

GALCERAN M T, MOYANO E, PUIGNOU L and PAIS P (1996), 'Determination of heterocyclic amines by pneumatically assisted electrospray liquid chromatography-mass spectrometry', *J Chromatogr A*, 730185–194.

GERMANY, MINISTRY OF ENVIRONMENT (1994), Cited in IPCS (1998).

GORDON R J and BRYAN R J (1973), 'Patterns in airborne polynuclear hydrocarbon concentrations at four Los Angeles sites', *Environ Sci Technol*, 7 1050–1053.

GRIEST W H and CATON J E (1983), 'Extraction of polycyclic aromatic hydrocarbons for quantitative analysis' in Bjorseth A (ed.), *Handbook of Polycyclic Aromatic Hydrocarbons*, New York, Marcel Dekker, 95–147.

GRIMMER G (1983), 'Chemistry', in Grimmer G (ed.), *Environmental Carcinogens: Polycyclic aromatic hydrocarbons*, Boca Raton, FL, CRC Press, pp. 27–60.

GRIMMER G and BOEHNKE H (1975), 'Polycyclic aromatic hydrocarbon profile analysis of high-protein foods, oils and fats by gas chromatography', *J Assoc Off Anal Chem*, 58 725–733.

GROB K, KAELIN I and ARTHO A (1991), 'Coupled LC-GC: the capacity of silica gel (HP)LC columns for retaining fat', *J High Resol Chromatogr*, 14 373–376.

GUILLEN M D, SOPELANA P and PARTEARROYO M A (2000a), 'Determination of polycyclic aromatic hydrocarbons in commercial liquid smoke flavorings of different compositions by gas chromatography-mass spectrometry', *J Agric Food Chem,* 48 126–131.

GUILLEN M D, SOPELANA P and PARTEARROYO M A (2000b), 'Study of several aspects of a general method for the determination of polycyclic aromatic hydrocarbons in liquid smoke flavourings by gas chromatography-mass spectrometry', *Food Addit Contam*, 17(1) 27–44.

GUILLEN M D, SOPELANA P and PARTEARROYO M A (2000c), 'Polycyclic aromatic hydrocarbons in liquid smoke flavorings obtained from different types of wood, effect of storage in polyethylene flasks on their concentration', *J Agric Food Chem,* 48 5083–5087.

HAMMOND E D, SELIKOFF I J and LAWTHER P O (1976), 'Inhalation of B[a]P and cancer in man', *Ann NY Acad Sci*, 271 116–124.

HANUS J P, GUERRERO H, BIEHL E and KENNER C T (1979), 'High pressure liquid chromatographic determination of polynuclear aromatic hydrocarbons in oyster', *J Assoc Off Anal Chem*, 62 29–35.

HECHT S S, LAVOIE E, AMIN S, BEDENKO V and HOFFMANN D (1980), 'On the metabolic activation of the benzofluoranthenes, in Bjorseth A and Dennis A J (eds), *Polynuclear Aromatic Hydrocarbons: Chemistry and biological effects*, Columbus, OH, Battelle Press, 417–433.

HERBES S E (1981), 'Rates of microbial transformation of polycyclic aromatic hydrocarbons in water and sediments in the vicinity of coal-coking waste water discharge', *Appl Environ Microbiol,* 41 20–28.

HERMANN M (1981), 'Synergistic effects of individual polycyclic aromatic hydrocarbons on the mutagenicity of their mixtures', *Mutat Res*, 90 399–409.

HERMANN M, DURAND J P, CHARPENTIER J M, CHAUDE O, HOFNUNG M, PETROFF N, VANDECASTEELE J P and WEILL N (1980), 'Correlations of mutagenic activity with polynuclear aromatic hydrocarbon content of various mineral oils', in Cooke M and Dennis A J (eds), *Polynuclear Aromatic Hydrocarbons: Chemical analysis and biological fat*, Columbus, OH, Battelle Press, 899–916.

HUSAIN A, NAEEMI E, DASHTI B, AI-OMIRAH H and AL-ZENKI S (1997), 'Polycyclic aromatic hydrocarbons in food products originating from locally reared animal in Kuwait', *Food Addit Contam*, 14(3) 295–299.

IARC (1972), 'Certain polycyclic aromatic hydrocarbons and heterocyclic compounds', *IARC Monographs on the Evaluation of the Carcinogenic Risk of Chemicals to Humans*, Lyon, International Agency for Research on Cancer, Vol. 3.

IARC (1983), 'Polynuclear aromatic compounds, Part 1 Chemical, environmental and experimental data', *IARC Monographs on the Evaluation of the Carcinogenic Risk of Chemicals to Humans,* Lyon, International Agency for Research on Cancer, Vol. 32.

IARC (1987), 'Overall Evaluation of Carcinogenicity', *IARC Monographs on the Evaluation of the Carcinogenic Risk of Chemicals to Humans: An Updating of IARC Monographs*, Volumes 1 to 42, Supplement 7.

IUPAC (1987), 'Recommended method for a thin-layer-chromatographic screening method for the determination of benzo(a)pyrene in smoked food', *Pure Appl Chem,* International Union of Pure and Applied Chemistry, 59 1735–1738.

JACOB J and GRIMMER G (1979), 'Extraction and enrichment of polycyclic aromatic hydrocarbons (PAH) from environmental matter, in Egan H, Castegnaro M, Bogovski P, Kunte H and Walker E A (eds), *Environmental Carcinogens: Selected methods of analysis. Volume 3: Analysis of polycyclic aromatic hydrocarbons in environmental samples,* Lyon, International Agency for Research on Cancer (IARC Scientific Publications No. 29), 79–89.

JARVENPAA E, HUOPALAHTI R and TAPANAINEN P (1996), 'Use of supercritical fluid extraction-high performance liquid chromatography in the determination of polycyclic aromatic hydrocarbons from smoked and broiled fish', *J Liq Chrom Technol*, 19(9) 1473–1482.

JOE F L JR, SALEMME J and FAZIO T (1984), 'Liquid chromatographic determination of trace residues of polynuclear aromatic hydrocarbons in smoked foods', *J Assoc Off Anal Chem*, 67(6) 1076–1082.

JONES K C, STRATFORD J A, WATERHOUSE K S and VOGT N B (1989), 'Organic contaminants in Welch soils, Polynuclear aromatic hydrocarbons', *Environ Sci Technol,* 23 540–550.

KARL, H. and LEINEMANN M (1996), 'Determination of polycyclic aromatic hydrocarbons in smoked fishery products from different smoking kilns', *Z Lebensm Unters Forsch*, 202 458–464.

KATZ M, HEDDLE J A and SALAMONE M F (1981), *Mutagenic activity of polycyclic aromatic hydrocarbons and other environmental pollutants*, Columbus, OH, Battelle Press, 519–528.

KAYALI-SAYADI M N, RUBIO-BARROSO S, CUESTA-JIMENEZ M P and POLO-DIEZ L M (1998), 'Rapid determination of polycyclic aromatic hydrocarbons in tea infusion samples by high-performance liquid chromatography and fluorimetric detection based on solid-phase extraction', *Analyst,* 123 2145–2148.

KENNAWAY E L (1930), 'Further experiments on cancer producing substances', *Biochem J*, 24 497–504.

KORENAGA T, KAJIHARA T and TSUKIYAMA Y (1999), 'Determination and dynamic analysis of polycyclic aromatic hydrocarbons in soil and plant samples', *BUNSEKI KAGAKU (Anal Sci)*, 48(69) 631–636.

LANDRUM P F, NIHART S R, EADIE B J and HERCHE L R (1987), 'Reduction bioavailability of organic contaminants to the amphipod *Pontoporeia hoyi* by dissolved organic matter of sediment intestitial waters', *Environ Toxicol Chem*, 6 11–20.

LARSEN J C and LARSEN P B (1998), 'Chemical Carcinogens', in Hester R E, and Harrison R M (eds), *Air Pollution and Health*, issues in Environmental Sciences and Technology, The Royal Society of Chemical, Cambridge.

LARSSON B and SAHBERG G (1982), 'Polycyclic aromatic hydrocarbons in lettuce. Influence of a highway and an aluminium amelter', in Cooke M, Fisher A J (eds), *Polynuclear Aromatic Hydrocarbons: Physical and biological chemistry*, Columbus, OH, Battelle Press, 417–426.

LARSSON B K, ERIKSSON A T and CERVENKA M (1987), 'Polycyclic aromatic hydrocarbons in crude and deodorised vegetable oils', *Journal of the American Oil Chemists Society*, 64 365–370.

LAWRENCE J F and WEBER D F (1984), 'Determination of polycyclic aromatic hydrocarbons in Canadian samples of processed vegetable and dairy products by liquid chromatography with fluorescence detection', *J Agric Food Chem*, 32 794–797.

LEBO J A, ZAJICEK J L, SCHWARTZ T R, SMITH L M and BEASLEY M P (1991), 'Determination of monocyclic and polycyclic aromatic hydrocarbons in fish tissue', *J Assoc Off Anal Chem*, 74(3) 538–544.

LEGRAVEREND C, HARRISON D E, RUSCETTI F W and NEBERT D W (1983), 'Bone marrow toxicity induced by oral benzo*[a]*pyrene: Protection resides at the level of the intestine and liver', *Toxicol Appl Pharmacol*, 70 390–401.

LEGRAVEREND T, GUENTHER M and NEBERT D W (1984), 'Importance of the route of administration for genetic differences in benzo[a]pyrene-induced in utero toxicity and teratogenicity', *Teratology*, 29 35–47.

LEWIS W M (1975), 'Polynuclear aromatic hydrocarbons in water', *Water Treat Exam,* 23 243–277.

LINTAS C, DE MATTHAEIS M C and MERLI F (1979), 'Determination of benzo(a)pyrene in smoked, cooked and toasted food products', *Food Cosmet Toxicol*, 17 325–328.

LLOYD J W (1971), 'Long-term mortality study of steelworkers, V. Respiratory cancer in coke plant workers', *J Occup Med,* 13 53–68.

LO M T and SANDI E (1978), 'Polycyclic aromatic hydrocarbons (polynuclear) in foods', *Res Rev*, 69 35–85.

LOFROTH G, TOFTGARD R, NILSSON L, AGURELL E and GUSTAFSSON J A (1984), 'Short-term bioassays of nitro derivatives of benzo *[a]*pyrene and Perylene', *Carcinogenesis*, 5 925–930.

LOPEZ-ABENTE G, SANZ-ANQUELA J M and GONZALEZ C A (2001), Consumption of wine stored in leather wine bottles and incidence of gastric cancer. *Arch Environ Health*, 56 559–561.

MACLURE K M and MACMAHON B (1980), 'An epidemiologic perspective of environmental carcinogenesis', *Epidemiol Rev*, 2 19–48.

MALCOLM H M and DOBSON S (1994), 'The calculation of an environmental assessment level (EAL) for atmospheric PAHs using relative potencies', London, Department of the Environment, 34pp (Report No. DoE/HMIP/RR/94/041).

MALISZEWSKA-KORDYBACH B (1996), 'Polycyclic aromatic hydrocarbons in agricultural soils in Poland: preliminary proposals for criteria to evaluate the level of soil contamination', *Appl Geochem,* 11 121–127.

MALISZEWSKA-KORDYBACH B (2000), 'Polycyclic aromatic hydrocarbons in agroecosystems-example of Poland', *Polycyclic aromatic hydrocarbons,* 21 287–295.

MALISZEWSKA-KORDYBACH B and SMRECZAK B (1998), 'Polycyclic aromatic hydrocarbons (PAH) in agricultural soils in eastern Poland', *Toxicol Environ Chem,* 66 53–58.

MAY W E and WISE S A (1984), 'LC determination of polycyclic aromatic hydrocarbons in air particulate extracts', *Anal Chem*, 56(2) 225–232.

MAZUMDAR S, REDMOND C K and SOLLECITO W (1975), 'An epidemiological study of exposure to coal tar pitch volatiles among coke oven workers', *J Air Pollut Control Assoc* 25 382–389.

McCANN J, CHOI E, YAMASAKI E and AMES B N (1975), 'Detection of carcinogens as mutagens in the Salmonella/microsome test: Assay of 300 chemicals', *Proc Natl Acad Sci USA*, 72 5135–5139.

McCLURE P and SCHOENY R (1995), 'Evaluatin of a component-based relative potency approach to cancer risk assessment for exposure to PAH', *Fifteenth international symposium on polycyclic aromatic compounds: Chemistry, biology and environmental impact.* Ispara, Joint Research Centre European Commission, Belgirate, Italy, p. 161.

McGILL A S, MACKIE P R, PARSONS E, BRUCE C and HARDY R (1982), 'The polynuclear aromatic hydrocarbon content of smoked foods in the United Kingdom', in Cooke M, Dennis A J and Fisher G L (eds), *Polynuclear aromatic hydrocarbons: Physical and biological chemistry*, Columbus, OH, Battelle Press, 491–499.

MENICHINI E, BOCCA A, MERLI F, IANNI D and MONFREDINI F (1991a), 'Polycyclic aromatic hydrocarbons in olive oils on the Italian market', *Food Addit Contam*, 8(3) 363–369.

MENICHINI E, DOMENICO A DI and BONANNI L (1991b), 'Reliability assessment of a gas chromatographic method for polycyclic aromatic hydrocarbons in olive oil', *J Chromatogr*, 555 211–220.

MENZIE C A, POTOCKI B B and SANTODONATO J (1992), 'Exposure to carcinogenic PAHs in the environment', *Environ Sci Technol*, 26 1278–1284.

MOCHIZUKI E, KOBAYASHI H and NAKAYAMA A (1987), 'Simplified analysis of polycyclic aromatic hydrocarbons in water with Sep-Pak reversed phased cartridges', *Yamanashi-ken Eisei Kogai Kenkyusho Nenpo (Annual Rep Yamanashi Pref Inst Publ Hlth),* 31 8–11.

MONTIZAAN G K, KRAMERS P G H, JANUS J A and POSTHUMUS R (1989), 'Integrated criteria document PAH: Effects of 10 selected compounds', Appendix to Report No.

758474011. Bilthoven, National Institute of Public Health and Environmental Protection, 180 pp (Re-publication in March 1989 of addendum to Report No. 758447007).

MORET S and CONTE L S (1998), 'Off-line LC-LC determination of PAHs in edible oils and lipidic extracts', *J High Resol Chromatogr*, 21 253–257.

MORET S, BORTOLOMEAZZI R, REBECCA S and CONTE L S (1996a), 'Determinazione HPLC degli idrocarburi policiclici aromatici negli oli di oliva: comparazione di alcuni metodi di estrazione e purificazione (HPLC evaluation of polycyclic aromatic hydrocarbons in olive oils: A comparison of some extraction and clean up method', *Riv Ital Sost Grasse* 73 141–146.

MORET S, GROB K and CONTE L S (1996b), 'On-line solvent evaporator for coupled LC systems: further development', *J High Resol Chromatogr*, 19 434–438.

MORET S, GROB K and CONTE L S (1996c), 'On-line high-performance liquid chromatography-solvent evaporation-high-performance liquid chromatography-capillary gas chromatography-flame ionization detection for the analysis of mineral oil polyaromatic hydrocarbons in fatty foods', *J Chromatogr A*, 750 361–368.

MORET S, PIANI B and BORTOLOMEAZZI R (1997a), 'HPLC determination of polycyclic aromatic hydrocarbons in olive oils', *Z Lebensm Unters Forsch*, 205 116–120.

MORET S, GROB K and CONTE LS (1997b), 'Mineral oil polyaromatic hydrocarbons in foods, e.g. from jute bags, by on-line LC-solvent evaporation (SE)-LC-GC-FID', *Z Lebensm Unters Forsch*, 204 241–246.

MORET S, CONTE L and DEAN D (1999), 'Assessment of polycyclic aromatic hydrocarbon content of smoked fish by means of a fast HPLC/HPLC method', *J Agric Food Chem*, 47 1367–1371.

MORET S, DUDINE A and CONTE L S (2000), 'Processing effects on the polyaromatic hydrocarbon content of grapeseed oil' *J Assoc Off Anal Chem*, 77(12) 1289–1292.

MORET S, CERICCO V and CONTE L S (2001), 'On-line solvent evaporator for coupled normal phase-reversed phase high-performance liquid chromatography systems: heavy polycyclic aromatic hydrocarbons analysis', *J Microcolumn Separations*, 13(1) 13–18.

MOTTIER P, PARISOD V and TURESKY R J (2000), 'Quantitative determination of polycyclic aromatic hydrocarbons in barbecued meat sausages by gas chromatography coupled to mass spectrometry', *J Agric Food Chem*, 48 1160–1166.

MUKERJEE S, ELLENSON W D, LEWIS R G, STEVENS R K, SOMERVILLE M C, SHADWICK D S and WILLIS R D (1997), 'An environmental scoping study in the lower Rio Grande Valley of Texas: III Residential microenvironmental monitoring for air, house dust, and soil', *Environm Intern*, 23(5) 657–673.

MUSIAL C J and UTHE J F (1986), 'Rapid semimicro method for determination of polycyclic aromatic hydrocarbons in shellfish by automated gel permeation/liquid chromatography', *J Assoc Off Anal Chem*, 69(3) 462–466.

NAF C, BROMAN D and BRUNSTROM B (1992), 'Distribution and metabolism of polycyclic aromatic hydrocarbons (PAHs) injected into eggs of chicken (*Gallus domesticus*) and common eider duck (*Somateria mollissima*)', *Environ Toxicol Chem*, 11 1653–1660.

NAKAGAWA T, SESHIMO A, YAMAMOTO C, SATO Y and KAWAMURA T (1991), 'Study of oral intakes of polycyclic aromatic hydrocarbons (PAHs) in life environment', *Ann Rep Yokohama Inst Health*, 30 113–116.

NAKANO M and FUKUSHIMA M (1994), 'Formation of polycyclic aromatic hydrocarbons

(PAHs) in lamb during roasting', *SYOKUHIN EISEIGAKU ZASSHI (J Food Hyg Soc Japan)*, 35(1) 41–45.

NEBERT D W, PUGA A and VASILIOU V (1993), 'Role of the Ah receptor and the dioxin-inducible [Ah] gene battery in toxicity, cancer, and signal transduction', *Annals of the New York Academy of Science,* 685 624–640.

NEMOTO S, TAKATSUKI S, MATSUDA R, SAKAI K and TOYODA M (1998), 'Analysis for petroleum-related contaminants in seafoods by GC', *SYOKUHIN EISEIGAKU ZASSHI (J Food Hyg Soc Japan),* 39(1) 31–38.

NISBET I C T and LaGOY P K (1992), 'Toxic equivalency factors (TEFs) for polycyclic aromatic hydrocarbons (PAHs)', *Regul Toxicol Pharmacol*, 16 290–300.

OBANA H, HORI S, TANAKA R and KASHIMOTO T (1984), 'Dietary intakes of polycyclic aromatic hydrocarbons', *SYOKUHIN EISEIGAKU ZASSHI (J Food Hyg Soc Japan)*, 25(1) 35–40.

OBERLY T J, BEWSEY B J and PROBST G S (1984), 'An evaluation of the L5178YTK +/- mouse lymphoma forward mutation assay using 42 chemicals', *Mutat. Res*, 125 291–306.

OBUCHI A, AOYAMA H, HORI A and OBUCHI H (1984), 'Determination of polycyclic aromatic hydrocarbons in disel exhaust particularte matter and diesel fuel oil', *J Chrom*, 312 247–259.

OHNISHI Y, KINOUCHI T, TSUTSUI H, UEJIMA M and NISHIFUJI K (1986), 'Mutagenic nitropyrenes in foods', in Hayashi Y, Nagao M, Sugimura T, Takayama S, Tomatis L, Wattenberg L W and Wogan G N (eds), *Diet, Nutrition and Cancer*, Tokyo, Japan Scientific Societies Press, 107–118.

PERFETTI G A, NYMAN P J, FISHER S, JOE JR F J and DIACHENKO G W (1992), 'Determination of polycyclic aromatic hydrocarbons in seafood by liquid chromatography with fluorescence detection', *J Assoc Off Anal Chem*, 75 872–877.

PFANNHAUSER W (1991), 'Polycyclic aromatic hydrocarbons (PAH) in food and selected vegetables in Austria', *Mitt Geb Lebensmittelunters Hyg*, 82 66–79.

PFEFFER H U (1994), 'Ambient air concentrations of pollutants at traffic-related sites in urban areas of North Rhine-Westphalia Germany', *Sci Total Environ*, 146/147 263–273.

PHARM SOC JAP (2000), 'Analytical methods for food contaminants', in *Method of Analysis in Health Science'*, Tokyo, Pharmaceutical Society of Japan, 489–491.

PLATT K L, PFEIFFER E, PETROVIC P, FRIESEL H, BEERMANN D, HECKER E and OESCH F (1990), 'Comparative tumorigenicity of picene and dibenz [a,h] anthracene in the mouse', *Carcinogenesis*, 11 1721–1726.

POTT P (1775), 'Surgical observations relative to the cancer of the scrotum', Reprinted in *Natl Cancer Institute Monographs*, 1973 10 7–13.

POTTHAST K (1977), 'Polycyclic aromatic hydrocarbons in smoked meat products. An application method'. *Acta Alimentaria Polonica*, 3 195–201.

POTTHAST K and EIGNER G (1975), 'A new method for the rapid isolation of polycyclic aromatic hydrocarbons from smoked meat products', *J Chromtogr*, 103 173–176.

PURCHASE I F H, LONGSTAFF E, ASHBY J, STYLES J A, ANDERSON D, LEFEVRE P A and WESTWOOD F R (1976), 'Evaluation of six short term tests for detecting organic chemical carcinogens and recommendations for their use', *Nature*, 264 624–627.

RENE J J, VREULS J, DALLUGE U and BRINKMAN A TH (1999), 'Gas chromatography time-of-flight mass spectrometry for sensitive determination of organic micro-contaminants', *J. Microcolumn Separations*, 11(9) 663–675.

RICE J E, COLEMAN D T, HOSTED T J, LAVOIE E J, McCAUSTLAND D J and WILEY J C (1985),

'Identification of mutagenic metabolites of indeno[1,2,3-*cd*]pyrene formed *in vitro* with rat liver enzymes', *Cancer Res*, 45 5421-5425.

ROBINSON J L, JOHN J, SAFA A L, KIRKES K A and GRIFFITH P E (1987), 'Evaluation of disposable cartridges for trace enrichment from aqueous solutions', *J Chrom*, 402 201–210.

ROSENKRANZ H S and HOWARD P C (1986), 'Structural basis of the activity of nitrated polycyclic aromatic hydrocarbons', in Ishinishi N, Koizumi A, McClellan R O, Stober W (eds), *Carcinogenic and Mutagenic Effects of Diesel Engine Exhaust*, Amsterdam, New York, Oxford, Elsevier Science Publishers, 141–168.

SANDER L C and WISE S A (1997), *NIST Special Publication 922, Polycyclic Aromatic Hydrocarbon Structure Index*, available at http://ois.nist.gov/pah/

SANDERS M (1995), 'Distribution of polycyclic aromatic hydrocarbons in oyster (*Crassostrea Virginica*) and surfacee sediment from two estuaries in South Carolina', *Arch Environ Contam Toxicol*, 28 397–405.

SANTODONATO J, HOWARD P and BASU D (1981), 'Health and ecological assessment of polynuclear aromatic hydrocarbons', *J Environ Path Toxicol* , 5 1–376.

SCHLEMITZ S and PFANNHAUSER W (1996), 'Monitoring of nitropolycyclic aromatic hydrocarbons in food using gas chromatography', *Z Lebensm Unter Forsch,* 203 61–64.

SCHNEIDER K, ROLLER R, KALBERLAH F and SCHUHMACHER-WOLZ U (2002), 'Cancer risk assessment for oral exposure to PAH mixtures', *J Appl Toxicol*, 22 73–83.

SHENDRIKOVA I A and ALEKSANDROV V A (1974), 'Comparative characteristics of penetration of polycyclic hydrocarbons through the placenta in the fetus in rats', *Bull Exp Biol Med*, 77 77–79.

SHIRAISHI Y and SHIRATORI T (1981), 'Estimation of intake of benzo(a)pyrene by Japanese from the analysis of meals', *SYOKUHIN EISEIGAKU ZASSHI (J Food Hyg Soc Japan)*, 22(5) 436–440.

SIMKO P and BRUNCOVA B (1993), 'Lowering of polycyclic aromatic hydrocarbons concentration in a liquid smoke flavour by sorption into polyethylene packaging', *Food Addit Contam*, 10(2) 257–263.

SIMMON V F, ROSENKRANZ H S, ZEIGER E and POIRIER L A (1979), 'Mutagenic activity of chemical carcinogens and related compounds in the intraperitoneal host-mediated assay', *J Natl Cancer Inst*, 62 911–918.

SPEER K and MONTAG A (1988), 'Polycyclische aromatische Kohlenwasserstoffe in nativen pflanzlichen Ölen', *Fat Sci Technol*, 90 163–167.

SPEER K, STEEG E, HORSTMANN P, KUHN TH and MONTAG A (1990), 'Determination and distribution of polycyclic aromatic hydrocarbons in native vegetable oils, smoked fish products, mussels and oysters, and bream from the River Elbe', *J High Resol Chromatogr*, 13 104–111.

STAVRIC B, LAU BP-Y, MATULA T I, KLASSEN R, LEWIS D and DOWNIE R H (1997), 'Mutagenic heterocycric aromatic amines (HAAs) in processed food flavour samples', *Food and Chemical Toxicology*, 35(2), 185–197.

STRANDBERG B, BERGQVIST P A and RAPPE C (1998), 'Dialysis with semi-permeable membranes as an efficient lipid removal method in the analysis of bioaccumulative chemicals', *Anal Chem*, 70(3) 526–533.

TAKAHASHI G (1974), 'Distribution and metabolism of benzo(a)pyrene in fetal mouse', *Bull Chest Dis Res Inst Kyoto Univ*, 7 155–160.

TAKEDA S (2001), 'Analysis of hazardous chemicals by capillary electrophoresis', *BUNSEKI KAGAKU (Anal Sci)*, 50(11) 721–731.

TAMAKAWA K, TAKAHASHI Y, MISHIMA Y, SEKI T and TSUNODA A (1985), 'Mutagenicity and benzo[a]pyrene contents in soils in Sendai city: Influences of particulate substances produced studded tires of automobiles', *EISEI KAGAKU (J Hyg Chem)*, 31(5) 329–333.

TAMAKAWA K, OHGANE Y, KATOH Y, MISHIMA Y and SEKI T (1986), 'Simplified analysis of polycyclic aromatic hydrocarbons in daily diet with Sep-Pak silica cartridge', *EISEI KAGAKU (J Hyg Chem)*, 32(6) 475–477.

TAMAKAWA K, AIHARA Y, MISHIMA Y, SEKI T and TSUNODA A (1987a), 'Analysis of polynuclear aromatic hydrocarbons in roadside deposits containing asphalt dust', *KOUGAI TO TAISAKU (J Env Pollt Cont)*, 23(14) 1367–1372.

TAMAKAWA K, KATOH Y, OHGANE Y, MISHIMA Y, SEKI T and TSUNODA A (1987b), 'Daily dietary intakes of polycyclic aromatic hydrocarbons', *EISEI KAGAKU (J Hyg Chem)*, 33(1) 66–70.

TAMAKAWA K, AIHARA Y, TAKAHASHI Y and SEKI T (1988), 'Seasonal variations of mutagenic activities of airborne particulates Influences of asphalt dust produced by studded tires use of automobiles', *Taikiosen Gakkaishi (J Japan Soc Air Pollut)*, 23(3) 143–150.

TAMAKAWA K, SEKI T and TSUNODA A (1992), 'HPLC detection of polycyclic aromatic hydrocarbons', in Nollet L M L (ed.), *Food Analysis By HPLC*, New York, Marcel Dekker, 697–711.

TATATSUKI K, SUZUKI S, SATO N and USHIZAWA I (1985), 'Liquid chromatography determination of polycyclic aromatic hydrocarbons in fish and shellfish', *J Assoc Off Anal Chem*, 68 945–949.

TATENO T (1990), 'Polycyclic aromatic hydrocarbons produced from grilled vegetable', *SYOKUHIN EISEIGAKU ZASSHI (J Food Hyg Soc Japan),* 32(3) 271–276.

TATENO T (2000), 'Polycyclic aromatic hydrocarbons concentration in seasoning' *Bulletin of Tokyo Kasei University*, 40 91–94.

TATENO T and KAGEYAMA Y (1999), 'Determination of polycyclic aromatic hydrocarbons in milk commercially available in Tokyo and in raw milk from cattle farm', *SYOKUHIN EISEIGAKU ZASSHI (J Food Hyg Soc Japan)*, 40(1) 90–97.

THORSTEINSSON T (1967), 'Polycyclic hydrocarbons in commercially and home-smoked food in Iceland', *Cancer,* 23 455–457.

TOKIWA H (1992), 'Mutagenicity and carcinogenicity of nitrated polycyclic aromatic hydrocarbons', *J Japan Soc Air Pollut*, 27 73–84.

TOKIWA H and OHNISHI Y (1986), 'Mutagenicity and Carcinogenicity of nitroarenes and their sources in the environment', *CRC Crit Rev Toxicol*, 17 23–60.

TOKIWA H, MORITA K, TAKEYOSHI H, TAKAHASHI K and OHNISHI Y (1977), 'Detection of mutagenic activity in particulate air pollutants', *Mutat Res*, 48 237–248.

TOMKINS B A, JENKINS R A, GRIEST W H, REAGAN R R and HOLLADAY S K (1985), 'LC determination of benzo[a]pyrene in total particularte matter of cigarette smoke', *J Assoc Off Anal Chem*, 68(5) 935–940.

TONG C, BRAT V S, TELANG S, LASPIA, M F, FAZIO M, REISS B and WILLIAMS G M (1983), 'Effects of genotoxic polycyclic aromatic hydrocarbons in rat liver culture systems', in Cooke M and Dennis A J (eds), *Polynuclear Aromatic Hydrocarbons: Formation; metabolism,and measurement*, Columbus, OH, Battelle Press, 1189–1203.

TSUJI I, KOIDE K, MORIYAMA H, TANABE K and MATSUSHITA H (1985), 'Analysis of polynuclear aromatic hydrocarbons in shellfishes, seabottom sediments and sea water by high performance liquid chromatography', *SYOKUHIN EISEIGAKU*

ZASSHI (J Food Hyg Soc Japan), 26(1) 50–55.

TUOMINEN J P, PYYSALO H S and SAURI M (1988), 'Cereal products as a source of polycyclic aromatic hydrocarbons', *J Agric Food Chem*, 36, 118–120.

UK (2002), 'PAHs in the UK diet: 2000 total diet study samples (Number 31/02)', *Food Survey Information Sheet,* The United Kingdom Food Standard Agency, available at http://www.foodstandards.gov.uk/multimedia/pdfs/31pah.pdf

US EPA (1978), *Ambient water quality criteria: Naphthalene,* Washington DC, p. B/6 (PB-296 786).

US EPA (1990), 'Determination of benzo(a)pyrene and other polynuclear aromatic hydrocarbons in indoor air', in Winbery W T Jr, Forehand L, Murphy N T, Ceroli A, Phinney B and Evans A (eds), *Compendium of methods for the determination of air pollutants in indoor air, US Environmental Protection Agency, Method IP-7,* Research Triangle Park, North Carolina, pp. 550–639.

US EPA (1993), 'Provisional guidance for quantitative risk assessment of polycyclic aromatic hydrocarbons', US Environmental Protection Agency, Office of Health and Environmental Assessment, Environmental Criteria and Assessment Office, Cincinnati, Ohio, EPA/600/R-93/089 PB94-116571.

US EPA (1999), US Environmental Protection Agency. Integrated Risk Information System (IRIS). Evidence for Human Carcinogenicity Weight of Evidence Characterization, available at http://www.epa.gov/ngispgm3/iris/.

VAESSEN H A M G, SCHULLER P L, JEKEL A A and WILBERS A A M M (1984), 'Polycyclic aromatic hydrocarbons in selected foods, Analysis and occurence', *Toxicol Environ Chem*, 7 297–324.

VAESSEN H A M G, JEKEL A A and WILBERS A A M M (1988), 'Dietary intake of polycyclic aromatic hydrocarbons', *Toxicol Environ Chem,* 16 281–294.

VAN STIJIN F, KERKHOFF M A T and VANDEGINSTE B G M (1996), 'Determination of polycyclic aromatic hydrocarbons in eadible oils and fats by on-line donor-acceptor complex chromatography and high-performance liquid chromatography with fluorescence detection', *J Chromatogr A*, 750 263–273.

VOUTSA D and SAMARA C (1998), 'Dietary intake of trace elements and polycyclic aromatic hydrocarbons via vegetables grown in an industrial Greek area', *The Science of the Total Environment*, 218 203–216.

VREULS J J, JONG G DE and BRINKMAN U A (1991), 'On line coupling of liquid chromatography, capillary gas chromatography and mass spectrometry for the determination and identification of polycyclic aromatic hydrocarbons in vegetable oils', *Chromatograhia*, 31 113–118.

WANG G, LEE A S, LEWIS M, KAMATH B and ARCHER R K (1999), 'Accelerated solvent extraction and gas chromatography/mass spectrometry for determination of polycyclic aromatic hydrocarbons in smoked food samples', *J Agric Food Chem*, 47 1062–1066.

WEISBURGER J H (2001), 'Antimutagenesis and anticarcinogenesis, from the past to the future', *Mutation Research,* 480–481 23–35.

WINKLER E, BUCHELE A and MUELLER O (1977), 'Verfahren zur Bestimmung des Gehaltes an policyclischen aromaticshen Kohlenwasserstoffen in Mais mit Hilfe der Kapillargaschromatographie', *J Chromatogr*, 138 151–164.

WISE S A, BENNER B A, CHESLER S N, HILPERT L R, VOGT C R and MAY W E (1986), 'Characterization of the polycyclic aromatic hydrocarbons from two standard reference material air particulate samples', *Anal Chem*, 58(14) 3067–3077.

WOOD A L, BOUCHARD D C, BRUSSEAU M L and RAO P S C (1990), 'Cosolvent effects on sorption and mobility of organic contaminants in soil', *Chemosphere*, 21 575–587.

WOOD A W, CHANG R L, LEVIN W, RYAN D E, THOMAS P E, LEHR R E, KUMAR S, SARDELLA D J, BOGER E, YAGI H, SAYER J M, JERINA D M and CONNEY A H (1981), 'Mutagenicity of the bayregion diol-epoxides and other benzo-ring derivatives of dibenzo(a,h)-pyrene and dibenzo(a,i)pyrene', *Cancer Res*, 41 2589–2597.

WYNDER E L and HOFFMANN D (1967), *Tobacco and Tobacco Smoke*, New York, Academic Press.

WYNDER E L and GORI G B (1977), 'Contribution of the environment to cancer incidence: an epidemiologic exercise', *J Natl Cancer Inst*, 58 825.

XIA L, ZHU M, TAO F and HU Z (1988), 'HPLC determination of PAHs in drinking water by switching column and fluorescence wavelength program technique', *Fenxi Huaxue (Analytical Chemistry)*, 16(2) 147–149.

YAMAGIWA K and ICHIKAWA K (1918), 'Experimental study of the pathogenesis of carcinoma', *J Cancer Res*, 3 1–29.

20

Dioxins and polychlorinated biphenyls (PCBs)

L. A. P. Hoogenboom, RIKILT – Institute of Food Safety, The Netherlands

20.1 Introduction

Food products may contain environmental contaminants at levels that can affect human health. At present dioxins and other persistent organic pollutants are a group of compounds that causes great concern. This is based not only on the persistence and accumulation of these compounds in our food chain, but also on the small to non-existent margin between toxicological guidelines on safe human intakes and actual exposure of humans to these compounds. Due to various measures, levels of PCBs and dioxins in food and humans have started to decline. However, more recently it was shown that levels of other persistent compounds, in particular brominated flame retardants have started to increase in food and human samples, causing concern about possible future effects. Although the environment may contribute to the exposure in particular cases, the major part comes from food. Products of animal origin, including fish, contribute most to the intake. This chapter presents the current situation on the toxicity of these compounds, the tools to detect their presence in the food chain and current exposure levels.

20.2 Dioxins and PCBs

Dioxins is a generic name for two groups of compounds, the polychlorinated dibenzofurans (PCDFs) and the polychlorinated dibenzo-p-dioxins (PCDDs) (Fig. 20.1). These compounds are characterized by a planar structure and a varying number of chlorine atoms. In practice only the 2,3,7,8–substituted congeners are metabolically resistant and thus accumulate in biological systems.

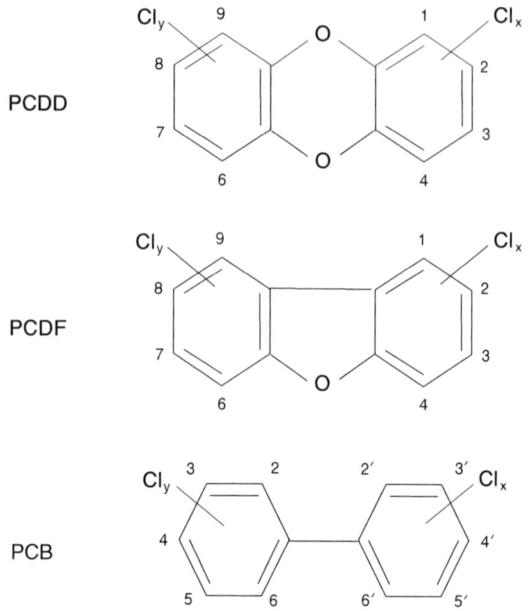

Fig. 20.1 Structures of polychlorinated dibenzo-p-dioxins (PCDD), dibenzofurans (PCDF), and polychlorobiphenyls (PCB). The most toxic congener is 2,3,7,8–tetrachlorodibenzo-p-dioxin (TCDD). The other toxic six PCDD and ten PCDF congeners contain at least 4 chlorine atoms and always at the 2, 3, 7 and 8 positions. The 12 toxic PCBs contain 4 or more chlorine atoms and none (non-ortho) or only one (mono-ortho) of them at the 2, 2′, 6, or 6′ position.

In addition to dioxins, it has been shown that 12 out of 209 PCB-congeners may also have a planar structure and resemble dioxins in their stability and biological effects.

Dioxins were first identified as a possible threat to the food chain during the early 1960s. Large numbers of chickens died from a disease called chicken edema disease after consuming contaminated feed (Sanger *et al.*, 1958; Schmittle *et al.*, 1958; Higginbotham *et al.*, 1968; Firestone, 1973). The feed contained fat prepared from cowhides that had been treated with chlorinated phenols. It took about ten years to identify dioxins as the causative factor in chicken edema disease, which can partly be explained by the fact that these compounds were new to researchers on environmental contaminants, but also by the very great toxic potency and hence the low levels required for toxic effect. Other major incidents like the Yu-Sho and Yu-Cheng rice oil contaminations in Japan and Taiwan in 1968 and 1979 respectively, and the Seveso incident in Italy in 1976 confirmed the considerable toxicity of these compounds at relatively low levels. The rice oil incidents were caused by leakage of PCB oil, used as heat transfer fluid, into the oil (Kuratsune *et al.*, 1972, Hsu *et al.*, 1985). Only later did it become apparent that the PCB oil also contained large amounts of PCDFs, which might be responsible for at least part of the observed effects. In the late 1980s another important source was detected: the incineration of municipal waste (Olie *et al.*, 1977). In several countries including the Netherlands it was shown that this resulted in elevated levels of dioxins on grass and as a result in milk from dairy cows (Liem *et al.*, 1991). Large investments were made to reduce the emission of dioxins from MWIs with the result that dioxin levels in milk decreased over time.

More recent incidents with PCBs and dioxins have shown that these compounds still pose a major threat to the food chain. In the US, dioxins were detected in ball clay used in feed for chickens and cat fish (Hayward *et al.*, 1999, Ferrario *et al.*, 2000). In Europe, citrus pulp used for animal feed was shown to be contaminated, resulting in moderately increased levels in milk (Malisch, 2000). A much larger incident, however, was the chicken crisis in Belgium involving an estimated 200–300 kg PCB oil that contaminated 60 tons of fat used for the production of animal feed (Bernard *et al.*, 1999; Hoogenboom *et al.*, 1999; Larebeke *et al.*, 2001). Again chickens were affected most, showing decreased egg hatching and symptoms resembling chicken edema disease. At least in Europe, this resulted in strict regulations on these compounds (EC, 2001, 2002). As a result several novel sources were elucidated like kaolinic clay, cholin chloride, sequestered minerals and dried grass and bakery meal, in all cases products used in animal feed.

Dioxins are produced as by-products in the synthesis of certain chemicals, like the wood preserving agent pentachlorophenol and the herbicide 2,4,5–trichlorophenoxyacetic acid (Agent Orange). However, they may also be present in heated PCB oil and formed during incineration of plastics and other waste. Each source may produce its own specific congener pattern. Figure 20.2 shows the congener patterns of dioxins in the most recent food and feed incidents, starting with the Brazilian citrus pulp incident in 1998. The patterns are presented as the relative contributions of each congener to the TEQ level. The patterns are very typical for the source and can actually be used to identify a source. The use of lime originating from a PVC production plant for neutralization and water removal of citrus pulp led to another typical pattern (Malisch, 2000). In the case of the PCB contamination of Belgian feed, oxidation resulted primarily in the formation of PCDFs. In the case of the cholin chloride for example, the contamination was traced back to the mixing with PCP-treated wood, showing the typical pattern of higher chlorinated dioxins (Llerena *et al.*, 2003). The most recent incident in the Netherlands resulted from the use of waste wood for drying of bakery waste and showed a pattern resembling that of burned painted wood (Wunderli *et al.*, 2000). These cases demonstrate that dioxins may result from a variety of different sources.

20.2.1 PCBs

PCBs are a group of 209 different congeners, which have been produced as technical mixtures (e.g. Arochlor 1254) and have been used in large amounts as heat transfer fluids, hydraulic lubricants and dielectric fluids for capacitors and

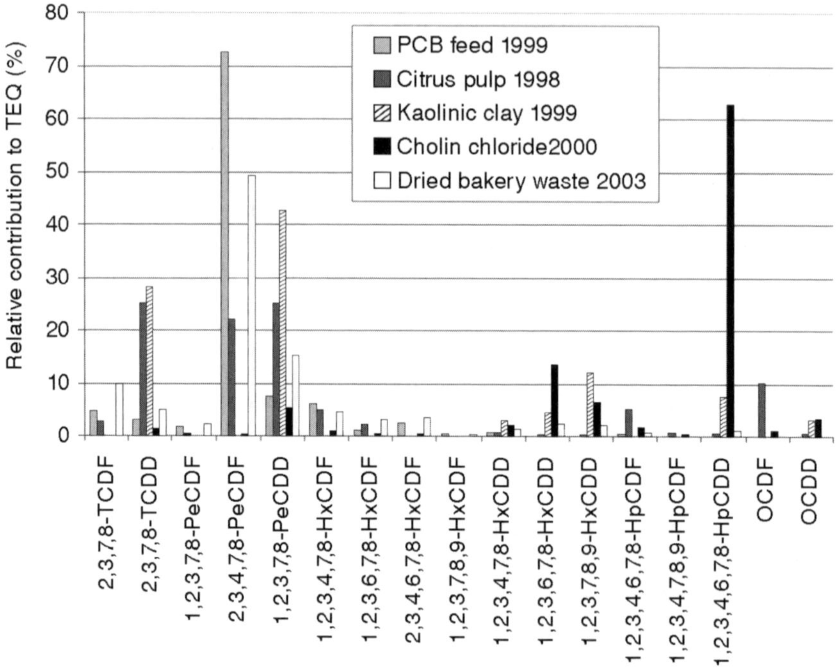

Fig. 20.2 Congener patterns of the most recent contaminations of the food chain, expressed as the relative contribution to the TEQ level.

transformers (Safe, 1994). Although these uses are now generally prohibited, the main potential problems are in the disposal of old electrical equipment and the persistence of PCB residues in the environment. Twelve of the PCB congeners have a planar structure and similar properties to dioxins. Other PCBs have been shown to affect brain development (Schmidt, 1999) and appear to be responsible for the tumour promotion effects of these mixtures (Plas *et al.*, 2001). In addition metabolites of non-dioxin-like PCBs interfere with the homeostasis of vitamin A and thyroid hormones (Safe, 1994).

In practice, the consumer will be exposed to a mixture of dioxins, dioxin-like PCBs and other PCBs, and the toxicology of these mixtures is very complex. As a result, no exposure limits for non-dioxin-like PCBs have been established thus far, although there are limits for PCBs in food. In order to avoid difficulties in analysing all 209 congeners, it is customary to analyse only seven so-called indicator PCBs that represent the different technical mixtures. These include PCBs 28, 53, 101, 138, 153 and 180 as well as PCB 118, which is a dioxin-like mono-ortho PCB. It is important to realise that the total amount of PCBs in a technical mixture may be three to four times fold higher than the amounts of these indicator substances. This relative contribution may change in animal-derived products due to selective absorption, metabolism, carry-over and accumulation of the different congeners.

20.3 Assessing the toxic effects of dioxins and dioxin-like PCBs

Dioxins and dioxin-like PCBs bind to the so-called Ah receptor present in mammalian cells, thus resulting in the transcription of a large number of genes. These genes include those encoding for biotransformation enzymes like cytochrome P450 1A and 1B and glucuronyl-transferases, as well as genes involved in the growth regulation of cells (Guo *et al.*, 2004). In laboratory animals, exposure to TCDD results in liver tumours in female rats, and at lower levels of exposure in effects on the immune and reproductive systems, as well as impaired learning (WHO, 2000). Another typical effect is endometriosis, a symptom where cells from the endometrium grow in sites outside the uterine cavity. This effect has been observed in Rhesus monkeys exposed for 4 years to doses of 5 and 25 ng TCDD/kg in the diet (Rier *et al.*, 1993). The effect only became apparent after an additional 10 years on clean feed. There are also effects observed in humans exposed accidentally to these compounds like chloracne, neurodevelopmental delays and neurobehavioural effects, and an increased risk of diabetes and certain cancer types like soft tissue sarcomas and liver cancer (WHO, 2000).

Based on these effects, the World Health Organisation (WHO) and the EU Scientific Committee on Food (SCF) have set very low exposure limits, of respectively 2 pg TEQ/kg bw/day (WHO, 2000) and 14 pg TEQ/kg bw/week (SCF, 2001). These limits include the 17 toxic 2,3,7,8–chlorinated PCDDs and PCDFs as well as 12 planar PCBs. The expression of limits on a weekly basis acknowledges the fact that the toxic effects are normally not a result of a single exposure, but the systematic increase of body burdens due to continuous intake of these compounds and their storage in body fat. The great toxicity of dioxins and PCBs is thought to be jointly due to their effects at low levels, their lipophilic nature and their resistance to metabolic degradation, resulting in accumulation in the body. Eventually this may result in body burdens that are higher than safe levels, thus resulting in the adverse effects described above. One of the few mechanisms leading to a significant reduction in body burden levels is the excretion of these compounds in breast milk. Similarly in food-producing animals, dioxins can be transferred into milk and eggs.

20.3.1 The TEQ principle

Levels of dioxins and dioxin-like PCBs are normally expressed in TEQs (Toxic Equivalents). This refers to the use of the so-called TEQ principle, whereby the concentrations of the different congeners are multiplied by a toxic equivalency factor (TEF), expressing their toxicity relative to the most toxic congener 2,3,7,8-tetrachlorodibenzo-p-dioxin (TCDD) (Berg *et al.*, 1998). Most of the toxicological data have been obtained from studies with TCDD, the most toxic congener. Other dioxins and dioxin-like PCBs are not equally toxic. At the same time there is strong evidence that the effects of the different congeners are

Table 20.1 TEF values as assigned by the WHO in 1997

Compound	TEF value
PCDDs	
2,3,7,8–TCDD	1
1,2,3,7,8–PeCDD	1
1,2,3,4,7,8–HxCDD	0.1
1,2,3,6,7,8–HxCDD	0.1
1,2,3,7,8,9–HxCDD	0.1
1,2,3,4,6,7,8–HpCDD	0.01
OCDD	0.0001
PCDFs	
2,3,7,8–TCDF	0.1
1,2,3,7,8–PeCDF	0.05
2,3,4,7,8–PeCDF	0.5
1,2,3,4,7,8–HxCDF	0.1
1,2,3,6,7,8–HxCDF	0.1
1,2,3,7,8,9–HxCDF	0.1
2,3,4,6,7,8–HxCDF	0.1
1,2,3,4,6,7,8–HpCDF	0.01
1,2,3,4,7,8,9–HpCDF	0.01
OCDF	0.0001
Non-ortho PCBs	
3,4–3′4′ PCB (77)	0.0001
3,4,5–4′ TeCB (81)	0.0001
3,4–3′4′5′ PCB (126)	0.1
3,4,5–3′4′5′ PCB (169)	0.01
Mono-ortho PCBs	
2,3,4–3′,4′ PeCB (105)	0.0001
2,3,4,5–4′ PeCB (114)	0.0005
2,4,5–3′,4′ PeCB (118)	0.0001
3,4,5–2′,4′ PeCB (123)	0.0001
2,3,4,5–3′,4′ HxCB (156)	0.0005
2,3,4–3′,4′,5′ HxCB (157)	0.0005
2,4,5–3′,4′,5′ HxCB (167)	0.00001
2,3,4,5–3′,4′,5′ HpCB (189)	0.0001

additive. In order to deal with this particular problem, the so-called TEQ approach has been introduced. The different congeners have been assigned a so-called TEF value, which is a weighted value, based on the differential effects in various experiments. TEF values are consensus factors agreed upon by international scientists involved in the field. The last time these TEF values were evaluated was during a WHO workshop in The Netherlands in 1997. These values are shown in Table 20.1. It was agreed to evaluate the TEF values every five years, depending on new data from toxicological studies. As a result the TEQ levels in food may change dramatically if the TEF value of a congener that contributes significantly is changed. The last revision of the TEF for

PeCDD from 0.5 to 1 caused, for example, an estimated increase of 15% in the TEQ levels.

At present the major concern may be on the mono-ortho PCBs for which the TEF values might be too high (WHO, 2000). This may be related to the difficulty in obtaining sufficient material of high purity to assess the *in vivo* effects relative to TCDD. In vitro studies with mono-ortho compounds indicate that the actual TEF values may have to be reduced. This may have particular consequences for food products where this group of compounds has a relatively high contribution to the TEQ level, such as eel from polluted rivers, for example.

In principle, a compound should have the following properties to obtain a TEF value:

- a compound must show a structural relationship to the PCDDs and PCDFs
- a compound must bind to the Ah receptor
- a compound must elicit Ah receptor-mediated biochemical and toxic responses
- a compound must be persistent and accumulate in the food chain.

Many other compounds have been shown to have affinity for the Ah receptor, including polyaromatic hydrocarbons and a number of plant secondary metabolites, but these compounds failed to pass the other criteria. Other compounds like the polybrominated dioxins and PBBs might be considered for a TEF value, but adequate studies are missing for the assignment of a TEF value.

An important issue is whether the effects of different dioxins and dioxin-like PCBs, but also other Ah receptor agonists are actually additive or whether there may also be antagonistic activity. Furthermore, Safe (1995, 1998) was one of the first to point out the often very high levels of Ah receptor agonists in certain foods of plant origin. However, there is a substantial difference between these compounds, and dioxins and PCBs, since these plant-derived compounds are often metabolised completely before entering the bloodstream. Certain flavonoids are rapidly conjugated in the gut wall, thus losing their biological activity. Further studies are required to reveal which naturally-occurring compounds may actually retain their activity in the blood. In addition, it is thought that the toxicity of dioxins is due not to the occasional intake of a relatively high level, but the increase in body burden above a certain threshold, thus resulting in a continuous stimulation of the Ah receptor pathway. It remains to be elucidated whether natural Ah receptor agonist may reach effective concentrations and cause the related effects.

20.4 Analytical methods and current exposure levels

Because of the low limits for food and feed, dioxins can at present only be analysed by high resolution GC/MS (HRGC/HRMS). In addition, an extensive clean-up is required starting with the extraction of fat and its subsequent removal by gel permeation chromatography (GPC) or acid silica. Pesticides and other lipophilic substances need to be removed by subsequent clean-up steps. In order to account for possible recovery losses in the different column and evaporation steps, ^{13}C-labelled standards are added at the first step. Individual dioxins are identified by retention time and mass, and quantified. Using the TEF values, the levels are transferred into TEQs and summed into one figure. This can also be done for the non-ortho and mono-ortho PCBs. The levels are normally reported as lower bound and/or upper bound levels, thereby dealing with the levels of non-detected congeners. When reported as upper bound levels, as required by current legislation in the EU, the levels of non-detected congeners are equal to the detection limits.

The intensive clean-up and associated equipment is very costly. Furthermore, sample throughput is relatively small, causing further problems during situations as during the Belgian dioxin crisis in 1999. Therefore, there is a major need for cheap and high-throughput screening methods that can be used to select potentially contaminated samples and, equally important, to clear negative samples. Initial assays were based on the induction of cytochrome P450 enzymes in hepatoma cells or freshly isolated hepatocytes. These cells contain the different steps of the Ah receptor pathway. Elevated levels of these enzymes are detected by the increased metabolism of ethoxyresorufin into resorufin (EROD activity). However, the assay is potentially sensitive for false-negative results, since the enzyme has a number of inhibitors. Therefore novel assays, like CALUX, were developed based on cells with reporter genes like that encoding for the firefly enzyme luciferase. Following exposure to dioxin-like compounds, the cells start to synthesise luciferase which can easily be detected by a light-producing assay. Compared to HRGC/HRMS, the assay requires only a very simple clean-up, usually based on acid silica. However, the assay does not allow the use of internal standards. As a result the clean-up must be simple and highly reproducible, and proper control samples must be included in each test series to control for recovery and possible contaminants in the chemicals used for clean-up. Under these conditions the assay has been proven its usefulness for controlling dioxins (Hoogenboom, 2002). Recently, the EU has set guidelines for the performance of analytical methods within a laboratory. HRGC/HRMS was established as the reference method.

The analysis of the so-called indicator PCBs and, in fact, also the mono-ortho PCBs does not require the same sensitivity due to the much higher levels. In practice, GC with either ECD or MS/MS detection is used. As a result this analysis is much cheaper and more analytical capacity is in general available. In specific cases, like during the Belgian dioxin/PCB crisis in 1999 and possibly also in the case of, for example, eels from polluted rivers, indicator PCB analysis might actually be used as a screening tool for samples. The major problem is that this might result in a more general application and that dioxins from other non-PCB like sources are overlooked.

20.4.1 Current exposure to dioxins and PCBs

Several studies have shown that at present, the exposure of part of the population in Western countries to dioxins and dioxin-like compounds exceeds the exposure limits set by the WHO and SCF (Liem *et al.*, 2000). A recent study in the Netherlands showed that the median of the lifelong intake of dioxins and dioxin-like PCBs by the Dutch population at present is 1.2 pg TEQ/kg bw. Dioxins and PCBs contributed to a similar extent to the exposure. The 90th percentile was 1.9 pg TEQ/kg bw and it was estimated that 8% of the population exceeded the current exposure limits (Baars *et al.*, 2004). In the same study, the median and 90th percentile for the estimated intake figures for indicator PCBs were respectively 5.6 and 10.4 ng/kg bw/day. Dairy products, meat, oils and fats, fish and vegetable products contributed 27, 23, 17, 16 and 13% respectively to the exposure of dioxin-like compounds. Similar figures were obtained for the indicator PCBs, although fish showed a 10% higher contribution. Slightly higher intake levels for dioxins only were obtained by Llobet *et al.* (2003) for the Catalonia region in Spain, showing an average intake of 1.4 pg TEQ/kg bw/day. The higher intake might be explained by the higher consumption of fish products that contributed for 31% to the intake. In a recent study from Japan the relative contribution of fish products was even higher, being more than 50% of the average daily intake of respectively 1.6 and 3.2 pg TEQ/kg bw/day for dioxins and the sum of dioxins and dioxin-like PCBs (Tsutsumi *et al.*, 2001).

It is important to note that in general the intake levels have decreased during the last decades, due to various measures to control the major sources. In the Netherlands the intake of dioxins and dioxin-like PCBs decreased from about 8 and 4 pg TEQ/kg bw/day in 1978 and 1984 to respectively 2.2 and 1.2 TEQ/kg bw/day in 1990 and 1999 (Baars *et al.*, 2004). This decreased intake is also reflected in the levels detected in human milk, which also showed a marked decrease in the various countries. Apart from incidental high exposures, the major impact of an incident like the one in Belgium in 1999 is that these efforts are temporarily diminished.

Consumers with certain preferences may have an increased intake of dioxins and PCBs. It has been shown for example, that eel from contaminated rivers may contain relatively high levels of dioxins and dioxin-like PCBs (Hoogenboom *et al.*, 2004). As a result the frequent consumption of such eel may result in elevated exposure. Unfortunately, the same may be true for people consuming eggs from free-range chickens. These eggs may contain levels up to 10 pg TEQ/g fat or more and therefore contribute to a significant exposure.

In order to further reduce the intake of the population, the EU has developed a strategy for further reducing exposure. This includes the establishment of residue limits for food products: 1 ng TEQ/kg fat for pork, 2 ng TEQ/kg fat for poultry, and 3 ng TEQ/kg fat for beef, milk and eggs (EC, 2001). In addition limits have been set for animal feed (0.75 ng TEQ/kg) and their ingredients (0.75–6 ng/kg TEQ) (EC, 2002). At the moment planar dioxin-like PCBs are included in the exposure limits but not yet in the EU food and feed limits. Based on more detailed information on current levels of these PCBs, the EU limits will be adapted in the near future.

20.5 Brominated flame retardants

Flame retardants are compounds used to decrease the flammability of plastics and thereby the risk of fire. Several classes of compounds have been or are being used, like the polybrominated biphenyls (PBBs), the polybrominated diphenylethers (PBDEs), tetrabromobisphenol A and hexabromocyclododecane (HBCD) (Fig. 20.3). PBBs are no longer produced and have been replaced by other compounds. PBDEs have been, and still are, produced in the Netherlands, France, Great Britain, The United States and Japan, primarily as the tetra-, penta-, octa- and deca-mixtures (de Boer, 2000). The penta-mixture contains primarily tetra- and penta-BDEs, the octa-mixture hepta- and octa-BDEs and the decamixture deca-PBE. High quantities are added to plastics like polyurethane foam. TBBP-A is used as an additive in electronic equipment (circuit boards). The use of the deca PBDE mixture has been forbidden in Europe since 2003 but the deca-mixture is still used.

PBBs were involved in one of the most tragic accidents in food-producing animals, being the Michigan incident, which occurred in the autumn of 1973 (Carter, 1976). The feed additive Nutrimaster (magnesium oxide) was accidentally substituted with FireMaster FF-1, a flame-retardant based on polybrominated biphenyls (PBBs). Total PBB intakes as high as 250 grams per cow in about 16 days were estimated, initially resulting in symptoms like body-

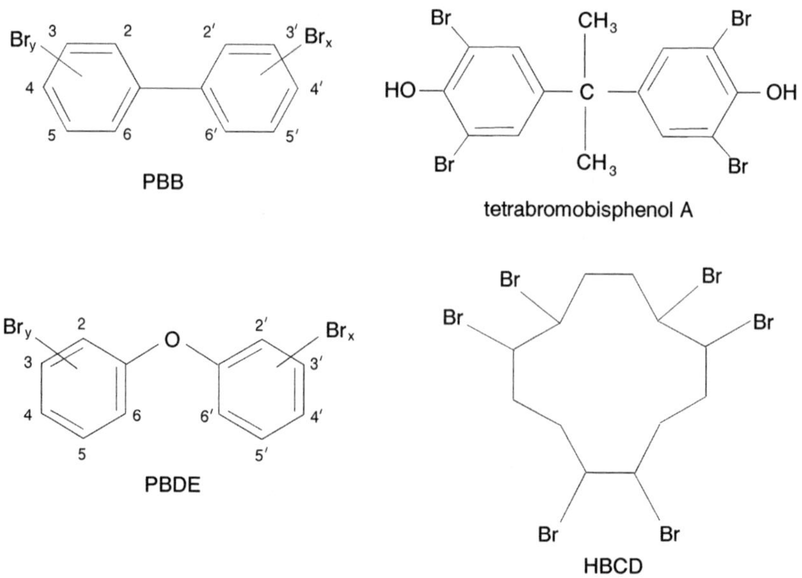

Fig. 20.3 Structures of the most important polybrominated flame retardants. In the case of the PBDEs, congeners numbered 47, 99, 100, 153, 154 and 209 correspond to respectively 2,4,2′,4′-tetraBDE, 2,4,5,2′,4′-pentaBDE, 2,4,6,2′,4′-pentaBDE, 2,4,5,2′,4′,5-‘hexaBDE, 2,4,5,2′,4′,6′-hexaBDE and 2,3,4,5,6,2′,3′,4′,5′,6′-decaBDE.

weight loss, a decreased milk production and a very typical effect on hoof growth. Fries (1985) estimated that up to 250 kg of FireMaster was fed to livestock, of which 125 kg was eliminated through the faeces and 94 kg ended up in human foods before regulation. Elevated levels of PBBs can still be measured in the milk of women in the affected area. In general, the use of PBBs has stopped and these compounds do not appear to be a major concern any more. However, this may not be the case for the PBDEs and HBCD.

20.5.1 Toxicity of flame retardants

In general the data on the toxicity of the PBDEs is rather limited (Darnerud *et al.*, 2001). The decabrominated compound has been tested extensively, showing that the compound is not mutagenic or genotoxic (Hardy, 2002). There are, however, indications for weak carcinogenic effects in livers of male mice. Preliminary reports on the potential binding of the non-planar compounds to the Ah receptor (Meerts *et al.* 1998; Brown *et al.* 2001), can probably be attributed to impurities, most likely brominated dioxins. This is shown by more recent data from studies with purified standards (Peters *et al.*, 2003). This contradiction may be explained by the presence of brominated dioxins in the test compounds, but at the same time there are strong indications that these compounds are also present in the technical products used in practice. Furthermore, they may be formed during combustion of PBDEs (Sakai *et al.*, 2001). Although data on the toxicity of bromodioxins are rather limited, Birnbaum *et al.* (2003) concluded that they are similarly toxic as their halogenated counterparts. Based on the criteria described above, including their their mechanism of action, they should be included in the TEQ principle and may in practice be added to the dioxins and dioxin-like PCBs present in food. Whether these compounds would actually contribute to a significant extent to the TEQ levels is unclear since very limited data are available on their presence in food. More data are available on the PBDEs and several recent studies have estimated the current exposure to these compounds.

In the case of PBDEs there are indications for an increased sensitivity of the foetus. As in the case of non-dioxin-like PCBs, exposure of young animals to the pentabromo congener BDE-99 (0.8 and 12 mg/kg bw/day) results in decreased learning and behavioural disturbance at a later age (Eriksson *et al.*, 2001a). Comparable effects, but to a lesser extent, were observed for the tetrabromo congener BDE-47, whereas TBBP-A showed no effects. Effects on behaviour have also been reported for the decabromo congener BDE-209 (Eriksson *et al.* 2001b). Similar to certain non-dioxin-like PCBs, PBDEs can affect the homeostasis of thyroid hormones. The LOAEL for this effect of the pentabromo BDE is around 1 mg/kg bw/day. Using a factor of 10, a NOAEL of 0.1 mg/kg bw was calculated by Darnerud *et al.* (2001).

The toxicity of HBCD has been investigated by the producers and are summarised in an EPA report (ACC, 2001; Hardy, 2001). HBCD consists of three stereo isomers (α, β, γ) which contribute 6, 8 and 80% respectively. The metabolism in rats is very extensive and more than 80% of a radiolabelled substance was excreted during the first 72 hours. The alpha congener was the relatively most persistent congener in the tissues. There are no indications that HBCD is mutagenic, genotoxic or carcinogenic. Exposure of rats exposed for 28 or 90 days resulted in reversible effects on liver size, as well as histological effects on liver and thyroid. There was also a decrease in thyroid hormone (T4) levels in the blood. The LOAEL was around 300 mg/kg bw/day, the NOAEL at 100 mg/kg bw/day. As in the case of PCBs and dioxins, these effects could be caused by induction of liver enzymes, resulting in an increased degradation of T4.

20.5.2 Analysis of flame retardants

Most of the brominated flame retardants like the PBBs and PBDEs can be analysed by GC using ECD or MS detection. In particular the BDE 209 may cause problems and requires specific measures. HBCD, being a mixture of three different congeners, can be analysed by LC/MS. Bromodioxins require HRGC/HRMS analysis.

20.5.3 Exposure to flame retardents

Darnerud *et al.* (2001) estimated the average exposure in Sweden at 51 ng/day based on market basket samples. This study was based on the congeners 47, 99, 100, 153 and 154. Using the same congeners Ryan and Patry (2001), Lind *et al.* (2002) and Wijesekera *et al.* (2002) calculated intakes for the Canadian, Swedish and British population of respectively 44, 41 and 91 ng/day. Bocio *et al.* (2003) calculated from the total diet study mentioned above for dioxins (Llobet *et al.*, 2003), a slightly higher intake for the Catalonian population being around 90 ng/day. An even higher intake was calculated by Winter-Sorkina *et al.* (2003) for the Dutch population, being around 213 ng/day. In these studies it was shown that fish, pork and beef contributed most to the intake. PBDEs have also been detected in human blood and milk in the lower ng/g lipid levels, thus being much lower than levels of PCBs. Although levels have increased over the last decades, there are some indications that at least for PBDEs these levels have reached their maximum and started to decline (Sjödin *et al.*, 2003).

Winter-Sorkina *et al.* (2003) also estimated the average daily intake of HBCD in the Netherlands and came to a figure of 190 ng/day. This figure was similar to the one estimated by Lind *et al.* (2002) for the average daily intake in Sweden, being around 162 ng/day with a 95th percentile of 332 ng/day.

Based on the NOAEL of 100 g/kg bw/day mentioned above, it is clear that the margin between the current average exposure around 1 ng/kg bw/day and the toxicological relevant intake is several orders of magnitude. The margin for HBCD was even higher. However, this margin wil be less for frequent consumers of products containing higher levels. Furthermore, the toxicological data are still scarce and results from ongoing research, in particular with respect to early development, may result in a lower NOAEL.

20.6 Abbreviations

2,4,5-T:	2,4,5-trichlorophenoxyacetic acid
AHH:	arylhydrocarbon hydroxylase
bw:	body weight
EROD:	ethoxyresorufin-O-deethylase
GC-ECD:	Gas chromatography-Electron capture detection
HBCD:	hexabromocyclododecane
HpCDD:	heptachlorodibenzo-p-dioxin
HpCDF:	heptachlorobenzofuran
HxCDD:	hexachlorodibenzo-p-dioxin
HxCDF:	hexachlorobenzofuran
MWI:	municipal waste incinerator
OCDD:	octachlorodibenzo-p-dioxin
OCDF:	octachlorobenzofuran
PBB:	polybromobiphenyls
PBDEs:	polybromodiphenylethers
PCBs:	polychlorobiphenyls
PCDD:	polychlorinated dibenzo-p-dioxins
PCDF:	polychlorinated dibenzofurans
PCP:	pentachlorophenol
PeCDD:	pentachlorodibenzo-p-dioxin
PeCDF:	pentachlorobenzofuran
SCF:	Scientific Committee on Food
TCDD:	2,3,7,8-tetrachlorodibenzo-p-dioxin
TCDF:	2,3,7,8-tetrachlorobenzofuran
TEF:	Toxic equivalency factor
TEQ:	Toxic equivalents
WHO:	World Health Organisation
ww:	wet weight

20.7 References

ACC (2001). 'Data summary and test plan for hexabromocyclododecane (HBCD)', at www.epa.gov/chemrtk/cyclodod/c13459.pdf

BAARS A J, BAKKER M I, BAUMANN R A, BOON P E, FREIJER J I, HOOGENBOOM L A P, HOOGERBRUGGE R, KLAVEREN J D, LIEM A K D, TRAAG W A and VRIES J DE (2004), 'Dioxins, dioxin-like PCBs and non-dioxin-like PCBs in foodstuffs: occurrence and dietary intake in the Netherlands', *Toxicology Letters* (in press).

BERG M VAN DEN, BIRNBAUM L S, BOSVELD A T C, BRUNSTRÖM B, COOK PH, FEELEY M, GIESY J P, HANBERG A, HASEGAWA R, KENNEDY S W, KUBIAK T, LARSEN J C, LEEUWEN F X R VAN, LIEM A K D, NOLT C, PETERSON R E, POELLINGER, L, SAFE, S, SCHRENK, D, TILLITT, D, TYSKLIND, M, YOUNES, M., WÄRN, F and ZACHAREWSKI, T (1998), 'Toxic Equivalency Factors (TEFs) for PCBs, PCDDs, PCDFs for humans and wildlife', *Environmental Health Perspectives*, 106, 775–792.

BERNARD A, HERMANS C, BROECKAERT F, POORTER G DE, COCK A DE and HOINS G (1999), 'Food contamination by PCBs and dioxins; an isolated episode in Belgium is unlikely to have affected public health', *Nature*, 401, 231–232.

BIRNBAUM L S, STASKAL D F and DILIBERTO J J (2003), 'Health effects of polybrominated dibenzo-p-dioxins (PBDDs) and dibenzofurans (PBDFs)', *Environment International*, 29, 855–860.

BOCIO A, LLOBET J M, DOMINGO J L, CORBELLA J, TEIXIDÓ A and CASAS C (2003), 'Polybrominated diphenyl ethers (PBDEs) in foodstuffs: human exposure through the diet', *J. Agric. Food Chem.*, 51, 3191–3195.

BROWN D J, VAN OVERMEIRE I, GOEYENS L, DENISON M S and CLARK G C (2001), 'Analysis of brominated flame retardants and brominated dibenzodioxins and biphenyls for Ah receptor activation using the CALUX bioassay', *Organohalogen Comp.*, 54, 12–15.

CARTER, L.J. (1976), 'Michigan's PBB incident : chemical mix-up leads to disaster', *Science*, 192, 240–243.

DARNERUD P O, ERIKSEN G S, JÓHANNESSON T, LARSEN P B and VILUKSELA M (2001), 'Polybrominated diphenyl ethers: occurrence, dietary exposure, and toxicology', *Environm. Health Persp. Suppl.* 109, 49–68.

DE BOER J, HORST A VAN DER and WESTER P G (2000) 'PBDEs and PBBs in suspended particulate matter, sediments, sewage treatment plant in- and effluents and biota from the Netherlands', *Organohalogen. Comp.*, 47, 85–88.

EC (2001), 'Council regulation (EC) No 2375/2001 of 29 November 2001 amending Commission Regulation (EC) No 466/2001 setting maximum levels for certain contaminants in foodstuffs', *Official Journal of the European Communities*, L321, 1–5.

EC (2002), 'Council directive 2001/102/EC of 27 November 2001 amending Directive a999/29/EC on the undesirable substances and products in animal nutrition', *Official Journal of the European Communities*, L6, 45–49.

ERIKSSON P, JAKOBSSON E and FREDERIKSSON A (2001a), 'Brominated flame retardants: a novel class of developmental neurotoxicants in our environment?', *Environm. Health Persp.*, 109, 903–908.

ERIKSSON P, VIBERG H, ANKARBERG E, JAKOBSSON E, ÖRN E and FREDERIKSSON A (2001b), 'Polybrominated diphenyl ethers (PBDEs): a novel class of environmental neurotoxicants in our environment', *Proceedings of the second international workshop on brominated flame retardants, BFR* 2001, pp 71–73.

FERRARIO J P, BYRNE C J and CLEVERLY D H (2000), '2,3,7,8–Dibenzo-p-dioxins in mined clay products from the United States: evidence for possible natural origin', *Environmental Science and Technology*, 34, 4524–4532.

FIRESTONE D (1973), 'Etiology of chick edema disease', *Environmental Health Perspectives*, 5, 59–66.

FRIES, G.F. (1985), 'The PBB episode in Michigan: an overall appraisal', *CRC Critical Reviews in Toxicology*, 16, 105–156.

GUO J, SARTOT M, KARAYALAS, MEDVEDOVIC M, KANN S, PUGA A, RYAN P and TOMLINSON C G (2004), 'Expression of genes in the TGF-β signalling pathway is significantly deregulated in smooth muscle cells from aorta of aryl hydrocarbon receptor knockout mice', *Toxicolpgy and Applied Pharmocology*, 1994, 79–89.

HARDY M L (2001), 'Regulatory status and environmental properties of brominated flame retardants undergoing risk assessment in the EU: DBDPO, OBDPO, PeBDPO and HBCD', *Polymer Degradation and Stability* 64, 545–556.

HARDY M L (2002) 'The toxicology of the three commercial polybrominated diphenyl oxide (ether) flame retardants', *Chemosphere*, 46, 757–777.

HAYWARD D G, NORTRUP D, GARDNER A and CLOWER M (1999), 'Elevated TCDD in chicken eggs and farm-raised catfish fed a diet with ball clay from a Southern United States mine', *Environmental Research Section A*, 81, 248–256.

HIGGINBOTHAM G R, HUANG A, FIRESTONE D, VERRETT J, RESS J and CAMPBELL A D (1968), 'Chemical and toxicological evaluations of isolated and synthetic chloro derivatives of dibenzo-p-dioxin', *Nature*, 220, 702–703.

HOOGENBOOM L A P (2002), 'The Combined use of the CALUX bioassay and the HRGC/HRMS method for the detection of novel dioxin sources and new dioxin-like compounds', *Environmental Science and Pollution. Research*, 9, 9–11.

HOOGENBOOM L A P, TRAAG W A and MENGELERS M J B (1999), 'The Belgian dioxin crisis; involvement of RIKILT', poster presented at Dioxin '99 in Venice, Italy.

HOOGENBOOM L A P, TRAAG W A, HOOGERBRUGGE R, BAUMANN B, PORTIER L, WEG G VAN DER and VRIES J DE (2004), 'The use of the CALUX-bioassay and indicator-PCBs for screening of elevated levels of dioxins and dioxin-like PCBs in eel'. *Food Add. Contam.* (submitted).

HSU S T, MA C I, HSU S K, WU S S, HSU N H and YEH C (1985), 'Discovery and epidemiology of PCB poisoning in Taiwan: a four-year follow-up', *Environmental Health Perspectives* 59, 5–10.

KURATSUNE M, YOSHIMURA T, MATSUZAKA J and YAMAGUCHI A (1972), 'Epidemiologic study on Yusho, a poisoning caused by ingestion of rice oil contaminated with a commercial brand of polychlorinated biphenyls', *Environmental Health Perspectives,* 1, 119–128.

LAREBEKE N VAN, HENS L, SCHEPENS P, COVACI A, BAYENS J, EVERAERT K, BERNHEIM J L, VLIETINCK R and POORTER G DE (2001), 'The Belgian PCB and dioxin incident of January-June 1999: exposure data and potential impact on health', *Environmental Health Perspectives*, 109, 265–273.

LIEM A K D, HOOGERBRUGGE R, KOOTSTRA P R, VAN DER VELDE E G and DE JONG A P J M (1991), 'Occurrence of dioxins in cow's milk in the vicinity of municipal waste incinerators and a metal reclamation plant in the Netherlands', *Chemosphere*, 23, 1975–1984.

LIEM A K D, FÜRST P and RAPPE C (2000), 'Exposure of populations to dioxins and related compounds', *Food Additives and Contaminants*, 4, 241–259.

LIND Y, AUNE M, ATUMA S, BECKER W, BJERSELIUS R, GLYN A and DARNERUD P O (2002) 'Food intake of the brominated flame retardants PBDEs and HBCD in Sweden', *Organohalogen Comp.*, 58, 181–184.

LLERENA J J, ABAD E, CAIXACH J and RIVERA J (2003) 'An episode of dioxin contamination in feedingstuff: the choline chloride case', *Chemosphere*, 53, 679–683.

LLOBET J M, DOMINGO J L, BOCIO A, CASAS C, TEIXIDÓ A and MÜLLER L (2003), 'Human exposure to dioxins through the diet in Catalonia, Spain: carcinogenic and non-carcinogenic risk', *Chemosphere*, 50, 1193–1200.

MALISCH R (2000), 'Increase of the PCDD/F-contamination of milk, butter and meat samples by use of contaminated citrus pulp', *Chemosphere*, 40, 1041–1053.

MEERTS I, LUIJKS E, MARSH G, JAKOBSSON E, BERGMAN A and BROUWER A (1998), 'Polybrominated diphenylethers (PCBEs) as Ah-receptor agonists and antagonists', *Organohalogen Compounds*, 37, 147–150.

OLIE K, VERMEULEN P L and HUTZINGER O (1977), 'Chlorodibenzo-p-dioxins and chlorodibenzofurans are trace components of fly ash and flue gas of some municipal incinerators in the Netherlands', *Chemosphere*, 8, 455–459.

PETERS A K, SANDERSON J T, BERGMAN A and BERG M VAN DEN (2003) 'Induction and inhibition of cytochrome P450 1A1, 1B1, and ethoxyresorufin-O-deethylation activity by polybrominated diphenyl ethers (PBDE) in MCF7 cells', *Organohalogen Comp.*, 61, 100–103.

PLAS S A VAN DER, SUNDBERG H, BERG H VAN DEN, SCHEU G, WESTER P, JENSEN S, BERGMAN A, DE BOER J, KOEMAN J H and BROUWER A (2001), 'Contribution of planar (0-1 ortho) and non-planar (2–4 ortho) fractions of Arochlor 1260 to the induction of altered hepatic foci in female Spague-Dawley rats', *Toxicoogy and Applied Pharmacology*, 169, 255–268.

RIER S E, MARTIN D C, BOWMAN R E, DMOWSKI W P and BECKER J L (1993), 'Endometriosis in Rhesus monkeys (Macata mulatta) following chronic exposure to 2,3,7,8 tetrachlorodibenzo-p-dioxin', *Fundamental and Applied Toxicology*, 21, 433–441.

RYAN J K and PATRY B (2001) 'Body burdens and food exposure in Canada for polybrominated diphenyl ethers (BDEs)', *Organohalogen Comp.*, 51, 226–229.

SAFE S H (1994), 'Polychlorinated biphenyls (PCBs): environmental impact, biochemical and toxic responses, and implications for risk assessment', *Critical Reviews in Toxicology*, 24, 87–149.

SAFE S H (1995) 'Human dietary intake of arylhydrocarbon (Ah) receptor agonists: mass balance estimates of exodioxins and endodioxins and implications for health assessment', *Organohalogen Comp.*, 26, 7–13.

SAFE S H (1998) 'Development validation and problems with the Toxic Equivalency factor approach for risk assessment of dioxins and related compounds', *L. Anim. Sci.*, 76, 134–141.

SAKAI S, WATANABE J, HONDA Y, TAKATSUKI H, AOKI I, FUTAMATSU M and SHIOZAKI K (2001), 'Combustion of brominated flame retardants and behavior of its byproducts', *Chemosphere* 42, 519–531.

SANGER V L, SCOTT L, HAMDY A, GALE C and POUNDEN W D (1958), 'Alimentary toxemia in chickens', *Journal of the American Veterinary Medical Association*, 133, 172–176.

SCF (2001), 'Opinion of the Scientific Committee on Food on the risk assessment of dioxins and dioxin-like PCBs in food. Scientific Committee on Food report CS/CNTM/DIOXIN/20 final', http://europa.eu.int/comm/food/fs/sc/scf/out90_en.pdf.

SCHMIDT, C.W. (1999), 'Poisoning young minds', *Environmental Health Perspectives*, 107, 302–307.

SCHMITTLE S C, EDWARDS H M and MORRIS D (1958), 'A disorder of chickens probably due to a toxic feed-preliminary report', *Journal of the American Veterinary Medical Association*, 132, 216–219.

SJÖDIN A, PATTERSON D G and BERGMAN A (2003) 'A review on human exposure to brominated flame retardants-particularly polybrominated diphenyl ethers', *Environment International*, 29, 829–839.

TSUTSUMI T, YANAGI T, NAKAMURA M, KONO Y, UCHIBE H, IIDA T, HORI T, NAKAGAWA R, TOBIISHI K, MATSUDA R, SASAKI K and TOYODA M (2001), 'Uptake of daily intake of PCDDs, PCDFs, and dioxin-like PCBs from food in Japan', *Chemosphere*, 45, 1129–1137.

WHO (2000), 'Consultation on assessment of the health risk of dioxins; re-evaluation of the tolerable daily intake (TDI): executive summary', *Food Additives and Contaminants*, 17, 223–240.

WIJESEKERA R, HALLIWELL C, HUNTER S and HARRAD S A (2002) 'A preliminary assessment of UK human exposure to polybrominated diphenyl ethers (PBDEs)',

Organohalogen Comp., 55, 239–242.

WINTER-SORKINA R DE, BAKKER M I, DONKERSGOED G VAN and KLAVEREN J D VAN (2003), 'Dietary intake of brominated flame retardants by the Dutch population', RIVM-report 310305001/2003, Bilthoven, The Netherlands.

WUNDERLI S, ZENNEGG M, DOLEZAL I S, GUJER E, MOSER U, WOLFENSBERGER M, HASLER P, NOGER D, STUDER C and KARLAGANIS G (2000), 'Determination of polychlorinated dibenzo-p-dioxins and dibenzo-furans in solid residues from wood combustion by HRGC/HRMS', *Chemosphere*, 40, 641–649.

21

Detecting organic contaminants in food: the case of fish and shellfish

S. van Leeuwen and J. de Boer, Netherlands Institute for Fisheries Research

21.1 Introduction: the problem of organic contaminants

Over the last two decades, organic contaminants in the environment and food have gained much attention from scientists, policy makers, manufacturers and environmental non-governmental organisations. From a food safety point of view, crises on contaminants like the Belgian dioxin crisis (1999), in which polychlorinated biphenyls (PCBs) entered the food chain as a result of using PCB-contaminated oil for production of feed, have increased consumers' concern on contaminants in their food. Fish and shellfish are susceptible to contamination with undesired substances that have entered the aquatic environment prior to, during or after use and production of these substances.

The importance of contaminants with regard to the health of humans is normally based on the following criteria: persistence; bioaccumulation and toxic effect. Another aspect that should be taken into account is the production volume of the chemicals. A very toxic substance may be of relatively low importance when its production volume is very limited. The production and use of some of the contaminants discussed in this book, such as PCBs, was stopped years ago, whereas substances with comparable properties and behaviour are still produced and used in high quantities, like polybrominated diphenyl ethers (PBDEs).

This chapter will discuss concentrations of a wide range of organic contaminants in fish and shellfish. Furthermore, the sources and contamination of fish will be discussed as well as general principles of analysis. Finally, future trends and sources for further information are briefly addressed.

21.2 Sources of organic contaminants

Organic contaminants originate from a variety of sources. With the exception of halogenated dibenzo-p-dioxins (PCDDs) and – furans (PCDFs) and polycyclic aromatic hydrocarbons (PAHs), most organic contaminants have originally been manufactured as formulations for specific applications. In most cases these formulations are complex mixtures with varying degrees of halogenation, depending on the physicochemical properties required by the application.

Most manufactured contaminants are made from the chlorination (or bromination) of the parent hydrocarbon in the presence of an appropriate catalyst. The production, properties and usage of each group of contaminants have been extensively reviewed and is well documented (Brinkman and de Kok, 1980; WHO, 1992, 1994a, b; Erickson, 1997). The primary sources of these compounds are in many cases interdependent, and examples are now discussed.

21.2.1 Direct manufacture for use in either open or closed systems

Various compounds and formulations have been manufactured for use in open systems such as additives in plastics or sealed systems as transformers. This group comprises PCBs, polychlorinated terphenyls (PCTs), polybrominated biphenyls (PBBs), PBDEs, polychlorinated alkanes (PCAs) and polychlorinated naphthalenes (PCNs). These contaminants span a wide application range including use as plasticisers, flame retardants, lubricants, in cutting oils in metal works, dielectric fluids, paper coatings and printing inks. For example, PBDEs are generally applied as flame retardants in materials to prevent them from catching fire (de Boer, 2000a, b, c), whereas PCAs find their application as, for example, plasticiser in polyvinyl chloride (PVC), rubber paintings and as extreme pressure lubricant in the metal working industry (Slooff *et al.*, 1992; Muir *et al.*, 2000; Poremski *et al.*, 2001).

Musk compounds find their application as synthetic fragrances in personal care products and alkyl phenolic compounds (and their ethoxylates) originate from application as, for example, detergents (Staples *et al.*, 1998).

21.2.2 Impurities in manufacture and subsequent use of the primary product

PCDDs are present as impurities in pentachlorophenol (PCP) used as a wood preservative, and in herbicides such as Agent Orange which is used as a defoliant. PCNs and polybrominated naphthalenes (PBNs) are present as impurities in PCB and PBB manufacture, respectively. In addition, PCDDs and PCDFs are present as impurities in the high temperature chlorination manufacture of other chlorinated contaminants. Unlike the PBDEs, the chlorinated homologues (PCDEs) are not manufactured directly for commercial use, but they are an impurity of technical chlorophenols primarily produced as wood preservatives.

21.2.3 Formation through the disposal of other contaminants

PCDDs and PCDFs are formed in the incineration of material containing PCBs, PCNs and PVC. PCDDs and PCDFs are not manufactured and have no commercial use. They are formed as by-products of incineration of waste products, combustion of sewage sludge and fires containing chlorinated materials such as PCBs, PVC, PCP and PCDEs (Fiedler *et al.*, 1990). Most of these compounds are formed in the incineration process when the temperature is not sufficient to completely destroy the parent compounds. A similar process occurs with brominated flame retardants (BFRs) such as PBBs and PBDEs from which polybrominated dibenzodioxins (PBDDs) and dibenzofurans (PBDFs) are formed (Sakai *et al.* 2001).

21.2.4 Direct manufacture for use as pesticides

Organochlorine pesticides (OCPs) have been produced mainly for agricultural applications. The group of OCPs comprises a variety of compounds like aldrin, dieldrin, lindane, DDT, toxaphene and hexachlorobenzene (HCB).

21.3 Organic contaminants in fish

21.3.1 Accumulation of organic contaminants in fish

The main source of contaminants is via uptake through the aquatic food web to fish and shellfish. Due to the lipophilicity of most of the contaminants, these substances are well absorbed in the lipids of fish. The uptake can take place either directly from the surrounding water or by uptake from food (bio-accumulation) (Geyer *et al.*, 2000), leading to higher concentrations in fish compared with their food or surrounding water. Concentrations can increase further when the fish serves as food for other (bigger) carnivorous species, leading to biomagnification (Geyer *et al.*, 2000) in the food chain.

For farmed fish the main source of contamination is the feed, which can be composed of potentially contaminated ingredients like fish meal and fish oil. Fish oil originating from European waters shows dioxin concentrations about 10 times higher compared with oil originating from the Pacific (SCAN, 2000). In particular, the diet of carnivorous species contains substantial amounts of fish oil and meal, leading up to 98% of relative contribution of fish oil and fish meal to the contamination of fish with dioxins (SCAN, 2000). A recent study showed considerable levels of dioxins, PCBs, toxaphene and OCPs in European farmed salmon which are likely to relate to the elevated levels of these contaminants in European salmon feed (Hites *et al.*, 2004).

The lipophilic contaminants are generally very persistent and fish show limited ability to eliminate these contaminants by diffusion or by transformation (e.g. in the liver followed by excretion). An exception are the PAHs which are metabolised in the gall-bladder and subsequently excreted (Baussant *et al.*, 2001) and are therefore generally not found in fish. However, shellfish have no ability to metabolise PAHs and therefore these substances accumulate in shellfish.

21.3.2 Polycyclic aromatic hydrocarbons (PAHs)

As described above, PAHs do not normally occur in fish and are, therefore, of no importance with respect to human health. Shellfish, however, metabolise PAHs only to a minor extent and therefore accumulate PAHs.

There is no recent data on concentrations of PAHs in Dutch mussels (see Table 21.1), but data from 1991 shows concentrations up to 6.8 μg/kg wet weight (ww) for the sum of 13 PAHs and concentrations below 1 μg/kg ww for the carcinogenic benzo(a)pyrene. PAH concentrations reported from the Mediterranean are extremely high as they are expressed on a dry weight (dw) basis (see Table 21.1). There is only limited data available from scientific publications and therefore, the current situation concerning PAHs in mussels and other shellfish is not clear, which shows the need for new data.

21.3.3 Polychlorinated biphenyls (PCBs)

The group of PCBs is a complex mixture, consisting of 209 congeners. A representative selection of congeners, the seven so-called indicator PCBs (CB 28, 52, 101, 118, 138, 153 and 180) are regularly analysed in fish samples and are often included in monitoring programmes. Therefore, a vast amount of data is available (see Table 21.2).

Eel samples from polluted areas in the Netherlands like Haringvliet, river Meuse, river Rhine and Western Scheldt show high concentrations of PCBs up to 730 μg/kg ww for CB 153, occasionally exceeding Dutch maximum residue limits (MRLs) (Anon., 1984). Fish originating from other places than the contamination hot spots (e.g. industrialised areas and polluted rivers) generally show significantly lower concentrations. Marine fish generally show lower concentrations compared with freshwater fish due to dilution of the more contaminated river effluents (Atuma *et al.*, 1996; Ylitalo *et al.*, 1999; Leonards *et al.*, 2000).

For farmed salmon there was no clear difference in PCB concentrations compared with wild salmon from Scotland. Concentrations of PCBs in farmed salmon were both higher and lower than the investigated wild salmon samples (Jacobs *et al.*, 2001a, b). This was also observed for OCPs and PBDEs in farmed and wild salmon (Jacobs *et al.*, 2001a, b). Clearly, concentrations in farmed salmon depend very much on the origination of fish oil and fish meal used in the feed. Fish oil and meal from the Pacific generally contain lower concentrations of contaminants compared with fish oil from Europe (SCAN, 2000). In another study the concentrations of contaminants (including PCBs) were significantly higher in European salmon compared to salmon from North America (Hites *et al.*, 2004).

Since the production and use of PCBs stopped in the early 1980s, temporal trends show clearly declining PCB concentrations in freshwater and marine fish up to a

Table 21.1 Typical concentrations of PAHs in fish and shellfish (μg/kg)

Country	Location	Year	Species	BaP*	DahA	BaA	BbF	BkF	IP	Ch	Fluo	P	Py	ww/dw**	References
The Netherlands	Various	1991	Mussels	0.6	< 1	1.2	4.7	1.2	1.1	1.9	6.4		6.8	ww	LAC (1991)
Italy	Mediterranean Sea	1999	Mussels	7–127		5.7–250	12–218	14–98		19–262	67–924	21–436	29–351	dw	Piccardo *et al.* (2001)
France	Mediterranean Sea	1995	Mussels	0.2–9.7	0.24–2.9***	0.11–16	2–39****		0.62–7.5	3.6–142	1.2–20	7.4–86	1.2–53	dw	Baumard *et al.* (1998)

* BaP: benzo(a)pyrene, DahA: dibenzo(a,h)anthracene, BaA: benzo(a)anthracene, BbF: benzo(b)fluoranthene, BkF: benzo(k)fluoranthene, IP: indeno(1, 2, 3-c,d)pyrene, Ch: chrysene, Fluo: fluoranthene, P: phenanthrene: Py: pyrene
** ww: wet weight and dw: dry weight
*** Including dibenzo[a, c]anthracene
**** Including benzo[j]fluoranthene and benzo[k]fluoranthene

Table 21.2 Typical concentrations of PCBs in fish (μg/kg)

Country	Year	Species	CB 28	CB 52	CB 101	CB 118	CB 138	CB 153	CB 180	Sum	ww/dw	References
Sweden	1992–93	Various Eel	< 0.05–0.38 0.81	< 0.05–2.3 5.4	0.09–7.9 19	0.07–6.6 30	0.25–13 50	0.35–20 69	0.08–4.8 19		ww	Atuma *et al.* (1996)
Barents and Greenland Sea	1991–92	Various	ND–1.8	0.1–8.2	0.5–42	0.3–16	1.3–29	0.2–22	0.7-6.8	6.0–113 (11)*	dw	Ali *et al.* (1997)
Netherlands	1999	Eel	<0.7–12	1.5–110	1.7–160	2.5–160	6.3–390**	9.0–730	2.9–270		ww	de Boer *et al.* (2000a)
Netherlands	2000	Various marine and freshwater	< 0.1–8.7	< 0.1–42	< 0.1–77	< 0.1–77	0.04–130	< 0.1–200	< 0.1–74		ww	Leonards *et al* (2000)
UK, Mersey estuary, Liverpool Bay	1990–92	Various vertebrates	0.2–1.1	0.1–1.9	0.7–3.7		3–4.5	2.7–4.9	1.2–2.2		ww	Leah *et al.* (1997)
West of UK	1991–94	Mackerel			5.0–8.7	ND-6.8	4.8–17	5.7–22	1.3–5.6		ww	Karl and Lehman (1997)
USA, Great Lakes	1993?	Various		1.4–6.9		3.3–8.5	8.9–20	3.5–19	4.0–10***			
USA, San Francisco Bay	1994	Various fish from anglers								17–638****	ww	Fairey *et al.* (1997)
USA, North/South Atlantic and Monterey Bay	1992–98	Various	0.3–9.1	0.9–36	3.1–70	3.2–56	13–176	7.6–234	9.6–90	50–1400 (24)	lw	Froeschesies *et al.* (2000)
USA, Altantic/ Pacific coast	1993–94	Various			0.39–14	0.28–5.5	ND-7.8	0.43–19	0.20–6.0		ww	Ylitalo *et al.* (1999)
North America, Europe	2001–02	Farmed salmon								Up to 55 (n = ?)	ww	Hites *et al.* (2004)

ND: not detected; * In brackets: number of summarised congeners; ** Sum CB 138 and CB 163; *** Sum CB-180 and CB 193; **** Expressed as the sum of Arochlors 1248, 1254, 1260 and 5460 factor of four in North-America and Europe (Picer and Picer, 1994; de Vault *et al.*, 1996; Roose *et al.*, 1998; de Boer *et al.*, 2000a). From Table 21.2 it is clear that CB 138 and CB 153 are the predominant congeners in fish samples.

21.3.4 Polychlorinated dibenzodioxins (PCDDs) and -furans (PCDFs) and dioxin-like PCBs (dl-PCBs)

The availability of data within the European Union (EU) on dioxins has increased considerably after the Belgian dioxin crisis in 1999. Following this crisis, legislation on dioxins in food and feed has become active in the EU since 1 July 2002. The MRLs for fish and fish oil for human consumption are 4 pg PCDD/F-toxic equivalents (TEQ)/g ww and 1.5 pg PCDD/F-TEQ/g lw, respectively. Dioxin-like PCBs (dl-PCBs) are not included in this MRL, but will be included in legislation in the future (2004).

Biological samples often contain a complex mixture of PCDD/Fs and dl-PCBs. 2, 3, 7, 8–TCDD is the most potent dioxin-congener with a the toxic equivalency factor (TEF) of 1 and the potency of other congeners or dl-PCBs is equal or lower. The concentration of individual congeners multiplied by their TEF factors results in the total concentration of dioxins and dl-PCBs, expressed in TEQs (van den Berg *et al.*, 1998). The TEQ principle has been discussed in more detail in Chapter 20.

The data from the SCOOP assessment (see Table 21.3) show that most fish samples were well below the EU MRL, although a crab sample from Sweden and Baltic salmon showed concentrations of 10.2 and 7.0 pg TEQ/g product, respectively (SCOOP, 2000). Data on dl-PCBs was limited probably due to the fact that accurate methods of analysis have only become available in the last 5–10 years (Hess *et al.*, 1995). High concentrations of dioxins and dl-PCBs were also found in pike perch from the Netherlands, farmed salmon and tuna from the Mediterranean (Leonards *et al.*, 2000), herring from Scotland (Parsley *et al.*, 1998) and some samples from Asia (Sakurai *et al.*, 2000; Jeong *et al.*, 2001).

Eel from several polluted main rivers in the Netherlands showed high concentrations of dioxins and dl-PCBs up to 7.9 and 44 pg TEQ/g ww, respectively, whereas in lakes and smaller rivers concentrations were considerably lower (van Leeuwen *et al.*, 2002). Concentrations of dioxins and (dl-)PCBs in farmed eel were within the range of the wild eel samples (van Leeuwen *et al.*, 2002). Concentrations of dioxins and dl-PCBs in farmed eel and imported eel were below the EU MRL. The dl-PCBs in the eel samples contributed significantly more (average *ca.* 80%) to the total TEQ compared with the contribution of dioxins. Also in fish other than eel dl-PCBs generally predominantly contribute to the total TEQ, although contribution figures have a wider range (from *ca.* 50–95%) (Leonards *et al.*, 2000). As far as future EU legislation is concerned, it is not yet clear how future MRLs will evolve when dl-PCBs are included in legislation (expected by the end of 2004).

Table 21.3 Typical concentrations of PCDDs, PCDFs and dioxin-like PCBs in fish and shellfish (ng TEQ/kg)

Country	Year	Species	WHO / I	PCDD/F	PCB	Sum	lw/ww	References
Denmark	1995-99	Various	I	0.01–1.6			ww	SCOOP (2000)*
Finland		Trout, farmed		0.74	1.5			
Norway		Crab		10.2				
Sweden		Various		0.13–7.0**	0.23–9.1**			
UK		Various		0.03–2.1	0.07–6.2			
Italy		Various		0.1–0.86				
Netherlands	2002	Eel, freshwater	WHO	0.21–7.9	0.7–44	0.89–52		van Leeuwen *et al.* (2002)
		Eel, farmed		0.9–3.1	2.8–7.7	3.9–11		
North Sea	2000	Various marine and freshwater fish	WHO	0.01–3.9	0.02–33	0.03–37	ww	Leonards *et al.* (2000)
Scotland	1995–96	Cod, haddock, plaice, whiting	WHO	0.01–0.52	0.01–0.85	0.02–1.3	ww	Parsley *et al.* (1998)
		Salmon		0.57–0.99	1.3–3.0	2.2–3.9		
		Mackerel		0.14–1.7	0.34–6.0	0.48–7.5		
		Herring		0.34–3.8	0.46–10	6.8–14		
Italy, Adriatic Sea	1997–98	Various	I	0.07–1.1			ww	Bayarri *et al.* (2001)
Japan, Tokyo bay	1995	Various fish	I	0.32–2.1			ww	Sakurai *et al.* (2000)
		Japanese cockle		3.6				
		Crab		2.6				
Korea, Main river systems	1999–00	Crucian		ND–4.1			ww	Jeong *et al.* (2001)
		Minnow		ND–1.1				
Korea, market fish	1999	Various		0.013–0.58			ww	Ok *et al.* (2001)
Korea, major cities	2000?	Various salt water and shellfish	WHO	0.001–2.9	0.001–6.7		ww	Choi *et al.* (2001)
North America, Europe	2001–02	Salmon, farmed	WHO			1–3.3	ww	Hites *et al.* (2004)

* National average concentrations of 1995–1999 data
** High concentrations originate from Baltic salmon

21.3.5 Polybrominated diphenyl ethers (PBDEs) and other brominated flame retardants (BFRs)

Although concentrations of PBDEs in fish have been determined since the late 1970s (de Boer and Dao, 1993), considerable data have only recently become available due to an increased awareness of the environmental impact of PBDEs (Luross *et al.*, 2002; Rice *et al.*, 2002; de Boer *et al.*, 2003; Hale *et al.*, 2003). From Table 21.4 it is clear that, generally, concentrations of the tetra- and penta-BDEs are predominant over concentrations of higher brominated BDEs, due to the use of the penta-mixture mainly consisting of tetra and penta-BDEs (de Boer, 2000b).

The concentration of the various BDEs in freshwater and marine fish ranges from the mid ng/kg to mid μg/kg range. Generally, when levels are transformed to a wet weight (or product) basis, it can be concluded that the levels in fish from the Great Lakes (Canada) and the Baltic Sea are higher compared to levels in samples from other locations. Among the Great Lakes, Lake Ontario showed considerably higher levels than the other lakes, which might be explained by possible local point sources in the heavily urbanised lake basin (Luross *et al.*, 2002).

De Boer and Allchin (2001) established temporal trends of PBDEs in eel originating from the Haringvliet-East in the Netherlands and found an approximate eight-fold decrease in concentrations of BDE 47 from 1979 to 1999 (*ca.* 1200 to *ca.* 150 μg/kg lw). On the other hand, exponential increases of tetra-, penta- and hexa-BDE concentrations were detected between 1981 and 2000 in ringed seals in the Canadian Arctic (Ikonomou *et al.*, 2002), reflecting the continuing production and use of high volumes of the technical penta-BDE mixture in North America (Alcock *et al.*, 2003; Hale *et al.*, 2003).

Jacobs *et al.*, (2001a) determined 9 BDE congeners in 13 samples of farmed and wild salmon (Norway, Scotland, Ireland and Belgian market) and found concentrations ranging from 5.0 to 43 μg/kg ww BDE 47 in wild salmon, whereas farmed samples contained BDE 47 at little lower concentrations of 3.1 to 29 μg/kg ww.

Only limited data is available on hexabromocyclododecane (HBCD) concentrations in fish. Concentrations in herring from the Baltic Sea and freshwater locations from Sweden showed considerable concentrations comparable to BDE concentrations. Close to point sources, high concentrations of up to 8 mg/kg lw were detected (Sellstrom *et al.*, 1998). Only recently, data on stereoisomers of HBCD has become available as a result of an isomer specific high performance liquid chromatography-electrospray ionisation-mass spectrometry (LC-ESI-MS) method of analysis (Morris *et al.*, 2003; Tomy *et al.*, 2003).

HBCD has a substantial potential for bioaccumulation. As production continues, it may be expected that HBCD will be found at considerable concentrations in seafood and freshwater fish. Tetrabromobisphenol-A (TBBP-A) data in biota are scarce because laboratories have just established methods for this flame retardant. TBBP-A has the highest production volume of all

Table 21.4 Concentrations of PBDEs and HBCD in fish and shellfish ($\mu g/kg$)

Country	Year	Species	BDE-47	BDE-99	BDE-100	BDE-153	BDE-154	Sum*	HBCD	lw/ww/dw	References
The Netherlands	1999	Flounder	0.5–20	<0.01–4.6		<0.02-<1				dw	de Boer *et al.* (2003)
		Bream	0.2–130	<0.01–<0.8		<0.9-4.1					
		Mar. Mussel	0.9–4.3	0.3–1.6		<0.1-<0.2					
		Freshw. Mussel	0.7–17	0.4–11		<0.1-1.5					
UK**	?	Eel, trout						4.9–235 (6)	20–3216	ww	Allchin and Morris (2003)
Greenland	?	Sculpin, liver	1.7–7.8							ww	
Sweden, Baltic Sea	2000?	Herring	5.8–21	1.2–8.0	1.1–3.9	0.16–1.2	0.23–1.2		4.3–36	lw	Nylund *et al.* (2001)
Sweden, freshwater***	1995	Pike	40–2000	33–1600	9.3–1000			49–4600 (3)	<50–8000	lw	Sellstrom *et al.* (1998)
Norway	?	Trout, char	0.06–8.3	0.04–8.0						ww	Schlabach *et al.* (2001)
		Burbot, liver	9.7–1044	11–911						ww	
Scotland	1999	Salmon, wild and farmed	15–43	2.8–14	2.4–9.9	ND–1.3	ND–3.6	24.6–85 (9)		lw	Jacobs *et al.* (2001)
Norway			0.4	0.7	ND	ND	ND	1.1			
Ireland	2001	Wild and farmed	5.0–26	1.3–5.6	1.1–7.9	ND	ND–1.3	8.4–52			
			3.1–10	ND–1.6	ND–2.8	ND–0.2	ND	3.1–19			
Japan	1998	Various edible marine fish****	1.2–38	0.13–2.4	0.12–1.5	0.018–1.7	0.21–1.7				Akutsu *et al.* (2001)
USA	1999	Various freshwater fish	1.3–4.0	0.48–0.50	0.44–0.49	0.4–1.0	0.43–1.89	5.3–14 (8)		ww	Rice *et al.* (2002)
Canada, Great Lakes	?	Lake trout	16–58	2.0–14	2.5–5.7	0.89–4.9				ww	Luross *et al.* (2002)
USA, Lake Ontario	?	Sculpin, trout							1–3 α-HBCD 0.3–0.7 γ-HBCD	ww	Tomy *et al.* (2003)

* In brackets the number of summed congeners
** River Skerne, affected by a sewage treatment plant
*** River Viskan, affected by possible point sources
**** Including conger eel, flounder, gray mullet, horse mackerel, red sea bream, sea bass and yellowtail

brominated flame retardants. However, due to its more polar character and the covalent binding to plastic in its applications (de Wit, 2002), it will presumably be present at lower concentrations in seafood.

21.3.6 Polychlorinated naphthalenes (PCNs)

PCN mixtures theoretically consist of 75 congeners, although the technical mixtures produced in the past show a different composition due to a different degree of chlorination (Järnberg, 1997). Although individual congeners can be detected, the data reported here are the total PCN concentrations (sum of individual congeners). Typical concentrations determined in fish during the last decade are mentioned in Table 21.5.

Fish from the Baltic Sea and from Sweden showed substantial PCN concentrations. Järnberg found very high concentrations of PCNs up to 360 μg/kg lw in pike assuming that nearby point sources of PCNs contaminated the analysed fish (Järnberg *et al.*, 1997). Baltic fish showed large variation, from 0.54 to 290 μg/kg lw and generally high compared with pg/g-concentrations (ww) found in tuna and swordfish from the Mediterranean (Kannan *et al.*, 2001a). Concentrations in fish from the USA were in the range of 0.019 μg/kg ww (Kannan *et al.*, 2000) to 33 μg/kg ww (Falandysz, 1998).

21.3.7 Polychlorinated terphenyls (PCTs)

Technical PCT mixtures are very complex as theoretically 8557 PCT congeners exist (Remberg *et al.*, 1998). It is not possible to detect individual congeners (as with PCBs) and therefore concentrations of total PCTs are reported (de Boer, 2000b). Literature data must be treated with great care because of the large variation in analytical procedures and calculation methods used.

The available dataset on PCT concentrations in the environment is very limited compared with that on PCBs. Hale *et al.* (1990) determined very high concentrations of PCTs of up to 35 000 μg/kg ww in oysters from the Back River, Chesaspeake Bay, USA, close to a major US aeronautics research facility (see Table 21.6). Much lower concentrations were determined in (shell)fish samples collected from Spanish markets which contained concentrations from *ca.* 1 to 65 μg/kg ww and Bonito Tuna contained concentrations of *ca.* 63 to 260 μg/kg ww (Fernández *et al.*, 1998). Cod liver from the southern North Sea contained concentrations of 410 μg/kg, which were ten times higher compared with the northern part of the North Sea (de Boer, 1995). However, concentrations in twaite shad, herring were considerably lower. Eel caught in Dutch freshwater showed concentrations of 6 to 200 μg/kg ww. The highest concentrations were detected in main river systems such as the rivers Meuse and Rhine. A good relationship could be determined between the concentrations of PCBs and PCTs in biota (expressed on a lipid weight basis), roughly reflecting production volumes of PCBs and PCTs (de Boer, 1995).

Table 21.5 Typical concentrations of PCNs in fish (μg/kg)

Country	Year	Species	lw/ww	Concentration	References
Italy, Mediterranean	1999	Tuna	ww	7.0–22.6*	Kannan *et al.* (2001a)
		Swordfish		14.6–14.8*	
Sweden, freshwater	?	Pike	lw	130–360**	Järnberg *et al.* (1997)
		Pike, Cod, Burbot		2.6–15	
Sweden, Baltic sea		Herring		8.4–26	
Sweden, Baltic Sea	1991–93	Sculpin	lw	0.54–1.5	Lundgren *et al.* (2002)
Poland, Gulf of Gdansk, Baltic Sea	1992	Stickleback	lw	35–130	Falandysz *et al.* (1998)
	?	Fish	lw	8.9–290***	
Baltic sea	?	Herring	lw	0.98–26***	Falandysz (1998)
USA, Purvis Creek	1997	Crab, hepatopancreas	ww	13.3****	Kannan, *et al.* (1998)
		Mullet		6.1	
USA, Great Lakes	1996–97	Various	ww	0.019–26.4	Kannan *et al.* (2000)
USA, Saginaw Bay	?	Fish	lw	0.16–33	Falandysz (1998)

* ng/kg
** Possibly close to point sources
*** Tetra to hepta-CNs
**** Near former chlor-alkali plant

Table 21.6 Typical concentrations of PCTs in fish and shellfish ($\mu g/kg$)

Country	Location	Year	Species	Concentration	lw/ww	Standard used	References
The Netherlands	Various freshwater	1991–92	Eel	6–200	ww	A5442	de Boer (1995)
	Hollandse Yssel	1990	Pike perch	5			
	Southern North Sea	1992	Cod, liver	410			
	Northern North Sea			40			
	Southern North Sea	1991	Twaite shad	10			
	Doggersbank	1990	Plaice	1			
	Dutch coast	1991	Herring	3			
USA	Fresh water creek	1987–89	Oyster	400–35 000*	?	A5432	Hale *et al.* (1990)
Spain	Market samples	1996?	Mussel	9.8–18	ww	A5460	Fernández *et al.* (1998)
			Clams	1.2–24			
			Salmon	21–64			
			Tuna (bonito)	63–259			

* Near aerospace complex

21.3.8 Polychlorinated alkanes (PCAs)

PCAs are produced by the chlorination of a mixture of (branched) alkanes with different carbon numbers. In addition a varying degree of chlorination leads to tens of thousands of possible congeners (Muir *et al.*, 2000). The PCAs are subdivided into three groups with different carbon lengths and degrees of chlorination: short chain (SCCA, C10–C13); medium chain (MCCA, C14–C17) and long chain PCAs (C18–C20).

The limited data available is predominantly on concentrations of the SCCAs in fish (see Table 21.7). Generally, concentrations of SCCAs range from *ca.* 100 to 1700 μg/kg lw in fish muscle. Limited data on fish livers from Norwegian burbots show concentrations ranging from 226 to 3700 μg/kg lw.

The limited data hampers clear conclusions on contamination related to species, fat content of the fish and the fishing grounds the fish originates from. Moreover, the available data should be treated with great care for its limited accuracy due to the use of technical mixtures and the detection methods applied (as discussed later).

21.3.9 Organochlorine pesticides (OCPs)

Together with PCBs, OCPs have been analysed for a long time in several fish species. Therefore, a considerable amount of data on the OCPs in fish is available from different species and origin (see Table 21.8). OCPs are included in several national monitoring programmes.

The highest pollution concentrations of HCB, HCHs (sum) and DDTs (sum) are observed in eel from the Netherlands, flounder, perch and mussels from Estonia and Latvia, various fish from the Great Lakes, and also in farmed and wild salmon from Scotland. Fish from the Baltic area show considerable concentrations of α- and γ-HCHs (up to 255 μg/kg ww) and high concentrations of over 1 mg/kg ww of DDE and DDD (Olsson *et al.*, 2000; Roots, 2001). Mostly, DDE is predominant over DDD and DDT. The drin (aldrin, dieldrin) concentrations are generally below 1 μg/kg ww, except for some UK and US Great Lakes fish samples.

The highest concentrations of chlordane (sum) are found in the USA Great Lakes and perch from the Baltic area. With *ca.* nine per cent fat, the herring samples contained *ca.* 5 μg/kg ww chlordane, which is in the same range as fish from North-West European seas. Farmed salmon from Chile contained concentrations of < 0.1 μg/kg ww, whereas concentrations in Icelandic and Norwegian salmon ranged from 1.7—7.6 μg/kg ww (Karl *et al.*, 1998). The concentrations of OCPs in farmed salmon are rather high and are comparable with concentrations in fish originating from polluted waters (Jacobs *et al.*, 2001b). Temporal trends of DDT concentrations are declining (Picer and Picer, 1994; de Vault *et al.*, 1996).

21.3.10 Tris(4-chlorophenyl)methanol (TCPM) and tris(4-chlorophenyl)methane (TCPMe)

TCPM and TCPMe are globally spread contaminants which are found in fish, marine mammals and polar bears (de Boer, 2000c). There is only limited data

Table 21.7 Concentrations of PCAs in fish and shellfish ($\mu g/kg$)

Country	Year	Species	Conc.	Class	lw/ww	References
UK	1979?	Plaice, pouting, pike	<0.05–0.2*		ww	Campbell and McConnell (1980)
		Mussel	0.1–12.0*	C10-20		
		Plaice, pouting, pike	<0.05–0.2*	C20-30		
		Mussel	<0.1–0.1*			
UK	?	Freshwater fish	<100–5200	SCCA**		Nicholls *et al.* (2001)
Marmara Sea		Blue fish	405	C10-13	lw	Coelhan *et al.* (2000)
		Silver side	332			
Mediterranean		Sardine	903			
Atlantic		Angler	206			
		Cod	170			
		Shark	417			
		Sole	207			
North Sea		Herring	805			
Norway	2000?	Trout, Arctic char	108–1692	C10-13	lw	Borgen *et al.* (2001)
		Burbot, liver	226–3700			
USA, Detroit river/Lake Erie	1995	Perch	82	C14-17		Tomy and Stern (1999)
		Catfish	904			

* ppm, mussel close to outlet of PCA production plant
** Chain length not specified

Table 21.8 A selection of typical concentrations of OCPs in fish and shellfish (expressed in μg/kg)

Country	Year	Species	HCB	ΣHCH*	ΣDDT*	ΣCHLs*	Drins	ww/lw/dw	References
Netherlands	1999	Eel	1.2–81	3.5–199** <0.1–66 α <0.9–78 β <4.3–55 γ	11–164 7.2–89 DDE 4.2–62 DDD <0.7–29 DDT			ww	de Boer *et al.* (2000a)
Scotland	1999	Salmon, wild and farmed	13–44	ND–23 ND–6.8 α ND–8.7 β ND–	45–249 29–123 DDE 3.3–46 DDD 8.9–40 DDT			lw	Jacobs *et al.* (2001)
Norway		Salmon, farmed	ND	11	5.1				
Turkey Aegean Sea	1995	Red Mullet			0.86–4.5 DDD 10–18 DDE		0.10–0.61 Aldrin	ww	Kucuksezgin *et al.* (2001)
Greenland	1994–95	Mussel	0.01–0.1	0.2–0.5	0.2–0.8			ww	Dietz *et al.* (2000)
		Arctic char	0.6–1.0	0.4–0.6	2–20			ww	
Greenland, fresh	1994–95	Char	0.72	0.41 0.23 α 0.04 β 0.15 γ	4.0 3.4 DDE 0.13 DDD 0.32 DDT	4.8 0.41 oxy chl. 0.09 tr. chl. 0.54 cis chl. 2.3 tr. nona. 1.2 cis nona.	0.72 Dieldrin	ww	
Ireland	1993–96	Herring				1.5–2.4		ww	Karl *et al.* (1998)
Atlanto-Scandian						1.6–9.7			
South Norway						0.1–1.5			
North Sea						<0.1–5.1			
English Channel						2.2, 3.2			
Farmed Salmon						<0.1–7.6			
West coast UK****	1991–94	Mackerel***	1.3–2.6	0.6–1.8 α 0.6–1.3 γ	5.2–11 DDE		5.4–8.8 Dieldrin	ww	Karl and Lehmann (1997)
Latvia, Lake Burtnieku	1996	Perch	5.9–16	4.1–8.8 α 7.4–22 γ	40–1000 DDE 13–140 DDD	2.0–16 tr. nona.		ww	Olsson *et al.* (2000)

Table 21.8 Continued

Country	Year	Species	HCB	ΣHCH*	ΣDDT*	ΣCHLs*	Drins	ww/lw/dw	References
Estonia, marine	1998	Flounder		2.3–112 α 6.1–255 γ	10.1–1521 DDE 45–4130 DDD 14–47 DDT			lw	Roots (2001)
		Perch		2.1–31 α 2.2–74 γ	22–119 DDE 0.4–51 DDD 1.2–50 DDT				
	1998	Mussel		6.7–8.5 α 4.3–4.8 γ	45.8–74 DDE 7.4–13 DDD 24–44 DDT				
West-Baltic Sea	1990–91	Mussel	0.2–2.4	2.5–22	6.6–88 3.9–40 DDE 0.9–29 DDD 1.8–18 DDT			dw	Lee *et al.* (1996)
Southern Baltic	1991–93	Herring				49 6.0 oxy chl. 2.3 tr. chl. 14 cis chl. 12 tr. nona. 3.6 cis nona.		lw	Strandberg *et al.* (1998)
Alaska	?	Trout	0.46	0.56	2.7	1		ww	Allen-Gil *et al.* (1997)
USA, Great Lakes	?	Various commercial fish	0.22–9.3	0.28–23	1.1–124	0.94–45	0.24–41 Dieldrin	ww	Newsome and Andrews (1993)
Canada, Northwater Polynya	1998	Arctic cod		90 40 α 27 β 23 γ				ww	Moisey *et al.* (2001)

* Total concentrations. Concentrations of individual compounds specified if available
** Highest concentration originates from a polluted area close to a former lindane production site
*** Length class mentioned: 37–38 cm
**** Concentrations in mackerel from German Bight, from Norwegian coast and close to Shetlands were in the same range

Table 21.9 Concentrations of TCPMe and TCPM in fish and shellfish (μg/kg lipid weight)

Country	Location	Year	Species	TCPM	TCPMe	Reference
The Netherlands	Northern North Sea	1992	Cod liver	5.7	1.7	de Boer (1997)
	Southern North Sea	1993		40	ND	
	Southern North Sea	1987	Cod liver oil	51	3	
	Southern North Sea	1987	Mackerel oil	35	0.6	
	Wadden Sea	1994	Mussels	13	<6	
	Freshwater	1994	Eel	10–360	ND–37	
Italy?	Mediterranean Sea	1992	Tuna, perch, angler, mullet	<1	<1	
Poland	Baltic South coast	1991–95	Various	ND–11	ND–30	Falandysz *et al.* (1999)

available (see Table 21.9) on concentrations of TCPM and TCPMe in fish. TCPMe shows generally lower concentrations (factor 2 to 50) compared with TCPM, although samples from the Baltic Sea contained higher concentrations of TCPMe (up to 30 μg/kg lw) than TCPM (up to 11 μg/kg lw) (Falandysz *et al.*, 1999).

The only freshwater fish with relevant data reported in the literature was eel from different freshwater locations from the Netherlands showing concentrations up to 360 μg/kg. Due to the limited data on toxicity of these compounds (de Boer, 2000c) and the absence of fish data from other than European regions it is not possible to draw conclusions on the impact on human health of these contaminants.

21.3.11 Toxaphene

Although toxaphene consists theoretically of over 30 000 congeners, in environmental samples only a few hundred congeners are present. Initial reports were based on total toxaphene, but the increasing commercial availability of individual congeners and information on the persistency of specific congeners led to the determination of a selection of individual congeners (de Geus *et al.*, 1999; Whittle *et al.*, 2000; Vetter *et al.*, 2001).

A selection of typical toxaphene concentrations is shown in Table 21.10. The Great Lakes area in North America, known for their contamination with toxaphene, show considerably high concentrations, up to almost 2 mg/kg ww total toxaphene. The tolerable daily intake (TDI) of toxaphene, estimated to be 0.2 μg/kg/day can only be exceeded by regular consumers of highly contaminated fish (Berti *et al.*, 1998). In 1997 a European research project titled 'Investigation into the Monitoring, Analysis and Toxicity of Toxaphene (MATT)' was initiated. As a part of this programme, concentrations of the individual congeners Parlar no. 26, 50 and 62 were determined in a vast amount of samples in marine and freshwater fish in north-

Table 21.10 Concentrations of toxaphene in fish and shellfish (μg/kg wet weight)

Location	Year	Species	Individual congeners						Total Tox. (mg/kg ww)	References
			P26	P40	P41	P44	P50	P62		
Iceland	2000?	Cod, liver	10–18	6–9	3–4	20–35	11–12	10–14		Vetter *et al.* (2001)
Baltic Sea		Cod, liver	35–83	3–16	6–17	31–88	21–40	8–41		
Baltic Sea, Swedish coast		Salmon	2.22–10.5				2.8–16	0.39–3.0		Atuma *et al.* (2000)
Greenland	1994–95	Arctic char	0.67				1.8	0.64	0.013	Cleemann *et al.* (2000)
USA, Lake Michigan	1997–98	Various							0.15–1.2	Stapleton *et al.* (2001)
USA, Lake Superior	1998	Lake Trout	0.02	0.02	0.01	0.02	0.11	0.06	1.9	Whittle *et al.* (2000)
USA, Lower Rio Grande Valley	1997	Common carp							ND–0.31	Wainwright *et al.* (2001)

west European samples and arctic samples. Due to the global distillation effect, concentrations are higher in the colder regions (e.g. Barents Sea) compared to, for example, the Netherlands (de Boer *et al.*, 2004). The predominant congener contribution to the sum of P 26, 50 and 62 varies with the origin of the samples.

21.3.12 Nonylphenol (ethoxylate) compounds

Most of the reported data originates from fish caught in waters in industrialised/urbanised areas. Some of these waters may be influenced by sewage treatment plants (Vethaak *et al.*, 2002). No data is reported on fish from remote areas like the arctic regions. The data ranges from 5 μg/kg ww to 380 μg/kg dw for NP and up to 3100 μg/kg dw for its ethoxylates (see Table 21.11). The highest concentrations reported were detected in fish from the Glatt River in Switzerland, which is influenced by one nearby sewage treatment plant (Ahel *et al.*, 1993). The concentrations in fish from marine waters are relatively low.

Alkylphenols are known for their estrogenic potential (Odum *et al.*, 1997; Vethaak *et al.*, 2002). Although the bioaccumulative properties of alkylphenols are less strong than, for example, those of PCBs, the combination of the concentrations found and the estrogenic effects cause concerns about the occurrence of these compounds in fish.

21.3.13 Musk compounds

After their application in private households, musk compounds are dumped in the environment via sewage treatment plants. This is the main route for contamination of (freshwater) fish, which is shown by the high concentrations of musk compounds (up to 20.3 mg/kg lw for 1,3,4,6,7,8–hexahydro-4,6,6,7,8,8, hexamethylcyclopenta(g)-2–benzopyrane (HHCB)) in rainbow trout that originates from the River Stör, 3 km downstream of a sewage treatment plant (Table 21.12).

Eel samples from the Netherlands contained concentrations of musk xylene (MX) and musk ketone (MK) in the range of <0.5 to 45 μg/kg ww, with MX being predominant (de Boer and Webster, 1999). This is in the same range as observed PCB concentrations in similar samples. No data on HHCB and 7–acetyl-1,1,3,4,4,6, hexamethyltetrahydronaphthalene (AHTN) have been reported for Dutch samples. Data from German fish samples show that the polycyclic musk compounds are predominant compared with the nitro musks, which reflects the higher production and use figures discussed earlier (Rimkus, 1999). On the contrary, Canadian clam samples from Halifax harbour showed the highest concentrations of MK (Gatermann *et al.*, 1999).

21.3.14 Perfluorinated compounds (PFCs)

PFCs is a relatively new group of substances. Very little is known on the toxicity and fate of PFCs. Physicochemical properties and behaviour cannot be predicted

Table 21.11 Concentrations of nonylphenol (ethoxylates) in fish ($\mu g/kg$)

Country	Year	Species	NP	NP1EO	NP2EO	dw/lw/ww	References
Switzerland	1984–85	Various fish	150–380	180–3100	130–2300	dw	Ahel *et al.* (1993)
USA, Lake Mead	1999	Carp	184	242		ww	Snyder *et al.* (2001b)
UK, River Tyne	1997	Flounder	5–55	<LOD		ww	Lye *et al.* (1999)
Italy, Ortbetello lagoon	1998–99	Grass goby	0.12–1.6	28–508	0.3–48	ww	Corsi and Focardi (2002)
The Netherlands, various freshwater locations	1999–2001	Bream	30–160	150–500		ww	Vethaak *et al.* (2002)
The Netherlands, Wadden Sea		Flounder		100			
The Netherlands, harbour	1996	Flounder, liver	< 150			ww	de Boer *et al.* (2001b)

Table 21.12 Typical concentrations of musk compounds in fish and shellfish ($\mu g/kg$)

Country	Location	Year	Species	M-xylene	M-ketone	HHCB	AHTN	lw/ww/dw	References
The Netherlands	Meuse, Eijsden	1996	Eel	45	11			ww	de Boer and Wester (1996)
	Various			<3–17	4–33				
			Pike perch	<0.5	<0.5				
	Southern North Sea		Various	<2	<4				
			Shrimp, mussel	<0.5	<1				
Germany	Berlin	1996	Eel	1–79	1–380	15–4131	10–1408	ww	Fromme *et al.* (1999)
	River Ruhr	?				400, 600	500, 700	lw	Rimkus (1999)
	River Elbe	?	Pike perch	<10–90	10–70	600–3840	320–990		
	River Stor*	?	Brown trout	200, 240	1000, 1200	13700, 20300	10600, 13400		
North Sea		?	Shrimps	<10–10	20–430	<40–60	<40–60		
North Sea coast		?	Mussels	<10–20	10–30	<30–110	<30–60		
Canada		?	Various	ND–0.8	ND–140	ND–27	ND–6	ww	Gatermann *et al.* (1999)

* 3 km downstream a sewage treatment plant

Table 21.13 Concentrations of PFFs in fish and shellfish (μg/kg wet weight)

Country	Location	Year	Species	PFOS	PFOA	lw/ww/dw	References
USA	Michigan waters	1990s	Carp, Chinook salmon, brown trout and lake whitefish	7–300		ww	Giesy and Kannan (2001)
USA	Gulf of Mexico and Chesapeake Bay	1996–98	Oysters	<42–1225		dw	Kannan *et al.* (2002)
Belgium	Western Scheldt/North Sea	2001	Crab, shrimp	25–800		ww	van de Vijver *et al.* (2002)
Belgium	Western Scheldt/North Sea	2001	Plaice, bib	<10–111		ww	Hoff *et al.* (2003)
Canada	Toronto	2000	Common shiner, liver	2000-72 900*	6-91*	ww	Moody *et al.* (2002)
Japan	Tokyo Bay	2002	Var. fish, liver	3–7900		ww	Taniyasu *et al.* (2003)

* After accidental release of fire retardant foam

using models for lipophilic substances like PCBs as these compounds have both hydrophobic and oleophobic type properties and form a third phase in an octanol-water partitioning system which is normally used to predict lipophilicity (Moody and Field, 2000). PFCs have been applied for their water and fat repelling properties in, for example, coatings for cardboard food containers, in dirt repelling coatings for shoes, carpets and leather, and in aqueous fire-fighting foams. Some PFCs are used as a polymerisation aid in the production of Teflon.

Although limited data is currently available, it is expected that more information will become available on concentrations of PFOS and other fluorinated substances in fish in the near future. A selection of current data is given in Table 21.13. High concentrations of PFOS were found in fish and shellfish from the United States, up to 1225 μg/kg dw (Kannan *et al.*, 2002). High concentrations of PFOS were also found in Belgium (North Sea and Western Scheldt estuary) up to 800 μg/kg ww PFOS. Perfluorooctanoic acid (PFOA) and homologues of these surfactants were also determined in freshwater fish after an accidental release of fire-fighting foams (Moody *et al.*, 2002) (nd-2210 μg/l). Long chain PFCs (other than PFOS) were also determined in biota from the Canadian arctic at levels from < 0.5 to 230 μg/kg ww in fish livers.

These data show that PFOS is distributed on a global scale. Furthermore, other PFCs have also been detected in fish from various (remote) locations, although at lower levels compared to PFOS. Considering the lack of knowledge on the physical behaviour, toxicity, bioaccumulation and fate of these compounds on the one hand, and the high levels, global distribution and production volumes on the other, there is an urgent need for more research in the coming years.

21.4 Analysing particular organic contaminants in fish

21.4.1 Analysis of PCBs

The general procedure for analysis of lipophilic organic substances consists of the following basic steps: extraction; clean up and final determination of the compounds. Figure 21.1 shows the general scheme for the analysis of PCBs and other lipophilic compounds discussed in this chapter.

Extraction

PCBs are lipophilic, so the extraction methods are based on the isolation of the lipid fraction from the sample matrix (de Boer, 2001). Soxhlet extraction has been used for the extraction of PCBs from a wide variety of matrices including fish using mixtures of non- and medium-polar solvents (e.g. n-pentane/dichloromethane, 1:1, hexane/acetone, 1:1). The non-polar solvent extracts the PCBs from the triglycerides, the medium-polar solvent extracts the PCBs from the phospholipids or other more polar solvents (Hess *et al.*, 1995). Prior to the extraction the sample is macerated, homogenised and ground with dry sodium sulphate to bind the water present in the sample. Freeze-drying is not

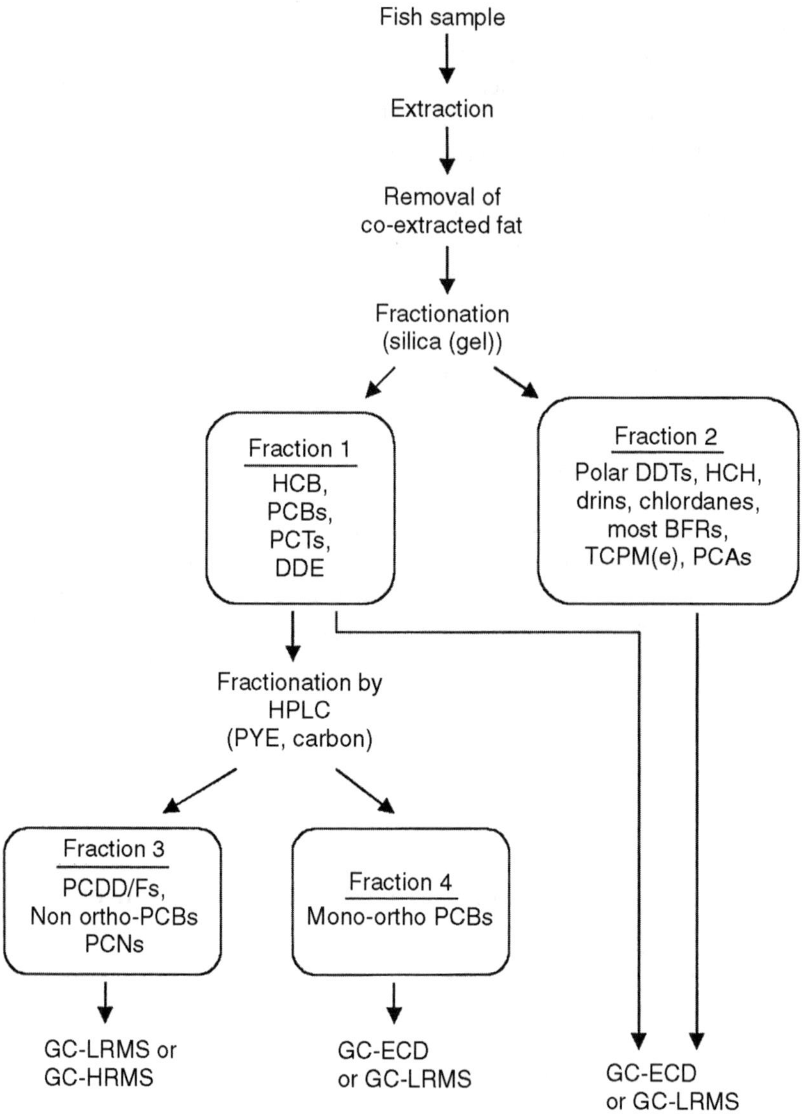

Fig. 21.1 General analysis scheme for the lipophilic organohalogen contaminants discussed in this chapter.

recommended as it may easily cause losses of the more volatile PCBs and may cause cross-contamination. Other extraction techniques used are supercritical fluid extraction (SFE), solid-phase extraction (SPE), accelerated solvent extraction (ASE), microwave assisted extraction (MAE) and cold extraction by Ultra-Turrax (de Boer, 2001).

Clean up
The clean up of the extracted lipid fraction consists of the removal of the lipids from the extract and fractionation in order to remove possible interfering compounds. The lipid removal is carried out by destructive methods (saponification of sulphuric acid treatment) or by non-destructive methods such as gel permeation chromatography (GPC) or alumina columns, with the latter being favoured over GPC for its efficient lipid removal (Hess *et al.*, 1995; de Boer, 2001). However, rigid gels are nowadays available for high performance GPC which result in improved separation. Subsequently, pre-fractionation is carried out in order to separate the PCBs from other compounds like organochlorine pesticides in order to reduce possible interferences during gas chromatographic separation of the PCBs. Silica gel columns or Florisil columns are frequently used and the process can be automated (Hess *et al.*, 1995; de Boer, 2001).

Determination
PCBs are a complex mixture, consisting of 209 different congeners. The method of choice is capillary gas chromatography (GC) since this technique enables the determination of individual compounds. The separation is carried out on capillary columns with a stationary phase that is providing enough selectivity. Stationary phases with varying polarity are used, such as CP-Sil-8 (95% methyl, 5% phenylpolysiloxane) or CP-Sil-19 (85% methyl, 7% phenyl, 7% cyanopropyl, 1% vinylpolysiloxane) providing different resolution, but no single column is able to separate all 209 congeners (de Boer *et al.*, 1992; Hess *et al.*, 1995; de Boer, 2001). Narrow bore columns (0.15 mm internal diameter) are preferred for their increased resolving power (de Boer and Dao, 1989). Multi-dimensional GC techniques may become more important in the near future for PCBs and complex mixtures of contaminants in general, as with that technique peak overlap can be almost completely avoided (Korytar *et al.*, 2002). Figure 21.2 shows the potential of comprehensive multi-dimensional GC (MDGC) by a nearly complete separation of a standard mixture of PCBs and WHO dioxins and furans. Electron capture detectors (ECD) and modern bench-top mass spectrometric detectors (MSD) are used, the latter being more selective than the ECD (Hess *et al.*, 1995; de Boer, 2001). Dl-PCBs require a more specific clean up, comparable to that of dioxins. They can be determined by low resolution MS.

21.4.2 Analysis of PCDDs, PCDFs and non-ortho substituted PCBs

The concentrations of dioxins and furans in samples occur at a 100–1,000-fold lower concentration than PCBs and therefore a high sensitivity and lower limits of detection are required (Liem, 1999). The analytical procedure should be highly selective as a distinction is required for dioxins, furans and dioxin-like PCBs from a multitude of other, co-extracted and possibly interfering compounds present at concentrations up to several orders of magnitude higher than the compounds of interest (Liem, 1999).

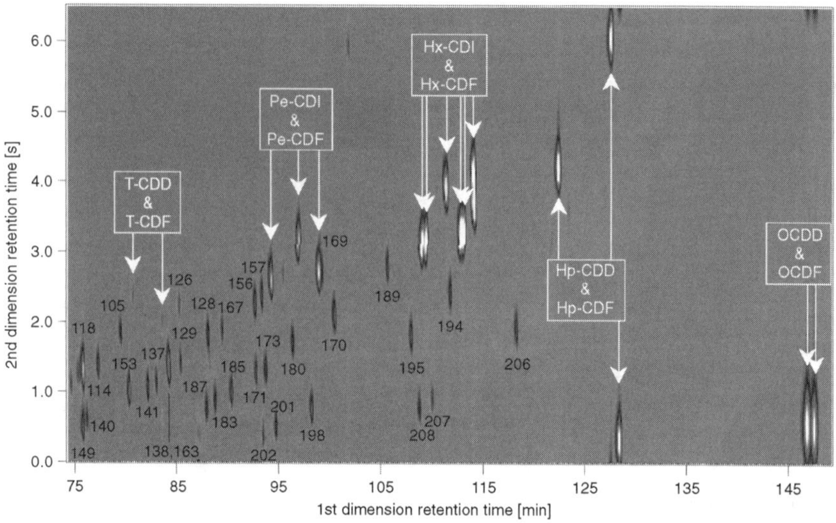

Fig. 21.2 GCxGC-μECD analysis of a mixture of 90 PCBs and 17 WHO PCDD/Fs with a HP-1-HT-8 column combination. Reprinted with permission from Korytar *et al.* (2002).

The pre-treatment and extraction procedure, as well as the removal of the lipids from the extract, is very similar to the PCB analytical procedure. Subsequently, the extract is applied to an additional fractionation step, carbon or PYE column (2-(1-pyrenyl)ethyldimethylsilyl) chromatography, retaining planar multi-ring compounds like non-ortho PCBs, PCDDs, PCDFs as well as other planar compounds (Hess *et al.*, 1995; Liem, 1999).

The final determination is carried out by GC-high resolution MS (GC-HRMS), which currently is the only technique able to provide the required selectivity and sensitivity (Liem and Theelen, 1997). However, currently instrumental techniques (GCxGC-ECD, GC-ion trap low resolution MS/MS) are being developed that might be able to provide the required selectivity and sensitivity (www.dioxins.nl).

21.4.3 Analysis of other contaminants

The PAH analysis is fairly straightforward and generally starts with alkaline saponification of the lipids and subsequent extraction of the PAHs with an organic solvent (Baumard *et al.*, 1998; Kelly *et al.*, 2000). The extract is further cleaned by alumina, silica gel or aminosilane chromatography (Baumard *et al.*, 1998; Kelly *et al.*, 2000; Piccardo *et al.*, 2001). The cleaned extract can be analysed by HPLC, using PAH tailor-made columns (establishing pi-pi interactions with the PAHs) and subsequent fluorescence detection (Kelly *et al.*, 2000; Piccardo *et al.*, 2001). On the other hand, GC-EI-MS is emerging for PAH analysis using apolar columns like HP-5 or CP-Sil 5 (Baumard *et al.*, 1998; Kelly *et al.*, 2000; Baussant *et al.*, 2001). GC-MS has specific advantages like the ability to detect non-fluorescent PAHs which cannot be analysed by HPLC-fluorescence detection, although both techniques are complementary to each other. Deuterated compounds are commercially available which can be used as internal standards in GC-MS quantification (Kelly *et al.*, 2000).

As shown in Fig. 21.1, most other lipophilic organohalogen contaminants can be determined using comparable extraction and clean-up strategies as being used for the analysis of PCBs and PCDD/Fs. However, specific adaptations are required for each group of contaminants depending on the complexity of the technical mixture (e.g. PCAs and PCTs), the possible thermal or chemical degradation of some contaminants (e.g. some OCPs and decaBDE) or the unknown behaviour during extraction and clean up (e.g. PFCs).

PBDEs, TBBP-A and HBCD can be determined by GC-ECD and GC-MS, although MS is preferred because use can be made of the prominent bromine clusters in the MS spectra. The fully brominated diphenyl ether (deca-BDE) is sensitive to deterioration by UV light and thermal heating in the GC oven and therefore measures should be taken to prevent losses of deca-BDE during analysis. De Boer *et al.*, (2001a) determine deca-BDE separately on a shorter column (15 m) to minimise deterioration of this thermo-labile compound. Recently, the individual stereoisomers of HBCD have also been analysed by HPLC-ESI-MS (Morris *et al.*, 2003).

Considering only 75 possible congeners, the gas chromatographic analysis of PCNs is fairly straightforward using non-polar columns like Ultra-1 which was able to separate 44 in a Halowax 1014 mixture, out of 75 possible congeners (Järnberg *et al.*, 1994). Detection is performed by NCI or EI-(HR)MS in the SIM mode, with electron ionisation (EI) being favoured as the responses are similar for all congeners (Jakobsson and Asplund, 2000).

The technical mixture of PCTs is very complex (8557 theoretical congeners). PCTs are found in the same fraction after silica gel elution as PCBs. Higher temperatures are required to elute them from GC columns because they have higher boiling points. Total determinations, using the technical Aroclor mixtures as standards, have been used (Wester *et al.*, 1996) as congener-specific determination is still not possible. Comprehensive MDGC may be a solution for this problem in the future.

Technical PCA mixtures consist of tens of thousands of congeners and separation of all individual congeners is impossible by single column GC and probably even not possible with multi-dimensional GC. Therefore, methods are developed that result in the sum of short-, medium- of long chain-CAs, based on comparison with one of the technical mixtures available (Muir *et al.*, 2000). The use of technical mixtures that do not match the pattern as observed in the sample decrease the quality of data reported (Coelhan *et al.*, 2000) and therefore data should be treated as semi-quantitative.

The methods for OCP determinations are similar to those for PCB analysis. Traditional methods for PCB and OCP clean up result in two fractions after the elution over the silica column (see section PCBs), one PCB fraction and one OCP fraction in which most pesticides are present. However, (a part of) trans-nonachlor, cis- and trans-chlordane, hexachlorobutadiene (HCBD), QCB, HCB,

OCS, p,p-DDE, o,p-DDE, PCA and PCTA may be found among the PCBs in the first fraction as well. Some OCPs (e.g. dieldrin, endrin and p,p-DDE) decompose under sulphuric acid and therefore, this clean-up step should be avoided when analysing these specific OCPs (de Boer and Law, 2003).

For TCPM and TCPMe, the extraction and clean-up procedure is similar to the OCP procedure. TCPM and TCPMe elute at relatively high oven temperatures (270—300 °C), which is comparable with the PCTs. Details on the analysis of these compounds can be found in a review by de Boer (2000c).

The very complex mixture of toxaphene, consisting of theoretically 32,768 possible congeners disables the complete separation of all individual congeners (de Geus, 2000). With the application of multi-dimensional GC an increased separation power was obtained resulting in 246 peaks (more than twice the number obtained in single column GC) (de Boer *et al.*, 1997). For the quantification of toxaphene often technical mixtures and levels are reported as total-toxaphene resulting in a possible mismatch between the congener profile present in the sample and the technical mixture (Vetter and Oehme, 2000; Breackevelt *et al.*, 2001). Although there is a lack of standards, a limited number (mixtures from) of individual congeners (e.g. Parlar nos. 26, 32, 40, 41, 44, 50 and 62) are commercially available (Vetter and Oehme, 2000). For this reason (a selection of) these individual congeners are generally reported.

The analysis of musk compounds is very similar to the methods applied for PCBs and OCPs, generally starting with (Soxhlet) extraction of the lipids from the sample, subsequent lipid removal by aluminum oxide or GPC (Fromme *et al.*, 1999; Rimkus, 1999). The PCBs and OCPs are removed from the extract by separation on silica gel column. The final determination is carried out by GC-ECD, GC-NPD, GC-EI-MS or GC-NCI-MS, whose specific (dis)advantages are discussed by Rimkus (1999).

Nonylphenol and short-chain nonylphenol ethoxylates (NP1EO and NP2EO) in fish can be analysed by both HPLC and GC. The analysis starts with extraction of the compounds from the matrix by Soxhlet extraction (Snyder *et al.*, 2001b) or steam distillation (Ahel *et al.*, 1993; Lye *et al.*, 1999; Snyder *et al.*, 2001), followed by GPC, alumina chromatography or silica chromatography for removal of the lipids (Lye *et al.*, 1999; Snyder *et al.*, 2001b; Tsuda *et al.*, 2001). Quantification is fairly straightforward and is performed by normal-phase HPLC and fluorescence detection (Ahel *et al.*, 1993; Snyder *et al.*, 2001b). GC-MS is also frequently employed for detection and quantification (Lye *et al.*, 1999; Snyder *et al.*, 2001b; Tsuda *et al.*, 2001).

The analysis of PFCs is not as 'straightforward' as the already complicated analysis for PCBs or PBDEs. As PFCs have surfactant properties, the behaviour of PFOS during sample treatment or determination is not yet completely understood, which makes the analysis susceptible to analytical mistakes and problems. Giesy and Kannan (2001) extracted biota samples after addition of water and a counterion and bufferd it at pH 10, following extraction with organic solvent (methyl-tert-butyl-ether). The separation was performed on a C18 HPLC column and detection was performed by electrospray(ESI)-MS (negative ion mode). Recoveries range typically from below 50% to over 150% showing that the method of analysis is not yet completely under control (Giesy and Kannan, 2001; Kannan *et al.*, 2001b, 2002; Taniyasu *et al.*, 2002; Hoff *et al.*, 2003). Moody *et al.* (2001) used a similar HPLC-ESI-MS method for determination of PFOS and related substances in water samples (Moody *et al.*, 2001). Derivatising and determination with GC has limited utility (Moody and Field, 2000).

21.5 Health issues for organic contaminants in fish

The toxic potency of the substances discussed varies considerably among the different contaminant groups. Dioxins have shown developmental and reproductive effects in rats and monkeys and have carcinogenic potency (Liem and Theelen, 1997; SCF, 2000). Within the EU a tolerable weekly intake (TWI) of 14 pg WHO-TEQ/kg bodyweight (bw)/week was advised by the EU Scientific Committee for Food (SCF). Fish generally shows highest concentrations of dioxins among other food items and therefore, humans with diets including a substantial amount of fish (Scandinavia, Southern European countries) have an increased chance to exceed the TWI of 14 pg PCDD/F-TEQ/kg bw/week. A new set of European maximum residue limit (MRL) values for food including fish and fish oil (4 pg PCDD/F-TEQ/g ww and 2 pg PCDD/F-TEQ/g fat, respectively) (Anon., 2001) became active on 1 July 2002. From Table 21.3 it is clear that only a limited amount of fish and shellfish samples exceeded the limit 4 pg PCDD/F-TEQ/g ww. It is anticipated that in 2004 the MRLs will be evaluated in the light of possible inclusion of the dl-PCBs.

PCBs, other than the dl-PCBs, have a tumour promotion potential (independent of the dioxin-type of toxicity) (van der Plas, 2000). Based on this observation, tolerable daily intake (TDI) of 300 ng/kg bw/day was calculated. Depending on the composition of the diet, this TDI can possibly be exceeded for consumers with fish rich diets or when highly contaminated fish is consumed. For PCBs several countries have limit values for the sum of indicator PCBs or for individual congeners. The Netherlands has congener specific limits up to 600 μg/kg PCB 153 in eel, whereas in Belgium currently a limit of 75 μg/kg for the sum of the indicator PCBs is discussed. The later limit could lead to considerable non-compliance for freshwater fish and some non compliance for marine fish.

Concerning toxaphene, Germany and Austria have set a MRL (0.1 mg/kg ww for three indicator congeners and the sum of toxaphene, respectively). Table 21.10 shows that samples from the Great Lakes exceed the total toxaphene MRL of Austria, whereas none of the samples from Germany, the Netherlands, Sweden and Ireland exceeded the MRL (de Boer *et al.*, 2004). The United States and Canada have set a TDI .

The toxicity of NP is not extensively investigated. However, estrogenic activity of NP was observed from an induction of a uterotropic response in rodents after exposure to NP (Odum *et al.*, 1997). It is not clear how these results should be interpreted for disrupting human hormonal systems and the impact on human health.

For some substances like PFOS and PCAs, very limited or no data is available on human toxicity and therefore the relevance cannot be expressed. However, based on the production volumes and use (in the past), there is some concern on the possible toxic potency of these substances.

In normal risk assessment approaches, the health effects of individual contaminants or a group of contaminants are evaluated. For example the MRLs for the WHO-PCDD/Fs are based on this approach (van den Berg *et al.*, 1998; EC, 2001). In a recent study on contaminants in farmed salmon samples, consumption advice was developed based on potential cancer risks and on the assumption of a risk additivity of dieldrin, toxaphene and PCBs. This resulted in strict recommendation of consumption of between less than one (European farmed salmon) to eight meals of (North America farmed) salmon per month (Hites *et al.*, 2004).

21.6 Future trends

A vast amount of data has been produced during the last two decades on concentrations of a wide range of contaminants in fish. Monitoring data show that concentrations of PCBs and OCPs are declining and, except for some hot spots, concentrations are generally below the applicable MRLs. This is mainly due to phasing out of the use of PCBs and OCPs and the controlled way of dismantling old transformers in order to prevent PCB-containing oils from entering the environment. Also other contaminants like PCNs, PCTs and toxaphene are not used any more and it is expected that concentrations are declining, although less research has been conducted for these contaminants, and monitoring data are not available.

BFR concentrations in fish reflect the ongoing production of these chemicals. Although the penta-mix related PBDEs show a decline in Europe (but not in the United States (de Wit, 2002)), other relatively new substances like HBCD and TBBP-A show considerable concentrations in fish. A temporal trend studied in guillemot samples shows an increasing trend from 1969 to 1997 (de Wit 2002). Furthermore, the toxicological importance of these compounds needs further research efforts. This is currently being assessed in several research studies in Europe.

Other contaminants still in use but with very little data are alkylphenols and their ethoxylates, musk compounds and PCAs. Future monitoring should also focus on these substances. Furthermore, PFOS and other fluorinated substances represent a group of contaminants of which very little is known. The unique properties (compared to lipophilic contaminants) hamper the prediction of concentrations in the environment, fate, toxicity and metabolism. Scientists should pay attention to this class of substances to fill the data gaps in order to evaluate environmental concentrations and health risks of these contaminants.

Recent crises on dioxins and BSE in food (Belgium, 1999) have generated consumer concern about undesired substances in their food. As a result, research and monitoring of contaminants in food in the European Union have intensified. It is therefore expected that more data will become available on contaminants in fish for legislative purposes and to evaluate positive and negative health aspects of fish consumption.

The farming of fish, of which volumes are increasing world-wide (FAO 2001), provides the possibility to control the concentrations of contaminants in the produced fish. Fish meal and fish oil from Chile and Peru show considerably lower concentrations of dioxins (SCAN, 2000) and therefore, by careful selection of these little contaminated ingredients for farmed fish diets the concentrations in the farmed fish can be kept low. Furthermore, the replacement of fish oil and fish meal by vegetable ingredients provides another possibility to reduce organic contaminant concentrations in farmed fish.

21.7 Sources of further information and advice

This chapter has focused mainly on concentrations of contaminants in fish. Information on other aspects of these contaminants like concentrations in other environmental compartments, toxicity research and evaluation, human intake and legislative aspects are not discussed within this framework. Some recent and extensive reviews on these subjects are mentioned below:

J. Paasvirta (2000), New Types of Persistent Halogenated Compounds. Springer-Verlag. 3, part K, Berlin, Germany. Contaminants discussed are: TCPM and TCPMe, PCTs, PBDEs, PCNs, PCAs and toxaphene.
G. Rimkus, Synthetic Musks in the Environment. Elsevier, Amsterdam, The Netherlands, in press.
Liem, A. K. D. and R. M. C. Theelen, 1997, Dioxins: chemical analysis, exposure and risk assessment, Thesis, University of Utrecht, The Netherlands

Information concerning legislation, safety and current monitoring can be obtained from the following websites:

www.epa.gov
www.who.int
www.europa.eu.int
www.efsa.eu.int

21.8 References

AHEL, M., J. MCEVOY and W. GIGER (1993), 'Bioaccumulation of the lipophilic metabolites of nonionic surfactants in freshwater organisms', *Environmental Pollution*, 79, 243–248.

AKUTSU, K., H. OBANA, M. OKIHASHI, M. KITAGAWA, H. NAKAZAWA, Y. MATSUKI, T. MAKINO, H. ODA and S. HORI (2001), 'GC/MS analysis of polybrominated diphenyl ethers in fish collected from the Inland Sea of Seto, Japan', *Chemosphere*, 44 (6), 1325–1333.

ALCOCK, R. E., A. J. SWEETMAN, K. PREVEDOUROS and K. C. JONES (2003), 'Understanding levels and trends of BDE-47 in the UK and North America: an assessment of principal reservoirs and source inputs'. *Environment International*, 29 (6), 691–698.

ALI, I. B., C. R. JOIRIS and L. HOLSBEEK (1997), 'Polychlorinated biphenyls in Barents and Greenland seas fish', *Bulletin of Environmental Contamination and Toxicology*, 58 (6), 885–892.

ALLCHIN, C. R. and S. MORRIS (2003), 'Hexabromocyclododecane (HBCD) diastereoisomers and brominated diphenyl ether congener (BDE) residues in edible fish from the rivers Skerne and Tees, U.K.', *Organohalogen Compounds*, 61, 41–44.

ALLEN-GIL, S. M., C. P. GUBALA, R. WILSON, D. H. LANDERS, T. L. WADE, J. L. SERICANO and L. R. CURTIS (1997), 'Organochlorine pesticides and polychlorinated biphenyls (PCBs) in sediments and biota from four US Arctic lakes', *Archives of Environmental Contamination and Toxicology*, 33, 378–387.

ANON. (1984), 'Regeling normen PCBs (Warenwet)', Staatscourant, 239 The Netherlands.

ANON. (2001), 'Council regulation (EC) No 2375/2001, 29 November 2001' European Commission.

ATUMA, S. S., C.-E. LINDER, A. WICKLUND-GLYNN, Ö. ANDERSSON and L. LARSSON (1996), 'Survey of consumption fish from Swedish waters for chlorinated pesticides and polychlorinated biphenyls', *Chemosphere*, 33 (5), 791–799.

ATUMA, S. S., A. BERGH, I. NILSSON and M. AUNE (2000), 'Toxaphene levels in salmon (*Salmo salar*) from the Baltic sea', *Chemosphere*, 41, 517–520.

BAUMARD, P., H. BUDZINSKI and P. GARRIGUES (1998), 'Polycyclic aromatic hydrocarbons in sediments and mussels of the Western Mediterranean Sea', *Environmental Toxicology and Chemistry*, 17 (5), 765–776.

BAUSSANT, T., S. SANNI, A. SKADSHEIM, G. JONSSON and J. F. BORSETH (2001), 'Bio-accumulation of polycyclic aromatic compounds: 2. modeling bioaccumulation in marine organisms chronically exposed to dispersed oil', *Environmental Science & Technology*, 20 (6), 1185–1195.

BAYARRI, S., L. T. BALDASSARRI, N. IACOVELLA, F. FERRARA and A. DI DOMENICO (2001), 'PCDDs, PCDFs, PCBs and DDE in edible marine species from the Adriatic Sea', *Chemosphere*, 43, 601–610.

BERTI, P. R., O. RECEVEUR, H. M. CHAN and H. V. KUHNLEIN (1998), 'Dietary exposure to chemical contaminants from traditional food among adult Dene/Metis in the western Northwest Territories, Canada', *Environmental Research*, 76 (2), 131–142.

BORGEN, A. R., M. SCHLABACH, R. KALLENBORN and E. FJELD (2001), 'Polychlorinated alkanes in freshwater fish', *Organohalogen Compounds*, 52, 75.

BREACKEVELT, E., G. T. TOMY and G. A. STERN (2001), 'Comparison of an individual congener standard and technical mixture for the quantification of toxaphene inenvironmental matrices by HRGC/ECNI-HRMS'. *Environmental Science & Technology*, 35, 3513–3518.

BRINKMAN, U. A. T. and A. DE KOK (1980), 'Production, properties and usage', in R. D. Kimbrough, *Halogenated Biphenyls, Terphenyls, Naphthalenes and related products, Topics in Environmental Health*, Amsterdam, Elsevier. 4, 1–40.

CAMPBELL, I. and G. MCCONNELL (1980), 'Chlorinated paraffins and the environment. 1. Environmental occurence', *Environmental Science & Technology*, 14 (10), 1209–1214.

CHOI, D., S. HU, K. WON and C. KIM (2001), 'Surveillance of the selected fish and shellfish for dioxins', *Organohalogen Compounds*, 51, 368–371.

CLEEMANN, M., F. RIGET, G. B. PAULSEN, J. DE BOER, J. KLUNGSOYR and P. AASTRUP (2000), 'Organochlorines in Greenland lake sediments and landlocked Arctic char (*Salvelinus alpinus*)', *The Science of the Total Environment*, 245, 173–185.

COELHAN, M., M. SARACI and H. PARLAR (2000), 'A comparative study of chlorinated alkanes as standards for the determination of C10–C13 polychlorinated paraffines in fish samples', *Chemosphere*, 40, 685–689.

CORSI, I. and S. FOCARDI (2002), 'Nonylphenols in a lagoon environment: p-nonylphenol and nonylphenol ethoxylates in fish tissue', *Bulletin of Environmental Contamination and Toxicology*, 68 (6), 908–914.

DE BOER, J. (1995), 'Analysis and biomonitoring of complex mixtures of persistent halogenated micro-contaminants', Thesis, Department of Chemistry, Free University, Amsterdam.

DE BOER, J. (1997), 'Environmental distribution and toxicity of tris(4-chlorophenyl)-methanol and tris(4-chlorophenyl)methane', *Rev Environmental Contaminant Toxicology*, 150, 95–106.

DE BOER, J. (2000a), 'Polybrominated biphenyls and diphenylethers', in J. Paasvirta, *New Types of Persistent Halogenated Compounds*, Berlin Heidelberg, Springer-Verlag. 3, part K: 62–95.

DE BOER, J. (2000b), 'Polychlorinated terphenyls', in J. Paasvirta, *New Types of Persistent Halogenated Compounds*, Berlin Heidelberg, Springer-Verlag. 3, part K: 43–59.

DE BOER, J. (2000c), 'Tris(4–chlorophenyl)methanol and tris(4–chlorophenyl)methane', in J. Paasvirta, *New Types of Persistent Halogenated Compounds*, Berlin Heidelberg, Springer-Verlag. 3, part K: 31–41.

DE BOER, J. (2001), 'Polychlorinated biphenyls', in W. Kleibömer, *Environmental Analysis*, Elsevier Science B.V. 237–262.

DE BOER, J. and C. ALLCHIN (2001), 'An indication of temporal trends in environmental PBDE levels in Europe', *Organohalogen Compounds*, 52, 13–17.

DE BOER, J. and Q. T. DAO (1989), 'The analysis of individual chlorobiphenyl congeners in fish extracts on 0.15 i.d. capillary columns', *Journal of High Resolution Chromatography*, 12, 755–759.

DE BOER, J. and Q. T. DAO (1993), 'Overview of bromodiphenyl ether data in aquatic biota and sediments', RIVO, Report no. C020/93, IJmuiden, The Netherlands.

DE BOER, J. and R. J. LAW (2003), 'Developments in the use of chromatographic techniques in marine laboratories for the determination of halogenated contaminants and polycyclic aromatic hydrocarbons', *Journal of Chromatography A*, 6, 1–2.

DE BOER, J. and P. G. WESTER (1999), 'Het voorkomen van nitromusks in Nederlandse visserijproducten', RIVO, Report no. C060/96, IJmuiden, The Netherlands.

DE BOER, J., Q. T. DAO and R. VAN DORTMOND (1992), 'Retention times of fifty one chlorobiphenyl congeners on seven narrow bore capillary columns coated with different stationary phases', *Journal of High Resolution Chromatography*, 15, 249–255.

DE BOER, J., H.-J. DE GEUS and U. A. TH. BRINKMAN (1997), 'Multidimensional gas chromatographic analysis of toxaphene'. *Environmental Science & Technology*, 31, 873–879.

DE BOER, J., H. PIETERS and S. P. J. VAN LEEUWEN (2000a), 'Verontreinigingen in aal en snoekbaars: monitorprogramma ten behoeve van de Nederlandse sportvisserij 1999', RIVO, Report no. C048/00, IJmuiden, The Netherlands.

DE BOER, J., A. VAN DER HORST and P. G. WESTER (2000b), 'PBDEs and PBBs in suspended particulate matter, sediments, sewage treatment plant in- and effluents and biota from the Netherlands', *Organohalogen Compounds*, 47, 85.

DE BOER, J., C. ALLCHIN, R. LAW, B. ZEGERS and J. P. BOON (2001a) 'Methods for the analysis of polybrominated dipheylethers in sediments and biota', *Trends in Analytical Chemistry*, 20 (10), 591–599.

DE BOER, J., T. E. VAN DER ZANDE, H. PIETERS, F. ARIESE, C. A. SCHIPPER, T. VAN BRUMMELEN and A. D. VETHAAK (2001b), 'Organic contaminants and trace metals in flounder liver and sediment from the Amsterdam and Rotterdam harbours and off the Dutch coast', *Journal of Environmental Monitoring*, 3, 386–393.

DE BOER, J., P. G. WESTER, *et al.* (2003), 'Polybrominated diphenyl ethers in influents, suspended particulate matter, sediments, sewage treatment plant and effluents and biota from the Netherlands', *Environmental Pollution*, 122 (1), 63–74.

DE BOER, J., P. E. G. LEONARDS, H. J. DE GEUS, P. G. WEITER, A. BROUWER, H. BESSELINK, E. NIXON, B. MCHUGH, G. G. RIMKUS, J. KLUNGSOYR and G. NESJE (2004), MATT – Investigation into the monitoring, analysis and toxicity of toxaphene in marine foodstuffs, Final report European Research project FAIR CT PL.96.3131.

DE GEUS, H.-J. (2000), 'Toxaphene: a challenging analytical problem'. *Journal of Environmental Monitoring*, 2, 503–511.

DE GEUS, H. J., H. BESSELINK, A. BROUWER, J. KLUNGSOYR, B. MCHUGH, E. NIXON, G. G. RIMKUS, P. G. WESTER and J. DE BOER (1999), 'Environmental occurance, analysis and toxicology of toxaphene compounds', *Environmental Health Perspectives*, 107 (1), 115–144.

DE VAULT, D. S., R. HESSELBERG, P. W. RODGERS and T. FEIST (1996), 'Contamination trends in lake trout and walleye from the Laurentian Great Lakes', *Journal of Great Lakes Research*, 22 (4), 884–895.

DE WIT, C. (2002), 'An overview of brominated flame retardants in the environment', *Chemosphere*, 46, 583–624.

DIETZ, R., F. RIGET, M. CLEEMANN, A. AARKROG, P. JOHANSEN and J. C. HANSEN (2000), 'Comparison of contaminants from different trophic levels and ecosystems', *The Science of the Total Environment*, 245, 221–231.

EC (2001), 'Council regulation (EC) No. 2375/2001 of 29 November 2001 amending Commission Regulation No. 466/2001 setting maximum levels for certain contaminants in foodstuffs', *Official Journal of the European Communities (L321/1).*

ERICKSON, M. D. (1997), *Analytical Chemistry of PCBs*, New York, CRC Press.

FAIREY, R., K. TABERSKI, S. LAMERDIN, E. JOHNSON, R. P. CLARK, J. W. DOWNING, J. NEWMAN and M. PETREAS (1997), 'Organochlorines and other environmental contaminants in muscle tissues of sportfish collected from San Francisco Bay', *Marine Pollution Bulletin*, 34 (12), 1058–1071.

FALANDYSZ, J. (1998), 'Polychlorinated naphthalenes: an environmental update', *Environmental Pollution*, 101, 77–90.

FALANDYSZ, J., L. STRANDBERG, B. STRANDBERG and C. RAPPE (1998), 'Polychlorinated naphthalenes in three-spined stickleback *Gasterosteus aculeatus* from the gulf of Gdansk', *Chemosphere*, 37 (9–12), 2473–2487.

FALANDYSZ, J., B. STRANDBERG, L. STRANDBERG and C. RAPPE (1999), 'Tris(4-

chlorophenyl)methane and Tris(4-chlorophenyl)methanol in sediment and food webs from the Baltic South coast', *Environmental Science & Technology*, 33 (4), 517–521.

FAO (2001), FAO yearbook, Fishery Statistics, Aquaculture production 1999, vol 88/2, FAO, Rome.

FERNÁNDEZ, M. A., L. M. HERNÁNDEZ, M. J. GONZÁNLEZ, E. ELJARRAT, J. CAIXACH and J. RIVERA (1998), 'Analysis of polychlorinated terphenyls in marine samples', *Chemosphere*, 36 (14), 2941–2948.

FIEDLER, H., O. HUTZINGER and C. TIMMS (1990), 'Dioxins: sources of environmental load and human exposure', *Toxicological and Environmental Chemistry*, 29, 157–243.

FROESCHEIS, O., R. LOOSER, G. M. CAILLIET, W. M. JARMAN and K. BALLSCHMITER (2000), 'The deep-sea as a final global sink of semivolatile persistent organic pollutants? Part I: PCBs in surface and deep-sea dwelling fish of the North and South Atlantic and the Monterey Bay Canyon (California)', *Chemosphere*, 40 (6), 651–660.

FROMME, H., T. OTTO, K. PILZ and F. NEUGEBAUER (1999), 'Levels of synthetic musks; bromocyclene and PCBs in eel (Anguilla anguilla) and PCBs in sediment samples from some waters of Berlin/Germany', *Chemosphere*, 39 (10), 1723–1735.

GATERMANN, R., J. HELLOU, H. HÜHNERFUSS, G. G. RIMKUS and V. ZITKO (1999), 'Polycyclic and nitro musks in the environment: a comparison between Canadian and European aquatic biota', *Chemosphere*, 38 (14), 3431–3441.

GEYER, H. J., G. G. RIMKUS, I. SCHEUNERT, A. KAUNE, K. W. SCHRAMM, A. KETTRUP, M. ZEEMAN, D. C. G. MUIR, L. G. HANSEN and D. MACKAY (2000), 'Bioaccumulation and occurence of endocrine-disrupting chemicals (EDCs), persistent organic pollutants (POPs), and other organic compounds in fish and other organisms including humans', in B. Beek, *Bioaccumulation*, Berlin Heidelberg, Springer-Verlag. 2, part J: 1–178.

GIESY, J. P. and K. KANNAN (2001), 'Global distribution of perfluorooctane sulfonate in wildlife', *Environmental Science & Technology*, 35 (7), 1339–1342.

HALE, R., J. GREAVES, K. GALLAGHER and G. G. VADAS (1990), 'Novel chlorinated terphenyls in sediments and shellfish of an estuarine environment', *Environmental Science & Technology*, 24, 1727–1731.

HALE, R. C., M. ALAEE, J. B. MANCHESTER-NEESVIG, H. M. STAPLETON and M. G. IKONOMOU (2003), 'Polybrominated diphenyl ether flame retardants in the North American environment', *Environment International*, 29 (6), 771–779.

HESS, P., J. DE BOER, W. P. COFINO, P. E. G. LEONARDS and D. E. WELLS (1995), 'Critical review of the analysis of non- and mono-*ortho*-chlorobiphenyls', *Journal of Chromatography A*, 703, 417–465.

HITES, R. A., J. A. FORAN, D. D. CARPENTER, M. C. HAMILTON, B. A. KNUTH and S. J. SCHWAGER (2004), 'Global assessment of organic contaminants in farmed salmon', *Science*, 303 (5655), 226–229.

HOFF, P. T., K. VAN DE VIJVER, W. VAN DONGEN, E. L. ESMNS, R. BLIST and W. M. DE COEN (2003), 'Perfluorooctane sulfonic acid in bib (Trisopterus luscus) and plaice (Pleuronectes platessa) from the Western Scheldt and the Belgian North Sea: Distribution and biochemical effects', *Environmental Toxicology and Chemistry*, 22 (3), 608–614.

IKONOMOU, M. G., S. RAYNE and R. F. ADDISON (2002), 'Exponential increases of the brominated flame retardants, polybrominated diphenyl ethers, in the Canadian arctic from 1981 to 2000', *Environmental Science & Technology*, 36 (9), 1886–1892.

JACOBS, M., A. COVACI and P. SCHEPENS (2001a), 'Investigation of polybrominated diphenyl ethers in Scottish and European farmed Atlantic salmon (*Salmo salar*), salmon aquaculture feed and fish oils', *Organohalogen Compounds*, 51, 239–242.

JACOBS, M., A. COVACI and P. SCHEPENS (2001b), 'Investigation of selected PCBs and organochlorine pesticides farmed Atlantic salmon (*Salmo salar*), salmon aquaculture feed and fish oil components of the feed', *Organohalogen Compounds*, 51, 314.

JAKOBSSON, E. and L. ASPLUND (2000). 'Polychlorinated naphthalenes (PCNs)', in J. Paasvirta, *New Types of Persistent Halogenated Compounds*. Berlin Heidelberg, Springer-Verlag. 3, part K: 97–126.

JÄRNBERG, U. (1997), 'Analytical methods for studying polychlorinated naphthalene congener profiles and levels in the environment', Thesis, Department of Analytical Chemistry and Institute of Applied Environmental Research, Stockholm University, Stockholm.

JÄRNBERG, U., L. ASPLUND, C. DE WIT, A.-L. EGEBÄCK, U. WIDEQVIST and E. JAKOBSSON (1997), 'Distribution of polychlorinated naphthalene congeners in environmental and source-related samples', *Archives of Environmental Contamination Toxicology*, 32, 232–245.

JEONG, G.-H., J.-C. YOU, C.-H. JOO and S.-E. JEON (2001), 'Distribution characteristics of 2, 3, 7, 8-substituted dioxins in the fresh water fishes from the major rivers in S. Korea', *Organohalogen Compounds*, 51, 247–250.

KANNAN, K., T. IMAGAWA, A. L. BLANKENSHIP and J. P. GIESY (1998), 'Isomer-specific analysis and toxic evaluation of polychlorinated naphthalenes in soil, sediment, and biota collected near the site of a former Chlor-Alkali plant', *Environmental Science & Technology*, 32, 2507–2514.

KANNAN, K., N. YAMASHITA, J. S. KHIM, R. M. DAY, C. L. SUMMER and J. P. GIESY (2000), 'Polychlorinated naphthalenes and polychlorinated biphenyls in fishes from Michigan waters including the Great lakes', *Environmental Science & Technology*, 34, 566–572.

KANNAN, K., S. CORSOLINI, T. IMAGAWA, S. FOCARDI and J. P. GIESY (2001a). Polychlorinated -naphthalenes, -biphenyls, -dibenzo-p-dioxins and -dibenzofurans in tuna, swordfish, cormorants and swallows from Italy. *Organohalogen Compounds*, 52, 374–377.

KANNAN, K., J. C. FRANSON, W. W. BOWERMAN, K. J. HANSEN, J. D. JONES and J. P. GRESY (2001b), 'Perfluorooctane sulfonate in fish-eating water birds including bald eagles and albatrosses', *Environmental Science & Technology*, 35 (15), 3065–3070.

KANNAN, K., K. J. HANSEN, T. L. WADE and J. P. GIESY (2002), 'Perfluorooctane sulfonate in oysters, Crassostrea virginica, from the Gulf of Mexico and the Chesapeake Bay, USA', *Archives of Environmental Contamination and Toxicology*, 42 (3), 313–318.

KARL, H. and I. LEHMANN (1997), 'Variation of organochlorine residues with length in the edible part of mackerel (*Scomber scombrus*) from different fishing grounds', *Archives of Fisheries Marine Research*, 45 (2), 135–147.

KARL, H., I. LEHMANN and K. OETJEN (1998), 'Levels of chlordane in fish muscle, -meal, -oil and -feed', *Chemosphere*, 36 (13), 2819–2832.

KELLY, C. A., R. LAW and H. S. EMERSON (2000), Methods for analysis for hydrocarbons and polycyclic aromatic hydrocarbons (PAH) in marine samples. CEFAS, Lowestoft.

KORYTAR, P., J. DE BOER, P. E. G. LEONARDS and U. A. T. BRINKMAN (2002), 'High-resolution separation of polychlorinated biphenyls by comprehensive two-dimensional gas chromatography', *Journal of Chromatography A*, 958, 203–218.

KUCUKSEZGIN, F., O. ALTAY, E. ULUTURHAN and A. KONTAS (2001), 'Trace metal and organochlorine residue levels in red mullet (*Mullus barbatus*) from the Eastern Aegean, Turkey', *Water Research*, 35 (9), 2327–2332.

LAC (1991), 'Jaarverslag 1991', Ministerie van LNV, Den Haag.

LEAH, R. T., M. S. JOHNSON, L. CONNOR and C. LEVENE (1997), 'Polychlorinated biphenyls in fish and shellfish from the Mersey Estuary and Liverpool Bay', *Marine Environmental Research*, 43 (4), 345–358.

LEE, K. M., H. KRUSE and O. WASSERMANN (1996), 'The patern of organochlorines in mussels *Mytilus edulis L.* from the West Baltic Sea', *Archives of Environmental Contamination Toxicology*, 31, 68–76.

LEONARDS, P. E. G., M. LOHMAN, M. M. DE WIT, G. BOOY, S. H. BRANDSMA and J. DE BOER (2000), 'Actuele situatie van gechloreerde dioxines, furanen en polychloorbifenylen in visserij-producten: quick and full-scan'. RIVO, Report no. C34/00, IJmuiden, The Netherlands.

LIEM, A. K. D. (1999), 'Basic aspects of methods for the determination of dioxins and PCBs in foodstuffs and human tissues', *Trends in Analytical Chemistry*, 18 (6), 429–439.

LIEM, A. K. D. and R. M. C. THEELEN (1997), 'Dioxins: chemical analysis, exposure and risk assessment', Thesis, University of Utrecht, Utrecht.

LUNDGREN, K., R. ISHAQ, B. VAN BAVEL, M. TYSKLIND and D. BROMAN (2001). Polychlorinated naphthalene levels and congener profiles in a benthic food chain in the Baltic sea. *Organohalogen Compounds*, 52, 370–380.

LUROSS, J. M., M. ALAEE, D. B. SERGEANT, C. M. CANNON, D. M. WHITTLE, K. R. SOLOMON and D. C. G. MUIR (2002), 'Spatial distribution of polybrominated diphenyl ethers and polybrominated biphenyls in lake trout from the Laurentian Great Lakes', *Chemosphere*, 46 (5), 665–672.

LYE, C. M., C. L. J. FRID, M. E. GILL, D. W. COOPER and D. M. JONES (1999), 'Estrogenic alkylphenols in fish tissues, sediments and waters from the U.K. Tyne and Tees estuaries', *Environmental Science & Technology*, 33, 1009–1014.

MOISEY, J., A. T. FISK, K. A. HOBSON and R. J. NORSTROM (2001), 'Hexachlorocyclohexane (HCH) isomers and chiral signatures of a-HCH in the Arctic marine food web of the Northwater Polynya', *Environmental Science & Technology*, 35, 1920–1927.

MOODY, C. A. and J. FIELD (2000), 'Perfluorinated surfactants and the environmental implications of their use as fire-fighting foams', *Environmental Science & Technology*, 34 (18), 3864–3870.

MOODY, C. A., W. C. KWAN, J. W. MARTIN, D. C. G. MUIR and S. A. MABURY (2001), 'Determination of perfluorinated surfactants in surface water samples by two independent analytical techniques: liquid chromatography/tandem mass spectrometry and 19F NMR', *Analytical Chemistry*, 73, 2200–2206.

MOODY, C. A., J. W. MARTIN, W. C. KWAN, D. C. G. MUIR and S. C. MABURY (2002), 'Monitoring perfluorinated surfactants in biota and surface water samples following an accidental release of fire-fighting foam into Etohicoke Creek', *Environmental Science & Technology*, 36 (4), 545–551.

MORRIS, S., C. R. ALLCHIN, P. BERSUDER, B. N. ZEGERS, J. J. H. HAFTKA, J. P. BOON, S. H. BRANDSMA, A. W. KRUIJT, I VANDER VEEN, J VAN HESSELINGEN and J. DE BOER (2003), 'A new LC-MS method for the detection and quantification of hexabromocyclododecane diastereoisomers and tetrabromobisphenol-A flame retardants in environmental samples', *Organohalogen Compounds*, 60, 436–439.

MUIR, D. C. G., G. A. STERN and G. T. TOMY (2000), 'Chlorinated paraffins', in J. Paasvirta, *New Types of Persistent Halogenated Compounds*, Berlin Heidelberg, Springer-Verlag. 3, part K: 204–236.

NEWSOME, W. H. and P. ANDREWS (1993), 'Organochlorine pesticides and polychlorinated biphenyl congeners in commercial fish from the great lakes', *Journal of AOAC International*, 76 (4), 707–710.

NICHOLLS, C. R., C. R. ALLCHIN and R. J. LAW (2001), 'Levels of short and medium chain length polychlorinated n-alkanes in environmental samples from selected industrial areas in England and Wales', *Environmental Pollution*, 114 (3), 415–430.

NYLUND, K., A. KIERKEGAARD, U. ERIKSSON, L. ASPLUND, A. BIGNERT and M. OLSSON (2001). Spatial distribution of some polybrominated diphenyl ethers and hexabromocyclododecane in herring (*Clupea harengus*) along the Swedish coast. The second international workshop on brominated flame retardants, Stockholm.

ODUM, J., P. A. LEFEVRE, S. TITTENSOR, D. PATON, E. J. ROUTLEDGE, N. A. BERESFORD, J. P. SUMPTER and J. ASHBY (1997), 'The rodent uterotrophic assay: Critical protocol features, studies with nonyl phenols, and comparison with a yeast estrogenicity assay', *Regulatory Toxicology and Pharmacology*, 25 (2), 176–188.

OK, G., S.-J. KIM, S.-H. JI and I.-S. LEE (2001), 'Polychlorinated dibenzo-*p*-dioxins and polychlorinated dibenzofurans in marked fish and meat samples in the market of Pusan city, Korea', *Organohalogen Compounds*, 51, 328–311.

OLSSON, A., K. VALTERS and S. BUREAU (2000), 'Concentrations of organochlorine substances in relation to fish size and trophic position: a study on perch (*Perca fluviatilis L.*)', *Environmental Science & Technology*, 34, 4878–4886.

PARSLEY, K., C. WRIGHT and S. THORPE (1998), 'PCDDs, PCDFs and PCBs in marine fish, salmon and fish fingers'. MAFF, Report no. FD97/66, United Kingdom.

PICCARDO, M. T., R. CORADEGHINI and F. VALERIO (2001), 'Polycyclic aromatic hydrocarbon pollution in native and caged mussels', *Marine Pollution Bulletin*, 42 (10), 951–956.

PICER, M. and N. PICER (1994), 'Levels and long-term trends of polychlorinated biphenyls and DDTs in mussels collected from the middle Adriatic coastal waters', *Chemosphere*, 29 (3), 465–475.

POREMSKI, H.-J., S. WIANDT and T. KNACKER (2001), 'Chlorinated paraffins – a further pop to consider?' *Organohalogen Compounds*, 52, 397–400.

REMBERG, G., P. SANDRA, W. NYIRY, N. WINKER and A. NIKIFOROV (1998), 'Calculation of the polychlorinated terphenyl congener distribution and gas chromatographic retention behaviour of selected single standards on four stationary liquid phases', *Fresenius Journal of Analytical Chemistry*, 362, 404–408.

RICE, C. P., S. M. CHERNYAK, L. BEGNOCHE, R. QUINTAL and J. HICKEY (2002), 'Comparisons of PBDE composition and concentration in fish collected from the Detroit river, MI and Des Plaines River, IL', *Chemosphere*, 49 (7), 731–737.

RIMKUS, G. G. (1999), 'Polycyclic musk fragrances in the aquatic environment', *Toxicology Letters*, 111, 37–56.

ROOSE, P., K. COOREMAN and W. YVYNCKE (1998), 'PCBs in cod (*Gadus morhua*), flounder (*Platichthys flesus*), bleu mussel (*Mytilus edulis*) and brown shrimp (*Crangon crangon*) from the Belgian continental shelf: relation to biological parameters and trend analysis', *Chemosphere*, 37 (9–12), 2199–2210.

ROOTS, O. (2001), 'Halogenated environmental contaminants in fish from Estonian coastal areas', *Chemosphere*, 43, 623–632.

SAKAI, S., J. WATANABE, Y. HONDA, H. TAKATSUKI, I. AOKI, M. FUTAMATSU and K. SHIOZAKI (2001), 'Combustion of brominated flame retardants and behavior of its byproducts', *Chemosphere*, 42 (5–7), 519–531.

SAKURAI, T., J.-G. KIM, N. SUZUKI, T. MATSUO, D.-Q. LI, Y. YAO, S. MASUNAGA and J. NAKANISHI

(2000), 'Polychlorinated dibenzo-p-dioxins and dibenzofurans in sediment, soil, fish, shellfish and crab samples from Tokyo Bay area, Japan', *Chemosphere*, 40, 627–640.

SCAN (2000), 'Opinion of the scientific committee on animal nutrition on the dioxin contamination of feedingstuffs and their contribution to the contamination of food of animal origin', European Commission, Brussels.

SCF (2000), Opinion of the SCF on the risk assessment of dioxins and dioxin-like PCBs in food, European Commission, Brussels.

SCHLABACH, M., E. FJELD and E. BREVIK (2001). Polybrominated diphenylethers and other persistent organic pollutants in Norwegian freshwater fish. The second international workshop on brominated flame retardants, Stockholm.

SCOOP (2000), 'Assessment of dietary intake of dioxins and related PCBs by the population of EU Member states', Directorate-General Health and Consumer Protection, European Commission, Brussels.

SELLSTROM, U., A. KIERKEGAARD, C. DE WIT and B. JANSSON (1998), 'Polybrominated diphenyl ethers and hexabromocyclododecane in sediment and fish from a Swedish river', *Environmental Toxicology and Chemistry*, 17 (6), 1065–1072.

SLOOFF, W., P. F. H. BONT, J. A. JANUS and J. A. ANNEMA (1992), 'Exploratory report chlorinated paraffins', RIVM. Report no. 710401016, Bilthoven, The Netherlands,.

SNYDER, S. S., T. L. KEITH, S. L. PIERENS, E. M. SYNDER and J. P. GIESY (2001a), 'Bioconcentration of nonylphenol in fathead minnows (*Pimepales promelas*)', *Chemosphere*, 44, 1697–1702.

SNYDER, S. S., D L. VILLENEUVE, E. M. SYNDER and J. P. GIESY (2001b), 'Identification and quantification method for nonylphenol and lower oligomer nonylphenol ethoxylates in fish tissues', *Environmental Toxicology and Chemistry*, 20 (9), 1870–1873.

STAPLES, C. A., J. WEEKS, J. F. HALL and C. G. NAYLOR (1998), 'Evaluation of aquatic toxicity and bioaccumulation of C8 and C9–alkylphenolethoxylates', *Environmental Toxicology and Chemistry*, 17 (12), 2470–2480.

STAPLETON, H. M., C. MASTERSON, J. SKUBINNA, P. OSTROM and J. E. BAKER (2001), 'Accumulation of atmospheric and sedimentary PCBs and toxaphene in a lake Michigan food web', *Environmental Science & Technology*, 35, 3287–3293.

STRANDBERG, B., L. STRANDBERG, P. A. BERGQVIST, J. FALANDYSZ and C. RAPPE (1998), 'Concentrations and biomagnification of 17 chlordane compounds and other organochlorines in harbour porpoise (*Phocoena phocoena)*and herring from the Southern Baltic Sea', *Chemosphere*, 37 (9–12), 2513–2523.

TANIYASU, S., K. KANNAN, Y. HERII and N. YAMASHITA (2002), 'The first environmental survey of perfluorooctanesulfonate (PFOS) and related compounds in Japan', *Organohalogen Compounds*, 59, 311–314.

TOMY, G. T. and G. A. STERN (1999), 'Analysis of C_{14}–C_{17} polychloro-n-alkanes in environmental matrices by accelerated solvent extraction – high resolution gas chromatography/electron capture negative ion high resolution mass spectrometry', *Analytical Chemistry*, 71 (21), 4860–4865.

TOMY, G. T., W. BUDAKOWSKI, T. HALLDORSEN, M. WHITTLE, M. KEIR and M. ALAEE (2003), 'Biomagnification of alpha- and gamma-hexabromocyclododecane congeners in a lake Ontario food web', *Organohalogen Compounds*, 61, 111–114.

TSUDA, T., A. TAKINO, K. MURAKI, H. HARADA and M. KOJIMA (2001), 'Evaluation of 4-nonylphenols and 4-tert-octylphenol contamination of fish in rivers by laboratory accumulation and excretion experiments', *Water Research*, 35 (7), 1786–1792.

VAN DEN BERG, M., L. BIRBAUM, A. T. C. BOSVELD, B. BRUNSTRÖM, P. COOK, M. FEELEY, J. P. GIESY, A. HANBERG, R. HASEGAVA, S. W. KENNEDY, T. KUBIAK, J. C. LARSEN, F. X. R. VAN LEEUWEN, A. K. D. LIEM, C. NOLT, R. E. PETERSON, L. POELLINGER, S. SAFE, D. SCHRENK, D. TILLITT, M. TYSKLIND, M. YOUNES, F. WAERN and T. ZACHAREWSKI (1998), 'Toxic equivalency factors (TEFs) for PCBs, PCDDs and PCDFs for humans and wildlife', *Environmental Health Perspectives*, 106, 775–792.

VAN DER PLAS, S. A. (2000), 'Tumour promotion by complex mixtures of polyhalogenated aromatic hydrocarbons (PHAHs) and the applicability of the Toxic Equivalency Factor (TEF) concept', Thesis, Wageningen University, Wageningen.

VAN DE VIJVER, K., P. HOFF, W. VAN DONGEN, E. ESMANS, R. BLUST and W. DE COEN (2002). PFOS in marine and estuarine organisms from the Belgian North Sea and Western Scheldt estuary. SETAC, Vienna.

VAN LEEUWEN, S. P. J., W. A. TRAAG, L. A. P. HOOGENBOOM, G. BOOIJ, M. LOHMAN, Q. T. DAO and J. DE BOER (2002), 'Dioxines, furanen en PCBs in aal – Onderzoek naar wilde aal, gekweekte aal, geïmporteerde en gerookte aal', RIVO, Report no. C034/02, IJmuiden, The Netherlands.

VETHAAK, A. D., G. B. J. RIJS, S. M. SCHRAP, H. RUITER, A. GERRITSEN and J. LAHR (2002), 'Estrogens and xeno-estrogens in the aquatic environment of the Netherlands', RIZA/RIKZ report 2002.001. Lelystad/Den Haag.

VETTER, W. and M. OEHME (2000), 'Toxaphene. Analysis and environmental fate of congeners', in J. Paasvirta, *New Types of Persistent Halogenated Compounds*. Berlin Heidelberg, Springer-Verlag. 3, part K: 237–287.

VETTER, W., U. KLOBES and B. LUCKAS (2001), 'Distribution and levels of eight toxaphene congeners in different tissues of marine mammals, birds and cod livers', *Chemosphere*, 43, 611–621.

WAINWRIGHT, S. E., M. A. MORA, J. L. SERICANO and P. THOMAS (2001), 'Chlorinated hydrocarbons and biomarkers of exposure in wading birds and fish of the lower Rio Grande valley, Texas', *Archives of Environmental Contamination Toxicology*, 40, 101–111.

WESTER, P. G., J. DE BOER and U. A. TH. BRINKMAN (1996) 'Determination of polychlorinated terphenyls in aquatic biota and sediment with gas chromotography/mass spectometry using negative chemical ionization', *Environmental Science and Technology*, 30, 473–480.

WHITTLE, D. M., R. M. KIRILUK, A. A. CARSWELL, M. J. KEIR and D. C. MACEACHEN (2000), 'Toxaphene congeners in the Canadian Great Lakes basin: temporal and spatial food web dynamics', *Chemosphere*, 40, 1221–1226.

WHO (1992), *PCBs and PCTs Health and Safety Guide*, Geneva, WHO.

WHO (1994a), *Brominated Biphenyls*, Geneva, WHO.

WHO (1994b), *Brominated Diphenyl Ethers*, Geneva, WHO.

YLITALO, G. M., J. BUZITIS and M. M. KRAHN (1999), 'Analyses of tissues of eight marine species from Atlantic and Pacific coasts for dioxin-like chlorobiphenyls (CBs) and total CBs', *Archives of Environmental Contamination and Toxicology*, 37 (2), 205–219.

22

Identifying allergenic proteins in food

E. N. Clare Mills, J. A. Jenkins, J. A. Robertson, Institute of Food Research, Norwich; S. Griffiths-Jones, Wellcome Trust Sanger Institute, Cambridge; and P. R. Shewry, Institute of Arable Crops Research, UK

22.1 Introduction: the nature of allergens and allergies

During normal functioning, the body produces molecules called antibodies (also known as immunoglobulins – Ig) to any foreign (i.e. non-self) molecules that it encounters. This so-called humoral immune response is part of the defence mechanism whereby the body deals with infectious agents such as viruses and bacteria. One particular kind of antibody, known as IgE, is generated as part of the normal immune reaction to parasitic infections, such as malaria. However, under certain circumstances predisposed individuals can develop IgE responses to environmental agents, such as pollen, dusts and foods. The macromolecules (usually proteins) recognised by the IgE are known as allergens and they trigger a response by cross-linking IgE molecules bound to the surface of basophile or mast cells, causing them to release pre-formed inflammatory mediators, including histamine. It is these mediators which actually cause the physiological changes which manifest themselves in an allergic reaction, and can be quite diverse in nature. The resulting symptoms can include respiratory (wheezing, shortness of breath), skin (rashes such as hives, eczema and atopic dermatitis) and gastrointestinal symptoms (vomiting, diarrhoea).

As IgE-mediated reactions generally occur quite rapidly following exposure, they are classified as a Type I hypersensitivity reaction and are quite distinct from food intolerances. The latter can take much longer (even days) to manifest themselves and may not necessarily have an immunological basis. One example of a food intolerance which actually results from the loss of a digestive enzyme is lactose intolerance. This means that individuals are unable to tolerate cows' milk and some derived products. Another is the gluten intolerance syndrome, coeliac disease, which is thought to involve the immune system but which does not involve the development of an IgE response to wheat. Whilst the gluten proteins which trigger it are not IgE-binding proteins, some workers refer to them as allergens, and they are treated as such in the WHO Codex Alimentarius Commission Food Labelling recommendations.

Only around seven types of foods are responsible for causing the majority of food allergies, of which four originate from plants and include peanuts, tree nuts, wheat, and soy (Bush and Hefle, 1996). These are thought to sensitise individuals via the gastrointestinal tract, and can often result in more severe symptoms, including anaphylaxis. In addition to such foods, several types of allergen found in fresh fruits and vegetables have been identified. However, allergies towards the latter seem to develop as a consequence of individuals first developing inhalant allergies to agents such as pollen and latex. Termed cross-reactive allergy syndromes, these arise because of the high levels of homology between the sensitising allergens found in pollen, latex and allergens in foods such as apples, peaches, pears, celery, etc. Although severe reactions to these allergens can occur, in general the cross-reactive allergy syndromes have a milder profile of symptoms than foods believed to sensitise via the oral route, with reactions often being confined to the oral cavity. This has resulted in the pollen-fruit/vegetable allergies being associated with the so-called oral allergy syndrome (OAS).

A summary of the relationships, structures and properties of the food allergens involved in these two types of allergy are given below, followed by a discussion of how such knowledge can assist in identifying potential allergens, an important part of identifying and managing allergenic risks posed by novel foods.

22.2 Types of plant food allergens and their characteristics

The explosion in information arising from sequencing of entire genomes has stimulated the development of powerful computer-based methods to compare the amino acid sequences and structures of proteins. Such approaches, coupled with the large number of allergens which have now been sequenced, have allowed us to determine the structural and evolutionary relationships of plant food allergens (Mills *et al.*, 2003). Such comparisons indicate that the vast majority of plant food allergens that sensitise via the gastrointestinal tract belong to only three major groups of plant proteins: the prolamin and cupin super-families, together with certain members of the cysteine protease family. In contrast inhalant allergens that can trigger food allergies are more diverse, being spread across a larger number of protein families, with one family, known as the Bet v 1 family after the major inhalant allergen in birch pollen, dominating.

Many of the allergens are also so-called pathogenesis-related (PR) proteins, the expression of which is switched on as part of a plant's defence response following infection by microbes and fungi, in addition to abiotic stress (van Loon and van Strien, 1999). At present 17 different classes of PR proteins have been defined, of which around seven contain known food allergens (Hoffmann-Sommergruber, 2002). They encompass a number of types of biological activities, many of the proteins sharing more than one property, and include inhibitors of proteinases and α-amylases, polysaccharide hydrolases (including α-1,3-glucanases and endochitinases which hydrolyse fungal hyphae and/or insect cuticles), proteins which destabilise cell membranes causing membrane leakage (including thionins, 2S albumins, thaumatin-related proteins, and non-specific lipid transfer proteins [nsLTPs]) and an ability to bind chitin and other polysaccharides (including lectins, hevein and endochitinases). Many have a functional role in disrupting the growth of, for example, fungal hyphae as they penetrate the plant tissue at the site of infection. The relationship between allergenic potential and PR family membership is intriguing and whilst as yet no precise relationship has been defined, many are small proteins resistant to denaturation at low pH and proteolysis *in vitro* (Hoffman-Sommergruber, 2002).

22.2.2 Plant food protein allergen families sensitising via the gastrointestinal tract

Prolamin superfamily

This family comprises the alcohol-soluble (prolamin) storage proteins of cereals, the 2S storage albumins, non-specific lipid transfer proteins (nsLTP) and cereal inhibitors of α-amylase and/or trypsin. All but the nsLTPs are seed proteins, and family members share a characteristic skeleton of cysteine residues, containing characteristic Cys Cys and Cys X Cys motifs, where X represents any other residue. The skeleton contains either eight (2S albumins ns LTPs) or ten (α-amylase/trypsin inhibitors) cysteine residues, which form three or four intra-chain disulphide bonds respectively, and is broadly described by the following formula:

$$\begin{aligned}&\mathrm{Cys} - (\mathrm{X} = 7 - 13) - \mathrm{Cys} - (\mathrm{X} = 8 - 26) - \mathrm{Cys} - \mathrm{Cys} - (\mathrm{X} = 8 - 30)\\&-\mathrm{Cys} - \mathrm{X} - \mathrm{Cys} - (\mathrm{X} = 20 - 48) - \mathrm{Cys} - \mathrm{Cys}\end{aligned}$$

In the prolamin storage proteins this skeleton has been disrupted by the insertion of a repetitive domain comprising one or two short motifs rich in proline and glutamine. Three-dimensional structures have been defined for the 2S albumin, nsLTP and α-amylase/trypsin inhibitors and demonstrate that these family members also share a related fold consisting of bundles of four α-helices stabilised by disulphide bonds. This structural motif is illustrated by the structure of the ns LTP allergen from maize, Zea m 14 shown in Fig. 22.1.

There is a widespread perception that cereals and wheat in particular, are important allergenic foods. However, whilst their role in the occupational allergy, bakers' asthma, and in the aetiology of coeliac disease is well defined,

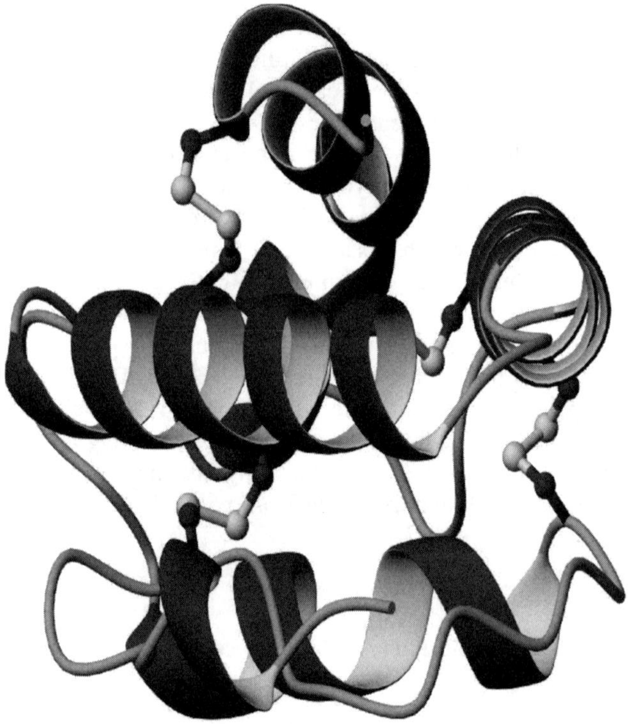

Fig. 22.1 Three-dimensional structure of a non-specific lipid transfer protein (nsLTP) allergen from maize illustrating the four α-helix motif characteristic of prolamin superfamily members. Ribbon representations of nsLTP based on the structure of Shin *et al.* (1995).

there is only limited information regarding their role in type I food allergy. Wheat prolamins have been shown to be IgE reactive (Maruyama *et al.*, 1998; Simonato *et al.*, 2001) and are involved in wheat-induced atopic dermatitis (Varjonen *et al.*, 1995, 2000; Tanabe *et al.*, 1996). They also seem to be involved in triggering exercise-induced anaphylaxis (EIA), a reaction that certain patients experience only on taking exercise following consumption of wheat containing foods (Palosuo *et al.*, 1999; Varjonen *et al.*, 1997).

In contrast the 2S albumins were among the first plant proteins to be described as allergens in cotton seed, over 50 years ago (Youle and Huang, 1981). These proteins can act as both occupational allergens, sensitising through inhalation of dusts, as well as acting as food allergens. 2S storage albumins have been identified as the major allergenic components in peanut (Ara h 2, 6, 7; Burks *et al.*, 1992, Kleber *et al.*, 1999), occur in oriental and yellow mustards (Bra j 1, Sin a 1; Menendez-Arias *et al.*, 1988; Monsalve *et al.*, 1993), oilseed rape (the napin, Bra n 1), castor bean (Ric c 1, 3), walnut (Jug r 1), and sunflower, sesame (Ses i 1; Pastorello *et al.*, 2001b and Ses i 2; Beyer *et al.*, 2002a), Brazil nut (Ber e 1; Pastorello *et al.*, 1998b), almond (Poltronieri *et al.*, 2002), and sunflower (Kelly *et al.*, 2000). It has also been reported that the 2S albumins of soy (Shibasaki *et al.*, 1980) and chickpea (Vioque *et al.*, 1999) are allergens.

The nsLTPs have an even wider distribution in plants than 2S albumins, with over 100 sequences being available from a variety of plant organs including seeds, fruit and vegetative tissues. Major allergens have been identified in peach (Pru p 3 [initially named Pru p 1]; Pastorello *et al.*, 1999a), apple (Mal d 3; Pastorello *et al.*, 1999b, Sanchez-Monge *et al.*, 1999) and maize (Zea m 14; Pastorello *et al.*, 2000) leading to the family being termed as 'pan-allergens' (Sanchez-Monge *et al.*, 1999). Like the 2S albumins, nsLTPs can sensitise both by inhalation and/or the oral route, as is illustrated by an individual who had an occupational allergy to spelt, the major allergen being the nsLTP, but experienced symptoms on consuming a variety of fruits (Pastorello *et al.*, 2001a). That nsLTP sensitisation can also occur via the lungs is also indicated by their being identified as pollen allergens (Duro *et al.*, 1996; Tejera *et al.*, 1999) but as yet there is no clear evidence of a link between sensitisation to pollen nsLTP and subsequent development of allergy to fruit.

The cereal α-amylase inhibitors can also sensitise individuals via the lungs giving rise to occupational allergies such as bakers' asthma (wheat, barley and rye) or via the gastrointestinal tract (wheat, barley and rice). The best characterised allergens of this group are the α-amylase inhibitors of rice grain with relative molecular weights (M_rs) of about 14,000–16,000 (Nakase *et al.*, 1996). More than ten different cDNA clones have been isolated indicating the presence of a multigene family (Alvarez *et al.*, 1995). The same allergens have been characterised in orally sensitised wheat allergic individuals, although only one M_r ~15,000 subunit was involved (James *et al.*, 1997). A M_r 16,000 beer allergen has also been described which originates from barley and appears to belong to the α-amylase inhibitor family (Curioni *et al.*, 1999), together with a major M_r 16,000 allergen in maize (Pastorello *et al.*, 2000).

Cupin superfamily

The cupins have a common basic β-barrel structure, the name 'cupin' being derived from the Latin for a small barrel or cask (Dunwell, 1998). The most important allergens identified in this superfamily are the 7S and 11S globulin seed storage proteins in which the cupin domain has been duplicated, and is exemplified by the allergenic soya globulin, proglycinin (Fig. 22.2). Both 11S and 7S globulins are oligomeric proteins, the 7S globulins usually existing as a trimeric complex of three subunits of M_r ~50,000, while the 11S globulins are typically hexameric with M_r ~60,000 subunits. The 11S globulin subunits are synthesised as a single chain and are post-translationally cleaved to give acidic and basic chains which remain associated by a single disulphide bond. Although the subunits of the two types of globulins have no obvious sequence similarity, they do have remarkably similar three-dimensional structures (Adachi *et al.*, 2001). Major allergens include the 7S and 11S globulins of soybean (Burks *et al.*, 1988; Rabjohn *et al.*, 1999), peanut (Ara h 1 and Ara h 3; Burks *et al.*, 1991, 1992), the 7S globulins of walnut (Jug r 2) (Teuber *et al.*, 1999), sesame (Beyer

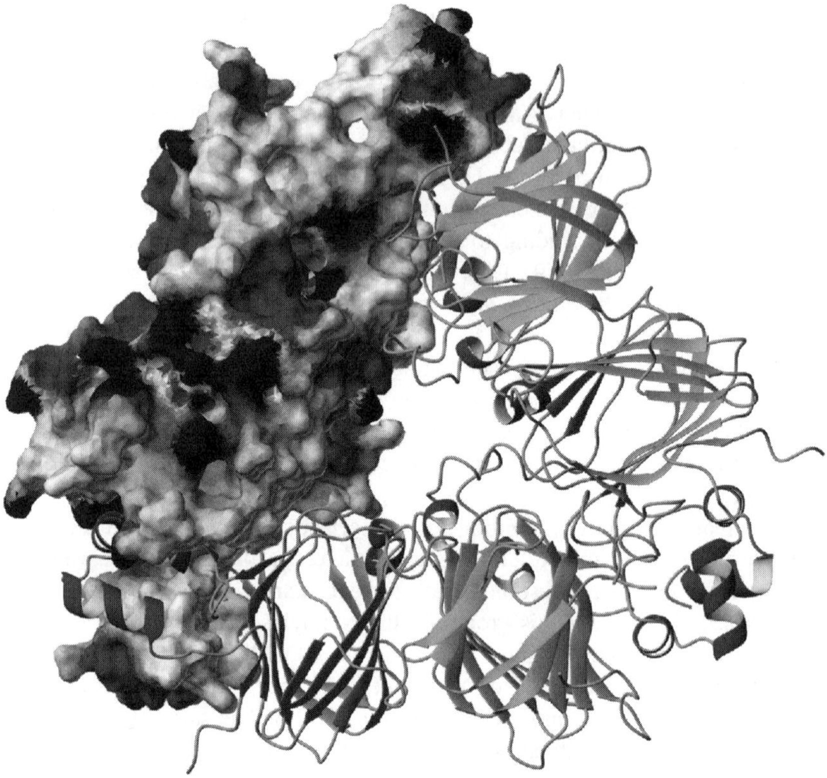

Fig. 22.2 Three-dimensional structure of the allergenic 11S globulin, proglycinin, from soybean illustrating the β-barrel motif characteristic of the cupin superfamily members. Ribbon representation of soybean proglycinin based on the structure of Adachi *et al.* (2001).

et al., 2002a), cashew nut (Ana c 1) (Wang *et al.*, 2002), one of the subunits of the proteolytically processed 7S globulin of lentil (Sanchez-Monge *et al.*, 2000), and hazelnut (Beyer *et al.*, 2002b). The 11S globulins have also been shown to be allergens in almond (also known as almond major protein, AMP) (Roux *et al.*, 2001) and implicated as allergens in coconut and walnut (Teuber and Petersen, 1999).

Cysteine protease superfamily

Cysteine proteases of the C1, or papain-like, family were originally characterised by having a cysteine residue as part of their catalytic site, which has now been extended to include conserved glutamine, cysteine, histidine and asparagine residues (Rawlings and Barrett, 1993). Whilst some family members share sequence homology, they may not have protease activity, a notable example being the P34 protein from soybean where the active site cysteine residue has been replaced with a glycine (Kalinski *et al.*, 1990).

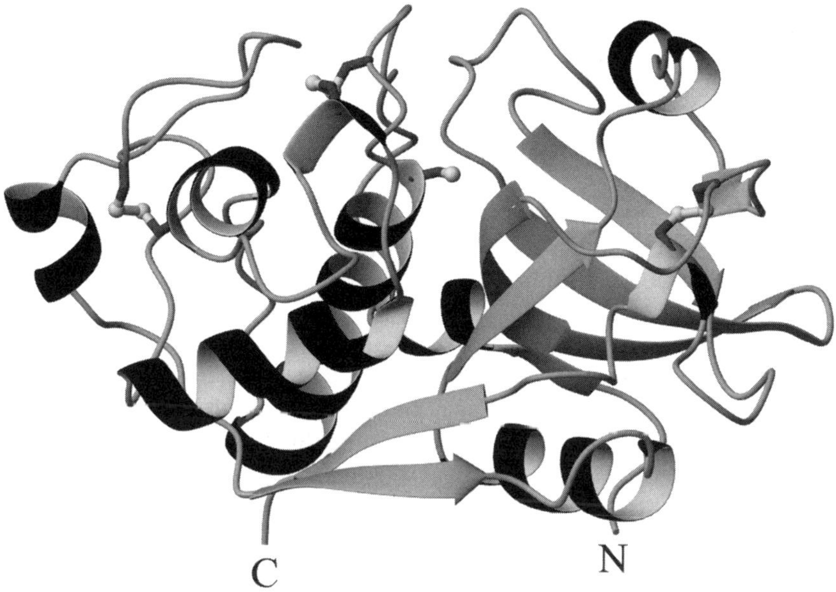

Fig. 22.3 Three-dimensional structure of the allergenic cysteine protease from kiwi fruit, actinidin. Ribbon representation of actinidin based on the structure of Baker (1980).

There are two major food allergens that belong to this family, the first of which to be identified was the major allergen from kiwi fruit, actinidin (Act c 1) (Pastorello *et al.*, 1998a; Fahlbush *et al.*, 1998; Möller *et al.*, 1997), the three-dimensional structure of which is shown in Fig. 22.3. Unlike other kiwi allergens, actinidin shows no IgE cross-reactivity with pollen proteins, implying that it acts to sensitise individuals via the GI tract rather than through inhalation (Pastorello *et al.*, 1996; Gall *et al.*, 1994). The second is the major allergen involved in soybean-induced atopic dermatitis (Ogawa *et al.*, 1993) known variously as Gly m Bd 30K, Gly m 1, or P34. Whilst initially identified as a 34kD oil body-associated protein, it is actually associated with the storage vacuoles of soybean (Kalinski et al., 1990), and becomes complexed with 7S globulin of soy, β-conglycinin (Ogawa *et al.*, 1993; Samoto *et al.*, 1996).

22.2.3 Inhalant allergens and cross-reactive allergy syndromes

The major birch pollen allergen, Bet v 1, is related to a class of putative plant defence proteins (PR10) and results in dietary reaction to proteins in a range of fruit (including Mal d 1 of apple and Pru av 1 of cherry) and vegetables (including Api g 1 of celery, Dau c 1 of carrot). Although the biological role of PR10 proteins has not been established, they are presumed to be defensive (Hoffman-Sommergruber, 2002). A further type of PR protein (PR-5) which is related to the sweet protein thaumatin is an allergen in fruits such as apple (Mal d 2) and cherry (Pru av 2). A second major pollen allergen, Bet v 2, is a profilin, a protein which binds to the actin cytoskeleton of cells. Sensitisation to this pollen protein results in allergic reactions to proteins in a wide range of fresh fruits and vegetables including fruits of the *Rosacea* such as apple (Mal d 1) together with other types of plant foods including celery (Api g 4), peanut (Ara h 5), soybean (Gly m 3), amongst many others. Inhalation of two other PR-type proteins from latex can also result in dietary allergy to related proteins in fruit and vegetables. These are PR-2/Hev b 2 (β1,3-glucanase) and PR-3/Hev b 6 (class II chitinases) which result in cross-reactive allergies to foods such as avocado, chestnut, banana, fig, kiwi and other foods.

22.2.4 Common properties of plant food allergens

Allergens found in foods, both of plant and animal origin that cause allergies as a result of oral sensitisation seem generally to be characterised by two properties, abundance in the food and/or structural stability. Thus, the major allergens of milk, egg, fish, and peanuts are all highly abundant, and can individually comprise up to 25–50% of the protein in the original food. Many allergens are stable proteins, resisting thermal denaturation and/or proteolysis and include cupin allergens (Mills *et al.*, 2002), members of the prolamin superfamily such as the nsLTPs (Douliez *et al.*, 2000), cows' milk β-lactoglobulin (Wal, 1998), cod parvalbumin (Bugajska-Scretter *et al.*, 1998) and hen egg ovomucoid (Cooke and Sampson, 1997). Many food allergens do share both these attributes, but certain proteins, such as the caseins, are both abundant and proteolytically labile proteins. Examples of the converse can also be found, with, for example, the nsLTPs which whilst they are very stable proteins, are not especially abundant.

One reason underlying such common characteristics may be that for a food allergen to sensitise an individual via the gastrointestinal tract it must possess properties which preserve its structure from degradation in the gastrointestinal tract. This would include resistance to low pH, proteolysis and surfactants such as bile salts, and would require that sufficient intact (or semi-intact) protein survives to be taken up by the gut and sensitise the mucosal immune system. However, allergens involved in cross-reactive allergy syndromes do not share such properties, having instead more in common with inhalant allergens to which they are homologous. Thus, they are readily soluble in physiological buffers, tend to be thermolabile and are readily broken down by proteases. Consequently, whilst they are able to elicit an allergic reaction, they are often unable to sensitise an individual through ingestion. Thus, fruit allergens belonging to the Bet v 1 family of proteins which are involved in the pollen-fruit allergy syndrome are considered to be 'incomplete' allergens, as ingestion of fruit itself does not stimulate an IgE response, but does trigger histamine release from mast cells loaded with IgE to the birch pollen allergen Bet v 1 (Alberse, 2000).

22.3 Identifying potentially allergenic proteins: bioinformatics

There is increasing interest in the use of bioinformatic approaches to identifying potentially allergenic proteins which are largely based on demonstrating a lack of similarity between a 'novel' protein and known allergens for a protein to be acceptable for consumption. Such bioinformatic approaches offer a fast and cheap way of eliminating potential allergens at an early stage in the selection of target genes in the development of GMOs for food use. In many cases they are being used to 'predict' protein allergenicity, although given our lack of understanding as to what precisely predisposes individuals to becoming allergic, and what makes some foods, such as peanut, more allergenic than others, this is not currently possible with any degree of certainty. In reality such computer-based '*in silico*' methods can only give some quantitative indication as to the similarity of a novel protein to a known allergen and are unable to give any indication of sensitisation potential *per se*. Nevertheless, such an objective means of assessing similarity of novel proteins to known allergens plays a useful part in assessing the allergenic potential of novel proteins.

One prerequisite for such an approach is the assembly of an appropriate database of allergen sequences. The term 'allergen' is used loosely in databases such as ExPasy and is largely dependent on the information supplied by an individual submitting a sequence. Consequently many known allergens that were sequenced 20 years ago do not include the term 'allergen' in their description, whilst others have it included because of their homology to known allergens, but lack data on clinical reactivity. It is thus very hard to automatically extract a set of allergen sequences from the general sequence databases (Gendel, 2002). As a consequence curated lists and databases, where sequences have been included with a clear definition as to their allergenicity, are more reliable and include that developed by the Allergen Nomenclature Committee (http://www.allergen.org/), one maintained at the US FDA (http://www.iit.edu/~sgendel/foodallr.htm; Gendel, 1998), and another hosted by the Food Allergy Research and Resource Programme (FARRP) at the University of Nebraska (http://www.allergenonline.com; Hileman *et al.*, 2002).

22.3.1 Pair-wise methods

A number of ways of identifying novel food protein allergens have been proposed, in order to rationalise the identification of novel proteins in foods. A joint FAO/WHO Expert Consultation on Foods Derived from Biotechnology (WHO-FAO, 2001) proposed a decision tree based on a preliminary screen using computational sequence analysis to identify proteins with sequence similarity to known allergens. The consultation considered that a novel protein would exhibit IgE cross-reactivity with a known allergen if it shared either 35% sequence identity (determined using a window of 80 amino acids and a suitable gap penalty), or an identical stretch of six contiguous amino acids. Previously

Metcalfe *et al.* (1996) had proposed a threshold of eight identical amino acids on the basis of the length of a T-cell epitope, although IgE binding sites can involve shorter sequences in an allergen (Becker and Reese, 2001). Subsequently the WHO-FAO 2001 consultation noted that an identity of six amino acids had a significant probability of occurring by chance and suggested that the significance of such matches should be verified using allergic sera. Gendel (2002) has also pointed out that using default values in alignment programs designed to detect evolutionary relationships may not find the short identical sequences postulated to result in cross-reactivity. He recommended that only identities should be scored and that the statistical significance of the alignment be ignored.

Such pair-wise screening for sequence homology is very effective at identifying proteins which belong to families with highly conserved sequences, such as the Bet v 1 family of pollen allergens (Breiteneder and Ebner, 2000), but is less effective when levels of sequence identity drop below 40%. It can also result in a large number of false positive allergens being identified, with almost 70% of sequenced rice proteins being identified as potential allergens using a peptide length of six residues. Hileman *et al.* (2002) tested different criteria for identifying potential allergens by comparing sequences of maize proteins (not known as allergens) with those of known allergens. Searches using a six amino acid window wrongly predicted that 41 out of 50 maize proteins were potential allergens and even an eight amino acid window predicted 7 out of 50. They recommend a comparison using the sequence comparison algorithm, FASTA, which identified only nine potential allergens from the maize proteins which shared >35% identity over 80 amino acids with known allergens, of which only six were similar over their entire length. In order to improve the precision other computational methods are being developed to 'predict' allergenicity. Recently a method based on a computerised learning system which extracts features from sequence alignments produced using another computer programme, FASTA3, and the k-Nearest-Neighbour (kNN) algorithm, has been developed which can correctly classify around 81% of allergens and 98% of non-allergens (Zorzet *et al.*, 2002).

22.3.2 Profile-based methods

A range of bioinformatics methods can be used for determining relationships between protein sequences, with family or profile-based methods having been shown to significantly out-perform pair-wise methods. The application of profile-based methods to the classification of food and related aero-allergens has shown that 78% could be classified into only seven protein families according to the Pfam database of protein families (Griffiths-Jones *et al.*; http://www.sanger.ac.uk/Software/Pfam/). Of around 1500 protein families in the *Arabidopsis thaliana* genome, fewer than 30 contain proteins homologous to allergens from other plant species. Such an analysis suggests that protein family membership can be used as a strong predictive risk factor for plant protein allergenicity, even when pair-wise similarity to other known allergens is low.

However, the process of allergenic risk assessment relies on information from a number of different sources, as we do not have a complete understanding of the molecular mechanisms of the aberrant IgE responses in food allergy. It is also complicated by our lack of adequate animal models for food allergenicity. Decision-tree approaches have been proposed to facilitate this assessment, initially by ILSI in conjunction with the Food Biotechnology Council in 1996 (ILSI (1996) with a revised version proposed by a joint FAO/WHO Expert Consultation on Foods Derived from Biotechnology (WHO-FAO, 2001). However, the third session of the FAO-WHO Codex Alimentarius Commission Ad Hoc Intergovernmental Task Force on Foods Derived from Biotechnology (ALINORM 03/34) decided in March 2002 not to elaborate the decision-tree approach. As no single criterion is sufficiently predictive of allergenicity, they recommended that the risk assessment process should adopt an integrated step-wise case-by-case approach which takes account of information of several types. Such information would be likely to include relationships between novel proteins and known allergens, defined using bioinformatics tools, as well as information regarding cross-reactivity defined using patient allergic sera, *in vitro* measures of protein digestibility and *in vivo* sensitisation using animal models. Despite their shortcomings, these are the best tools currently available that can be used to assess the allergenic potential of a novel protein.

22.4 Identifying potentially allergenic proteins: resistance to pepinolysis and IgE reactivity

A number of allergenic proteins, including those from peanut, soybean and cows' milk, have been reported to show remarkable resistance to digestion by pepsin when compared with non-allergenic proteins. In one study all of the allergenic proteins tested remained either undigested, or gave stable fragments, which persisted for 8–60 min (depending on the allergen), while the non-allergens were completely digested after less than 15 seconds (Astwood *et al.*, 1996). As peptides require a molecular weight of greater than 3,000 Daltons in order to stimulate an immune response, large stable fragments, as well as intact proteins, have the potential to act as sensitisers. Consequently resistance to pepsin digestion has become enshrined in the approaches used for assessing the allergenic potential of novel proteins. However, there is much debate as to its validity as the apparent stability of a protein can be very dependent on the experimental conditions employed.

An extension of the original work of Astwood *et al.* (1996), using a larger number of plant proteins, including some metabolic proteins with no history of food allergenicity, has thrown some doubt on the usefulness of pepsin resistance to predicting allergenicity (Yagami *et al.*, 2000; Fu *et al.*, 2002). Thus, using allergic sera from latex allergic patients, Yagami *et al.* (2000) found that cross-reactive allergens present in protein extracts of latex, avocado, kiwi and banana, were, in general, broken down rapidly by pepsin, with the potato allergens being more stable. Using sera from sufferers of oral allergy syndrome (where pollen is the main sensitising agent) these workers also found that the main allergens in melon and peach were also broken down rapidly by pepsin. However, these results are consistent with the hypothesis that sensitisation in such cross-reactive syndromes occurs via inhalation, the reactions to fruits tending to be confined to the oral cavity, and seldom being systemic, implying that the allergens are labile in the GI tract of man. This is also supported by the fact that nsLTP allergens, which are able to cause systemic symptoms and are thought to sensitise via the GI tract are resistant to pepsinolysis (Asero *et al.*, 2000). Fu and co-workers (2002), using purified proteins, found that of 22 allergens analysed, 12 were degraded almost instantly, and 5 very rapidly under the conditions employed, a similar proportion of non-allergens (8 out of 16 instantly broken down, 3 rapidly) showing similar instability. Both groups of proteins were more stable to simulated intestinal fluid containing pancreatin, a mixture of pancreatic enzymes, with only two allergens being broken down instantly, and five rapidly, whilst three non-allergens were broken down instantly and three were degraded rapidly.

As with all enzyme assays the results are strongly dependent on the substrate concentration and it is evident that changes in the substrate:protease ratio alter the apparent susceptibility of allergens to proteolysis and depending on the ratio of enzyme used the same protein can be shown to be either stable or labile to pepsin (Fu *et al.*, 2002). The pepsin digestion protocols that have been employed typically involve pepsin:substrate ratios in the range 1:5–1:10. Such ratios may be considered far in excess of those likely to be found in the stomach. For example, pepsin secretion in adults has been estimated between 20—30 k units of enzyme activity/24 h at 37 °C (Documenta Geigy, 1973), and from the activity in commercially available pepsin preparations used in digestion assays, this would be the equivalent of around 10 mg pepsin secreted/24 h. A typical adult dietary intake of protein around 75 g/24 h would give a ratio of ~3 mg protein/unit pepsin secreted compared to ~4 μg protein/unit pepsin used during digestion assays. Allowing for meal effects on secretion and gastric emptying and possible differences in pepsin activity under *in vivo* conditions, the ratios used during digestion assays are likely to remain orders of magnitude greater than ratios found *in vivo*.

Resistance to pepsinolysis as a diagnostic tool for allergens can be misleading since many non-allergens can also resist pepsin digestion. This is illustrated in Fig. 22.4 which shows the breakdown of the proteins, haemoglobin, β-casein and β-lactoglobulin under equivalent digestion conditions. Haemoglobin, not known to be an allergen, precipitates at acid pH and digestion of the resultant 'solid' substrate proceeds slowly. Constituent peptides with MW >3000 Daltons can persist for over 1 hour even when assayed at a 1:30 pepsin:substrate ratio, an enzyme ratio similar to the 1:10 ratio employed by Astwood *et al.* (1996). With the known cows' milk allergens, β-casein and β-lactoglobulin, β-casein also precipitates at acid pH and is digested similar to haemoglobin, whereas β-lactoglobulin remains in solution but is apparently little affected by

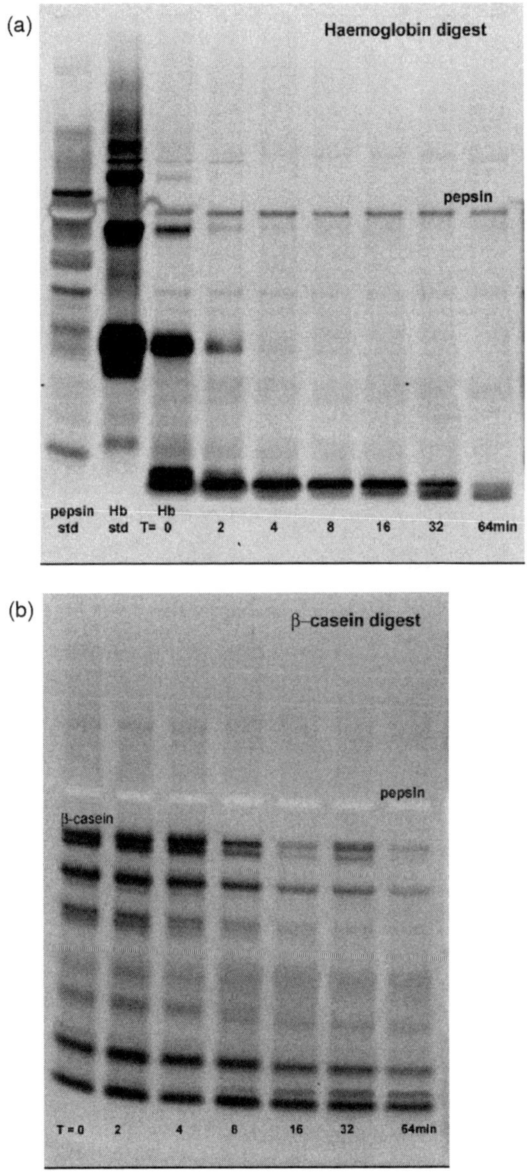

Fig. 22.4 SDS_PAGE analysis of the digestion of bovine haemoglobin (A), together with cows' milk β-casein (B) and β-lactoglobulin (C) using porcine pepsin. Digestion was performed using a pepsin:protein ratio of 20:1 (w:w); samples of digest were removed at 0, 2, 4, 8, 16, 32 and 64 min and the pH raised to neutrality to terminate digestion prior to SDS-PAGE analysis. Gels were stained with colloidal Coomasie Blue. Hb – haemoglobin; BLG – β-lactoglobulin. Pepsin standard is shown alongside the Hb digest and its position in digests is indicated.

(c)

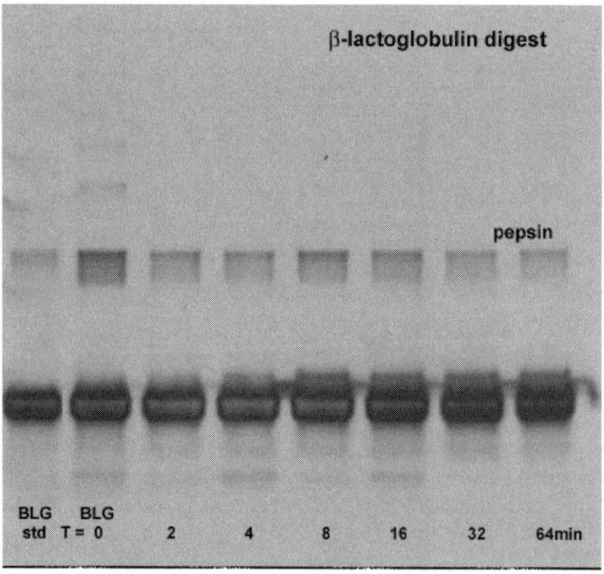

Fig. 22.4 (continued)

exposure to pepsin. At higher pH, under conditions for digestion with trypsin, β-casein becomes soluble and can be instantly digested to relatively low molecular weight peptides even at enzyme:substrate ratios of < 1:500. Thus, substrate availability as well as protein structure can be important in controlling digestion and this will affect using resistance to pepsinolysis as a reliable diagnostic tool to identify a food allergen.

The systems employed are also not physiological as they do not involve the pH titrations that occur *in vivo*, nor do they contain phospholipids and other enzymes, such as gastric lipase found in the human stomach (Gargouri *et al.*, 1989). Thus, the simulated intestinal fluid used by Fu *et al.* (2002) neither contained bile salts nor involved prior digestion of the proteins by pepsin, as is the case *in vivo*, where proteins first experience the low pH conditions of the stomach before entering the small intestine. So what is being measured when a protein's resistance to proteolysis is determined? At high substrate:protein ratios, rather than indicating the potential for a protein to be resistant to digestion *in vivo* in man, the pepsin digestion systems being employed are probably acting more as a bioassay of intrinsic protein stability resulting from the properties of its three-dimensional structure. Thus, at a molecular level proteolytic cleavage sites are well known to be more accessible to proteases when presented in more mobile regions of a protein, and this is especially true for pepsin, which has a preference for attacking peptide bonds in more mobile, flexible segments (Dunn and Hung, 2000). None of the currently published methods encompass the complexities of the environments experienced by food as it journeys down the human digestive tract.

As regards identifying allergens, it seems that a bioassay for 'stability' in terms of protein structure has some value, but needs to be interpreted in conjunction with other information, such as the similarity of proteins to known allergens, and sensitisation potential. None of the methods currently being used reflect stability to digestion *in vivo* and take no account of the structure of foods and the mechanical breakdown of that structure in the gut, which may afford protection to allergens and other food proteins in the digestive environment.

22.4.1 IgE reactivity and sensitisation potential of proteins

Identifying proteins which are closely related to previously identified allergens and which can consequently elicit a reaction in already sensitised individuals is more straightforward than assessing the potential of a new protein to actually sensitise an individual. Such an approach allows the identification of an allergen by checking the IgE reactivity of novel proteins using serological methods (such as immunoblotting and RAST) with panels of well-defined human allergic sera. These tests can be complemented by cross-reactivity studies using suitable antibody preparations from experimental animal sources to substantiate the potential for cross-reactivity. The WHO/FAO decision tree recommends that combinations of allergic sera are used from individuals with both food and inhalant (e.g. pollen) allergies, which in the case of GMOs for food use encompass allergies to both monocotyledonous and dicotyledonous plant species. There are concerns over the ethical aspects regarding the development and use of human allergic serum banks, as much of the serum collected by clinical researchers is bound by ethical consent which revolves around the benefits that accrue to the patients from any research. Clearly the benefits are less apparent when sera are used in such a risk assessment process.

Largely as a result of our current lack of knowledge regarding the mechanisms of food allergenicity, particularly regarding the sensitisation of non-allergic subjects, the positive predictability of the targeted serum screen is uncertain. As a consequence the sensitising potential still needs to be assessed using animal models. However, this too has considerable uncertainty as, despite much research, there is still no well validated animal model for oral sensitisation. In order to generate an IgE response towards a food generally requires either using an adjuvant in conjunction with oral dosing (such as cholera toxin, or the addition of polysaccharides such as carageenan), or a combination of both oral and intraperitoneal exposure (Penninks and Knippels, 2001) although another approach, simply to determine the inherent sensitising potential independently of the effects of the GI tract using parenteral administration of proteins has also been proposed (Dearman *et al.*, 2001). The choice of animal species and strain is also important. Dogs have been found to be more amenable to oral sensitisation than small mammals (Ermel *et al.*, 1997) but require larger doses and in some cultures the extensive use of dogs in toxicological assessments is less acceptable. The most widely used animal models are the mouse (using the high IgE responder strain Balb/c) and rats (especially the Brown Norway rat), and to a more limited extent guinea pigs (Penninks and Knippels, 2001; Dearman *et al.*, 2001). In general, mice and rats are more favoured as there is greater knowledge of their physiology and how it compares with that of man. However, whilst there are indications that not all proteins behave in a similar fashion in stimulating IgE and IgG responses in experimental animals, the predictive value of such behaviour in identifying potential allergens is still debated.

22.5 Future trends

Identifying new potential allergens, particularly those which have no structural or biological relationships with known allergens, cannot be done with a high degree of certainty. It is clear that not all foods are equally allergenic, yet the precise molecular basis for these differences remains unclear. There is little evidence that particular protein sequences or structures promote the development of IgE responses, although food allergens appear to be good antigens (i.e. able to stimulate an antibody response). There is some evidence from animal studies that, based on a limited number of allergens tested so far, allergens are intrinsically able to preferentially elicit an IgE response in experimental animals (Dearman and Kimber, 2001; Dearman *et al.*, 2001). It may also be that protein stability and resistance to digestion may play a role in determining the allergenic potential of proteins when sensitising via the GI tract. However, only when we have a greater understanding of the molecular pathology of food allergy which embraces both the aspects of food (allergen structure, interactions with the food matrix and the potential adjuvant effects of other food components) coupled with the genetic factors in man which predispose some individuals to becoming atopic, will it be possible to make a more completely reliable prediction of novel protein allergenicity. Until this information is available, allergen identification will continue to be an uncertain process, requiring a great deal of information on many different aspects of protein structure and properties and relying on comparisons with known food allergens.

22.6 Acknowledgements

ENCM, JAJ and JAR acknowledge the support of BBSRC through the competitive strategic grant, and through the EU (Allergest [QLK1-CT-2001-01239]; Informall [QLRT-2001-02284]).

22.7 References

ADACHI M, TAKENAKA Y, GIDAMIS AB, MIKAMI B, UTSUMI S (2001) 'Crystal structure of soybean proglycinin A1aB1b homotrimer', *J Mol Biol*, 305, 291–305.

ALBERSE RC (2000) 'Structural biology of allergens', *J Allergy Clin Immunol*, 106, 228–238.

ALVAREZ AM, ADACHI T, NAKASE M, AOKI N, NAKAMURA R, MATSUDA T (1995) 'Classification of rice allergenic protein cDNAs belonging to the α-amylase/trypsin inhibitor gene family', *Biochim. et Biophys. Acta*, 1251, 201–204.

ASERO R, MISTRELLO G, RONCAROLO D, DE VRIES SC, GAUTIER MF, CIURANA CL, VERBEEK E, MOHAMMADI T, KNUL-BRETTLOVA V, AKKERDAAS JH, BULDER I, AALBERSE RC, VAN REE R (2000) 'Lipid transfer protein: a pan-allergen in plant-derived foods that is highly resistant to pepsin digestion', *Int Arch Allergy Immunol*, 122, 20–32.

ASTWOOD JD, LEACH JN, FUCHS RL (1996) 'Stability of food allergens to digestion in vitro', *Nature Biotechnology*, 14, 1269–1273.

BAKER EN (1980) 'Structure of actinidin after refinement at 1.7 Å resolution', *J. Mol. Biol.*, 141, 441–484.

BECKER WM, REESE G (2001) 'Immunological identification and characterization of individual food allergens.', *J Chromatogr B Biomed Sci Appl*, 756,131–140.

BEYER K, BARDINA L, GRISHINA G, SAMPSON HA (2002a) 'Identification of sesame seed allergens by 2-dimensional proteomics and Edman sequencing: Seed storage proteins as common food allergens', *J Allergy Clin Immunol*, 110, 154–159.

BEYER K, GRISHINA G, BARDINA L, GRISHIN A, SAMPSON HA (2002b) 'Identification of an 11S globulin as a major hazelnut food allergen in hazelnut-induced systemic reactions', *J Allergy Clin Immunol*, 110, 517–23.

BREITENEDER H, EBNER C (2000) 'Molecular and biochemical classification of plant-derived food allergens', *J Allergy Clin Immunol*, 106, 27–36.

BUGAJSKA-SCRETTER A, ELFMAN L, FUCHS T, KAPIOTIS S, RUMPOLD H, VALENTA R, SPITZAUER S (1998) 'Parvalbumin, a cross-reactive fish allergen, contains IgE-binding epitopes sensitive to periodate treatment and Ca^{2+} depletion', *J Allergy Clin Immunol*, 101, 67–74.

BURKS AW, BROOKS JR, SAMPSON HA (1988) 'Allergenicity of major component proteins of soybean determined by enzyme-linked immunosorbent assay (ELISA) and immunoblotting in children with atopic dermatitis and positive soy challenge', *J. Allergy Clin. Immunol.*, 81, 1135–1142.

BURKS AW, WILLIAMS LW, HELM RM, CONNAUGHTON C, COCKRELL G, O'BRIEN T (1991) 'Identification of a major peanut allergen, *Ara h III*, in patients with atopic dermatitis and positive peanut challenges', *J Allergy Clin Immunol*, 88, 172–179.

BURKS AW, WILLIAMS LW, CONNAUGHTON C, COCKRELL G, O'BRIEN TJ, HELM RM (1992) 'Identification and characterization of a second major peanut allergen, *Ara h III*, with use of the sera of patients with atopic dermatitis and positive peanut challenge', *J Allergy Clin Immunol*, 90, 962–969.

BUSH RK, HEFLE SL (1996) 'Food allergens', CRC *Critical Reviews in Food Science and Nutrition*, 36 (Suppl), S119–163.

COOKE SK, SAMPSON HA (1997) 'Allergenic properties of ovomucoid in man', *J Immunol.*, 159, 2026–2032.

CURIONI A, SANTUCCI B, CRISTADO A, CANISTRACI C, PEITRAVALLE M, SIMONATO B, GIANNATTASIO M (1999) 'Urticaria from beer: an immediate hypersensitivity reaction due to a 10kDa protein derived form beer', *Clin. Exp. Allergy*, 29, 407–413.

DEARMAN RJ, KIMBER I (2001) 'Determination of protein allergenicity: studies in mice', *Toxicol Lett*, 120, 181–186.

DEARMAN RJ, CADDICK H, STONE S, BASKETTER DA, KIMBER I (2001) 'Characterisation of antibody responses to food proteins: influence of route of exposure', *Toxicol* 167,

217–231.

DOCUMENTA GEIGY (1973) Gastric Juice. In: Diem K, Lentner C (eds), *Scientific Tables*, 7th Edition, pp. 646–651, Geigy Pharmaceuticals Macclesfiejd

DOULIEZ J-P, MICHON T, ELMORJANI K, MARION D (2000) 'Structure, biological and technological function of lipid transfer proteins and indolines, the major lipid binding proteins from cereal kernels', *J Cereal Sci*, 32, 1–20.

DUNN BM, HUNG S-H (2000) 'The two sides of enzyme-substrate specificity: lessons from the aspartic proteinases', *Biochim Biophys Acta.*, 1477, 231–240.

DUNWELL JM (1998) 'Cupins: a new superfamily of functionally diverse proteins that include germins and plant storage proteins', *Biotechnol Genet Eng Rev*, 15, 1–32.

DURO G, COLOMBO P, COSTA MA, IZZO V, PORCASI R, DI FIORE R, LOCOROTONDO G, MIRISOLA MG, COCCHIARA R, GERACI D (1996) 'cDNA cloning, sequence analysis and allergological characterization of Par j 2.0101, a new major allergen of the *Parietaria judaica* pollen', *FEBS Letts.*, 399, 295–298.

ERMEL RW, KOCK M, GRIFFEY SM, REINHART GA, FRICK OL (1997) 'The atopic dog: a model for food allergy', *Lab Anim Sci*, 47, 40–49.

FAHLBUSH B, RUDESCHKO O, SCHUMANN C, STEURICH R, HENZGEN M, SCHLENVOIGT G, JAGER L (1998) 'Further characterisation of IgE-binding antigens in kiwi with particular emphasis on glycoprotein allergens', *J Investig Allergol Clin Immunol* 8, 325–332.

FU T-J, ABBOTT UR, HATZOS C (2002) 'Digestibility of food allergens and nonallergenic proteins in simulated gastric fluid and simulated intestinal fluid – a comparative study', *J Agric Food Chem.*, 50, 7154–7160.

GALL H, KALVERAM KJ, FORCK G, STERRY W (1994) 'Kiwi fruit allergy – A new birch pollen-associated food allergy', *J Allergy Clin Immunol*, 94, 70–76.

GARGOURI Y, MOREAU H, VERGER R (1989) 'Gastric lipases: biochemical and physiological studies', *Biochim Biophys Acta*, 1006, 255–271.

GENDEL S (1998) 'The use of amino acid sequence alignments to assess potential allergenicity of proteins using genetically modified foods', *Adv Food Nutr Res* 42, 45–62.

GENDEL SM (2002) 'Sequence analysis for assessing potential allergenicity', *Ann N Y Acad Sci.*, 964, 87–98.

HILEMAN RE, SILVANOVICH A, GOODMAN RE, RICE EA, HOLLESCHAK G, ASTWOOD JD, HEFLE S (2002) 'Bioinformatic methods for allergenicity assessment using a comprehensive allergen database', *Int Arch Allergy Immunol*, 128, 280–291.

HOFFMANN-SOMMERGRUBER K (2002) 'Pathogenesis-related (PR)-proteins identified as allergens', *Biochem Soc Trans*, 30, 930–935.

ILSI (1996) 'The safety assessment of novel foods', Guidelines prepared by ILSI Europe Novel Food Task Force, International Life Sciences Institute, European Branch, Brussels.

JAMES JM, SIXBEY JP, HELM RM, BANNON GA, BURKS AW (1997) 'Wheat α-amylase inhibitor: A second route of allergic sensitisation', *J Allergy Clin Immunol*, 99, 239–244.

KALINSKI A, WEISEMANN JM, MATTHEWS BF, HERMAN EM (1990) 'Molecular cloning of a protein associated with soybean seed oil bodies that is similar to thiol proteases of the papain family', *J. Biol. Chem.*, 265, 13843–13848.

KELLY JD, HLYWKA JJ, HEFLE SL (2000) 'Identification of sunflower seed IgE-binding proteins', *Int Arch Allergy Immunol*, 121, 19–24.

KLEBER JT, CRAMERI R, APPENZELLER U, SCHLAAK M, BECKER WM (1999) 'Selective cloning of peanut allergens, including profilin and 2S albumins, by phage display technology', *Int Arch All Immunol*, 119, 265–274.

MARUYAMA N, ICHISE K, KATSUBE T, KISHIMOTO T, KAWASE S-I, MATSUMURA Y, TAKEUCHI Y, SAWADA T, UTSUMI S (1998) 'Identification of major wheat allergens by means of the *Escherichia* coli expression system', *Eur J Biochem*, 255, 739–745.

MENENDEZ-ARIAS L, MONEO I, DOMINGUEZ J, RODRIGUEZ R (1988) 'Primary structure of the major allergen of yellow mustard (*Sinapis alba* L.) seed, Sin a I', *Eur J Biochem*, 177, 159–166.

METCALFE DD, ASTWOOD JD, TOWNSEND R, SAMPSON HA, TAYLOR SL, FUCHS RL (1996) 'Assessment of the allergenic potential of foods derived from genetically engineered crop plants', *Crit Rev Food Sci Nutr*, 36 Suppl: S165–186.

MILLS ENC, JENKINS J, MARIGHETO N, BELTON PS, GUNNING AP, MORRIS VJ (2002) 'Allergens of the cupin superfamily', *Biochem Soc Trans*, 30, 925–929.

MILLS ENC, MADSEN C, SHEWRY PR, WICHERS HJ (2003) 'Food allergens of plant origin – the relationship between allergenic potential and biological activity (PROTALL)', *Trends Food Sci Technol*, 14, 145–156.

MÖLLER M, PASHCKE A, VIELUF D, KAYMA M, VIETHS S, STEINHART H (1997) 'Characterization of allergens in kiwi fruit and detection of cross-reactivities with allergens of birch pollen and related fruits', *Food Agric. Immunol.*, 9, 107–121.

MONSALVE RI, GONZALEZ DE LA PENA MA, MENEZES-ARIAS L, LOPEZ-OTIN C, VILLALBA M, RODRIGUEZ R (1993) 'Characterization of a new oriental-mustard (*Brassica-juncea*) allergen Bra j I: detection of an allergenic epitope', *Biochem. J.*, 293: 625–632.

NAKASE M, ADACHI T, URISU A, MIYASHITA T, ALVAREZ AM, NAGASAKA S, AOKI N, NAKAMURA R, MATSUDA T (1996) 'Rice (*Oryza sativa* L.) α-amylase inhibitors of 14–16 kDa are potential allergens and products of a multigene family', *J. Agric. Food Chem.*, 44, 2624–2628.

OGAWA T, TSUJI H, BANDO N, KITAMURA K, ZHU Y-L, HIRANO H, NISHIKAWA K (1993) 'Identification of the soyabean allergenic proteins, Gly m Bd 30 K, with the soybean seed 34 kDa oil-body-associated protein', *Biosci Biotech Biochem*, 57, 1030–1033.

PALOSUO K, ALENIUS H, VARJONEN E, KOIVULUHTA M, MIKKOLA J, KESKINEN H, KALKKINEN N, REUNALA T (1999) 'A novel wheat gliadin as a cause of exercise-induced anaphylaxis', *J Allergy Clin Immunol*, 103, 912–917.

PASTORELLO EA, PRAVETTONI V, ISPANO M, FARIOLI L, ANSALONI R, ROTONDO F, INCORVAIA C, ASMAN I, BENGTSSON A, ORTOLANI C (1996) 'Identification of the allergenic components of kiwi fruit and evaluation of their cross-reactivity with timothy and birch pollens', *J Allergy Clin Immunol*, 98, 601–610.

PASTORELLO EA, CONTI A, PRAVETTONI V, FARIOLI L, RIVOLTA F, ANSALONI R, ISPANO M, INCORVAIA C, GIUFFRIDA MG, ORTOLANI C (1998a) 'Identification of actinidin as the major allergen of kiwi fruit', *J Allergy Clin Immunol*, 101, 531–537.

PASTORELLO EA, FARIOLI L, PRAVETTONI V, ISPANO M, CONTI A, ANSALONI R, ROTONDO F, INCORVAIA C, BENGTSSON A, RIVOLTA F, TRAMBAIOLI C, PREVIDI M, ORTOLANI C (1998b) 'Sensitization to the major allergen of Brazil nut is correlated with the clinical expression of allergy', *J Allergy Clin Immunol*, 102, 1021–1027.

PASTORELLO EA, FARIOLI L, PRAVETTONI V, ORTOLANI C, ISPANO M, MONZA M, BAROGLIO C, SCIBOLA E, ANSALONI R, INCORVAIA C, CONTI A (1999a) 'The major allergen of peach (*Prunus persica*) is a lipid transfer protein', *J Allergy Clin Immunol*, 103, 520–526.

PASTORELLO EA, PRAVETTONI V, FARIOLI L, ISPANO M, FORTUNATO D, MONZA M, GIUFFRIDA MG, RIVOLTA F, SCIBOLA E, ANSALONI R, INCORVAIA C, CONTI A, ORTOLANI C (1999b) 'Clinical role of a lipid transfer protein that acts as a new apple-specific allergen', *J Allergy Clin Immunol*, 104, 1099–1106.

PASTORELLO EA, FARIOLI L, PRAVETTONI V, ISPANO M, SCIBOLA E, TRAMBAIOLI C, GIUFFRIDA MG, ANSALONI R, GODOVAC-ZIMMERMANN J, CONTI A, FORTUNATO D, ORTOLANI C (2000) 'The maize major allergen, which is responsible for food-induced allergic reactions, is a lipid transfer protein', *J Allergy Clin Immunol*, 106, 744–751.

PASTORELLO EA, FARIOLI L, ROBINO AM, TRAMBAIOLI C, CONTI A, PRAVETTONI V (2001a) 'A lipid transfer protein involved in occupational sensitization to spelt', *J Allergy Clin Immunol*, 108, 145–146.

PASTORELLO EA, VARIN E, FARIOLI L, PRAVETTONI V, ORTOLANI C, TRAMBAIOLI C, FORTUNATO D, GIUFFRIDA MG, RIVOLTA F, ROBINO A, CALAMARI AM, LACAVA L, CONTI A (2001b) 'The major allergen of sesame seeds (*Sesamum indicum*) is a 2S albumin', *J Chromatogr B Biomed Sci Appl*, 756, 85–93.

PENNINKS AH, KNIPPELS LMJ (2001) 'Determination of protein allergenicity: studies in rats', *Toxicol*, 120, 171–180.

POLTRONIERI P, CAPPELLO MS, DOHMAE N, CONTI A, FORTUNATO D, PASTORELLO EA, ORTOLANI C, ZACHEO G (2002) 'Identification and characterisation of the IgE-binding proteins 2S albumin and conglutin gamma in almond (*Prunus dulcis*) seeds', *Int Arch Allergy Immunol*, 128, 97–104.

RABJOHN P, HELM EM, STANLEY JS, WEST CM, SAMPSON HA, BURKS AW, BANNON GA (1999) 'Molecular cloning and epitope analysis of the peanut allergen Ara h 3', *J Clin Invest*, 103, 535–542.

RAWLINGS ND, BARRETT AJ (1993) 'Evolutionary families of peptidases', *Biochem J*, 290, 205–218.

ROUX KH, TEUBER SS, ROBOTHAM JM, SATHE SK (2001) 'Detection and stability of the major almond allergen in foods', *J Agric Food Chem*, 49, 2131–2136.

SAMOTO M, MIYAZAKI C, AKASAKA T, MORI H, KAWAMURA Y (1996) 'Specific binding of allergenic soybean protein Gly m Bd 30K with α'- and α-subunits of conglycinin in soy milk', *Biosci Biotech Biochem*, 60, 1006–1010.

SÁNCHEZ-MONGE R, LOMBARDERO M, GARCIA-SELLÉS FJ, BARBER D, SALCEDO G (1999) 'Lipid-transfer proteins are relevant allergens in fruit allergy', *J Allergy Clin Immunol*, 103, 514–519.

SANCHEZ-MONGE R, PASCUAL CY, DIAZ-PERALES A, FERNANDEZ-CRESPO J, MARTIN-ESTEBAN M, SALCEDO G (2000) 'Isolation and characterisation of relevant allergens from boiled lentils', *J Allergy Clin Immunol*, 106, 955–961.

SHIBASAKI M, SUZUKI S, TAJIMA S, NEMOTO H, KUROUME T (1980) 'Allergenicity of major component proteins of soybean', *Int Arch Allergy Appl Immunol*, 61, 441–448.

SHIN DH, LEE JY, HWANG KY, KIM KK, SUH SW (1995) 'High-resolution crystal-structure of the nonspecific lipid-transfer protein from maize seedlings', *Structure*, 3, 189–199.

SIMONATO B, PASINI G, GIANNATTASIO M, PERUFFO AD, DE LAZZARI F, CURIONI A (2001) 'Food allergy to wheat products: the effect of bread baking and in vitro digestion on wheat allergenic proteins. A study with bread dough, crumb, and crust', *J Agric Food Chem*, 49, 5668–5673.

TANABE S, ARAI S, YANAGIHARA Y, TAKAHASHI K, WATANABE M (1996) 'A major wheat allergen has a Gln-Gln-Gln-Pro-Pro motif identified as an IgE-binding epitope', *Biochem Biophys Res Commun*, 219, 290–293.

TEJERA M, VILLALBA M, BATANERO E, RODRIGUEZ R (1999) 'Identification, isolation and characterisation of Ole e 7, a new allergen of olive tree pollen', *J Allergy Clin Immunol*, 104, 797–802.

TEUBER SS, PETERSEN WR (1999) 'Systemic allergic reaction to coconut (*Cocos nucifera*) in 2 subjects with hypersensitivity to tree nut and demonstration of cross-reactivity to legumin-like seed storage proteins: New coconut and walnut food allergens', *J Allergy Clin Immunol*, 103, 1180–1185.

TEUBER SS, DANDEKAR AM, PETERSON WR, SELLERS CL (1998) 'Cloning and sequencing of a gene enconding a 2S albumin seed storage protein precursor from English walnut (*Juglans regia*), a major food allergen', *J Allergy Clin Immunol*, 101, 807–814.

TEUBER S, JARVIS KC, DANDEKAR AM, PETERSON WR, ANSARI A (1999) 'Identification and cloning of a complimentary DNA encoding a vicilin-like proprotein, Jug r 2, from English walnut kernel (*Juglans regia*), a major food allergen', *J Allergy Clin Immunol*, 104, 1111–1120.

VAN LOON LC, VAN STRIEN EA (1999) 'The families of pathogenesis-related proteins, their activities and comparative analysis of PR-1 type proteins', *Physiol Mol Plant Pathol* 55, 85–97.

VARJONEN E, VAINIO E, KALIMO K, JUNTUNEN-BACKMAN K, SAVOLAINEN J (1995) 'Skin-prick test and RAST responses to cereals in children with atopic dermatitis. Characterization of IgE-binding components in wheat and oats by an immunoblotting method', *Clin. Exp. Allergy.*, 25, 1100–1107.

VARJONEN E, VAINIO E, KALIMO K (1997) 'Life-threatening, recurrent anaphylaxis caused by allergy to gliadin and exercise', *Clin. Exp. Allergy*, 27, 162–166.

VARJONEN E, VAINIO E, KALIMO K (2000) 'Antigliadin IgE – indicator of wheat allergy in atopic dermatitis', *Allergy*, 55, 386–391.

VIOQUE J, SANCHEZ-VIOQUE R, CLEMENTE A, PEDROCHE J, BAUTISTA J, MILLAN F (1999) 'Purification and partial characterization of chickpea 2S albumin', *J Agric Food Chem*, 47, 1405–1409.

WAL J-M (1998) 'Cow's milk allergens', *Allergy*, 53, 1013–1022.

WANG F, ROBOTHAM JM, TEUBER SS, TAWDE P, SATHE SK, ROUX KH (2002) 'Ana o 1, a cashew (*Anacardium occidental*) allergen of the vicilin seed storage protein family', *J Allergy Clin Immunol*, 110, 160–166.

WHO-FAO (2001) 'Evaluation of Allergenicity of Genetically Modified Foods', Report of the joint FAO/WHO expert consultation on allergenicity of foods derived from Biotechnology, 22–25th January 2001, pp. 1–26.

YAGAMI T, HAISHIMA Y, NAKAMURA A, OSUNA H, IKEZAWA Z (2000) 'Digestibility of allergens extracterd from natural rubber latex and vegetable foods', *J Allergy Clin Immunol*, 106, 752–762.

YOULE RJ, HUANG AHC (1981) 'Occurrence of low molecular weight and high cysteine containing albumin storage proteins in oilseeds of disperse species', *Am. J. Botany*, 68, 44–48.

ZORZET A, GUSTAFSSON M, HAMMERLING U (2002) 'Prediction of food protein allergenicity: a bioinformatic learnining systems approach', *In Silico Biol*, 2, 48–58.

23

Toxicological screening of paper and board packaging

A. von Wright, University of Kuopio, Finland

23.1 Introduction

In this chapter the toxicological screening methods that could potentially be applied to paper and board food packaging materials are briefly outlined. The chapter starts with an overview of the present regulatory status regarding the safety testing of fibre-based packaging materials within the European Union (EU). This forms a background for the perceived need for toxicological screening tests and for the general requirements that such tests should fulfil. A number of presently known short-term tests are evaluated in the light of these criteria. The few known instances where short-term toxicological screening tests have been applied to paper and board are reviewed. Ongoing research in this area is briefly presented, as well as the impact of the research on the emerging European legislation. Finally some relevant research institutes, available websites and other additional information are listed for further contacts.

23.2 Regulatory background

In the EU the legal foundations governing materials and articles coming into contact with food are contained in the Framework Directive 89/109/EEC which states

> Materials and articles must be manufactured in compliance with good manufacturing practice so that, under their normal or foreseeable conditions of use, they do not transfer their constituents into foodstuffs in quantities which could either endanger human health or bring about

an unacceptable change in the composition of the foodstuffs or deterioration in the organoleptic characteristics thereof.

While specific directives exist to address the safety aspects of plastics, ceramics and regenerated cellulose, there is, as yet, no specific directive for paper and board intended for food contact. It should be noted, however, that so far there has been no indication of actual harmful consequences associated with food packages consisting of these materials.

23.2.1 The present regulatory status of paper and board-based packaging materials

Paper and board are natural materials, which have a remarkably long history of safe use. Consequently there has been no great pressure to apply specific regulatory measures to ensure their harmlessness in various applications, although in some countries (i.e. France, Italy and Germany) the legislation and the guidelines directed to the industry are rather detailed, especially in the case of recycled fibres (Escabasse and Ottenio, 2002). Typically the existing regulations define the chemicals that are allowed in the manufacture of paper and board and set limits for various contaminants (heavy metals, pentachlorophenol, polychlorinated biphenyls, etc.) in the products. A specific concern of the use of recycled fibre is also reflected in the Council of Europe policy statement on paper and board for food contact.

23.2.2 The Council of Europe policy statement concerning paper and board materials for food contact

In the absence of specific EU directives, the Council of Europe (CoE) policy statement on paper and board materials and articles intended for food contact remains, so far, the most authoritative document guiding the regulatory practices in Europe (although, as noted above, more specific national regulations already exist in certain countries). The version of the statement published in December 2002 (Anon. 2002) contains the specific resolution on the subject, urging the Member States to take into account in their national laws and regulations the principles defined in the document. It is specifically stated that paper and board should not transfer their constituents to foodstuffs in quantities which could endanger human health or cause an unacceptable change or organoleptic deterioration. Further, good manufacturing practice is required, the microbiological quality should be guaranteed, paper and board should not release antimicrobial substances, and specific limits for cadmium, lead and mercury, as well as for pentachlorophenol are defined. Instructions on testing conditions and on good manufacturing practice are given in specific technical documents attached to the policy statement. Aspects on the use of recycled fibres in the food contact material are given special attention in a separate technical document, the content of which is described in more detail below.

The Council of Europe guidelines on the use of recycled paper and board, limits for harmful substances
In the CoE guideline it is stated that some additional requirements are needed to ensure the safety of food contact materials and articles made of recycled fibre, due to the presence of printing inks, adhesives and other substances in the starting material. Aspects that should be considered include the source of recovered paper and board, the processing technologies applied to remove contaminants and the intended use of the product.

The recovered paper and board which is not considered suitable for use as raw materials include waste paper and board from hospitals, paper and board that has been in contact with garbage, stained sacks that have contained chemicals or foodstuffs, certain covering materials, carbonless copy paper, certain types of household waste paper (used kitchen towels, handkerchiefs, etc.) and PCB-containing materials.

Specific requirements for the end products include tests and migration limits for various types of toxic or harmful compounds such as Michler's ketone (4,4 bis(dimethylamino)benzophenone), 4,4 bis(diethylamino) benzophenone (DEAB), diisopropylnapthalenes (DIPNs) phthalates, solvents, partially hydrogenated terphenyls (HTTP), azo colourants, fluorescent whitening agents, primary aromatic amines, polycyclic aromatic hydrocarbons (PAH) and benzophenone. The amounts of these substances should either be below the detection limits or, in some cases (DIPN, HTTP, solvents) as low as can reasonably be achieved. For benzophenone a specific migration limit of 0.1 mg/dm^2 is defined. The requirements generally apply to products intended to be used in contact with aqueous and/or fatty foodstuffs or also with dry, non-fatty foodstuffs (requirements for DIPNs, HTTP, phthalates and solvents).

23.3 Requirements for toxicological testing

While there is no actual indication of major risks for public health due to fibre-based packaging materials, the increased safety consciousness of both consumers and legislators may lead to situations in which streamlining the regulatory framework on the safety of paper and board products, whether based on virgin or recycled fibre, becomes actual. In the present regulations the emphasis is on the chemical analysis of eventual contaminants and to some degree on the microbiological quality, and no requirements of toxicological safety testing apparently exist, yet. However, the potential usefulness of such tests has been indicated in various documents (Escabasse and Ottenio, 2002; the CoE resolution cited below).

The CoE resolution, when defining the end-product requirements for food contact materials made from recycled fibre, makes the following statement:

> Chemical or toxicological screening tests for possible unknown toxic substances are desirable. However, at present the implementation of chemical screening tests for unknown substances might not be feasible.

Furthermore, the knowledge about the applicability of toxicological screening tests for paper and board is insufficient for the time being although it should be noted that studies are in progress to establish the validity of these tests for paper and board. The use of these chemical or toxicological screening tests on paper and board should be evaluated and should be recommended in the future where necessary, based on new developments and results in this field.

In the following sections some requirements for toxicological screening tests applicable for paper and board are outlined, the presently available tests are briefly reviewed, and some examples of the actual applications of toxicological test to paper and board are given (Section 23.5).

23.3.1 The types of toxicological tests and test conditions required

The toxicological tests required for routine screening of food contact materials should, naturally, have endpoints relevant to consumer safety. In addition, they should be cheap, not labour intensive, and easy to perform for a large number of samples. They should also be validated and recognised by regulatory bodies. These criteria automatically exclude traditional animal testing either for acute, subacute or chronic toxicity, and also most of the presently known short-term or *in vitro* tests fall short of fulfilling all of them. However, some experience of either individual short-term tests or their combinations to assay extracts of paper and board is starting to emerge (Section 23.5).

An additional aspect that should be considered is the preparation of samples for testing. Extraction methods should take into account the types of food (aqueous, dry, fatty) with which the paper and board would interact in real-life situations, as well as such factors as the duration and the temperature conditions of the contact. The selection of the food simulants used for extraction can also be critical. While most of the biological tests are compatible with water extracts, solvents like ethanol or iso-octane are regularly used in immigration tests for the extraction of lipophilic compounds. These are usually not very well tolerated by the various biological systems and cell types used in *in vitro* tests. This limits the amount of extractants that can reasonably be tested, and increases the need for solvent controls in the assays. Change of solvents or concentrating the samples by evaporation may lead to problems with solubility, loss of volatile compounds, and unforeseen chemical interactions. Thus, the development of realistic extraction methods, compatible with the test systems used, should proceed in parallel with the eventual choice of biological tests for toxicological screening.

23.4 Cytotoxicity tests

Several types of *in vitro* tests are routinely applied to study the harmful effects at either cellular level (cytotoxicity tests) or on the genetic material (genotoxicity tests). For research purposes the cytotoxicity tests have been valuable screening tools, and in certain cases they can give valuable information on the structure-function relationships and mechanisms of toxicity. However, so far their use in regulatory toxicology has been relatively limited, the emphasis still being on whole animal studies. Several genotoxicity tests, on the other hand, have been thoroughly standardised, validated and included in various recommended guidelines for toxicity testing (i.e. OECD Guidelines on Genetic Toxicology Testing, 471–486).

In general, permanent mammalian cell lines of variable sources are utilised in the most common cytotoxicity tests. Although there are variations in the details of the test protocols, the cell cultures are usually directly exposed to the test agent in the growth medium, and after a certain exposure time, the resulting toxicity is measured. The endpoints can simply be cell death or growth inhibition, which can be detected by various methods, such as measuring the total protein content (TPC), using differential staining (i.e. neutral red uptake, NRU) or following the ability of the exposed culture to grow and form cellular colonies (CFA). These tests can be used to screen both pure chemicals and complex mixtures isolated from food or various environmental samples (Stammati *et al.*, 1999; von Wright *et al.*, 1992).

In addition to measuring cell death and growth inhibition, which usually do not give much information about the mechanisms of toxicity, cytotoxicity tests with a clear targeted function can sometimes be used. An example is the use of MTT (a tetrazolium salt), which stains blue because of the reaction with the mitochondrial enzyme succinate dehydrogenase. Thus the assay is very sensitive to mitochondrial poisons, although it can also be used to measure general cytotoxicity (Mosmann, 1983).

23.4.1 Tests for sublethal toxic effects

Cell death is a very drastic endpoint usually preceded by various other deleterious effects in the cell. With certain types of short-term tests it is possible to detect some of these effects, and thus gain information of non-lethal toxicity, which, however, could be relevant for the safety aspects. These tests can be based on certain enzymatic activities or other specific targeted functions in the cell. Some examples are presented below.

When hepatic cell lines that have retained their ability to respond to foreign compounds by the induction of specific drug metabolising enzymes (cytochrome P450 variants, such as CYP1A1) are used, this enzymatic activity can be measured and used as an indicator of toxicity (Sanderson *et al.*, 1996; Koistinen *et al.*, 1998).

RNA synthesis is a basic function of living cells, and its rate can be influenced by various factors. Measurement of the cellular RNA synthesis rate after exposure to the test agent by following the incorporation of radio-labelled uridine provides an indication of the toxicity of the sample (Fauris *et al.*, 1985). The method, originally designed for human HeLa S_3 cells, is particularly useful for water samples, since the cell culture medium can be constituted using the test sample as a base. However, the test can also be used by simply diluting the test agent into the growth medium. The test is used as an official test for bottled drinking water in France.

An example of the use of a highly specialised cell type to study targeted toxic effects on the cellular metabolism is the recently developed boar spermatozoon motility inhibition test (Andersson *et al.*, 1998). The motility of a spermatozoon depends on the integrity of mitochondrial functions, and thus the action of toxins affecting the energy metabolism is very rapidly detected as reduction of motility. Other endpoints that can be measured are plasma membrane integrity, astrosome function, and total cellular ATP and NAD reduction. This test has been particularly useful in the detection of certain types of bacterial toxins from various environmental and food sources.

A bacterial assay based on the inhibition of light emission of a bioluminescent bacterium *Vibrio fisheri* (ISO-standard 11348–1, 1998), originally developed to test the toxicity of industrial effluents, gives an indication of the effects of the test agent on the oxidative metabolism of the cell. As a bacterial assay its advantages are rapidity and relatively low costs, but naturally the differences between bacterial and mammalian systems make the interpretation of the results even more difficult than with other short-term tests.

The availability of recombinant DNA techniques has also made it possible to design cellular lines or microbial strains with highly specific properties for certain types of toxicity tests. In CALUX test, designed to respond specifically to dioxins, a recombinant mouse cell line, in which the activity of a luciferase enzyme causing bioluminescence is under a control element responding to an AhR receptor. This receptor is specific to dioxin-like compounds, and when combined with a dioxin it activates a cascade in the cell, leading in this case to induction of luciferase, the activity of which can be measured (Amakura *et al.*, 2003). Another example is the use of recombinant yeast cells in which the β-galactosidase gene is under a control element containing an oestrogen receptor. When the hormone or hormone-like compound reacts with the receptor, the enzyme is activated and the activity can be measured spectrophotometrically (Routledge and Sumpter, 1996).

23.5 Genotoxicity tests

As already pointed out above, genotoxicity tests represent an exceptionally high level of standardisation and official recognition among the short-term toxicological tests. This reflects the fact that the target of most genotoxic agents, DNA, is similar in all various life forms, and an agent that affects DNA in a bacterium, is likely to do so in humans too.

Due to their well-established status, good descriptions of the standard tests can be found in various textbooks and laboratory manuals (e.g. Preston and Hoffman, 2001). The *in vitro* genotoxicity tests can be roughly divided into point mutation tests, cytogenetic tests measuring chromosomal anomalies and tests for DNA damage and repair.

23.5.1 Point mutation tests

The best known point mutation test is the Ames *Salmonella* assay or Ames test. The assay was developed in the early 1970s and was later updated by the introduction of novel tester strains (Maron and Ames, 1983). The test is based on a number of *Salmonella* strains that are histidine auxotrophs, or mutated so that they cannot synthesise histidine and consequently cannot grow without an external source of this amino acid. If the strains are exposed to a mutagenic agent that reverses the original mutation, a revertant colony emerges on a solid test medium devoid of external histidine. The number of these revertant colonies is the measure of the mutagenic potential of the test agent. A mammalian microsome fraction (usually isolated from induced rat liver) is routinely included in the test to mimic the mammalian drug metabolism and activation of certain mutagens.

Point mutation tests have also been developed for cultured mammalian cells (de Marini *et al.*, 1989). These tests are based on the mutational resistance to otherwise cytotoxic agents (i.e. TK or HPRT mutations, conferring resistance to trifluorothymidine and 6-thioguanine, respectively). Compared to Ames test and other bacterial assays, they are, however, more laborious and time-consuming.

23.5.2 Mammalian cytogenetic tests

In mammalian cytogenetic tests the changes in the chromosome number and structure (as seen in a typical metaphase plate), resulting from genotoxic action, are microscopically monitored (Galloway *et al.*, 1994). The chromosome aberrations include gaps and breakages, deletions and chromatid exchanges. These kinds of analysis can be done both *in vitro* using cultured cells and *in vivo* by exposing experimental animals to the test agent and subsequently collecting suitable cells (peripheral lymphocytes, bone marrow cells) for analysis.

Because of the time and skills needed to analyse metaphase chromosomes, micronucleus tests are increasingly used as a simpler cytogenetic assay. The test is based on the presence of chromosomal fragments or whole chromosomes that have not been incorporated into a daughter nucleus at mitosis. Typically they can be seen as a stained body outside the cell nucleus in an interphase cell. The number of induced micronuclei is a measure of the genotoxic activity of the test agent (Miller *et al.*, 1998). Also this test can be performed both *in vitro* using cell cultures and *in vivo* by exposing experimental animals to the test agent and subsequent harvesting and analysis of suitable cells. In *in vivo* experiments the polychromatic lymphocytes are frequently used, since the micronuclei are naturally very easy to detect against the anucleate background (Hayashi *et al.*, 2000).

23.5.3 Tests for DNA damage and repair

The uses of bacterial mutants that are deficient in DNA repair functions and thus particularly sensitive to DNA damaging agents are routinely used to screen potential mutagens in assays that are usually based on differential killing. If a repair-deficient microbial strain is more sensitive to the lethal effects of the test agent than its repair-proficient but otherwise isogenic control strain, one of the targets of the test agents is probably DNA (Hamasaki *et al.*, 1992).

In mammalian cells the traditional assay for DNA repair has been the test of unscheduled DNA repair, in which the repair of damaged DNA is detected by autoradiography after incorporation of radio-labelled nucleotides into the newly synthesised DNA at the site of the damage (Madle *et al.*, 1994). A novel mammalian assay that measures directly the DNA damage is the so-called Comet assay or single-cell gel electrophoresis. The test is based on the fragmentation of the nuclear DNA as a result of genotoxic action. When a cell is subjected to electrophoresis after exposure to the test agent, the DNA fragments migrate in the electric field and can be seen as a 'comet tail' after staining with a fluorescent dye. The test can be applied to hepatocytes retaining their ability to metabolically activate mutagens (Uhl *et al.*, 2000).

23.6 Applying tests to paper and board

So far there have been relatively few published reports on the application of *in vitro* toxicological tests to extracts of paper and board. The published results relate to the use of the photobacterium test, RNA synthesis inhibition or to a battery of different test systems. The outcomes of these trials are summarised below.

23.6.1 Paper and board extracts in bacterial bioluminiscence assay

The bioluminiscence assay test has been included in the purity and toxicity assays of fibre-based products (Sipiläinen-Malm *et al.*, 1997; Jokinen *et al.*, 2001). In the latter study samples of pulp and food contact board were systematically evaluated using water extracts obtained from homogenised material. According to the results the light intensity curves were highly repeatable, the same samples giving consistently similar responses. However, regarding the toxicity, the results were difficult to interpret, because the samples often produced a pattern of variable photoemission induction and inhibition, depending on the concentration. The main practical result was that each board grade had a typical and highly stable response in the test, and this could be used as a quality control parameter for the stability of the production conditions.

23.6.2 RNA synthesis inhibition caused by paper and board water extracts

Fauris *et al.* (1998) made a systematic survey on six paper and fifteen board samples from different European countries using the RNA synthesis inhibition test for the toxicity screening. The samples represented both recycled (ten samples) and virgin fibres, among the latter both chemical and mechanical pulps were represented. The recycled fibres represented the four categories according to the CEN 1994 standard (category A represents raw materials consisting of unprinted or uncoloured paper, categories B, C and D represent increasing use of printed or coloured raw materials, D being made totally from mixed paper and board of variable origin). In the analysis of water soluble matter and in the preparation of water extracts, CEN standard procedures were used. The substances that were analysed from the actual samples included total and organic chlorine, pentachlorophenol, total sulphur and nitrogen, formaldehyde, glyoxal, heavy metals Cd, Pb and Cr, bacterial endotoxins and aflatoxin. GC analysis of the Tenax-absorbed material from the samples was also performed. According to the results the cytotoxicity of the samples ranged form very high (RNA synthesis rate 17% of the control) to non-toxic (RNA synthesis rate 94%). The same range of toxicities was found in samples representing both recycled products and virgin fibres. Among the latter, the toxic samples (RNA synthesis rate 60% or less of the control) represented mechanical pulps. The toxicities of the samples did not correlate with any individual analysed chemical component. Instead, there was a correlation between the toxicity and the numbers of peaks in the GC-chromatogram.

23.6.3 Extracts of recycled paper in a toxicological test battery

Binderup *et al.* (2002) have evaluated three different categories of recycled fibre-based food contact papers in a test battery consisting of a standard cytotoxicity test on human skin fibroblasts, Ames test for genotoxicity, recombinant yeast test for estrogenic activity and CALUX test for the detection of dioxin-like activity. The recycled papers were compared to virgin fibre (paper A). Paper B represented a product consisting of 40% virgin fibre, 40% recycled material from unprinted newspaper cuttings and 20% de-inked paper from newspapers and magazines. Papers C and D were derived from newspapers and magazines, D being de-inked. The samples were extracted both with 99% ethanol and water following the relevant CEN standards. The extracts were monitored for migrants using GC-IR-MS or GC-HRMS. The papers were also subjected for microbiological analyses (total aerobic bacteria, aerobic and anaerobic spore formers, *Bacillus cereus/thuringensis*, yeasts and moulds).

In the test, applied ethanol extracts showed more toxicity than water extracts and also contained higher amounts of material in the chemical analysis. Sample A produced least extractants, and was also least cytotoxic. Among the recycled products, sample C was the most toxic in the cytotoxicity assay. None of the extracts gave a positive effect in the Ames test, and all were too cytotoxic to the recombinant yeast cell line to produce meaningful results. Signs of dioxin-like activity were detected in all ethanol extracts, sample C showing the highest positive response, while with samples A and B this activity was non-significant. With water extracts a weak positive response was observed with samples B, C and D.

23.7 Conclusions and future trends

There is a wide variety of different *in vitro* tests that could be applied to extracts of food contact paper and board. However, there are few published reports of their use for this purpose, and at present it is not possible to form a consistent picture of their general applicability. The outcomes of the two most comprehensive studies published so far (Fauris, 1998; Binderup, 2002) illustrate this point. While both studies agree that the toxicity is correlated with the chemical complexity of the paper and board and apparently not attributable to any single compound alone, the different samples and different test systems applied make these two studies difficult to compare. While both studies show that *in vitro* tests can be applied to paper and board products, they also show that application of different tests and testing conditions could lead to a rather different interpretation of the results.

As has been stated in Section 23.3, CoE has recognised the potential value of toxicity tests as a method to ensure the safety of the food contact paper and board. In order to be of use to consumers, industry and regulators, the proposed tests should be evaluated, standardised and validated. This requires that same paper and board samples would be tested simultaneously using different test systems in order to discover eventual correlations or discrepancies between the results obtained. Also the relevance of positive results should be carefully evaluated in the light of whether they really reflect any toxicological risks to consumers or whether they can be regarded as artefactual. As pointed out in Section 23.3.1, proper and realistic sample preparation is also essential for toxicological testing to be meaningful.

In an ideal case the industry and regulators could have available a selection of validated short-term *in vitro* tests with sufficient historical background for the safety assessment. This would reduce the need for extensive chemical analysis of the products and would circumvent the practical impossibility of applying traditional toxicological tests routinely to paper and board for food contact. The tests should have relatively broad toxicological endpoints so that many types of harmful compounds could be detected, but the test battery could be complemented with highly specialised tests for specific types of chemical or biological risks (special assays for microbial toxins, endocrine distruptors, hormone-like compounds, etc.). An additional demand, from the practical point of view, is that the set-up and performance of at least some of the tests should be feasible in an industrial, quality control laboratory, and that a large number of samples could be processed in a relatively short time. The use of the photobacterium test to screen the stability of the products and production conditions (see Section 23.6.1 above) illustrates the point.

In order to answer those needs specified above, a collaborative effort (BIOSAFEPAPER) has been undertaken in the fifth EU framework programme. In this project, scheduled to last until the end of 2005 and coordinated by the University of Kuopio, Finland, nine European research institutes and 16 industrial partners aim at establishing a test battery with relevant toxicological endpoints and allowing a decision-tree approach to ensure consumer safety. An important aspect of the undertaking is also the development of extraction procedures compatible with the tests and reflecting real-life conditions. As the project is considered as a pre-normative research effort, special emphasis is devoted to the translation of the toxicological data to risk assessment, to the provision of a scientific basis for safety recommendations on fibre-based food contact materials and to the dissemination of the results to various stakeholders (industry, regulatory bodies, consumers). More detailed information on the project and its progress can be seen on the project homepage (http://www.uku.fi/biosafepaper/).

23.8 References

AMAKURA Y, TSUTSUMI T, NAKAMURA M, KITAGAWA H, FUJINO J, SASAKI K, TOYODA M, YOSHIDA T and MAITANI T (2003) Activation of the aryl hydrocarbon receptor by some vegetable constituents determined using in vitro reporter gene assay. *Biol Pharm Bull.* 26, 532–539.

ANDERSSON MA, MIKKOLA R, HELIN J, ANDERSSON MC and SALKINOJA-SALONEN M (1998) A novel sensitive bioassay for detection of *Bacillus cereus* emetic toxin and related depsipeptide ionophores. *Appl. Environ. Microbiol.* 64, 1338–1343.

ANON. (2002) Policy statement concerning paper and board materials and articles intended to come into contact with foodstuffs. Public Health Committee: Committee of Experts on Materials Coming into Contact with Food, Council of Europe.

BINDERUP M-L, PEDERSEN GA, VINGGAARD AM, RASMUSSEN ES, ROSENQUIST H and CEDERBERG T (2002) Toxicity testing and chemical analysis of recycled fibre-based paper for food contact. *Food Addit. Contam.* 19, 13–28.

DE MARINI DM, BROCKMAN HE, DE SERRES FJ, EVANS HH, STANKOWSKI LF and HSIEAW JR (1989) Specific-locus mutations induced in eukaryotes (especially mammalian cells) by radiation and chemicals: a perspective. *Mutat Res.* 220, 11–29.

ESCABASSE J-Y and OTTENIO D (2002) Food-contact paper and board based on recycled fibres: regulatory aspects-new rules and guidelines. *Food. Addit. Contam.* 19, 79–92.

FAURIS C, DANGLOT C and VILAGINÈS (1985), Rapidity of RNA synthesis in human cells. A highly sensitive parameter for water cytotoxicity evaluation. *Water Res.* 19, 677–684.

FAURIS C, LUNDSTRÖM H and VILAGINÈS (1998) Cytotoxicological safety assessment of papers and boards used for food packaging. *Food Addit.* Contam. 15, 716–728.

GALLOWAY SM, AARDEMA MJ, ISHIDATE M JR, IVETT JL, KIRKLAND DJ, MORITA T, MOSESSO P and SOFUNI T (1994) Report from working group on in vitro tests for chromosomal aberrations. *Mutat Res.* 312, 241–261.

HAMASAKI T, SATO T, NAGASE H and KITO H (1992) The genotoxicity of organotin compounds in SOS-chromotest and rec-assay. *Mutat Res.* 280, 195–203.

HAYASHI M, MACGREGOR JT, GATEHOUSE DG, ADLER ID, BLAKEY DH, DERTINGER SD, KRISHNA G, MORITA T, RUSSO A and SUTOU S (2000) In vivo rodent erythrocyte micronucleus assay. II. Some aspects of protocol design including repeated treatments, integration with toxicity testing, and automated scoring. *Environ Mol Mutagen.* 35, 234–252.

ISO 11348-1 (1998) Water quality-Determination of the inhibitory effect of water samples on the light emission of *Vibrio fisheri* (Luminescent bacteria test) Part 1: Method using freshly prepared bacteria.

JOKINEN K, SAVOLAINEN M and SÖDERHJELM L (2001) Photobacterium test for evaluation of toxicity of fibrous products, *Pap. Puu*, 83, 332–335.

KOISTINEN J, SOIMASUO M, TUKIA K, OIKARI A, BLANKENSHIP A and GIESY JP (1998) Induction of EROD activity in hepa-1 mouse hepatoma cells and estrogenicity in MCF-7 human breast cancer cells by extracts of pulp mill effluents, sludge, and sediment exposed to effluents. *Environmen. Toxicol. Chem.* 17, 1499–1507.

MADLE S, DEAN SW, ANDRAE U, BRAMBILLA G, BURLINSON B, DOOLITTLE DJ, FURIHATA C, HERTNER T, MCQUEEN CA and MORI H (1994) Recommendations for the performance of UDS tests in vitro and in vivo. *Mutat Res.* 312, 263–285.

MARON DM and AMES BN (1983) Revised methods for the Salmonella mutagenicity test. *Mutat Res.* 113, 173–215.

MILLER B, POTTER-LOCHER F, SEELBACH A, STOPPER H, UTESCH D and MADLE S (1998) Evaluation of the in vitro micronucleus test as an alternative to the in vitro chromosomal aberration assay: position of the GUM Working Group on the in vitro micronucleus test. Gesellschaft für Umwelt-Mutations-Forschung. *Mutat Res.* 410, 81–116.

MOSMANN T (1983) Rapid colorimetric assay for cellular growth and survival: application to proliferation and cytotoxicity assays. *J. Immunol. Meth.* 65, 55–63.

OECD GUIDELINES FOR TESTING OF CHEMICALS (2001): guidelines 471–486 (Genetic Toxicology Testing), Paris, OECD.

PRESTON RJ and HOFFMAN GR (2001) Genetic toxicology. In Klaassen CD, *Casarett's and Doull's Toxicology, The Basic Science of Poisons*, New York, McGraw-Hill, 321–350.

ROUTLEDGE EJ and SUMPTER JP (1996) Estrogenic activity of surfactants and some of their degradation products assessed using a recombinant yeast screen. *Environ. Toxicol. Chem.* 15, 241–248.

SANDERSON JT, AARTS JMMJG, BROUWER A, FROESE KL, DENISON MS and GIESY JP (1996) Comparison of Ah Receptor-Mediated Luciferase and Ethoxyresorufin-O-deethylase Induction in H411E Cells: Implications for Their Use as Bioanalytical Tools for the Detection of Polyhalogenated Aromatic Hydrocarbons. *Toxicol. Appl. Pharmacol.* 137, 316–325.

SIPILÄINEN-MALM T, LATVA-KALA K, TIKKANEN L, SUIHKO ML and SKYTTÄ E (1997) Purity of recycled fibre-based materials. *Food Addit. Contam.* 14, 695–703.

STAMMATI A, BONSI P, ZUCCO F, MOEZELAAR R, ALAKOMI H-L and VON WRIGHT A (1999) Toxicity of selected plant volatiles in microbial andmammalian short-term assays. *Food Chem.Toxicol.* 37, 813–823.

UHL M, HELMA C and KNASMULLER S (2000) Evaluation of the single cell gel electrophoresis assay with human hepatoma (Hep G2) cells. *Mutat Res.* 468, 213–225.

VON WRIGHT A, RAATIKAINEN O, TAIPALE H, KÄRENLAMPI S and MÄKI-PAAKKANEN J (1992) Directly acting geno- and cytotoxic agents from a wild mushroom *Dermocybe sanguinea*. *Mutati. Res.* 269, 27–33.

24

Detecting metal contamination

R. Montoro and D. Vélez, Instituto de Agroquímica y Tecnología de Alimentos (CSIC), Spain

24.1 Introduction

During much of the twentieth century, scientific progress took priority over environmental safety. The impressive development of technology and its negative impact on the food chain reduced public confidence in the healthiness of foods. As a result, the general public is now more alert to metal contamination in foods. The metals and metalloids present in the earth's crust, soils, water, atmosphere and biosphere, and consequently in foods, are stable compounds, persisting in the environment, having a slow rate of elimination, accumulating in tissues, and capable of undergoing transformations that increase their toxicity. Among them, lead, cadmium, arsenic and mercury are the ones that cause most problems to the food industry, and, although various countries have established legislation regulating their concentrations, they are still sometimes a danger for consumer health. This chapter comments on the analytical methodologies most commonly used at present for trace element determination. They include quantification not only of total contents but also of their chemical species. Comments will also be made about future trends.

24.2 Methods of preparing food samples for analysis

The determination of metals in foods requires prior preparation of the sample. Except for liquid samples, this generally involves the elimination of organic matter by a dry or wet ashing procedure. Other procedures, less aggressive but efficacious in isolating the analyte from food, have also been employed (slurries, alkaline solubilization, enzymolysis).

24.2.1 Dry ashing

This procedure involves incineration of the sample at a specific temperature. It is simple, cheap and safe, and requires minimal operator attention. It is a sample preparation technique compatible with the various instrumental quantification techniques because it allows the ash to be dissolved in the appropriate acid. It also allows the use of relatively large quantities of sample, up to 25 g.[1] The key factor in the dry ashing procedure is the avoidance of losses of analyte at the temperature selected for mineralization, which requires optimization of the method for each food/analyte combination.

After dry ashing procedures with temperatures ranging between 450ºC and 600ºC, Cd and Pb have been analyzed in a great variety of foods (flour,[1] tomato,[2] soy, vinegar, wine, malt, rice and hops,[3,4] mushrooms,[5] infant cereal,[6] spices,[7] biscuits,[8] hard and soft wheat[9] and liver paste, apple sauce, minced fish, wheat bran and milk powder[10]). With the exception of the analysis of spices, the samples were placed in the muffle without ashing aids. In some cases the composition of the matrix itself may act as a self-modifier and prevent volatilization of the analyte.

For As, dry ashing can involve analyte losses during heating owing to the formation of volatile chlorides and oxychlorides of As. A suitable quantity of ashing aids [MgO alone or with $Mg(NO_3)_2$][11–19] avoids these losses, allowing reliable determination of As in colour additives,[17] beverages,[15,16] sugar,[14] vegetables,[18] and seafood products.[11–13,19] The mineralization conditions are variable, and although a muffle temperature of 750ºC[17] has been employed in colour additives, for most foods 500ºC[12–15] has not been exceeded. Dry ashing techniques are not used in the case of Hg.

24.2.2 Wet digestion

These techniques combine the use of strong oxidizing acids and temperature to destroy the organic matter. Nitric acid alone or combined with other acids such as H_2SO_4, HF or $HClO_4$, and sometimes with H_2O_2, acts as an oxidizing agent.

The traditional systems for wet digestion of samples use Teflon or glass beakers heated by a hot plate or sand bath. The quantity of sample that can be digested is low, and large volumes of reagents are necessary. These traditional systems have been replaced by the use of microwaves, currently the equipment most employed as a heat source for wet digestion methods. A microwave system substantially reduces digestion times, use of reagents and contamination during the process. The digestion can be done in a multimode microwave oven or in a monomode (focused) microwave oven. Closed vessels and open vessels can be used in both cases.

Wet digestion in traditional systems has been used for Cd or Pb determination in vegetables,[2,20–25] fish,[20,21,26–30] wine,[31] meat,[20,25,27,28] cows' milk[32] and total diet.[33] Open-vessel microwave digestion in a monomode (focused) microwave oven has been employed to determine Cd and Pb in algae and cabbage.[22] Closed-vessel microwave digestion in a multimode microwave oven has been used extensively for determination of Cd and/or Pb in fish,[34–41] vegetables,[36,42] meat,[36,37,42–44] honey,[45] wheat bran[36] and milk powder.[36]

In the case of As, open wet digestion with traditional systems has been applied to tea,[46] coffee,[46] seafood products,[47–51] vegetables,[12, 46,49] wine and beer.[16] Pressurized decomposition in an autoclave has also been used to determine As in food.[46] This procedure does not break down organoarsenical compounds, and therefore, when HG-AAS is going to be used for quantification, the autoclaved solution requires an additional decomposition for full conversion of As to the inorganic form. The High Temperature and High Pressure Asher (HPA) system has been used to determine As in certified marine samples and foodstuffs[52,43] but a temperature of 320ºC is necessary to break up the stable arsenic species.[53]

When the microwave alternative is used for the analysis of As, the modality most commonly applied is the closed-vessel multimode microwave, which has the drawback indicated in the wet digestion procedures mentioned earlier: the maximum attainable temperatures of 200 to 270ºC are often insufficient for complete decomposition of organoarsenic compounds, using HNO_3 as the only oxidant. Consequently, in the case of foods with a high proportion of organic arsenic compounds (seafood products), direct reading of the digest by hydride generation atomic absorption spectrometry (HG-AAS) provides concentrations lower than the real value. This drawback can be overcome by using inductively coupled plasma mass spectrometry (ICP-MS)[54] or electrothermal atomic absorption spectrometry ETAAS[55] for the quantification. Open-vessel microwave digestion in a monomode (focused) microwave oven coupled to ICP-MS[56] and hydride generation atomic fluorescence spectrometry (HG-AFS)[57] has been used to determine total As in seafood products.

For Hg, wet digestion using open flask,[58,59] pressurized systems[58,60–62] or microwave digestors [60,61,63–66] has been employed. Because Hg is a very volatile element, wet digestion in open vessels, even at low temperature, may cause losses of Hg. Losses during digestion can be avoided by using closed teflon vessels under pressure.

24.2.3 Direct sample introduction

Although solution nebulization is the most common method for introducing samples into atomic spectrometers, methods involving minimal sample handling have also been employed.

Solid sampling

This procedure has some advantages (reduction of sample preparation and risk of sample contamination), but it presents difficulties related to sample introduction, micro-weighing, calibration, sample inhomogeneity and poor precision. Various approaches have been described for analysis of foods. Micro-amount samples of rice, oyster and pepperbush have been analyzed using a tungsten boat furnace sample cuvette technique to digest the sample and generate Cd vapour, which is quantified by ICP-MS.[67] Thermal treatment of the sample using the double-vaporization mode of the two-step atomizer with a purged vaporizer has been used for analysis of Cd and Pb in potatoes, wheat, bovine liver, milk powder and grass-cereal mixtures.[68] Arsenic has been directly determined in sugars by ETAAS.[69]

Liquid sampling

In the case of liquid foods, direct analysis of Cd and Pb has also been described for edible oils and fat,[70,71] honey[45] and brandies.[72] Arsenic has been determined directly in wine and beer.[15,16] Analysis time and the risk of sample contamination are considerably decreased, and methods for routine analyses have been proposed.

Slurries

This technique substantially reduces sample preparation time. It is currently coming to the fore in the analysis of Cd and Pb in foods. Triton X-100, ethanol, plant glue (surfactants), HNO_3, H_2O_2 and/or chemical modifiers can be added to obtain a suspension. Manual stirring, magnetic stirring or ultrasonic stirring (bath or probes) can be employed for slurry preparation.[73–86]

The slurry approach has been used to determine As in baby foods[87] and seafood.[88,89] Both studies used nitric acid, Triton X-100 and matrix modifier for preparation of the slurries. In the case of baby foods, H_2O_2 and silicon antifoam were also added. Slurry sampling has also been used for the determination of Hg in seafood,[89–91] baby foods[90] and food colorants.[92] Various procedures have been described: aqueous slurries with the addition of glycerol to achieve a uniform particle distribution,[93] aqueous slurries in the presence of EDTA, which subsequently acts as chemical modifier,[83] and obtaining of slurries in the presence of nitric acid and Triton X-100.[90–92]

Ultrasound-assisted extraction

This sample treatment permits quantification of analytes in the supernatant obtained after ultrasound-assisted treatment. In comparison with the conventional slurry technique, it does not require the use of stirring systems or stabilizing agents, it produces lower background signals and it improves accuracy and precision by eliminating sedimentation and volumetric errors inherent in the slurry technique.[94] Nitric acid has frequently been reported as an efficient extractant. Methods have been optimized with excellent results for determination of Pb and/or Cd[84,94–96] and As[88] in seafood.

24.2.4 Other procedures

There are other methods for isolating the analyte from the food and some of these are mentioned in the references. Alkaline solubilization with tetramethylammonium hydroxide has been used for fish sample preparation before quantification of Cd and Pb[97] and Hg.[98] An alkaline digestion using NaOH and

L-cysteine has been described for Hg.[58] Oxidative UV photolysis using hydrogen peroxide as oxidizing agent has been used for preparation of samples of wine[99] and honey[100] prior to quantification of Cd and Pb. In the case of As, enzymatic hydrolysis with a protease obtained from *Streptomyces griseus* has been described for As determination, with quantitative recoveries in mussel samples.[101]

24.3 Analytical methods for metal detection

24.3.1 Flame atomic absorption spectrophotometry

Among the analytical methodologies most commonly used for decades for the detection of trace elements, flame atomic absorption spectrophotometry (FAAS) is remarkable for its selectivity, speed and fairly low operational cost. Background correction is achieved by the use of a continuum source or Zeeman effect correction, which simultaneously measures total absorbance and non-specific absorbance, allowing immediate correction of the absorbance measure. The technique's lack of sensitivity for determination of low quantities of Cd, Pb, As and Hg in food can be alleviated by the used of various strategies:

- atom trapping
- a flow injection (FI) or continuous flow on-line preconcentration step
- sequential injection
- cold vapour generation (CVAAS)
- hydride generation (HG).

The application of atom trapping in FAAS preconcentrates the analyte atoms within the flame before measurement. This methodology offers simplicity, speed, lower analytical cost and less risk of contamination and has been applied to the determination of Pb in liqueurs,[102] and Cd in vegetables[2] and flour.[1] The current state of the art for other elements is discussed in an excellent paper.[103] Preconcentration systems[20,21,27,28,29,39–41] are performed in minicolumns by means of ion exchange or sorbent extraction techniques, and the preconcentrated analyte is eluted with an appropriate reagent into the nebulizer-burner system of an AAS. Preconcentration is also possible by means of on-line coprecipitation-dissolution, with high tolerance for interference from matrix elements, and optimum analytical features. Particular advantages are: low consumption of reagents, sample and time, less risk of sample contamination and ease of automation.[29,39] An automated sequential injection on-line solvent extraction-back extraction procedure was developed for the determination of Cd in sea lettuce.[23]

CVAAS is the method of choice for Hg determination because of its high sensitivity, absence of spectral interference, relatively low operation cost and simplicity. This technique has been extensively used for the determination of Hg from liquid, digested or slurry samples of food: fish,[60,62,63,65,91,98,104–107] vegetables[61,105] and milk powder.[105] The determination of Hg is based on the generation of elemental Hg vapour at room temperature, as it is the only element that is found in an atomic vapour state at room temperature. Organomercury compounds must be destroyed and converted to inorganic Hg before determination. FI-CV-AAS is the strategy least often used for Cd determination in foods. The food samples analyzed so far – rice powder[24] and Antarctic krill[84] – are few, but the methods proposed achieve low detection limits and good precision.

In the case of As, the sensitivity of the AAS technique is increased by introducing into the flame volatile covalent hydrides generated from aqueous solutions of the samples by means of a reducing agent. Hydride generation coupled to atomic absorption (HGAAS) allows a good preconcentration of the analyte and chemical separation of the As from potential matrix interferences, and it has the advantage of being cheaper in terms of both equipment and maintenance. HGAAS coupling is one of the techniques most commonly used for the determination of As in foods.[13,18,92]

In the case of Pb, there has been a little interest in HG determination. The procedure has been further developed by trapping the hydride on the inside of a graphite furnace atomizer. The procedure was used for the determination of Pb in calcium supplements. In the case of Cd, CdH_2 is formed when tetrahydroborate is introduced into an acidified solution of cadmium. The procedure is called cold vapour because CdH_2 is unstable at room temperature. A procedure has been developed for accurate determination of Cd by cold vapour in NIST SRM 1515 apple leaves.[108]

24.3.2 Electrothermal atomic absorption spectrometry

In view of the very low levels of Cd and/or Pb in food samples, ETAAS has been considered one of the best techniques for the determination of these elements. Numerous articles have been published on the analysis of Cd and/or Pb by ETAAS.[6,25,31,37,38,68,70,71,75,78,80,86,97,109,110] However, some difficulties may be encountered as a result of high volatility, which restricts ashing temperatures, and hence some chemical concomitants may not be readily eliminated at this step. Consequently, the remaining matrix constituents may produce high background absorption levels. In order to overcome this problem a large number of matrix modifiers have been proposed to provide analyte isoformations, and background correctors such as Deuterium Lamp, Zeeman or Smith-Hieftje are employed.

For many years As has been considered a difficult element for determination with ETAAS. However, as a result of recent advances in the technique, elimination or minimization of interferences due to structured background and spectral line overlap has been achieved. The combined use of transverse heated ETAAS and longitudinal Zeeman background correction has been successfully applied for the determination of As in seafood.[88] There are very few publications in which ETAAS is used for Hg determination in food samples. Baby food, seafood and colourants have recently been analyzed with this methodology by introducing the samples into the atomizer as slurries.[90,93] This, together with a fast program, avoids the Hg volatilization losses that can take place in a prior digestion. Other authors use slurries in a cold vapour batch mode generation system coupled with ETAAS.[93] The use of slurries avoids digestion of the sample and consequent losses of Hg.

24.3.3 Inductively coupled plasma atomic emission spectrometry (ICP-AES)

Even with modern equipment, the determination of Pb and Cd by ICP-AES does not often permit detection of low concentrations of Cd and Pb in foods. Dry ashing digestion is a classical alternative approach in order to improve, or not excessively impair, the detection limits obtained by ICP-AES. Research into the determination of As by ICP-AES has basically followed a combination of the technique of HG with ICP. The instrumental detection limits improve by at least an order of magnitude over those obtained with conventional nebulization. For determination of total Hg in food there are few applications of ICP-AES.[105]

24.3.4 Inductively coupled plasma mass spectrometry (ICP-MS)

With this analytical technique it is possible to achieve the limits of detection required for determination of Cd and Pb in foods, although it is not free from spectroscopic and matrix interference. In recent years, isotope dilution (ID) has been used for trace element quantification by ICP-MS. For very low Cd concentrations, the sensitivity at low resolution is much higher for double focusing ICP-MS than for quadrupole (Q) ICP-MS.[43,44,111] For As, one problem associated with determination using ICP-MS is polyatomic interference at mass-to-charge ratio (m/z) 75. The chloride ion present in biological samples combines with the plasma gas to form $^{40}Ar^{35}Cl^{+}$, which is detected together with As. One of the recent methods introduced to eliminate these polyatomic interferences is the use of collision and reaction cells, inserted before the ion optics and quadrupole filter of the ICP-MS spectrometer. Helium, hydrogen, ammonia and methane have been widely used as collision/reaction gases.[112] For the determination of total Hg there are few applications.[59,64,112] Some of these methods use the slurry approach to avoid sample digestion.

Electrothermal vaporization (ETV) is one of the sample introduction techniques currently employed in ICP-MS. It is an alternative to conventional pneumatic nebulization and offers the possibility of analyzing solid samples. Slurry sample ETV-ICP-MS has been applied to the analysis of food samples, although it is not free from problems associated with spectroscopic and non-spectroscopic interferences, residue accumulation in the furnace, analyte loss during transportation and poor reproducibility. It has been applied to the determination of Pb and/or Cd in fish,[34,67,73,82,83] milk powder,[85] bovine muscle,[73] egg powder,[73] rice and pepperbush,[67] As and Hg in fish[112] and Cd, Pb and Hg in fish.[94]

24.3.5 Spectrophotometric methods

There are very few articles published since 1996 in which spectrophotometry is applied to the analysis of Cd and Pb in foods. Two papers describing the synthesis and subsequent use of two new chromogenic reagents, both for the determination of Pb, might contribute to a revival of this analytical technique. The samples to which these methods were applied are malt extract, rice, hops, soy, vinegar and grape wine.[3,4]

24.3.6 Electroanalytical methods

Of the many electroanalytical techniques that exist, those most frequently described in the literature for the analysis of Cd, Pb and As in food are differential pulse anodic stripping voltammetry[32,99,100,113–115] and differential pulse cathodic stripping voltammetry,[99,114,116] with a single reference to the use of derivative potentiometric stripping[9] for analysis of Cd and Pb. The advantages of stripping voltammetry compared with non-electroanalytical techniques include: the ability to measure various trace elements simultaneously and determine the analyte without prior treatment of the sample, low maintenance cost and high sensitivity and selectivity. Some authors do the determination directly in the sample (refined beet sugar,[113] common salt,[114] whisky samples[115]), whereas in other articles there is a pre-treatment by dry ashing (hard and soft wheat),[9] wet ashing (cows' milk),[32] or oxidative UV photolysis (honey, wine).[99,100]

24.3.7 Neutron activation analysis

The technique is generally regarded as being very accurate and sensitive, but it is time-consuming and expensive and not generally used in analytical laboratories. This method requires little sample preparation, and has been used for total Hg determination in mussel certified reference materials, with results that do not differ statistically from those found using other analytical methods.[61] It has also been used for total As determination in seaweed.[117]

24.3.8 Atomic fluorescence spectrometry (AFS)

In recent years, the development of commercially available AFS instrumentation has provided a powerful tool for the determination of As and its species at ultratrace levels. In comparison with HGAAS or CVAAS, HGAFS offers advantages in terms of sensitivity and lower equipment cost. There is likely to be an increase in applications of As[15,16] and Hg.[58,60] AAS and AFS are sensitive to the interference of volatile nitrogen oxides formed as a reduction product of nitric acid during sample decomposition. This interference can be eliminated by resting the sample solution for one day after the digestion steps, purging with argon, or reducing the oxides by means of sulphamic acid or urea.[61,63]

24.4 Cadmium speciation in food

In animal tissues of vertebrates and many invertebrates (molluscs, crustaceans and insects) most of the Cd is bound to metallothioneins (MTs). In plants, Cd is at least partially complexed by several metal-binding complexes such as organic acids, metallothioneins and phytochelatins (PCs), these last-named being the main metal-binding proteins in higher plants. MTs are cysteine-rich polypeptides, and PCs (designated γ-EC peptides) are short glutathione-related peptides consisting of repetitive γ-glutamylcysteine units with a carboxyl-terminal glycine (γ Glu-Cys)$_n$ Gly.

Differences in Cd availability from different foodstuffs will certainly have a great impact on risk evaluation of dietary Cd and on estimation of tolerable Cd levels in different types of food products. Metabolism of Cd is dose dependent. At low dietary Cd doses, Cd is probably released from dietary CdMT after passage through the intestinal tract and uptake via the intestinal mucosa, and then follows the same disposition pathway as inorganic Cd. Current recommendations on Cd levels in foods of animal origin thus appear to be adequate as long as the Cd concentration in the diet is low. Despite this encouraging news, it must be remembered that vegetable foods are an even more important source of dietary Cd intake than animal foods. It is not known to what extent the metabolism of the Cd-phytochelatins of plants is comparable to that of Cd-metallothionein; this area needs further research attention.[118]

There is a distinct lack of data describing the form or chemical species in which Cd occurs in different foodstuffs. There are no reports of characterization studies of Cd-MTs and Cd-PCs in foods. Only one systematic approach based on the coupling of high resolution size-exclusion chromatography (SEC) with Q-ICP-MS detection has been developed, applied to the speciation of Cd-PCs in maize plant extracts.[119] The separation conditions were optimized using a series of standards prepared by incubation of cadmium with purified PCs. The method was validated by comparing the results obtained by SEC-ICP-MS with those obtained by reverse phase HPLC with post-column derivatization of phytochelatins.

24.5 Lead speciation in food

The harmful effects of organolead compounds are considered to be much greater than those of inorganic lead. The toxicity of alkyllead diminishes in the sequence R_4 Pb > R_3 Pb^+ > R_2 Pb^{2+} ($R = C_2H_5 > CH_3$). Tetraalkyllead (TAL) compounds, ten times more harmful than inorganic lead, can penetrate the skin and biological membranes and be readily absorbed through the lungs. In the environment, TAL pollutants are degraded by ozone and hydroxyl radicals into trialkyllead ions, whereas in biological systems dealkylation occurs through reactions with thiol groups in proteins and enzymes.[120]

Practically no work has been devoted to organolead speciation in foodstuffs.[120–122] The reason for this may be the low quantities of these chemical forms that were found in the studies carried out previously. Corroborating this, Szpunar and co-workers reported that the organolead fraction in wine accounted for only 0.1 to 1% of the total lead.[122] This may have made organolead compounds in food irrelevant from the toxicological point of view and focused studies on total lead, although speciation has occasionally shifted towards other kinds of biomolecules. With regard to the determination of individual inorganic lead compounds, although some authors say that it cannot be done by means of conventional techniques,[120] there are now studies on environmental samples in which both inorganic and organolead compounds are quantified by capillary GC-AAS, using a system of preconcentration onto diphenylthiocarbazone-anchored polymeric microbeads.[123]

24.6 Mercury speciation in food

As in the case of arsenic, determination of total mercury alone is no longer acceptable, as only partial information about the toxicological impact of mercury species can be obtained. Compounds of inorganic mercury can be much more toxic than the metal itself. Inorganic Hg is found as mercurious Hg(I) and mercuric Hg(II) cation. The greater part of the Hg(II) absorbed is concentrated in the kidneys, where it causes severe damage to the brush border membranes. The result is kidney failure.

The organic species appear in nature in the form of methyl mercury (MeHg), dimethylmercury (Me_2Hg) and ethylmercury (EtHg).[124] The biological effects of organic mercury are much more severe than those of either metallic or inorganic mercury.[125] The central nervous system is the target for organic mercury toxicity. MeHg has been listed as one of the six most dangerous chemicals in the environment by the International Program for Chemical Safety.[125] Numerous recent studies have concluded that, owing to its lipophilic nature, MeHg is accumulated in the animal and human food chain more easily than the inorganic forms,[124] and it has therefore been recognized as a major environmental pollution issue and health hazard for humans.

24.6.1 Sample treatment

Various procedures have been described for the isolation of mercurial species from food samples. As in the case of arsenic, the preservation of the organic moiety is the prerequisite of a successful leaching/digestion procedure prior to speciation analysis. Over the years, various procedures have been developed for this purpose: leaching with HCl or HCl-NaCl,[63,106,126] saponification with NaOH or KOH,[58,60,126] solubilization using TMAH,[127–129] and distillation in the presence of H_2SO_4-NaCl or H_2SO_4-KCl.[60,126,127,130–132] Microwaves with open-vessel microwave focused digestion or multimode microwave irradiation have recently been used in the acceleration of methods for MeHg extraction from biological samples.[126,133] Microwave-assisted leaching has been shown not only to reduce the time necessary for leaching but also to increase recoveries. Finally, the Westöö extraction procedure, a method that involves extraction from acidic media with benzene or toluene, has undergone various modifications since its first use in the late 1960s.[126,134,135] The Westöö extraction procedure with some modifications is the MeHg extraction procedure recommended by the US Environmental Protection Agency, even though it is quite time-consuming.[124]

24.6.2 Analytical methodologies for separation of mercury species

The analytical techniques most frequently applied for the determination of Hg species generally involve a chromatographic system (gas, liquid) or capillary electrophoresis for separation combined with suitable specific, sensitive element detectors. An excellent paper on mercury speciation has been published recently.[124]

Gas chromatography

The methods mainly used for the determination of individual mercury species are based on gas chromatography (GC) separation with detection by electron capture (ECD), AAS, microwave-induced plasma atomic emission detector (MIP-AED), ICP-MS being one of the preferred approaches for Hg detection. Separation of species by GC requires derivatization because of the thermal instability of Hg species in the inlet system and/or in the GC column.[136] To be amenable to GC separation they must be converted to non-polar, volatile and thermally stable species. The derivative chosen needs to retain the structure of the element-carbon bonds to ensure that the original moiety remains conserved.[137] The most common derivatization procedures used are hydride generation with sodium borohydride ($NaBH_4$), aqueous-phase ethylation with sodium tetraethylborate ($NaBEt_4$), and Grignard alkylation. Sodium tetraphenyl borate ($NaBPh_4$) has also been used, as it is more suitable for liquid-liquid extraction.[136] These derivatization procedures are indispensable but may cause problems in the quantification of mercury species, such as impurities in the ethylation reagent, identified as a major source of error, especially if large amounts of inorganic mercury are present; the ethyl mercury generated masks the natural compound present in the samples.

The GC-ECD hyphenated system has been used successfully for the analysis of MeHg in an intercomparison/certification exercise of mussel homogenate reference material and in certified reference materials.[58] There are descriptions of the use of GC-CV-AFS for MeHg quantification in fish samples.[58,60,126,138] Quartz furnace atomic absorption spectrometry (QF-AAS) has also been used as a detector in fish tissue Hg speciation. It provides derivatization by hydride generation or ethylation, preconcentration by cryotrapping, separation by packed column gas chromatography and detection by quartz furnace atomic absorption spectrometry.[139] The coupling of GC to MIP-AED has also been used in the analysis of Hg species in grains, cereal products, fruits, vegetables[140] and fish.[136,141,142] Glow discharge (GD) atomic emission spectrometry (AES) with a radio frequency (rf) source has also been used successfully as a detector. Hyphenated systems involving GC-rf-GD-AES[143] and GC-rf-hollow cathode-GD-AES[144] following a Grignard derivatization reaction have been described for Hg speciation in fish reference samples. The ICP-MS detector has also been used.[141,145–147] GC-low pressure-ICP-MS was employed for determination of MeHg in a fish reference material, with results close to the certified value when an alkaline digestion of the sample was used.[148]

Multicapillary gas chromatography (MCGC) has also been used for Hg speciation. The basic and unique features of a multicapillary column are the high speed of separation at large sample injection volumes and the exceptionally high range of volumetric velocities of the carrier gas at which the column retains its high efficiency. This makes MCGC ideally suited for plasma source detection leading to a coupled technique with a tremendous potential for speciation analysis.[149] This chromatography has been coupled to MIP-AES[150] and ICP-MS[149,151] with excellent results for MeHg speciation in fish samples.

Liquid chromatography

With HPLC the species do not require derivatization for efficient separation, which simplifies sample pretreatment by reducing the number of preparation steps, and it also reduces the inherent risks of contamination and creation of artifacts. In addition, HPLC instrumentation allows for on-line enrichment of species by using a preconcentration column. This step can be performed in parallel to mercury detection. Ion exchange chromatography has been applied for MeHg speciation in certified reference materials of seafood samples. The organic Hg is not retained in anion exchange (Dowex in Cl form), and the MeHg in the eluate is measured by CVAAS after decomposition to inorganic Hg by acid digestion and UV irradiation.[60,126] For HPLC separation, reversed phase columns are used most frequently, particularly RPC18. For preconcentration and for separation in the RPC18 column, mercury species need to form complexes with one of the following reagents: salts of quaternary ammonium halide, dithiocarbamates,[106,128,130–132] L-cysteine[152] and 2–mercaptoethanol.[133,152,153]

Capillary electrophoresis

Capillary electrophoresis (CE) has shown a notable capacity for the resolution and analysis of organomercury compounds in food samples. Compared with GC or HPLC methods, CE shows several advantages, including high resolving power, rapid and efficient separations, minimal reagent consumption and the possibility of separations with only minor disturbances of the equilibrium existing between the different species.[134] Other advantages are small volume sample requirements, minimal buffer consumption and rapid sample throughput.[129] After isolation of Hg species from food samples and prior to their separation by CE, it is necessary for the species to form stable complexes during electrophoretic migration. Cysteine is one of the reagents most commonly used for complexation of inorganic and organic mercury species. For separation, an alkaline pH is selected.[134] With regard to detection, in the

CE-ICP-MS system the efficiency of the nebulizer is a critical point.[129] Good sensitivity is obtained with on-line volatile species generation,[134] which provided results in good agreement with certified values for MeHg contents in certified reference materials. Dithizone sulphonate has also been used to form complexes with Hg species in the analysis of fish and crab samples.[135] For inorganic mercury and MeHg, a CE-ICP-MS methodology in which derivatization is not necessary has recently been optimized and applied to determination in seafood certified reference materials.[129]

Solid-phase microextraction (SPME)
This procedure is employed for MeHg determination in fish samples. It has been coupled to ICP-MS,[146] using a simple thermal desorption gas introduction interface consisting of a heated glass-lined splitless-type GC injector. This arrangement was placed directly at the base of the torch to minimize the length of the transfer line, providing fast desorption and high sample introduction efficiency. This system provides a new approach, with results for fish reference samples that are in good agreement with certified values.

24.7 Arsenic speciation in food

The arsenic species present in foods differ widely in their degrees of toxicity. This, together with their different metabolization, has made speciation studies essential in order to ascertain the real risk to human health that exposure to As implies. As(III) and As(V) are the most toxic species and are grouped together under the name of inorganic arsenic (AsI), classified by the International Agency for Research on Cancer as a carcinogen to humans. The organic species present in foods are of variable toxicity. Monomethylarsonic acid (MMA), dimethylarsinic acid (DMA), tetramethylarsonium ion (TMA^+) and tetramethylarsonium oxide (TMAO) have a toxicity lower than that of AsI. Arsenobetaine (AB) and arsenocholine (AC) are considered harmless.[154] With respect to arsenosugars, the study of their toxicity has not been carried out in depth, and only the low cytotoxicity of arsenosugar glycerol-ribose has been demonstrated.[155] Unceasing progress in analytical techniques suggests that the number of arsenic species identified in biological samples will increase in forthcoming years, thereby contributing to increased knowledge of the cycle of arsenic in nature.

24.7.1 Sample treatment

At present, complete extraction of the arsenic species present in a sample is a challenge. Arsenic compounds cover a wide range of polarities, and the extraction conditions ideal for one compound may be quite unsuitable for another.[156] In general, the suitability of each combination of extractant and extraction method is strongly influenced by the kind of food analyzed, and even for foods of the same kind very different extraction efficiencies have been found. The extraction process used must not bring about modifications of the arsenic species.

Solvent extraction

A methanol/water mixture is most frequently used for extraction of the organic species from foods. Other extractants that have been used are water, methanol, methanol/chloroform, citric acid, tetramethylammonium hydroxide, phosphoric acid and trifluoroacetic acid. Extraction is generally performed by traditional methods, such as mechanical shaking and sonication. Microwave-assisted extraction,[51,56,157–159] accelerated solvent extraction,[160] Kjeldahl[161] and Soxhlet extraction[51] have also been used with good results.

The extraction of As(III) and As(V) differs from the procedures described for the organic species. There is no consensus about the appropriate extraction method. As(III) strongly bonded to thiol groups in proteins is not extracted quantitatively with organic solvents and agitation, as has been shown by As(III) recovery assays carried out with real samples of fish.[162] On the other hand, three different extraction methods applied to rice flour CRM provided different concentrations of As(III) and As(V), with the peculiarity that the sum of As(III) and As(V) coincided in the three methods.[163] Partial reduction of As(V) to As(III) during the extraction process has also been shown.[162,163] For all these reasons it is advisable to quantify inorganic arsenic [As(III) + As(V)] and not the individual species. So far, studies that have shown quantitative extraction of inorganic arsenic have used HCl,[13,18,19,162] trifluoroacetic acid[163] or amylase[164] to hydrolyze the samples.

Enzymatic extraction

Trypsin or pancreatin have been used for quantitative extraction of arsenic species in baby foods containing fish.[54] Trypsin is suitable, but not pancreatin, the presence of which in the extract causes co-elution of some species.[54] Enzymes have also been used as a first stage of the extraction process. For example, in apples[164] and rice[163] an overnight α-amylase treatment has been used prior to sonication with organic solvents.

24.7.2 Methods for separation of arsenic species

After extraction of arsenic species from the food matrix and before their detection, an intermediate step is required in which the various arsenic species are separated.

High performance liquid chromatography

HPLC has become the most frequently used separation technique. It allows the creation of hyphenated systems because of the ease with which it can be coupled to HG-AAS, HG-AFS and ICP-MS. HPLC allows arsenic species separation on the basis of various mechanisms, which include size exclusion, cation and anion exchange, reversed phase and ion pairing. Most studies use anionic exchange columns. In recent years, the increase in the number of arsenic species identified in foods has made chromatographic separation much more complicated. The use of two-dimensional systems has now become the most valid approach in order to avoid chromatographic overlapping of species.

The kind of food studied determines what arsenic species are present and therefore the difficulty of their chromatographic separation. Bivalves, algae and mushrooms are the most complex samples because the arsenosugars that they contain present problems of overlapping with other arsenic species in customary working conditions. Raber et al.[165] make an elegant approach to the resolution of overlapping problems when there are arsenosugars in the samples. Madsen and co-workers[166] achieved a satisfactory separation of 12 standards of arsenic species [4 arsenosugars, As(III), As(V), MMA, DMA, TMAO, AB, AC and TMA^+] using anion-exchange and cation-exchange chromatography, although they did not succeed in detecting the species mentioned when they applied the chromatographic separation procedure to real samples. In fish, eight standard arsenic species were separated using two chromatograph columns.[167–169] From the first injection of the sample in an anion-exchange column, As(III), DMA, MMA and As(V) were determined. From a second injection in a cation-exchange column, the species AB, TMAO, AC and TMA^+ were separated and quantified. The same arsenic species were separated by making a single injection of the sample and using a column-switching system between an anion-exchange column and a cation-exchange column.[170] Recently, with the use of a three-step gradient elution in a cation exchanged HPLC-ICP-MS system, 23 arsenic species were separated with excellent selectivity in one analytical run.[171] Application of the separations mentioned to real samples may not provide such good results.

Capillary electrophoresis

CE coupled to indirect fluorescence detection,[172] UV detection,[173,174] ICP-MS[175] or ICP time-of-flight MS[176] has been applied for arsenic speciation of standards,[173,176] water,[174,175] soils, leachate and urine,[175] but there are no reports of its use for arsenic speciation in foodstuffs. The coupling with the greatest future is CE with ICP-MS. Major limitations that prevent more widespread use are the complicated coupling of the two techniques, the discrepancy between flow rates and the insufficient detection capability, resulting from the use of extremely small volumes.

24.7.3 Detection systems for the determination of arsenic species

Inductively coupled plasma-mass spectrometry

The HPLC-ICP-MS coupling is simple; the typical flow rate in HPLC (1 ml min^{-1}) is compatible with the uptake rate requirements of most commercial nebulizers. Moreover, elution of the mobile phase of the column is performed at atmospheric pressure, which is ideal for the ICP-MS sample introduction system. Studies using the HPLC-ICP-MS hyphenated system have described the on-line addition of isopropanol to the chromatograph eluate to reduce polyatomic interference, $^{40}Ar\ ^{35}Cl^{+}$ while also increasing the sensitivity of As determination.[52] An appropriate choice of chromatographic conditions can also help to avoid this interference, eluting $^{40}Ar\ ^{35}Cl^{+}$ with a retention time different from that of the arsenic species of interest.[52,168] Methanol forms part of many of the mobile phases employed, and the carbon created by its combustion may block the injector and cone orifices. The addition of oxygen to the nebulizer gas flow is one of the best solutions.[177] Finally, quadrupole-based instruments, working under 'cool plasma' conditions or by applying a collision cell, and double focusing sector field mass spectrometers minimize or avoid spectral interferences. Despite the drawbacks mentioned, HPLC-ICP-MS is the hyphenated technique most commonly used for the analysis of arsenic species in foods: fish,[51,52,56,157,158,160,161,169,178] algae,[165,166,179] meat,[52] cereals,[52,163] vegetables,[52,159,180] apples[164] and baby foods.[54]

Inductively coupled plasma-atomic emission spectrometry
This technique has a larger working range, but its instrumental limits of detection (LOD) are not good enough for many environmental and clinical applications, and it suffers from various interferences. Arsenic speciation studies in seafood products using HPLC-ICP-AES have shown that this technique is suitable for the determination of major compounds such as AB in marine organisms, but not for minor species of arsenic.[181] Axially-viewed ICP-AES has been shown to improve LODs by at least a factor of two.[182] Consequently, hyphenated HPLC-ICP-AES may be a reliable alternative for speciation analysis when very low detection limits are not required.

Atomic absorption spectrometry
AAS coupled to HG is the only AAS alternative used for As speciation in food. For the organoarsenic species that do not generate hydrides or do so with low efficiency, post-column derivatization is required. This process is performed by means of on-line thermo-oxidation (microwave, heated bath) or photo-oxidation (UV light) using an oxidant, generally $K_2S_2O_8$. In comparison with HPLC-ICP-MS, HPLC-HG-AAS has the advantage of being cheaper in terms of both equipment and maintenance. Although its limits of detection are slightly higher than those obtained by ICP-MS, they are suitable for quantification of arsenic species in most food matrices. Fish are the main kinds of food analyzed with this technique.[170,181,183,184]

Atomic fluorescence spectrometry
In recent years HG-AFS has been used considerably for detection of arsenic species. For some organoarsenical species, thermo-oxidation or photo-oxidation prior to HG-AFS is necessary. This technique has been used to detect arsenic species in seafood products[161,170,185] and beer.[15]

Neutron activation analysis
Neutron activation analysis (NAA) has been used in As speciation studies in seafood and mushrooms.[184] The off-line detection carried out by HPLC and NAA is the main disadvantage, because it hampers analysis of samples containing complex mixtures of arsenic species.

24.8 Future trends

The economic interdependence of different countries throughout the world resulting from increases in exports and imports of goods and services, together with the rapid expansion of technology, points to the need either to impose new legislative regulations or to harmonize and agree on existing regulations. This has led to a revival of interest in trace elements in foods, not only from the commercial viewpoint, which is known to provide a stimulus for all change, but also in other related areas, such as nutrition and toxicology. Aspects for future consideration which could help to improve international trade and inter-company competitiveness within the context of globalization, while always protecting the health of the consumer, are set out below. Some essential basic research needs are also described.

Validated methods having specified accuracy and precision, ruggedness, operating range, selectivity, susceptibility to interferences and limits of detection and determination are needed.[186] This can only be achieved by laborious interlaboratory collaborative studies and the use of well-characterized samples and reference materials. Quality assurance and quality control programmes and sampling (sample preservation and storage) protocols should also be fully appreciated.

New instrumentation, sample preparation techniques and sample introduction methodologies currently at the forefront of research but excluded from use in routine must make their way into the hands of laboratory personnel.[108] Reduction of waste production and reagent consumption is desirable, together with an advance in research on clean methodologies.

Automation with direct solids and slurry sampling approaches, as well as through more extensive use of on-line chemical manifolds and FI techniques, to minimize sample consumption and contamination and perform matrix separation-analyte concentration functions is needed.[186]

Development of fast, low-cost and, if possible, non-destructive methods to allow manufacturers and monitoring organisations to carry out rapid product control are needed. The availability of methods which could be developed at screening level would allow substantial reductions in the analytical workload of the laboratory and make it possible to act quickly in emergency situations.

Structural information about species is needed, since no molecular information is available from conventional plasma sources. The combination of liquid chromatography with electrospray/ionspray sources for measurement of fragments of ion patterns generates structural information which can be used to deduce species identity in the absence of standards.[108]

Chemometric data treatment methods must be developed for routine use. The possibility of combining some of the mentioned techniques with artificial intelligence programming such as neural networks may lead to the realization of a new form of smart instrumentation capable of fully automating component analyte detection and quantification.[187]

Species information is strongly needed. The advances achieved in the development of analytical methods should be used to increase knowledge of the chemical species present in food for human consumption. This task, although arduous and not highly valued by the scientific community, is a present necessity. It will be difficult to legislate about contents of species in foods in the absence of an extensive database that makes it possible to decide the basic concentrations that are customary in a product and concentrations that could be considered anomalous.[188]

Studies of possible modifications that the most significant species may undergo during the process of industrial manufacture, transport, storage and cooking must be carried out.

Total Diet studies are needed as a further stage in risk characterization. With such studies it is possible to evaluate the exposure of a specific population to a toxic (total contents and/or chemical species) in the form in which it is ingested (through processed, raw or cooked foods).

There is a need for *in vivo* or *in vitro* bioavailability studies, both for total contents and for chemical species. The information generated could provide feedback for legislation.

Multidisciplinary speciation studies in foods must be carried out. As the techniques available become more sophisticated, and almost certainly more expensive, further developments will depend on collaboration not only between researchers and institutes, but between countries too.[189]

24.9 References

1 ZHANG D Q, LI C M, YANG L L, SUN H W, 'Determination of cadmium in flour by atom trapping flame atomic absorption spectrometry using derivative signal processing', *Anal Chim Acta*, 2000 **405**(1–2) 185–190.

2 ZHANG D Q, LI C M, YANG L L, SUN H W, 'Determination of cadmium in vegetables by derivative flame atomic absorption spectrometry with the atom trapping technique', *J Anal At Spectrom,* 1998 **13**(10) 1155–1158.

3 LI Z, ZHU Z, CHEN Y, HSU C G, PAN J, 'Spectrophotometric determination of lead in biological samples with dibromo-*p*-methyl-methylsulfonazo', *Talanta*, 1999 **48**(3) 511–516.

4 FANG G, MENG S, ZHANG G, PAN J,'Spectrophotometric determination of lead in foods with dibromo-*p*-methyl-bromosulfonazo', *Talanta*, 2001 **54**(4) 585–589.

5 IŞILOĞLU M, YILMAZ F, MERDIVAN M, 'Concentrations of trace elements in wild edible mushrooms', *Food Chem*, 2001 **73**(2) 169–175.

6 ROCA DE TOGORES M, FARRÉ R, FRIGOLA A M, 'Cadmium and lead in infant cereals electrothermal-atomic absorption spectroscopic determination', *Sci Total Environ,*

1999 **234**(1/3) 197–201.

7 ABOU-ARAB A A K, ABOU DONIA M A, 'Heavy metals in Egyptian spices and medicinal plants and the effect of processing on their levels', *J Agric Food Chem,* 2000 **48**(6) 2300–2304.

8 ACAR O, KILIÇ Z, TÜRKER A R, 'Determination of lead in cookies by electrothermal atomic absorption spectrometry with various chemical modifiers', *Food Chem,* 2000 **71**(1) 117–122.

9 LO COCO F, MONOTTI P, FIECCHI V, CECCON L, 'Determination of lead (II) and cadmium (II) in hard and soft wheat by derivative potentiometric stripping analysis', *Anal Chim Acta,* 2000 **409**(1–2) 93–98.

10 JORHEM L, 'Determination of metals in foods by atomic absorption spectrometry after dry ashing: NMKL collaborative study', *J AOAC Int,* 2000 **83**(5) 1204–1211.

11 DAMKRÖNGER G, GROTE M, JANSSEN E, 'Comparison of sample digestion procedures for the determination of arsenic in certified marine samples using the FI-HG-AAS technique', *Fresenius J Anal Chem,* 1997 **357**(7) 817–821.

12 ADELOJU S B, YOUNG T M, 'Assessment of constant current anodic stripping potentiometry for determination of arsenic in fish and water samples', *Anal Letters,* 1997 **30**(1) 147–161.

13 MUÑOZ O, DEVESA V, SÚÑER M, VÉLEZ D, MONTORO R, URIETA I, MACHO M L, JALÓN M, 'Total and inorganic arsenic in fresh and processed fish products', *J Agric Food Chem,* 2000 **48**(9) 4369–4376.

14 SÚÑER M A, DEVESA V, CLEMENTE M J, VÉLEZ D, MONTORO R, URIETA I, JALÓN M, MACHO M L, 'Organoarsenical species contents in fresh and processed seafood products', *J Agric Food Chem,* 2002 **50**(4) 924–932.

15 MARTÍNEZ A, MORALES-RUBIO A, CERVERA M L, DE LA GUARDIA M, 'Atomic fluorescence determination of total and inorganic arsenic species in beer', *J Anal At Spectrosc,* 2001 **16**(7) 762–766.

16 SEGURA M, MADRID Y, CÁMARA C, 'Evaluation of atomic fluorescence and atomic absorption spectrometric techniques for the determination of arsenic in wine and beer by direct hydride generation sample introduction', *J Anal At Spectrom,* 1999 **14**(2) 131–135.

17 HEPP N M, 'Arsenic determination in certifiable color additives by dry ashing followed by hydride generation atomic absorption spectrometry', *J AOAC Int,* 1999 **82**(2) 327–330.

18 MUÑOZ O, DÍAZ O P, LEYTON I, NÚÑEZ N, DEVESA V, SÚÑER M A, VÉLEZ D, MONTORO R, 'Vegetables collected in the cultivated Andean area of the Nothern Chile. Total and inorganic arsenic contents in raw vegetables', *J Agric Food Chem,* 2002 **50**(3) 642–647.

19 ALMELA C, ALGORA S, BENITO V, CLEMENTE M J, DEVESA V, SÚÑER M A, VÉLEZ D, MONTORO R, 'Heavy metals, total arsenic and inorganic arsenic contents of algae food products', *J Agric Food Chem,* 2002 **50**(4) 918–923.

20 LEMOS V A, SANTELLI R E, DE CARVALHO M S, FERREIRA S L C, 'Application of polyurethane foam loaded with BTAC in an on-line preconcentration system: cadmium determination by FAAS', *Spectrochim Acta Part B,* 1998 **55**(9) 1497–1502.

21 MELO M H A, FERREIRA S L C, SANTELLI R E, 'Determination of cadmium by FAAS after on-line enrichment using a mini column packed with Amberlite XAD-2 loaded with TAM', *Microchem J,* 2000 **65**(1) 59–65.

22 MEERAVALI N N, KUMAR S J, 'Comparison of open microwave digestion and

digestion by conventional heating for the determination of Cd, Cr, Cu and Pb in algae using transverse heated electrothermal atomic absorption spectrometry', *Fresenius J Anal Chem*, 2000 **366**(3) 313–315.

23 WANG J, HANSEN E H, 'Development of an automated sequential injection on-line solvent extraction-back extraction procedure as demonstrated for the determination of cadmium with detection by electrothermal atomic absorption spectrometry', *Anal Chim Acta*, 2002 **456**(2) 283–292.

24 LIU M, XU S, 'The determination of trace cadmium by flow injection cold vapor generation AAS', *At Spectrosc*, 1997 **18**(6) 195–201.

25 ACAR O, 'Determination of cadmium and lead in biological samples by Zeeman ETAAS using various chemical modifiers', *Talanta* 2001 **55**(3) 613–622.

26 YOSHINAGA J, MORITA M, EDMONDS J S, 'Determination of copper, zinc, cadmium and lead in a fish otolith certified reference material by isotope dilution inductively coupled plasma mass spectrometry using off-line solvent extraction', *J Anal At Spectrom,* 1999 **14**(10) 1589–1592.

27 DE PEÑA Y P, LÓPEZ W, BURGUERA M, BURGUERA J L, LÓPEZ-CARRASQUERO, CARRILLO M, 'Flow injection system for cadmium preconcentration on poly(octadecyl diitaconate) (PDI-18) and atomic absorption spectrometry detection', *Anal Chim Acta*, 2001 **438**(1–2) 259–266.

28 DE PEÑA Y P, GALLEGO M, VALCÁRCEL M, 'Fullerene: a sensitive and selective sorbent for the continuous preconcentration and atomic absorption determination of cadmium', *J Anal At Spectrom*, 1997 **12**(4) 453–457.

29 ALI A, YIN X, SHEN H, YE Y, GU X, '1,10–Phenanthroline as a complexing agent for on-line sorbent extraction/preconcentration for flow injection-flame atomic absorption spectrometry', *Anal Chim Acta,* 1999 **392**(2–3) 283–289.

30 VOEGBORLO R B, EL-METHNANI A M, ABEDIN M Z, 'Mercury, cadmium and lead content of canned tuna fish', *Food Chem,* 1999 **67**(4) 341–345.

31 FRESCHI G P G, DAKUZAKU C S, DE MORAES M, NÓBREGA J A, NETO J A G, 'Simultaneous determination of cadmium and lead in wine by electrothermal atomic absorption spectrometry', *Spectrochim Acta Part B*, 2001 **56**(10) 1987 1993.

32 INAM R, SOMER G, 'A direct method for the determination of selenium and lead in cow's milk by differential pulse stripping voltammetry', *Food Chem,* 2000 **69**(3) 345–350.

33 ZHANG Z W, SHIMBO S, OCHI N, EGUCHI M, WATANABE T, MOON C S, IKEDA M, 'Determination of lead and cadmium in food and blood by inductively coupled plasma mass spectrometry: a comparison with graphite furnace atomic absorption spectrometry', *Sci Total Environ,* 1997 **205**(2–3) 179–187.

34 CHANG C C, JIANG S J, 'Determination of copper, cadmium and lead in biological samples by electrothermal vaporization isotope dilution inductively coupled plasma mass spectrometry', *J Anal At Spectrom,* 1997 **12**(1) 75–80.

35 BRUHN C G, SAN FRANCISCO N A, NEIRA J Y, NÓBREGA J A, 'Determination of cadmium and lead in mussels by tungsten coil electrothermal atomic absorption spectrometry', *Talanta*, 1999 **50**(5) 967–975.

36 JORHEM L, ENGMAN J, 'Determination of lead, cadmium, zinc, copper, and iron in foods by atomic absorption spectrometry after microwave digestion: NMKL collaborative study', *J AOAC Int,* 2000 **83**(5) 1189–1203.

37 LIMA E C, BARBOSA F JR, KRUG F J, 'The use of tungsten-rhodium permanent chemical modifier for cadmium determination in decomposed samples of biological materials and sediments by electrothermal atomic absorption

spectrometry', *Anal Chim Acta*, 2000 **409**(1–2) 267–274.

38 CID B P, BOIA C, POMBO L, REBELO E, 'Determination of trace metals in fish species of the Ria de Aveiro (Portugal) by electrothermal atomic absorption spectrometry', *Food Chem,* 2001 **75**(1) 93–100.

39 ENRÍQUEZ-DOMÍNGUEZ M F, YEBRA-BIURRUN M C, BERMEJO-BARRERA M P, 'Determination of cadmium in mussels by flame atomic absorption spectrometry with preconcentration on a chelating resin in a flow injection system', *Analyst,* 1998 **123**(1) 105–108.

40 YEBRA M C, ENRÍQUEZ M F, CESPÓN R M, 'Preconcentration and flame atomic absorption spectrometry determination of cadmium in mussels by an on-line continuous precipitation-dissolution flow system', *Talanta* 2000 **52**(4) 631–636.

41 YEBRA M C, ENRÍQUEZ M F, GARCÍA A, MORENO-CID A, 'Determination of trace amounts of lead in mussels by flow-injection flame atomic-absorption spectrometry coupled with on-line minicolumn preconcentration', *Fresenius J Anal Chem,* 2001 **370**(1) 64–68.

42 CORREIA P R M, OLIVEIRA E, OLIVEIRA P V, 'Simultaneous determination of Cd and Pb in foodstuffs by electrothermal atomic absorption spectrometry', *Anal Chim Acta,* 2000 **405**(1–2) 205–211.

43 VALLES MOTA J P, ENCINAR J R, DE LA CAMPA M R F, ALONSO J I G, SANZ-MEDEL A, 'Determination of cadmium in environmental and biological reference materials using isotope dilution analysis with a double focusing ICP-MS: a comparison with quadrupole ICP-MS', *J Anal At Spectrom*, 1999 **14**(4) 1467–1473.

44 MOTA J P V, DE LA CAMPA M R F, ALONSO J I G, SANZ-MEDEL A, 'Determination of cadmium in biological and environmental materials by isotope dilution inductively coupled plasma mass spectrometry: effect of flow sample introduction methods', *J Anal At Spectrom,* 1999 **14**(2) 113–120.

45 BETTINELLI M, BARONI U, SPEZIA S, TERNI C, 'Determination of trace elements in honey using ETV-ICP-MS', *At Spectrosc*, 2000 **21**(6) 195–204.

46 FEDOROV P N, RYABCHUK G N, ZVEREV A V, 'Comparison of hydride generation and graphite furnace atomic absorption spectrometry for the determination of arsenic in food', *Spectrochim Acta Part B*, 1997 **52**(9–10) 1517–1523.

47 LOCATELLI C, TORSI G, 'Voltammetric trace metal determinations by cathodic and anodic stripping voltammetry in environmental matrices in the presence of mutual interference', *J Electroanal Chem*, 2001 **509**(1) 80–89.

48 LOCATELLI C, TORSI G, 'Determination of Se, As, Cu, Pb, Cd, Zn and Mn by anodic and cathodic stripping voltammetry in marine environmental matrices in the presence of reciprocal interference. Proposal of a new analytical procedure', *Microchem J*, 2000 **65**(3) 293–303.

49 KABENGERA C, BODART P, HUBERT P, THUNUS L, NOIRFALISE A, 'Optimization and validation of arsenic determination in foods by hydride generation flame atomic absorption spectrometry', *J AOAC Int*, 2002 **85**(1) 122–127.

50 ØYGARD J K, LUNDEBYE A K, JULSHAMN K, 'Determination of inorganic arsenic in marine food samples by hydrochloric acid distillation and flow-injection hydride-generation atomic absorption spectrometry', *J AOAC Int,* 1999 **82**(5) 1217–1223.

51 GÓMEZ ARIZA J L, SÁNCHEZ RODAS D, GIRÁLDEZ I, MORALES E, 'Comparison of biota sample pretreatments for arsenic speciation with coupled HPLC-HG-ICP-MS', *Analyst*, 2000 **125**(3) 401–407.

52 ZBINDEN P, ANDREY D, BLAKE C, 'A routine ion chromatography ICP-MS method for the analysis of arsenic species applicable in the food industry', *At Spectrosc,* 2000

21(6) 205–215.
53 FECHER P, RUHNKE G, 'Determination of arsenic and selenium in foodstuffs – Methods and errors', *At Spectrosc,* 1998 **19**(6) 204–206.
54 PARDO-MARTÍNEZ M, VIÑAS P, FISHER A, HILL S J, 'Comparison of enzymatic extraction procedures for use with directly coupled high performance liquid chromatography-inductively coupled plasma mass spectrometry for the speciation of arsenic in baby foods', *Anal Chim Acta*, 2001 **441**(1) 29–36.
55 JULSHAMN K, THORLACIUS A, LEA P, 'Determination of arsenic in seafood by electrothermal atomic absorption spectrometry after microwave digestion: NMKL1 collaborative study', *J AOAC Int*, 2000 **83**(6) 1423–1428.
56 DAGNAC T, PADRÓ A, RUBIO R, RAURET G, 'Optimisation of the extraction of arsenic species from mussels with low power focused microwaves by applying a Doehlert design', *Anal Chim Acta,* 1998 **364**(1–3) 19–30.
57 VILANÓ M, RUBIO R, 'Determination of arsenic in seafood by focused microwave digestion and hydride generation-atomic fluorescence detection', *J AOAC Int,* 2001 **84**(2) 551–555.
58 HOVART M, LIANG L, AZEMARD S, MANDIĆ V, VILLENEUVE J P, COQUERY M, 'Certification of total mercury and methylmercury concentrations in mussel homogenate (*Mytilus edulis*) reference material, IAEA-142', *Fresenius J Anal Chem,* 1997 **358**(3) 411–418.
59 SHUQIN C, HANGTING C, XIANJIN Z, 'Determination of mercury in biological samples using organic compounds as matrix modifiers by inductively coupled plasma mass spectrometry', *J Anal At Spectrom,* 1999 **14**(8) 1183–1186.
60 DONAIS M K, SARASWATI R, MACKEY E, DEMIRALP R, PORTER B, VANGEL M, LEVENSON M, MANDIC V, AZEMARD S, HORVAT M, MAY K, EMONS H, WISE S, 'Certification of three mussel tissue standard reference materials (SRM) for methylmercury and total mercury content' *Fresenius J Anal Chem,* 1997 **358**(3) 424–430.
61 LIPPO H, JAUHIAINEN T, PERÄMÄKI P, 'Comparison of digestion methods for the determination of total mercury in environmental samples by flow injection CV-AAS', *At Spectrosc,* 1997 **18**(3) 102–108.
62 GAWLIK B, DRUGES M, BIANCHI M, BORTOLI A, KETTRUP A, MUNTAU H, 'TUNA FISH (T-30) – A new proficiency testing material for the determination of As and Hg in seafood', *Fresenius J Anal Chem,* 1997 **358**(3) 441–445.
63 RÍO-SEGADE S, BENDICHO C, 'Selective reduction method for separate determination of inorganic and total mercury in mussel tissue by flow-injection cold vapor technique', *Ecotoxicol Environ Safety*, 1999 **42**(3) 245–252.
64 FENG X, WU S, WHARMBY A, WITTMEIER A, 'Microwave digestion of plant and grain standard reference materials in nitric and hydrofluoric acids for multi-elemental determination by inductively coupled plasma mass spectrometry', *J Anal At Spectrom,* 1999 **14**(6) 939–946.
65 CAPELO J L, LAVILLA I, BENDICHO C, 'Chemometric approach for the optimization of a flow injection manifold applied to the determination of total Hg in seafood by cold vapor AAS', *At Spectrosc,* 2000 **21**(6) 229–233.
66 MURPHY J, JONES P, HILL S, 'Determination of total mercury in environmental and biological samples by flow injection cold vapour atomic absorption spectrometry', *Spectrochim Acta Part B,* 1996 **51**(14) 1867–1873.
67 OKAMOTO Y, 'Furnace-fusion system for the direct determination of cadmium in biological samples by inductively coupled plasma atomic emission spectrometry using tungsten boat furnace-sample cuvette technique', *J Anal At Spectrom*, 1999

14(11) 1767–1770.

68 GRINSHTEIN I L, VILPAN Y A, SARAEV A V, VASILIEVA L A, 'Direct atomic absorption determination of cadmium and lead in strongly interfering matrices by double vaporization with a two-step electrothermal atomizer', *Spectrochim Acta Part B*, 2001 **56**(3) 261–274.

69 DAKUZAKU C S, FRESCHI G P G, DE MORAES M, NÓBREGA J A, NETO J A G, 'Direct determination of arsenic in sugar by GFAAS with transversely heated graphite atomizer and longitudinal Zeeman-effect background correction', *At Spectrosc*, 2001 **22**(2) 271–275.

70 VAN DALEN G, 'Determination of cadmium in edible oils and fats by direct electrothermal atomic absorption spectrometry', *J Anal At Spectrom*, 1996 **11**(11) 1087–1092.

71 KARADJOVA I, ZACHARIADIS G, BOSKOU G, STRATIS J, 'Electrothermal atomic absorption spectrometric determination of aluminium, cadmium, chromium, copper, iron, manganese, nickel and lead in olive oil', *J Anal At Spectrom,* 1998 **13**(3) 201–204.

72 CAMEÁN A M, MORENO I, LÓPEZ-ARTIGUEZ M, REPETTO M, GONZÁLEZ A G, 'Differentiation of Spanish brandies according to their metal content', *Talanta*, 2001, **54**(1) 53–59.

73 POZEBON D, DRESSLER V L, CURTIUS A J, 'Determination of trace elements in biological materials by ETV-ICP-MS after dissolution or slurry formation with tetramethylammonium hydroxide', *J Anal At Spectrom*, 1998 **13**(10) 1101–1105.

74 BERMEJO-BARRERA P, MOREDA-PIÑEIRO A, MOREDA-PIÑEIRO J, KAUPPILA T, BERMEJO-BARRERA A, 'Slurry sampling for electrothermal AAS determination of cadmium in seafood products', *At Spectrosc*, 2000 **21**(1) 5–9.

75 VIÑAS P, PARDO MARTÍNEZ M, CAMPILLO N, HERNÁNDEZ-CÓRDOBA M, 'Fast determination of lead and copper in dairy products by graphite furnace atomic absorption spectrometry', *J AOAC Int*, 1999 **82**(2) 368–373.

76 VIÑAS P, PARDO-MARTÍNEZ M, HERNÁNDEZ-CÓRDOBA M, 'Rapid determination of selenium, lead and cadmium in baby food samples using electrothermal atomic absorption spectrometry and slurry atomization', *Anal Chim Acta*, 2000 **412**(1–2) 121–130.

77 MEERAVALI N N, KUMAR S J, 'Rapid slurry atomization using transverse heated electrothermal atomic absorption spectrometry for the determination of cadmium, copper, manganese and lead in biological reference materials', *J Anal At Spectrom,* 1998 **13**(7) 647–652.

78 LIMA E C, KRUG F J, FERREIRA A T, BARBOSA F JR, 'Tungsten-rhodium permanent chemical modifier for cadmium determination in fish slurries by electrothermal atomic absorption spectrometry', *J Anal At Spectrom,* 1999 **14**(2) 269–274.

79 HUANG S J, JIANG S J, 'Determination of lead in fish samples by slurry sampling electrothermal atomic absorption spectrometry', *Analyst,* 2000 **125**(8) 1491–1494.

80 FUYI W, ZUCHENG J, 'Direct determination of cadmium in solid biological materials by slurry sampling electrothermal atomic absorption spectrometry with polytetrafluoroethylene as a chemical modifier', *Anal Chim Acta*, 1999 **391**(1) 89–94.

81 MIERZWA J, SUN Y C, CHUNG Y T, YANG M H, 'Comparative determination of Ba, Cu, Fe, Pb and Zn in tea leaves by slurry sampling electrothermal atomic absorption and liquid sampling inductively coupled plasma atomic emission spectrometry', *Talanta*, 1998 **47**(5) 1263–1270.

82 LI Y C, JIANG S J, 'Determination of Cu, Zn, Cd and Pb in fish samples by slurry sampling electrothermal vaporization inductively coupled plasma mass spectrometry', *Anal Chim Acta,* 1998 **359**(1–2) 205–212.

83 LIAO H C, JIANG S J, 'EDTA as the modifier for the determination of Cd, Hg and Pb in fish by slurry sampling electrothermal vaporization inductively coupled plasma mass spectrometry', *J Anal At Spectrom,* 1999 **14**(10) 1583–1588.

84 LIVA M, MUÑOZ-OLIVAS R, CÁMARA C, 'Determination of Cd in sonicate slurries and leachates of biological and environmental materials by FI-CV-AAS', *Talanta,* 2000 **51**(2) 381–387.

85 HO C Y, JIANG S J, 'Determination of Cr, Zn, Cd and Pb in milk powder by slurry sampling electrothermal vaporization inductively coupled plasma mass spectrometry', *J Anal At Spectrom,* 2002 **17**(7) 688–692.

86 VIÑAS P, PARDO-MARTÍNEZ M, LÓPEZ-GARCÍA I, HERNÁNDEZ-CÓRDOBA M, 'Slurry atomisation for the determination of arsenic, cadmium and lead in food colourants using electrothermal atomic absorption spectrometry', *J Anal At Spectrom,* 2001 **16**(10) 1202–1205.

87 VIÑAS P, PARDO-MARTÍNEZ M, HERNÁNDEZ-CÓRDOBA M, 'Slurry atomization for the determination of arsenic in baby foods using electrothermal atomic absorption spectrometry and deuterium background correction', *J Anal At Spectrom,* 1999 **14**(8) 1215–1219.

88 SANTOS C, ALAVA-MORENO F, LAVILLA I, BENDICHO C, 'Total As in seafood as determined by transverse heated electrothermal atomic absorption spectrometry-longitudinal Zeeman background correction: An evaluation of automated ultrasonic slurry sampling, ultrasound-assisted extraction and microwave-assisted digestion methods', *J Anal At Spectrom*, 2000 **15**(8) 987–994.

89 CHEN S F, JIANG S J, 'Determination of arsenic, selenium and mercury in fish samples by slurry sampling electrothermal vaporization inductively coupled plasma mass spectrometry', *J Anal At Spectrom*, 1998 **13**(7) 673–677.

90 VIÑAS P, PARDO-MARTÍNEZ M, LÓPEZ-GARCÍA I, HERNÁNDEZ-CÓRDOBA M, 'Determination of mercury in baby food and seafood samples using electrothermal atomic absorption spectrometry and slurry atomization', *J Anal At Spectrom,* 2001 **16**(6) 633–637

91 RÍO-SEGADE S, BENDICHO C, 'Slurry sampling combined with ultrasonic pretreatment for total mercury determination in samples containing inorganic and methylmercury by flow injection-cold vapor-atomic absorption spectrometry', *J Anal At Spectrom,* 1999 **14**(12) 1907–1912.

92 VIÑAS P, PARDO-MARTÍNEZ M, LÓPEZ-GARCÍA I, HERNÁNDEZ-CÓDOBA M, 'Rapid determination of mercury in food colorants using electrothermal atomic absorption spectrometry with slurry sample introduction', *J Agric Food Chem,* 2002 **50**(5) 949–954.

93 MOREDA-PIÑEIRO J, LÓPEZ-MAHÍA P, MUNIATEGUI-LORENZO S, FERNÁNDEZ-FERNÁNDEZ E, PRADA-RODRÍGUEZ, D, 'Direct mercury determination in aqueous slurries of environmental and biological samples by cold vapour generation – electrothermal atomic absorption spectrometry', *Anal Chim Acta*, 2002 **460**(1) 111–122.

94 LAVILLA I, CAPELO J L, BENDICHO C, 'Determination of cadmium and lead in mussels by electrothermal atomic absorption spectrometry using an ultrasound-assisted extraction method optimized by factorial design', *Fresenius J Anal Chem,* 1999 **363**(3) 283–288.

95 CAPELO J L, LAVILLA I, BENDICHO C, 'Ultrasound-assisted extraction of cadmium

from slurried biological samples for electrothermal atomic absorption spectrometry', *J Anal At Spectrom*, 1998 **13**(11) 1285–1290.

96 LIMA E C, BARBOSA JR F, KRUG F J, SILVA M M, VALE M G R, 'Comparison of ultrasound-assisted extraction, slurry sampling and microwave-assisted digestion for cadmium, copper and lead determination in biological and sediment samples by electrothermal atomic absorption spectrometry', *J Anal At Spectrom*, 2000 **15**(8) 995–1000.

97 SILVA R G L, WILLIE S N, STURGEON R E, SANTELLI R E, SELLA S M, 'Alkaline solubilization of biological materials for trace element analysis by electrothermal atomic absorption spectrometry', *Analyst,* 1999 **124**(12) 1843–1846.

98 TAO G H, WILLIE S N, STURGEON R E, 'Determination of total mercury in biological tissues by flow injection cold vapour generation atomic absorption spectrometry following tetramethylammonium hydroxide digestion', *Analyst,* 1998 **123**(6) 1215–1218.

99 BULDINI P L, CAVALLI S, SHARMA J L, 'Determination of transition metals in wine by IC, DPASV-DPCSV, and ZGFAAS coupled with UV photolysis', *J Agric Food Chem,* 1999 **47**(5) 1993–1998.

100 BULDINI P L, CAVALLI S, MEVOLI A, SHARMA J L, 'Ion chromatographic and voltammetric determination of heavy and transition metals in honey', *Food Chem,* 2001 **73**(4) 487–495.

101 BERMEJO-BARRERA P, FERNÁNDEZ-NOCELO S, MOREDA-PIÑEIRO A, BERMEJO-BARRERA A, 'Usefulness of enzymatic hydrolysis procedures based on the use of pronase E as sample pre-treatment for multi-element determination in biological materials', *J Anal At Spectrom*, 1999 **14**(12) 1893–1900.

102 SUN H W, YANG L L, ZHANG D Q, WANG W X, SUN J M, 'Determination of lead traces in water and liqueurs by derivative atom trapping flame atomic absorption spectrometry', *Fresenius J Anal Chem,* 1997 **358**(5) 646–651.

103 MATUSIEWICZ H, 'Atom trapping and in situ preconcentration techniques for flame atomic absorption spectrometry', *Spectrochim Acta Part B*, 1997 **52**(12) 1711–1736.

104 SAMANTA G, CHAKRABORTI D, 'Flow injection atomic absorption spectrometry for the standardization of arsenic, lead and mercury in environmental and biological standard reference materials', *Fresenius J Anal Chem,* 1997 **357**(7) 827–832.

105 ROSE M, KNAGGS M, OWEN L, BAXTER M, 'A review of analytical methods for lead, cadmium, mercury, arsenic and tin determination used in proficiency testing', *J Anal At Spectrom,* 2001 **16**(9) 1101–1106.

106 YIN X, FRECH W, HOFFMANN E, LÜDKE C, SKOLE J, 'Mercury speciation by coupling cold vapour atomic absorption spectrometry with flow injection on-line preconcentration and liquid chromatographic separation', *Fresenius J Anal Chem,* 1998 **361**(8) 761–766.

107 LOGAR M, HORVAT M, FALNOGA I, STIBILJ V, 'A methodological study of mercury speciation using Dogfish liver CRM (DOLT-2)', *Fresenius J Anal Chem,* 2000 **366**(5) 453–460.

108 TYSON J F, 'High-performance, flow-based, sample pre-treatment and introduction procedures for analytical atomic spectrometry: Plenary Lecture', *J Anal At Spectrom,* **1999** 14(2) 169–178.

109 BLAKE C, BOURQUI B, 'Determination of lead and cadmium in food products by graphite furnace atomic absorption spectroscopy', *At Spectrosc*, 1998 **19**(6), 207–213.

110 VIÑAS P, LÓPEZ-GARCÍA I, LANZÓN M, HERNÁNDEZ-CORDOBA M, 'Direct determination of lead, cadmium, zinc, and copper in honey by electrothermal atomic absorption spectrometry using hydrogen peroxide as a matrix modifier', *J Agric Food Chem,* 1997 **45**(10) 3952–3956.

111 MARTINO F A R, SÁNCHEZ M L F, SANZ MEDEL A, 'Total determination of essential and toxic elements in milk whey by double focusing ICP-MS, *J Anal At Spectrom,* 2000 **15**(2) 163–168.

112 NIEMELÄ M, PERÄMÄKI P, KOLA H, PIISPANEN J, 'Determination of arsenic, iron and selenium in moss samples using hexapole collision cell, inductively coupled plasma-mass spectrometry', *Anal Chim Acta,* 2003 **493**(1) 3–12.

113 SANCHO D, VEGA M, DEBÁN L, PARDO R, GONZÁLEZ G, 'Determination of zinc, cadmium and lead in untreated sugar samples by anodic stripping voltammetry', *Analyst,* 1997 **122**(7) 727–730.

114 ALI A M M, 'Determination of trace metal ions in common salt by stripping voltammetry', *J AOAC Int,* 1999 **82**(6) 1413–1418.

115 BARBEIRA P J S, STRADIOTTO N R, 'Anodic stripping voltammetric determination of Zn, Pb and Cu traces in whisky samples', *Fresenius J Anal Chem,* 1998 **361**(5) 507–509.

116 SANCHO D, VEGA M, DEBÁN L, PARDO R, GONZÁLEZ G, 'Determination of copper and arsenic in refined beet sugar by stripping voltammetry without sample pretreatment', *Analyst,* 1998 **123**(4) 743–747.

117 VAN HULLE M, ZHANG C, SCHOTTE B, MEES L, VANHAECKE F, VANHOLDER R, ZHANG X R, CORNELIS R, 'Identification of some arsenic species in human urine and blood after ingestion of Chinese seaweed *Laminaria*', *J Anal At Spectrom,* 2004 **19**(1) 58–64.

118 GROTEN J P, VAN BLADEREN P J, 'Cadmium bioavailability and health risk in food', *Trends Food Sci Technol,* 1994 **5**(2) 50–55.

119 VACCHINA V, POKEĆ K, SZPUNAR J, 'Speciation of cadmium in plant tissues by size-exclusion chromatography with ICP-MS detection', *J Anal At Spectrom,* 1999 **14**(10) 1557–1566.

120 BAXTER D C, FRECH W, 'Speciation of lead in environmental and biological samples – technical report', *Pure Appl Chem,* 1995 **67**(4) 615–648.

121 ŁOBIŃSKI R, DIRKX W M R, SZPUNAR-ŁOBIŃSKA J, ADAMS F C, 'Speciation analysis of organolead compounds by gas chromatography with atomic spectrometric detection', *Anal Chim Acta,* 1994 **286**(3) 381–390.

122 SZPUNAR J, PELLERIN P, MAKAROV A, DOCO T, WILLIAMS P, MEDINA B, ŁOBIŃSKI R, 'Speciation analysis for biomolecular complexes of lead in wine by size-exclusion high-performance liquid chromatography-inductively coupled plasma mass spectrometry', *J Anal At Spectrom,* 1998 **13**(8) 749–754.

123 SALIH B, 'Speciation of inorganic and organolead compounds by gas chromatography-atomic absorption spectrometry and the determination of lead species after pre-concentration onto diphenylthiocarbazone-anchored polymeric microbeads', *Spectrochim Acta Part B*, 2000 **55**(7) 1115–1127.

124 CARRO A M, MEJUTO M C, 'Application of chromatographic and electrophoretic methodology to the speciation of organomercury compounds in food analysis', *J Chromatogr A,* 2000 **882**(1–2) 283–307.

125 REILLY, C. *Metal contamination of food.* Its significance for food quality and human health. Blackwell Science Ltd, Oxford, UK, 2002.

126 TUTSCHKU S, SCHANTZ M M, HOVART M, LOGAR M, AKAGI H, EMONS H, LEVENSON M, WISE S A, 'Certification of the methylmercury content in SRM 2977 Mussel Tissue

(organic contaminants and trace elements) and SRM 1566b Oyster Tissue', *Fresenius J Anal Chem,* 2001 **369**(3–4) 364–369.
127 HINTELMANN H, FALTER R, ILGEN G, EVANS R D, 'Determination of artifactual formation of monomethylmercury (CH_3Hg^+) in environmental samples using stable Hg^{2+} isotopes with ICP-MS detection: Calculation of contents applying species specific isotope addition', *Fresenius J Anal Chem,* 1997 **358**(3) 363–370.
128 QVARNSTRÖM J, TU Q, FRECH W, LÜDKE C, 'Flow injection-liquid chromatography-cold vapour atomic absorption spectrometry for rapid determination of methyl and inorganic mercury', *Analyst,* 2000 **125**(6) 1193–1197.
129 TU Q, QVARNSTRÖM J, FRENCH W, 'Determination of mercury species by capillary zone electrophoresis-inductively coupled plasma mass spectrometry: a comparison of two spray chamber-nebulizer combinations', *Analyst*, 2000 **125**(4) 705–710.
130 FALTER R, ILGEN G, 'Coupling of the RP C18 preconcentration HPLC-UV-PCO system with atomic fluorescence detection for the determination of methylmercury in sediment and biological tissue', *Fresenius J Anal Chem,* 1997 **358**(3) 407–410.
131 EIDEN R, FALTER R, AGUSTIN-CASTRO B, SCHÖLER H F, 'Distillation, on-line RP C18 preconcentration and HPLC-UV-PCO-CVAAS as a new combination for the determination of methylmercury in sediments and fish tissue', *Fresenius J Anal Chem,* 1997 **357**(4) 439–441.
132 FALTER R, ILGEN G, 'Determination of trace amounts of methylmercury in sediment and biological tissue by using water vapor distillation in combination with RP C18 preconcentration and HPLC-HPF/HHPN-ICP-MS', *Fresenius J Anal Chem,* 1997 **358**(3) 401–406.
133 RAMALHOSA E, SEGADE S R, PEREIRA E, VALE C, DUARTE A, 'Microwave treatment of biological samples for methylmercury determination by high performance liquid chromatography-cold vapour atomic fluorescence spectrometry', *Analyst*, 2001 **126**(9) 1583–1587.
134 DA ROCHA M S, SOLDADO A B, BLANCO E, SANZ-MEDEL A, 'Speciation of mercury using capillary electrophoresis coupled to volatile species generation-inductively coupled plasma mass spectrometry', *J Anal At Spectrom*, 2001 **16**(9) 951–956.
135 HARDY S, JONES P, 'Capillary electrophoresis determination of methylmercury in fish and crab meat after extraction as the dithizone sulphonate complex', *J Chromatogr A,* 1997 **791**(1–2) 333–338.
136 PALMIERI H E L, LEONEL L V, 'Determination of methylmercury in fish tissue by gas chromatography with microwave-induced plasma atomic emission spectrometry after derivatization with sodium tetraphenylborate', *Fresenius J Anal Chem,* 2000 **366**(5) 466–469.
137 CORNELIS, R., CARUSO, J., CREWS, H., HEUMANN, K. *Handbook of elemental speciation. Techniques and methodology*. John Wiley & Sons Ltd. England, 2003.
138 LOGAR M, HORVAT M, FALNOGA I, STIBILJ V, 'A methodological study of mercury speciation using Dogfish liver CRM (DOLT-2)', *Fresenius J Anal Chem,* 2000 **366**(5) 453–460.
139 TSENG C M, DE DIEGO A, PINALY H, AMOUROUX D, DONARD O F X, 'Cryofocusing coupled to atomic absorption spectrometry for rapid and simple mercury speciation in environmental matrices', *J Anal At Spectrom*, 1998 **13**(8) 755–764.
140 MADSON M R, THOMPSON R D, 'Determination of methylmercury in food commodities by gas-liquid chromatography with atomic emission detection', *J AOAC Int,* 1998 **81**(4) 808–816.
141 TU Q, QIAN J, FRECH W, 'Rapid determination of methylmercury in biological

materials by GC-MIP-AES or GC-ICP-MS following simultaneous ultrasonic-assisted *in situ* ethylation and solvent extraction', *J Anal At Spectrom*, 2000 **15**(12) 1583–1588.

142 DIETZ C, MADRID Y, CÁMARA C, 'Mercury speciation using the capillary cold trap coupled with microwave-induced plasma atomic emission spectroscopy', *J Anal At. Spectrom*, 2001 **16**(12) 1397–1402.

143 ORELLANA-VELADO N G, PEREIRO R, SANZ-MEDEL A, 'Glow discharge atomic emission spectrometry as a detector in gas chromatography for mercury speciation', *J Anal At Spectrom*, 1998 **13**(9) 905–909.

144 ORELLANA-VELADO N G, PEREIRO R, SANZ-MEDEL A, 'Mercury speciation by capillary gas chromatography with radiofrequency hollow cathode glow discharge atomic emission detection', *J Anal At Spectrom*, 2000 **15**(1) 49–53.

145 HINTELMANN H, EVANS R D, 'Application of stable isotopes in environmental tracer studies – Measurement of monomethylmercury (CH_3Hg^+) by isotope dilution ICP-MS and detection of species transformation', *Fresenius J Anal Chem*, 1997 **358**(3) 378–385.

146 MESTER Z, LAM J, STURGEON R, PAWLISZYN J, 'Determination of methylmercury by solid-phase microextraction inductively coupled plasma mass spectrometry: a new sample introduction method for volatile metal species', *J Anal At Spectrom*, 2000 **15**(7) 837–842.

147 ARMSTRONG H E L, CORNS W T, STOCKWELL P B, O'CONNOR G, EBDON L, EVANS E H, 'Comparison of AFS and ICP-MS detection coupled with gas chromatography for the determination of methylmercury in marine samples', *Anal Chim Acta*, 1999 **390**(1–3) 245–253.

148 ROSENKRANZ B, O'CONNOR G, EVANS E H, 'Low pressure inductively coupled plasma ion source for atomic and molecular mass spectrometry: Investigation of alternative reagent gases for organomercury speciation in tissue and sediment', *J Anal At Spectrom*, 2000 **15**(1) 7–12.

149 SLAETS S, ADAMS F, PEREIRO I R, ŁOBIŃSKI R, 'Optimization of the coupling of multicapillary GC with ICP-MS for mercury speciation analysis in biological materials', *J Anal At Spectrom*, 1999 **14**(5) 851–857.

150 PEREIRO I R, WASIK A, ŁOBIŃSKI R, 'Determination of mercury species in fish reference materials by isothermal multicapillary gas chromatography with atomic emission detection after microwave-assisted solubilization and solvent extraction', *J Anal At Spectrom*, 1998 **13**(8) 743–747.

151 WASIK A, PEREIRO I R, DIETZ C, SZPUNAR J, ŁOBIŃSKI R, 'Speciation of mercury by ICP-MS after on-line capillary cryofocussing and ambient temperature multicapillary gas chromatography', *Anal Commun*, 1998 **35**(10) 331–335.

152 CHIOU C S, JIANG S J, DANADURAI K S K, 'Determination of mercury compounds in fish by microwave-assisted extraction and liquid chromatography-vapor generation-inductively coupled plasma mass spectrometry', *Spectrochim Acta Part B*, 2001 **56**(7) 1133–1142.

153 HARRINGTON C F, ROMERIL J, CATTERICK T, 'The speciation of mercury and organomercury compounds by high performance liquid chromatography atmospheric pressure ionization mass spectrometry', *Rapid Commun Mass Spectrom*, 1998 **12**(14) 911–916.

154 SHIOMI, K, Chapter 12 in *Arsenic in the Environment, Part II: Human Health and Ecosystem Effects*. Nriagu, J. O. (Ed.), John Wiley & Sons, Inc., New York, 1994, vol. 27.

155 KAISE T, OYA-OHTA Y, OCHI T, OKUBO T, HANAOKA K, IRGOLIC K J, SAKURAI T, MATSUBARA C, 'Toxicological study of organic arsenic compounds in marine algae using mammalian cell culture technique', *J Food Hyg Soc Jpn,* 1996 **37**(3) 135–141.
156 FRANCESCONI K A, 'Complete extraction of arsenic species: a worthwhile goal?', *App Organomet Chem*, 2003 **17**(9) 682–683.
157 ACKLEY K L, B'HYMER C, SUTTON K L, CARUSO J A, 'Speciation of arsenic in fish tissue using microwave-assisted extraction followed by HPLC-ICP-MS', *J Anal At Spectrom*, 1999 **14**(5) 845–850.
158 CHATTERJEE A, 'Determination of total cationic and total anionic arsenic species in oyster tissue using microwave-assisted extraction followed by HPLC-ICP-MS', *Talanta,* 2000 **51**(2) 303–314.
159 LARSEN E H, HANSEN M, GÖSSLER W, 'Speciation and health risk considerations of arsenic in the edible mushroom *Laccaria amethystina* collected from contaminated and uncontaminated locations', *Appl Organomet Chem,* 1998 **12**(4) 285–291.
160 MCKIERNAN J W, CREED J T, BROCKHOFF C A, CARUSO J A, LORENZANA R M, 'A comparison of automated and traditional methods for the extraction of arsenicals from fish', *J Anal At Spectrom*, 1999 **14**(4) 607–613.
161 GÓMEZ-ARIZA J L, SÁNCHEZ RODAS D, GIRÁLDEZ I, MORALES E, 'A comparison between ICP-MS and AFS detection for arsenic speciation in environmental samples', *Talanta*, 2000 **51**(2) 257–268.
162 MUÑOZ O, VÉLEZ D, MONTORO R, 'Optimization of the solubilization, extraction and determination of inorganic arsenic [As(III) + As(V)] in seafood products by acid digestion, solvent extraction and hydride generation atomic absorption spectrometry', *Analyst*, 1999 **124**(4) 601–607.
163 HEITKEMPER D T, VELA N P, STEWART K R, WESTPHAL C S, 'Determination of total and speciated arsenic in rice by ion chromatography and inductively coupled plasma mass spectrometry', *J Anal At Spectrom*, 2001 **16**(4) 299–306.
164 CARUSO J A, HEITKEMPER D T, B'HYMER C, 'An evaluation of extraction techniques for arsenic species from freeze-dried apple samples', *Analyst,* 2001 **126**(2) 136–140.
165 RABER G, FRANCESCONI K A, IRGOLIC K J, GOESSLER W, 'Determination of arsenosugars in algae with anion-exchange chromatography and an inductively coupled plasma mass spectrometer as element-specific detector', *Fresenius J Anal Chem*, 2000 **367**(2) 181–188.
166 MADSEN A D, GOESSLER W, PEDERSEN S N, FRANCESCONI K A, 'Characterization of an algal extract by HPLC-ICP-MS and LC-electrospray MS for use in arsenosugar speciation studies', *J Anal At Spectrom*, 2000 **15**(6) 657–662.
167 VAN ELTEREN J T, SLEJKOVEC Z, 'Ion-exchange separation of eight arsenic compounds by high-performance liquid chromatography – UV decomposition – hydride generation – atomic fluorescence spectrometry and stability tests for food treatment procedures', *J Chromatogr A* 1997 **789**(1–2) 339–348.
168 LARSEN E H, 'Method optimization and quality assurance in speciation analysis using high performance liquid chromatography with detection by inductively coupled plasma mass spectrometry', *Spectrochim Acta Part B*, 1998 **53**(2) 253–265.
169 FALK K, EMONS H, 'Speciation of arsenic compounds by ion-exchange HPLC-ICP-MS with different nebulizers', *J Anal At Spectrom,* 2000 **15**(6) 643–649.
170 SÚÑER M A, DEVESA V, MUÑOZ O, VÉLEZ D, MONTORO R, 'Application of column

switching in high-performance liquid chromatography with on-line thermo-oxidation and detection by HG-AAS and HG-AFS for the analysis of organoarsenical species in seafood samples', *J Anal At Spectrom,* 2001 **16**(4) 390–397.

171 SLOTH J J, LARSEN E H, JULSHAMN K, 'Determination of organoarsenic species in marine samples using gradient elution cation exchange HPLC-ICP-MS', *J Anal At Spectrom,* 2003 **15**(5) 452–459.

172 HUANG Y M, WHANG C W, 'Capillary electrophoresis of arsenic compounds with indirect fluorescence detection', *Electrophoresis*, 1998 **19**(12) 2140–2144.

173 GASPÁR A, SÓGOR C, POSTA J, 'Separation of organic and inorganic arsenic species by capillary zone electrophoresis', *Chromatogr Supp*, 2000 **51** S135–S138.

174 VAN DEN BROECK K, VANDECASTEELE C, 'Capillary electrophoresis for the speciation of arsenic', *Mikrochim Acta*, 1998 **128**(1–2) 79–85.

175 VAN HOLDERBEKE M, ZHAO Y N, VANHAECKE F, MOENS L, DAMS R, SANDRA P, 'Speciation of six arsenic compounds using capillary electrophoresis-inductively coupled plasma mass spectrometry', *J Anal At Spectrom,* 1999 **14**(2) 229–234.

176 COSTA-FERNÁNDEZ J M, BINGS N H, LEACH A M, HIEFTJE G M, 'Rapid simultaneous multielemental speciation by capillary electrophoresis coupled to inductively coupled plasma time-of-flight mass spectrometry', *J Anal At Spectrom* 2000 **15**(9) 1063–1067.

177 SUTTON K L, CARUSO J A, 'Liquid chromatography-inductively coupled plasma mass spectrometry', *J Chromatogr A,* 1999 **856**(1–2) 243–258.

178 LAI V W M, CULLEN W R, RAY S, 'Arsenic speciation in scallops', *Mar Chem*, 1999 **66**(1–2) 81–89.

179 GALLAGHER P A, SHOEMAKER J A, WEI X, BROCKHOFF-SCHWEGEL C A, CREED J T, 'Extraction and detection of arsenicals in seaweed via accelerated solvent extraction with ion chromatographic separation and ICP-MS detection', *Fresenius J Anal Chem*, 2001 **369**(1) 71–80.

180 VELA N P, HEITKEMPER D T, STEWART K R, 'Arsenic extraction and speciation in carrots using accelerated solvent extraction, liquid chromatography and plasma mass spectrometry', *Analyst*, 2001 **126**(7) 1011–1017.

181 AMRAN M B, LAGARDE F, LEROY M J F, 'Determination of arsenic species in marine organisms by HPLC-ICP-OES and HPLC-HG-QFAAS', *Mikrochim Acta*, 1997 **127**(3–4) 195–202.

182 CHAUSSEAU M, ROUSSEL C, GILON N, MERMET J M, 'Optimization of HPLC-ICP-AES for the determination of arsenic species', *Fresenius J Anal Chem*, 2000 **366**(5) 476–480.

183 SÚÑER M A, DEVESA V, CLEMENTE M J, VÉLEZ D, MONTORO R, URIETA I, JALÓN M, MACHO M L, 'Organoarsenical species contents in fresh and processed seafood products', *J Agric Food Chem,* 2002 **50**(4) 924–932.

184 ŠLEJKOVEC Z., BYRNE A.R., SMODIŠ B., ROSSBACH M, 'Preliminary studies on arsenic species in some environmental samples', *Fresenius J Anal Chem*, 1996 **354**(5–6), 592–595.

185 SÚÑER M A, DEVESA V, RIVAS I, VÉLEZ D, MONTORO R, 'Speciation of cationic arsenic species in seafood by coupling liquid chromatography with hydride generation atomic fluorescence detection', *J Anal At Spectrom,* 2000 **15**(11), 1501–1507.

186 STURGEON R E, 'Future of atomic spectrometry for environmental analysis', *J Anal At Spectrom,* 1998 **13**(5) 351–361.

187 PENNEBAKER F M, JONES D A, GRESHAM C A, WILLIAMS R H, SIMON R E, SCHAPPERT M F,

DENTON M B, 'Spectroscopic instrumentation in the 21st Century: excitement at the horizon – Plenary lecture', *J Anal At Spectrom,* 1998 **13**(9) 821–827.

188 EBDON L, PITTS L, CORNELIS R, CREWS H, DONARD O F X, QUEVAUVILLER PH (eds), *Trace element speciation for environment, food and health.* The Royal Society of Chemistry, Cambridge, UK, 2001.

189 CREWS H M, 'Speciation of trace elements in foods, with special reference to cadmium and selenium: is it necessary?', *Spectrochim Acta Part B*, 1998 **53**(2) 213–219.

25

Mycotoxins: detection and control

M. Miraglia, F. Debegnach and C. Brera, Italian National Institute for Health

25.1 Introduction

Microscopic filamentous fungi can develop on a wide variety of food commodities and, under suitable environmental conditions, can lead to the production of highly toxic chemical substances, commonly known as mycotoxins. The most widespread and studied mycotoxins are metabolites of some genera of moulds such as *Aspergillus, Penicillium* and *Fusarium*. Conditions influencing mycotoxin biosynthesis include climate and geographical location of crops, cultivation practices, storage, and type of substrate. Valuable reviews on mycotoxins formation were published by Krogh (1987), Smith *et al.* (1998) and CAST (Council for Agricultural Science and Technology) (2003). Mycotoxins are often not affected by food processing since toxins can residue partly on the outer surface, and partly in the inner portions of the grains (Brera *et al.*, 2004; Trigo-Stockli *et al.*, 2002; Meister, 2001; Peraica *et al.*, 2001; Rychlik and Schieberle, 2001; Heilmann *et al.*, 1999; Sydenham *et al.*, 1997; Baxter, 1996; Osborne *et al.*, 1996; Scott, 1996; Scudamore, 1996; Subirade, 1996). Examples of reduction of mycotoxin levels due to processing include roasting of coffee and alkaline treatments.

Mycotoxin toxicity has been extensively investigated for the most important toxins, such as aflatoxins (AFLs), ochratoxin A (OTA), and *Fusarium* toxins. Information derived from the toxicokinetics in animal models has also been obtained. Toxic effects are mainly related to genotoxicity, carcinogenicity, mutagenicity, teratogenicity and immunotoxicity. Mycotoxins are able to form adducts with various molecular receptors such as DNA, RNA, functional proteins, enzymatic co-factors and membrane constituents. Updated reviews on the most relevant mycotoxins are provided by WHO (World Health

Organization) (2002) and, at European level, by SCF (Scientific Committee for Food) (2002, 2001, 2000a,b,c, 1999).

Among the various xenobiotics affecting food and animal feed, mycotoxins were neglected for many years. At the present time, their impact on human and animal health has been recognized increasingly. It is estimated that a considerable amount (25%) of the available food and feed supply worldwide is to some extent contaminated by mycotoxins, posing a significant problem for global food security (Mannon, 1985). The number of food products susceptible to mycotoxin contamination is continuously increasing, ranging from cereals to grape products including wine, coffee, cocoa, dried fruits and spices.

Harmonized approaches for the risk analysis on mycotoxins are still far from being achieved in part due to strong conflicts between the interests of different groups of countries (producing, exporting, importing, developed and under development) and of stakeholders. Several international organizations, such as FAO (Food and Agricultural Organization), WHO and CODEX *Alimentarious* (FAO/WHO, 1995) have undertaken an active role.

Each of the three components of the risk analysis process (risk management, risk assessment and risk communication) play a part in the planning of analytical and control activities.

25.2 Types of mycotoxins found in food and animal feed

A number of major mycotoxins have been extensively investigated in such areas as toxicity, exposure, prevention, control and detection. In addition to the major mycotoxins, a considerable number of minor toxins are known to be produced naturally by moulds. For many of them information about outbreaks of disease or experimental data, indicating their possible negative impact on human or animal health, is also available. However, for most of them there is only very limited information on their occurrence in food. Basic information is given below on several of the major and minor mycotoxins. Further information can be obtained through the references cited.

25.2.1 Aflatoxins

Aflatoxins are known as severe human hepatocarcinogens and as substances with potential adverse effects on livestock health and productivity. These toxins are produced by species of *Aspergillus*, mainly *A. flavus* and *A. parasiticus*, particularly in hot and humid areas. Drought stress and insect injury represent the main cause of fungal contamination and aflatoxins production in the field, while humidity higher than 85% and temperatures above 25°C are favourable to the growth of fungi during storage (Diener, 1969). These fungi are ubiquitous, but they are more abundant in subtropical areas with a warm and humid climate at 26 to 35 latitude north and south from the equator. The production of aflatoxins shows a great increase, attributable in particular to *A. flavus,* at above average temperatures and below average rainfall. The presence of insects usually corresponds to high levels of aflatoxins especially in the presence of European corn borer (*Ostrinia nubilalis*).

Aflatoxins are substances that are chemically related to difuranocoumarin. Among the 17 aflatoxins isolated at present, only four are considered to be relevant, i.e. aflatoxins B_1, B_2, G_1 and G_2, as they are widespread and toxic. The G series contains a D lactone ring, while the B series contains a cyclopentenone ring, which is responsible for the major toxicity of the B series. Aflatoxins are crystalline substances, soluble in moderately polar organic solvents, such as chloroform, methanol, dimethysulfoxide, scarcely soluble in water (10-30 μg/ml) and unsoluble in non-polar organic solvents. Pure aflatoxins are destroyed by UV radiations, unstable at pH <3 and >10 and in the presence of oxidizing components. These toxins have native fluorescence, which is used for their analysis and for the sorting of contaminated units (as in the case of dry figs and peanuts).

Aflatoxins occur in a wide variety of commodities including cereals, oilseeds, nuts (such as peanuts, walnuts and Brazil nuts), dried fruits (especially figs), spices, desiccated coconuts and crude oils. Reviews on toxicity, metabolism, and epidemiological studies are provided by several authors (WHO, 2002; Fink-Gremmels, 1998; Wild, 1998) and by IARC, that classified aflatoxin B_1 in the group 1 (carcinogenic to humans) (IARC, 1993). Molecular structures of aflatoxins are presented in Fig. 25.1.

25.2.2 Ochratoxin A

A variety of moulds included in the genera *Aspergillus* (mainly *A. ochraceus*) and *Penicillium* (mainly *P. verrucosum*) are able to produce ochratoxins, with OTA being the most relevant toxin (Frisvad, 1989). Ochratoxin A has been shown to be a potential nephrotoxin in all animal species tested, with the exception of mature ruminants. Ochratoxin A is carcinogenic to rodents and possesses teratogenic, immunotoxic and suspected neurotoxic and genotoxic properties. Furthermore, it may be implicated in the human desease Balkan Endemic Nephropathy (BEN) and in the development of urinary tract tumours in humans. The International Agency for Research on Cancer classified OTA as a possible human carcinogen (group 2B) (IARC, 1993).

Ochratoxin A contamination in grapes and derived products, such as wine occurs mostly as *A. carbonarious* attacks. In general, at 24°C the optimal A_w (water activity) values for the toxin's production are in a 0.95–0.99 range, depending on the producers; in general, at optimal A_w the toxin can be produced in the range 12–37°C for *A. ochraceus* and 4–31°C for *P. verrucosum*. Ochratoxin A contaminated crops include cereals, such as barley and maize, wheat and oat, groundnuts, beans such as coffee and cocoa and pulses. In cereals, OTA is produced more frequently by *Penicillium* than *Aspergillus*, as it generally occurs as storage contamination. Grains contaminated by OTA are likely to contain additional fungal metabolites, such as citrinin and penicillic

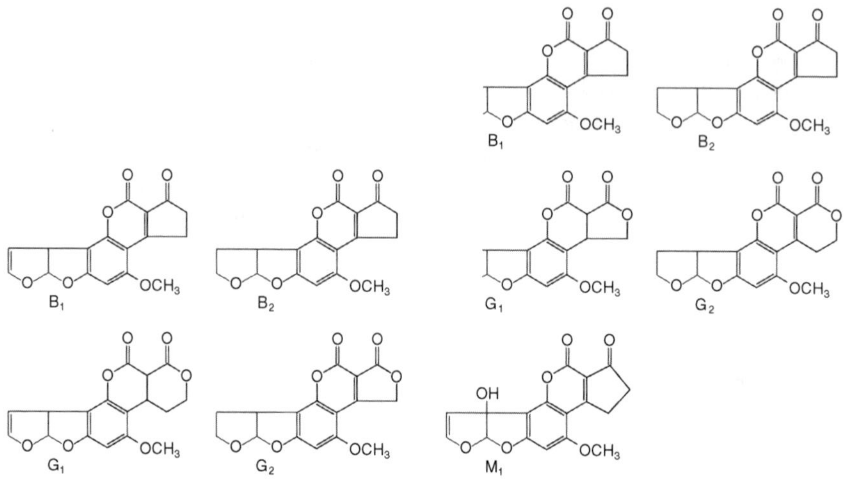

Fig. 25.1 Molecular structures of aflatoxins B_1, B_2, G_1, G_2 and M_1.

acid. In the past few years OTA has also been found contaminating other food products, including spices and beer (Task 3.2.7, 2002). Many researches have also reported the presence, in some case rather alarming, of OTA in human biological fluids such as serum and breast milk (Iavicoli *et al.*, 2002; Brera *et al.*, 2000; Palli *et al.*, 1999; Scott *et al.*, 1998; Ueno *et al.*, 1998). The molecular structure of ochratoxin A is presented in Fig. 25.2.

25.2.3 Trichothecenes

Trichothecenes are a wide group of mycotoxins produced by various species of different genera: *Fusarium, Myrothecium, Stachybotrys, Trichoderma, Cephalosporium, Trichothecium* and *Verticimonosporium* (Betina, 1993). Approximately 170 trichothecene mycotoxins are known. They are constituted by a system based on a common tetracyclic, sesquiterpenoid 12,13-epoxytrichothec-9-ene ring, and it is the epoxide group that is responsible for causing the toxicity (IPCS, 1990). Contamination occurs primarily in wheat, barley, rye and maize. Type A trichothecenes includes

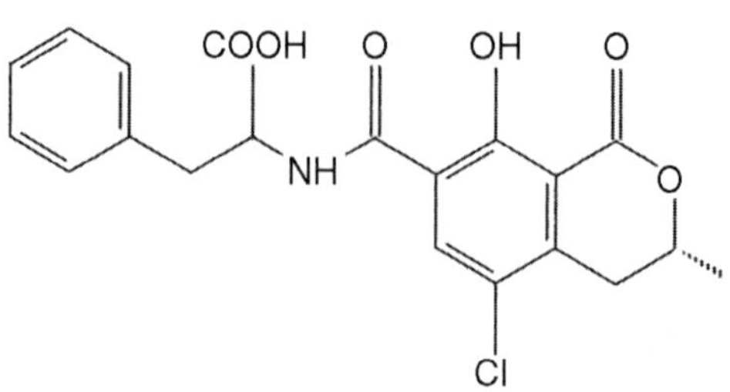

Fig. 25.2 Molecular structure of ochratoxin A.

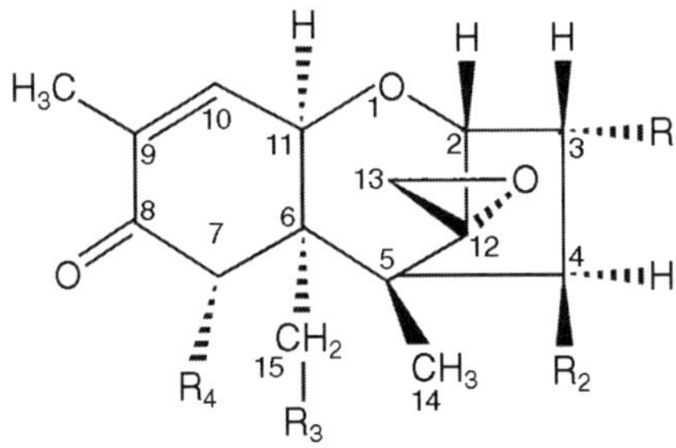

Fig. 25.3 Molecular structure of the main trichothecenes. R = OH or acyloxy group (most often acetoxy).

mainly T-2 toxin, HT-2 and diacetoxyscirpenol (DAS), while mycotoxins of type B mainly include 4-deoxynivalenol (DON), commonly known as vomitoxin, nivalenol (NIV), 3-acetyldeoxynivalenol (3-AcDON) and 15-acetyldeoxynivalenol (15-AcDON). Toxic effects include nausea, vomiting, visual disorder, vertigo, throat irritation and feed refusal in farm animals. Toxin T-2 has been demonstrated to be the most toxic, followed by DAS and NIV, with DON being the least toxic in acute toxicity studies, DON is, however, the most widespread in grains worldwide and therefore the most studied. Issues related to chemical and physical data, occurrence, toxicity, absorption, distribution and metabolism of trichothecenes are reviewed by WHO (WHO, 2002). Physicochemical data for some selected *Fusarium* toxins is given by Sydenham *et al.* (1996). The molecular structures of the main trichothecenes are shown in Fig. 25.3.

25.2.4 Patulin.

Patulin is a toxin usually related to apples and apple-derived products and it is produced by different species of the genera *Penicillium*, *Aspergillus* and *Byssochlamys*, of which *Penicillium expansum* is the most common species. Recent studies have revealed the toxin presence also in other fruits such as pears and peaches (Task 3.2.8, 2002; de Sylos and Rodrigues, 1999). From a chemical point of view patulin is a lactone, soluble in water, methanol, ethanol and acetone. It is a cytotoxic compound mediated by an increase in membrane permeability. It inhibits numerous enzymes *in vitro*, including DNA polymerase and RNA polymerase. Carcinogenic and mutagenic studies conducted up to the present are not sufficient to provide indications about these effects. In European countries maximum tolerable levels in fruit products, with particular reference to apples, were settled, the limit for baby food being considerably lower (10 μg/kg) than for general population (50 μg/kg) (Reg. EC, 2003; FAO, 1997). The molecular structure of patulin is given in Fig. 25.4.

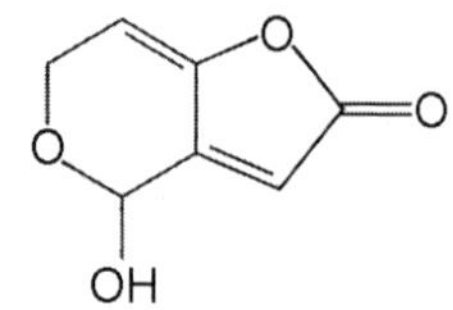

Fig. 25.4 Chemical structure of patulin.

25.2.5 Fumonisins

Fumonisins (FBs) are mycotoxins mainly produced by *Fusarium verticillioides* (Sacc.) Nirenberg (formerly *F. Moniliforme* Sheldon) and *Fusarium proliferatum*, which often occur in maize and maize-based food products at levels that could affect human and animal health. In particular, fumonisins have been shown to be hepatotoxic and nephrotoxic to most tested animal species and to cause leukoencephalomalacia in horses (Caramelli *et al.*, 1993; Wilson *et al.*, 1992), pulmonary oedema in swine (Harrison *et al.*, 1990) and hepatocarcinoma in rats (Gelderblom *et al.*, 1991). The US National Toxicology Program showed clear evidence of carcinogenic activity of fumonisin B_1 (FB_1) in male rats and female mice based on the increased incidence of renal tubule and hepatocellular neoplasms respectively (US NTP, 1999). On the basis of the toxicological evidence of fungal cultures containing high levels of fumonisins, the International Agency for Research on Cancer has classified *F. moniliforme* toxins as potentially carcinogenic to humans (class 2B carcinogens) (IARC, 2002). Most recently interest has focused on fumonisins as risk factor in oesophageal cancer. From a structural point of view fumonisins are correlated to the sphyngoid bases. The molecular structures of fumonisins are shown in Fig. 25.5.

25.2.6 Zearalenone

Zearalenone (ZEA) is a non-steroidal, estrogenic toxin produced mainly by *Fusarium graminearum, Fusarium culmorum* and *Fusarium sacchari*. This toxin is the second most frequent *Fusarium* metabolite after DON in maize. Zearalenone affects primarily the reproductive system of animals, this effect

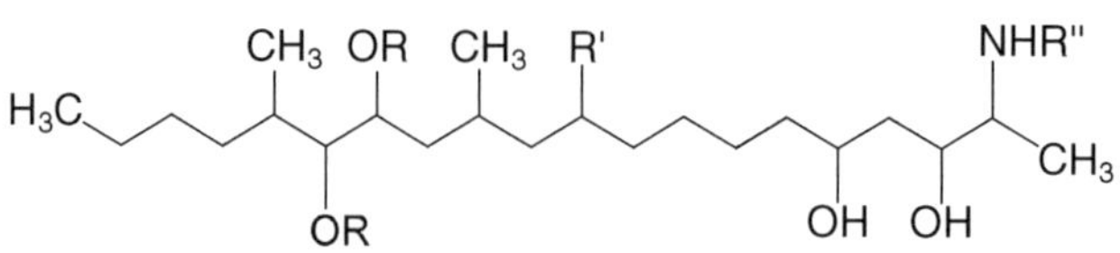

FB_1 R=$COCH_2CH(CO_2H)CH_2CO_2H$; R'=OH; R''=H

FB_2 R=$COCH_2CH(CO_2H)CH_2CO_2H$; R'=R''=H

Fig. 25.5 Molecular structures of fumonisins.

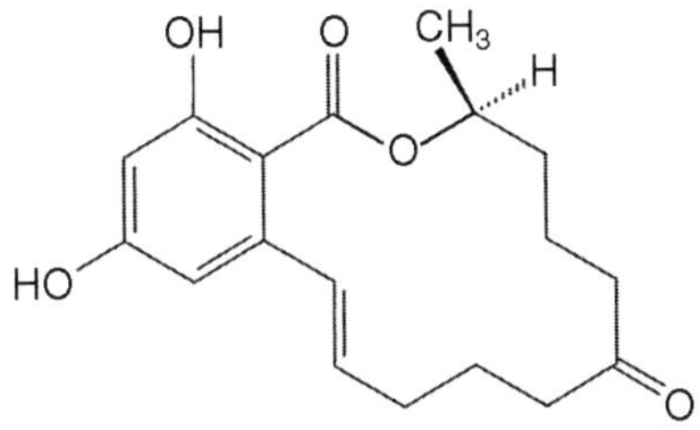

Fig. 25.6 The molecular structure of zearalenone.

being most evident in swine. Detailed information on zearalenone structure, molecular data, chemical and physical properties, occurrence and studies related to toxicity on animals and humans are reviewed by IARC (1993). The molecular structure of zearalenone is shown on Fig. 25.6.

25.2.7 Minor mycotoxins

- *Tremorgenic mycotoxins including penitrem.* Clinical signs in animals include muscle tremor, uncoordinated movements and general weakness.
- *Gliotoxin.* It is a highly immunosuppressive toxin produced by a wide variety of widespread moulds. Intoxication of camels is reported due to the ingestion of this toxin and it seems to be involved in human infections caused by *Candida albicans.*
- *Citreoviridin.* It causes paralysis, dyspnea, cardiovascular disturbances and loss of eyesight in experimental animals. It frequently co-occurs with aflatoxins and synergism is likely to occur.
- *Citrinin.* It co-occurs frequently with ochratoxin A, is nephrotoxic and its synergism with ochratoxin A has been demonstrated.
- *Sterigmatocyistin.* It is a precursor of the biosynthesis of aflatoxin B_1. It was detected in low concentration in green coffee, mouldy wheat and in the outer parts of mouldy cheese.
- *3-Nitropropionic acid.* It was detected in pasture and related to neurological disorders.
- *Fusaproliferin.* Preliminary studies indicate its toxic role, but no mammalian feeding studies have been conducted so far. It was detected in corn samples in Italy, Poland and United States.

Recent and valuable reviews on major and minor mycotoxins are available in CAST (2003) and in Miraglia (in press).

25.3 Risk management and control of mycotoxins in food

The risk management of mycotoxins implies, among others, activities that can be grouped under the general term 'control'. Control of mycotoxins includes various types of preventive and corrective actions to be carried out by the producers in order to implement regulations, establish legal limits, guidelines and control activities by the competent authorities.

25.3.1 Control through integrated management strategies

Since mycotoxins are seldom destroyed by technological processing and by cooking, prevention represents the most powerful tool for minimizing this kind of contamination. In order to manage the problem, an approach through integrated management strategies (IMS) should be used, taking into account all the stages in which contamination can occur i.e. production, handling and processing.

Therefore Hazard Analysis of Critical Control Point (HACCP) systems should in theory cover all the issues of the IMS for mycotoxins. Unfortunately, in practice, they often deal only with the processing steps as in the case of Council Directive 93/43/EEC of 14 June 1993 (Council Directive, 1993) on the hygiene of foodstuffs. The HACCP systems should indeed consider the overall production process and should give a basis for a responsible choice based on prevention and verification rather than on monitoring and analysis. The issue of HACCP for mycotoxins has been discussed by several authors (Lopez-Garcia, 2001; Brera *et al.*, 1996).

In order to manage effectively the impact of mycotoxins on human and animal health through prevention, it is very useful to gather global occurrence data within a risk management/risk assessment framework. The more accurate is the information on the occurrence of mycotoxins, the more targeted are the actions aimed at preventing the relevant moulds.

25.3.2 Occurrence

In order to gain a full and accurate picture of mycotoxin occurrence, information on frequency and levels of contamination by mycotoxins for the widest number of susceptible commodities in the largest number of countries should be compiled. Despite the huge amount of data available, the situation is far from complete. With this in mind one of the most important current initiatives is the GEMS Food Program (Global Environmental Monitoring System) (www.who.dk/foodsafety/Chemical/20020905_1). A recent and valuable review on the occurrence of mycotoxins in food and animal feed is available in the CAST Report (2003): data are grouped for potentially toxic genera/species found on different commodities, matrices in which mycotoxin contamination has been found, together with the resulting effects on animals and humans and occurrence of mycotoxins in processed food. At European level, the most recent database for the occurrence of some mycotoxins has been provided by the European Commission which has launched a number of valuable initiatives. Coordinated programmes were established for evaluating annually the occurrence in several commodities (ochratoxin A in cocoa and coffee, and aflatoxins in spices, groundnuts, pistachios and baby foods) and SCOOP. Tasks were run in the framework of the Scientific Cooperation for assessing the occurrence and exposure of the general population to several mycotoxins (aflatoxins, ochratoxin A, patulin and *Fusarium* toxins) (Task 3.2.10, 2003; Task 3.2.8, 2002; Task 3.2.7, 2002). As for OTA, it was recognized that even though cereals represent by far the largest contributor to exposure, other commodities also make a contribution (wine, vine fruits, coffee, cocoa, spices, beer), and others such as liquorice deserve further attention.

25.3.3 Preventive actions

Preventive actions for mycotoxins are commonly grouped in pre-harvest, harvest, storage, and post-harvest activities. The understanding of fungal ecology has been one of the most important milestones for the development of an integrated HACCP system: many initiatives have been undertaken in this respect and good results have already been achieved. An example worth mentioning is provided by the study carried out at international level on the problem of ochratoxin A contamination in coffee. Exhaustive research was carried out under the umbrella of FAO on the identification of critical control points for OTA contamination in coffee especially in the countries of origin. Research aimed at the prevention of mycotoxins was also largely supported in the framework of the European Commission's Quality of Life Research Programme. A list of the related websites is available at: http://www.lfra.co.uk/eman2/links.asp.

Pre-harvest prevention activities

A considerable amount of experimental research has been conducted to highlight parameters and practices aimed at preventing/minimizing mould infection and/or mycotoxin contamination on a large number of commodities and for a large number of fungi. Valuable reviews are available on this topic, including the CAST Report (2003), which considers pre-harvest control strategies individually for *Aspergillus, Fusarium,* Ergot and *Stachybotrys*, and the CODEX on ochratoxin A, patulin and aflatoxins in pistachio.

Pre-harvest prevention activities depend strongly on the species and the crops. For aflatoxin contamination in corn, adverse environmental factors such as high temperature and drought stress (Payne, 1998) can hardly be managed. A marked improvement can be achieved using good agricultural practices (GAP), such as appropriate fertilization and irrigation, crop rotation, use of pesticides, weed control, appropriate planting/harvesting time, and minimization of insect attack. Breeding practices can be used for developing resistance to mould infestation, and progress in genomics can contribute greatly in this area. The use of modern biotechnology represents a promising tool for the prevention of mycotoxin contamination. In this respect, genetically modified plants, with new inserted genes for the prevention of mould attack, are under study. Furthermore, indications are already available that some of the currently authorized insect resistant GM plants are less prone to aflatoxin and *Fusarium* contamination, probably due to the reduced number of damaged grains, since damaged grains are more susceptible to mycotoxin contamination. However, further research is necessary to investigate this issue.

The role of low input agricultural practices on mycotoxin contamination also has to be clarified. The lack of pesticide treatments should, in theory, enhance the moulding of the crop, but low input agricultural practices can hamper fungi infestation through enhanced resistance of the plant. To investigate this further, in the sixth Framework Programme (FP6), the research project SAFEFOOD, has been launched.

Harvest, post-harvest and storage prevention activities

As mentioned above, damage to kernels can enhance mycotoxin contamination, and in some cases the separation of mouldy units is not always sufficient to reduce the mycotoxin contamination very much. The control of humidity (water activity; A_w) represents by far the most effective prevention action in post-harvest and storage stages; however, factors such as insect, rodents or bird attack, or spots of moisture, or heat can promote mycotoxin, contamination. These can be prevented by several strategies including the use of appropriate pesticides, and various physical means, including modified atmosphere.

25.3.4 Control and legal limits

At present the setting of maximum residue limits (MRLs) for mycotoxins is a hotly debated issue at international level. In the CODEX Food Additives and Contaminants Committee, the issue has been discussed for more than ten years and valuable documentation has been put forward, but at the present moment there is still a lack of agreement on MRLs for mycotoxins, thus representing a serious impediment to harmonization in trade. In addition, while most industrialized countries recognize the need to set limits for mycotoxins, many developing countries have not yet taken action on this. Among the factors that can influence limits are the toxicology of, and exposure to the toxin, the need for sufficient food supply, legislation in other countries and the import–export relationship. In addition, other factors that should be taken into account are the influence of technological procedures on the fate of mycotoxins, the level of occurrence in commodities, the level of impact on human health, the contribution to the level of exposure for the selected commodities, and the availability of sampling and analytical methods suitable for the limit.

Many valuable surveys have been published on the issue of worldwide regulation on mycotoxins, starting from the first complete review published by FAO (1997). Rapid evolution in the field has meant there is a continuous need for updating: FAO is preparing a revised document that is expected to be published in 2004 and that will review the mycotoxin regulations worldwide in more than 100 countries.

During the last few years the European Commission has put in force a number of Regulations (Commission Regulation, 2003a,b, 2002) setting maximum limits for several mycotoxins (aflatoxins, ochratoxin A, patulin) in different foodstuffs (cereals, dried fruits, nuts and milk for AFLs, cereals and vine fruits for ochratoxin A and apple products for patulin). Limits for *Fusarium* toxins in cereals and for the above mentioned mycotoxins in additional matrices are expected in the near future.

25.4 Sampling for mycotoxins

Mycotoxin contamination of foods and animal feeds is commonly heterogeneously distributed throughout a bulk. Therefore, precautions must be taken in the sampling procedure so as to obtain a reliable and representative estimate of the concentration of a mycotoxin in a given lot. The error associated with sampling is much larger than the error associated with the sample preparation and analysis of the test portion. It should be considered that even extremely accurate methods of analysis do not correct the sampling error. The enforcement of the European Directive 98/53 (Commission Directive, 1998) fixed the procedures for sampling aflatoxins in some food categories such as cereals, dried fruits and milk. More recently, by adopting as a basis Directive 98/53 on aflatoxins, some other European Directives on other food commodities and other mycotoxins have been put in force, namely, Directive 2002/27/CE (Commission Directive, 2002b), amending Directive 98/53/EC, laying down the sampling methods and the methods of analysis for the official control of the levels for certain contaminants in foodstuffs covered sampling procedures for aflatoxins in spices, Directive 2002/26/EC (Commission Directive, 2002a) for ochratoxin A in cereals and dried vine fruits, and Directive 2003/78/EC (Commission Directive, 2003) for patulin in fruit products. Another Directive dealing with the sampling procedures for mycotoxins in baby foods is being considered. The rationale of these Directives is based on the adoption of a compromise between statistical and pragmatic approaches.

The implementation of these Directives is posing several questions in terms of the feasibility of the sampling plans, of the assigning of the duties, namely who does what, and the waste handling. Whitaker *et al.* (2001) recently developed a method for evaluating the performance of sampling plans for fumonisins in maize.

25.4.1 Feasibility of the sampling plan

The feasibility of the sampling procedures raises the most problematic issues. In particular, difficulties and needs can be summarized as follows:

- Depending on the lot size, extremely large time periods will be requested for implementing the whole procedure.

- High related costs have to be sustained by the importer; it has been calculated that an average of US$ 7,000 is necessary.
- Personnel safety issues must be rigorously observed.
- Occasionally, high time ranges for the delivery of the aggregate sample to the appointed laboratory for official control.
- The availability of functional facilities at the harbours has to be guaranteed in terms of masks, gloves, palettes, probes, suitable containers for the collection of samples, strategic points for sampling.

The need to draw in most cases, 30 kg of aggregate sample from at least 100 incremental samples, entails different procedures according to the various situations in which sampling has to be performed. Two particular situations have to be considered in the main: dynamic and static situations.

In the *dynamic situation*, representing the easiest circumstance, it is wise to carry out sampling procedures during the off-loading from ships or containers. Incremental samples should be taken at predefined intervals of time in such a way as to cover all the off-loading time. Only in this way can a reliable and representative aggregate sample be obtained. In sampling in *static situation,* as for commodities in containers, silos and lorries, additional inconveniences are to be considered. In particular, with containers it is necessary to remove all the bags or sacks or packages from each single container before performing the sampling procedure, and to re-load the container with the items after the sampling process. More specifically, the following drawbacks can be taken into consideration.

- Fulfilling the requirement of Directive 98/53 '... under the condition that the sub lot can be separated physically, each lot must be subdivided into sub lots. Taking into account that the weight of the lot is not always an exact multiple of the weight of the sub lots, the weight of the sub lot may exceed the mentioned weight by a maximum of 20% ...' can be troublesome due to the difficulty in separating the sub lots physically.
- The off-loading of the units to be sampled (sacks, packages, etc.) from the containers represents one of the most crucial drawbacks for a reliable and effective sampling procedure since it is a time-consuming process
- The sampling from containers require an open space area when implementing the procedure. In this case, therefore, atmospheric conditions can significantly lengthen the time required for the whole process.
- Availability of probes of different length to draw increments at specific sampling points.
- Difficult accessibility to the sampling points (especially for silos).
- The safety of the employed personnel.

25.4.2 Sampling at retail

Directive 98/53 does not provide any detailed information about sampling procedures for retail samples. At present, general information on the need to collect as much data as possible on homogeneous aggregate samples by following an unspecified procedure is given in the directive. However, it should be noted that market samples of lot sizes below 0.1 ton can follow the procedure described for retail samples.

An additional key point for the official control analysis is the preparation of the aliquots. Given the extremely heterogeneous nature of mycotoxins throughout a lot, all the increments have to be gathered, thoroughly mixed, and ground, in order to form the aggregate sample. Only after this process can the aggregate sample be subdivided into aliquots that are representative of the lot.

25.4.3 Sample preparation

A further key point is to maintain the representativeness from the lot to the test aliquot. It is well known that the sample preparation variance can be reduced both by increasing the test aliquot size and by increasing the degree of comminuting. To date, one of the more appropriate methodologies for obtaining an homogeneous test aliquot is to slurry the aggregate sample with water by using ratios typically of 1:1.25, 1:1.5, 1:2 depending on the matrix.

25.5 Standardization of methods for detecting mycotoxins

In the past five years much has been achieved in the standardization in methodologies for the detection of mycotoxins. This is especially important given the need to have harmonized tools for the detection of these toxins in food matrices. The related requirement is the availability of validated methods and this need has pushed the European Commission to support collaborative trials aimed at covering the principal and more critical issues in this area.

In addition, in agreement with the provision requested by ISO 17025, the use of certified reference materials, the need to participate in interlaboratory studies for proficiency testing purposes, the use of recovery factors and other provisions are strongly recommended (ISO/IEC/EN 17025). Specific criteria for the selection of methods of analysis for mycotoxins are given in CEN Standard N195. In particular, repeatability, reproducibility, recovery, extraction solvents, applicability and food types are covered. Performance criteria are given for aflatoxin B_1, total aflatoxins including M_1, ochratoxin A, patulin, fumonisin B_1 and B_2, deoxynivalenol, nivalenol, HT-2 toxin, T-2 toxin and zearalenone.

The use of Certified Reference Materials (CRMs) as pivotal tools for the evaluation of precision and accuracy is rather limited at the moment in the mycotoxin area, but their number is currently increasing. At present, CRMs for mycotoxins include aflatoxins, aflatoxin M_1 in milk powder, aflatoxin B_1 in defatted peanut meal and in compound feed, ochratoxin A in wheat, and deoxynivalenol in corn and wheat. All CRMs for mycotoxins can be purchased from the Institute for Reference Materials and Measurements (IRMM – http://

www.irmm.jrc.be_). As for the Reference Materials, a wider selection of various mycotoxins in many food matrices are available at the Central Science Laboratory (CSL) through the Food Analysis Performance Assessment Scheme (FAPAS – http://ptg.csl.gov.uk/fapas.cfm). Currently several international organizations deal with the standardization and harmonization of methods, their work being influenced by the final target of the analysis (trade/protection of health/research). Trade issues fall under the CODEX Alimentarius umbrella, aimed not only at protecting consumers' health, but also at ensuring fair practices in the food trade; CODEX work also aims at promoting coordination of all the work undertaken by international governmental and non-governmental organizations. Standards for aflatoxin B_1 in peanuts, aflatoxin M_1 in milk and cheese, and patulin in apple juices are currently under consideration.

Protection of health is a major concern in the standardization activities of WHO, EU, ISO, AOAC and FAO. Validated quantitative, semi-quantitative and screening methods are currently available for several mycotoxins in various food matrices. The main aim is to harmonize along general principles the performance of analytical methodologies characterized by reliability and trueness. In this respect, a big effort has been made over the past decade by the European Commission, and a large number of validated methods have been provided so far. Validation studies are necessary to provide a reliable reference for the implementation of control activities and for compliance with national and international regulations. A strong limitation is that they are expensive, time-consuming, and in some cases do not lead to the desired results. For this reason, single-laboratory validation studies can also be undertaken in order to work in compliance with ISO 17025 (ISO, 1999; ISO/IEC/EN 17025). For the development of method validation and single-laboratory validation, the guidelines from AOAC and IUPAC/ISO/CODEX (Thompson *et al.*, 1999) are strongly recommended.

A matter of debate in the diagnostic of mycotoxins is the use of recovery factors in reporting the analytical measurements. An important document dealing with this matter is the harmonized guidelines IUPAC/ISO/AOAC/CODEX (IUPAC, 1997) for the use of recovery in analytical measurement. These guidelines outline the theoretical framework for those analyses where the loss of analyte during the analytical procedure is considered unavoidable. In this respect the main issues that still need to be harmonized are:

- the validity of methods for estimating the recovery of the analyte from the matrix
- whether the recovery estimate should be used to correct the raw data in the test result.

Currently, uncertainty of analytical measurement also represents a crucial point in the analysis of mycotoxins. The definition of the uncertainty is given by the ISO as: 'A parameter, associated with the result of a measurement, that characterizes the dispersion of the values that could reasonably be attributed to the measure'. Actually, the evaluation of uncertainty is quite a complex matter and the adoption of a harmonized approach for its measurement is still under debate. Currently, Eurachem model (bottom-up), AMC-RSC method (top-down), NMKL approach, and Horwitz equation as an approximate evaluation, are currently useful tools for the calculation of uncertainty. Recently, a SCOOP Task, namely SCOOP 9.1 (Task 9.1, 2002), dealing with the issue of uncertainty has been finalized by the EU. In the final report, areas where inconsistency among countries has been demonstrated or where further clarification is required for avoiding possible inconsistency were pointed out.

25.6 The range of analytical methods for mycotoxins

Analytical methods for mycotoxins are mainly based on thin layer chromatography (TLC), high performance liquid chromatograpy (HPLC) or enzyme linked immunosorbent assay (ELISA). Other techniques such as gas chromatography (GC), gas chromatography-mass spectrometry (GC-MS), liquid chromatograpy-mass spectrometry (LC-MS), capillary electrophoresis (EC), are also extensively used. An excellent review on methods for mycotoxin analysis was published by FAO (1990), and annual updating on analytical methods are provided by the General Referee Report, Committee on Natural Toxins, published in the *Journal of AOAC International*. The issue of analytical methodology is also reviewed by Miraglia (in press).

Although biological and immunoenzymatic methods have received increasing attention during the last decade for the determination of mycotoxins, chemical and immunochemical assays have been mostly preferred especially in industrialized countries for their characteristics including a low limit of detection and a high specificity. A short description of the main techniques used in the analysis of mycotoxins is given, grouping them on the basis of their characteristics.

25.6.1 Screening methods

Screening methods allow the testing of a large number of samples, but the confirmation of positive ones is recommended. A high reliability of the screening methods is based on a low number of false positives, as well as on a low percentage of false negatives (less than 5%). These techniques meet one of the needs of food industry production, namely the availability of rapid methods allowing the 'on-line control' of mycotoxins in food. Biosensors and kits based on dipstick techniques are promising methodologies based on immunochemical reactions (Anklam *et al.*, 2002).

Enzyme-linked immunosorbent assay (ELISA)

Enzyme-linked immunosorbent assay-based methods are user-friendly methods at relatively low cost for the screening of a high number of samples. However, the disadvantage of this technique is the possibility of obtaining false positives when a cross-reaction happens, as well as false negatives when very low levels of contamination are to be checked. Therefore the ELISA methods are suggested as low cost screening methods prior to confirmatory analysis, in order to lower the costs considerably, when a high number of samples has to be analysed (Anklam *et al.*, 2002). The World Health Organization (WHO) provides the criteria for the acceptance/validation of immunoassay based kits and of other protein binding systems (WHO, 1980).

ELISA methods are available for aflatoxins, fumonisins, ochratoxin A, zearalenone; many immunochemical methods are given for trichothecenes (Morgan, 1989; Candlish, 1991; Park and Chu, 1996). The limits of detection greatly depend on the mycotoxins being evaluated and on specific kit (for example 0.05 ng/ml for aflatoxin M_1, 0.5 μg–200 μg/kg for fumonisins).

An ELISA method for aflatoxins in corn and for zearalenone in corn, wheat and feed (Agri-screen method) has been tested by an interlaboratory study and accepted as AOAC Official method (AOAC Int., 2000). ELISA methods are not available for patulin as specific monoclonal antibodies have not been developed.

New techniques for rapid methods

Biosensors are devices that use biological components to react with or bind to a target molecule and thus transduce this event into a detectable signal. The advantages of this technology may include more rapid assays, reusable sensor elements, and the capacity for continuous monitoring. The use of biosensors for the detection of aflatoxins is rapidly increasing, including disposable DNA electrochemical biosensors (Marrazza *et al.*, 1999), handled immunoaffinity fluorimetric biosensors (Carlson *et al.*, 2000) and biosensors based on lipid films and liposomes (Nikolelis *et al.*, 1999).

The biosensor is termed as an immunosensor in which the biological component is an antibody or an antibody fragment. The immunosensors for chemical contaminants may be classified according to the transduction element, which can be an optical, an electrochemical or a piezoelectric signal.

In fibre-optical immunosensors monoclonal antibodies are covalently coupled to an optical fibre (Maragos and Thompson, 1999); an antibody-bound glass prism surface uses surface plasmon resonance (SPR) for the direct detection of fumonisin B_1 (Mullet *et al.*, 1998). Other immunosensors are electrochemical sensors, which are based on potentiometric or amperometric measurements (Patel, 2002). The principle of fluorence polarization immunoassay was used for the determination of DON in wheat (Maragos *et al.*, 2002a,b). Non-destructive techniques include near or mid-infrared spectroscopic methods (Kos, 2001; Petterson, 2001) and Fourier transform infrared photo-acoustic spectroscopy (FTIR-PAS). These techniques couple the rapidity with the possibility to detect many mycotoxins simultaneously (Schneider, 1995; van der Gaag *et al.*, 2003).

In the past few years this last requirement has been desirable for confirmation methods, especially with control and monitoring purposes, in which a high number of analyses with high reliability in a short time is requested. This possibility would also be useful to obtain information on the exposure to many mycotoxins and on the effect of combined exposure to human health.

25.6.2 Confirmatory methods

Thin layer chromatography (TLC)

Even though the use of TLC methods in this context has decreased steadily over the past few years, this analytical technique is still routinely employed, especially in developing countries. Thin layer chromatography methods allow for a precise determination, at a level not lower than 2 ng/g; their disadvantages include the use of solvents that are considered to be ecological hazards.

TLC techniques have been reviewed and updated for the analysis of selected *Fusarium* toxins (Krska *et al*., 2001); a TLC-based method for deoxynivalenol in barley and wheat is included in the Official Methods of Analysis of AOAC; TLC-based methods adopted as AOAC Official methods also include those for aflatoxins in peanuts and corn, for aflatoxin M_1 in milk and cheese, for aflatoxin B_1 and M_1 in liver, for ochratoxin A in barley and in green coffee, for deoxynivalenol in wheat, for sterigmatocystin in barley and wheat, and for zearalenone in corn.

The proposed use of TLC in combination with immunoaffinity columns (IACs) represents a promising application that can improve the performance characteristics of the TLC-based methods (Stroka *et al*., 2000). An improvement in the technique includes the use of a microcomputer interfaced with a fluorodensitometer to simplify data handling (Whitaker *et al*., 1990). New detection techniques for TLC have also been developed as alternatives to traditional TLC scanners; the principles are based on the use of a semiconductor-based detection cell (SeBaDeC) or of a modified office scanner. As the cost of commercial office scanners is very low, these are of special interest for the quantification of mycotoxins when other instruments are not available, such as in developing countries, in which this technique still represents the most economical method for the analysis of trichothecenes (Stroka and Anklam, 2002a).

High Performance Liquid Chromatography (HPLC)

A wide variety of methods for most mycotoxins are based on HPLC, the methodology of choice for aflatoxins, ochratoxins, fumonisins, patulin and zearalenone. Fluorescence detection is used for ochratoxin A, aflatoxins and fumonisins, usually as derivative compounds. UV detection is used for zearalenone, deoxynivalenol (Truksess *et al*., 1996) and patulin (MacDonald, *et al*., 2000). HPLC-based methods are used increasingly, especially given improved processing times using IACs in the clean-up step. Advantages of HPLC methods include excellent performance characteristics, low detection levels (as low as 0.1 ng/g) and safety for the operator.

Before HPLC quantification, the mycotoxin should be extracted from the matrix by shaking the sample with the appropriate solvent, often the solvent being a mixture of water and an organic solvent in suitable proportion. In the subsequent clean-up step, the sample is purified and prepared for HPLC analysis; for most mycotoxins the clean-up step consists of two different approaches, the use of solid-phase extraction (SPE) cartridges and the use of immunoaffinity columns (IAC). The major advantages of SPE are mainly the possibility to regenerate the cartridge for further analysis and a very cheap cost. Disadvantages are a potentially low reproducibility of different batches of columns and/or possible low repeatability within a single batch. On the other hand the use of antibody-based immunoaffinity columns recently led to a considerable increase of reliability of results due to the high selectivity of this technique. Other advantages are the reduced time of analysis and the possibility, in proper conditions, to analyse more than one sample at a same time. Generally, the extract is purified by an immunoaffinity column containing antibodies specific for the mycotoxin under examination. The summarized procedure is quite similar for all the mycotoxins that can be analysed with the HPLC technique.

Association of Analytical Communities Official methods (AOAC Int., 2000) using HPLC include the Mycosep® clean-up procedure for aflatoxins in corn, almonds, Brazil nuts, peanuts and pistachio nuts; and the immunoaffinity column and post-column derivatization with pyridinium bromide perbromide (PBPB) for the determination of aflatoxin B_1 and total aflatoxins in peanut butter, pistachio paste, fig paste and paprika powder (Garner *et al.*, 1993). Other kinds of derivatization for aflatoxin analysis include post-column derivatization with iodine (Tunistra and Haasnoot, 1983) and with electrochemically generated bromide (Kobra Cell) (Kok *et al.*, 1986a, b), photolytic derivatization (Papadopoulou-Bouraoui *et al.*, 2002) and a pre-column derivatization with trifluoroacetic acid (TFA) (Beebe, 1978).

Methods for the determination of OTA by HPLC, mainly based on fluorescence detection, are also available. Since OTA shows native fluorescence, usually no derivatization step is required for the detection of this toxin. For confirmation purposes three methods are usually adopted, based on methylation (Cantafora *et al.*, 1983; Uchiyama *et al.*, 1985), an ammonia derivative formation (Micco *et al.*, 1995) and by LC-MS confirmation (Abramson, 1987; Ominski *et al.*, 1996).

Patulin is also usually determined by HPLC. According to the validated AOAC method the sample is extracted with ethyl acetate, employing the enzyme pectinase for ameliorating the performance of the method (MacDonald *et al.*, 2000). An LC method uses extraction and clean-up steps with a combination of Extrelut and Florisil cartridges (Herry and Leméayer, 1996). The use of SPE was also reported (Trucksess and Tang, 1999). In the reverse-phase LC the quantification of patulin is performed with UV detection (276 nm). GC/MS methods are also reported operating both without (Llovera *et al.*, 1999), and with various derivatizing agents (Rupp and Turnipseed, 2000; Roach *et al.*, 2000).

Notwithstanding, trichothecenes are frequently analysed by GC methods for HPLC, in particular an HPLC method was developed by Trucksess *et al.* (1996) for DON in wheat finished products. For the application of HPLC in the analysis of zearalenone, the method of Bennett *et al.* (1985) has also been adopted as an official method by AOAC (AOAC Int., 2000). Other methods based on HPLC and fluorescence detection are reported by Tanaka *et al.* (1993) and by Siedel *et al.* (1993).

Liquid chromatography with fluorescence detection remains the method of choice for the determination of fumonisins (Sydenham *et al.*, 1992; Ross *et al.*, 1990). An AOAC-IUPAC collaborative study with a liquid chromatographic method, based on the use of solid-phase extraction (SPE) cartridges and ortho-phthaldialdehyde (OPA) as derivatizing agent, was accepted as an official method of analysis (AOAC Int., 2000). In the final version the method is suitable for the determination of FB_1, FB_2 and FB_3. A method with an immunoaffinity column, based on clean-up and OPA plus 2-mercaptoethanol as derivative agent, was recently submitted to a collaborative study (Solfrizzo, 2000). A novelty in the clean up of fumonisins employing SAX (Strong Anion Exchange) + C18 was presented by Moller and Gustavsson (2000).

In the last few years, for fumonisin analysis, emphasis has also been given to capillary electrophoresis (Hines *et al.*, 1995), to evaporative light-scattering detection (Wilkes *et al.*, 1995; Plattner, 1995) and to mass spectrometry (Musser, 1996a,b; Seo *et al.*, 1996; Plattner *et al.*, 1996; Josephs, 1996; Meredith *et al.*, 1996), even though these techniques are generally useful for confirmatory but not for analytical work to be performed on a routine basis.

A wide number of HPLC methods for the analysis of various mycotoxins were tested by collaborative studies, to evaluate their effectiveness, and periodically reported on Methods Committee Reports published on Journal of AOAC International. Such methods include the liquid chromatographic method for the determination of patulin in clear and cloudy apple juices and apple puree (MacDonald *et al.*, 2000), the determination of aflatoxin B_1 in baby food (infant formula) by immunoaffiniy column clean-up and post-column bromination (Stroka and Anklam, 2002b), the determination of ochratoxin A in roasted coffee (Entwisle *et al.*, 2001).

Gas Chromatography (GC)

Gas chromatography-based methods represent the most widely employed technique for the determination of trichothecenes, as DON and NIV, since these compounds do not absorb strongly in the UV visible range and are non-fluorescent. In particular the gas chromatography and capillary column GC represent the most developed and used analytical techniques for the determination of multiple trichothecenes. Heptafluorobutyryl (HFB), trimethylsilyl (TMS) and trifluoroacetyl derivatives are frequently used, coupled with electron capture detection (ECD); however MS should be employed for confirmation of the peaks. A GC method (Heisel, 1986) has been collaboratively tested in barley and malt and accepted by the American Society of Brewing Chemists in its *Methods of Analysis*, 8th edn. Available methods for trichothecenes also include the Scott and Ware methods (Scott *et al.*, 1986; Ware *et al.*, 1984).

As for DON, determination methods have also been developed involving supercritical fluid chromatography (Young, 1992). In comparison with LC, supercritical fluid chromatography is characterized by sharper peaks and faster analysis times, similar to those obtained by capillary GC. The GC method for the determination of deoxynivalenol in wheat is reported by AOAC Official methods (AOAC Int., 2000).

Gas chromatography coupled with mass spectrometry could be used for the confirmation of patulin in apple juice (Roach *et al.*, 2000). Due to the low sensitivity, poor recovery and high level of imprecision, gas chromatography mass selective detection methods are not recommended as screening methods, while they fit better as confirmation tool as in the case of ochratoxin A in wine and beer (Soleas *et al.*, 2001).

Capillary Electrophoresis (CE)

Capillary electrophoresis is an analytical technique more and more extensively used in food analysis, its main advantages being reduction of organic solvents, small sample volume, increased efficiency and resolution. However, due to the rather high detection limit, the technique is not generally suitable for the determination of low concentration of mycotoxins. As for patulin, due to the lack of monoclonal antibodies for the step of immunoaffinity clean-up, the determination by capillary electrophoresis, as carried out by Tsao and Zhou (2000), presents the advantage of a relatively low limit of detection (3.8 μg/l).

Liquid Chromatography-Mass Spectrometry (LC-MS).

McFadden and Schueler (1969) performed the analysis of aflatoxins B_1, B_2, G_1, and G_2 by ion reconstruction at m/z 313, 315, 329, and 331 for the four aflatoxins respectively, by using a moving belt interface. Tiebach *et al.* (1985) used a direct liquid induction (DLI) interface with a reversed-phase microbore LC system, and obtained positive-ion chemical ionisation (PCI) and negative ion chemical ionisation (NCI) spectra for aflatoxin M_1 and reconstructed ion chromatograms for aflatoxins B_1, B_2, and M_1 (Tateo *et al.*, 1998).

A liquid chromatography/mass spectrometry method was reported by Cappiello *et al.* (1995) The chromatographic separation was performed with a reversed-phase packed capillary column coupled with a modified particle beam interface, capable of handling flow rates of microlitres per minute.

A rapid determination of fumonisin B_1 is performed without any clean-up or purification step using a straightforward HPLC-electrospray mass specrometry screening method (Hartl *et al.*, 1999). Determination and confirmation of aflatoxins B_1 and B_2, using aflatoxin M_1 as an internal standard, in several food products such as figs and peanuts, has been achieved by coupling with mass spectrometry. Due to the interference in the mass chromatograms, the quantification of aflatoxins using MS has proved unsatisfactory (Vahl and Jørgenson, 1998). LC-MS instruments using APCI (atmospheric pressure chemical ionization) interfaces or electrospray have recently been employed for the determination and identification of trichothecenes, including deoxynivalenol, at trace levels (Razzazi-Fazeli *et al.*, 1999; Plattner and Maragos, 2003; Laganà *et al.*, 2003).

25.7 Dealing with mycotoxins in developing countries

In many developing countries, agriculture represents the main sources of food and income, export markets to developed countries being especially important. For geographical and climatic reasons in many of those countries crops are highly susceptible to mycotoxin contamination thus impairing not only the health of the population but also the economic value of the exported crops.

As previously described, at the moment, in many developed countries, maximum tolerable levels have been characterized for specific mycotoxins in food destined for human and animal consumption. However, limits have not yet been set in many developing countries, and, in order to reach acceptable quality standards suitable for export requirements, those countries should be assisted by means of adequate training courses, in developing their ability to prevent and control mycotoxin contamination.

The main target for these countries is to limit mycotoxin contamination in the field by means of good agriculture practice, that have to be established on the basis of the specific geographical conditions and crop. In addition to prevention during crop cultivation, harvest and storage steps should be considered as critical control points. As for the relevance of control analysis in developing countries, it is crucial to set out a plan for the foodstuffs intended for export, together with the implementation of monitoring plans on the product destined for the internal market. The effectiveness of analytical controls depends on the availability of equipment and on the capability of the personnel. More often in developing countries methods of screening such as ELISA kits, are preferred, since they have low costs and do not require any qualified staff. These methods are not sufficiently accurate as screening methods, due to the occurrence of false positive answers and therefore they should be coupled with suitable confirmatory methods. It is of utmost importance that the ability of developing countries should also include the implementation of good sampling procedures.

25.8 References

ABRAMSON D (1987), 'Measurement of ochratoxin A in barley extracts by liquid chromatography-mass spectrometry', *J. Chromatog.*, 391, 315–320.

ACAR JALE (1998), 'The effects of processing technology on the patulin content of juice during commercial apple juice concentrate production', *Z Lebensm Unters Forsch A* 207, 328–331.

ANKLAM E, STROKA J, BENKE A (2002), 'Acceptance of analytical methods for implementation of EU legislation with a focus on mycotoxins', *Food Control* 13, 173–183.

AOAC INTERNATIONAL (2000), *Official Methods of Analysis* 17th edn, vol. II. Cunniff P, Arlington, VA, AOAC Int., 49, 1–60.

BAXTER E D (1996), 'The fate of ochratoxin A during malting and brewing', *Food Addit. Contam.*, 13, 23–24.

BEEBE R M (1978), 'Reverse-phase HPLC determination of aflatoxins in foods', *J. Ass. Off. Anal. Chem. Int.* 61, 1347–1352.

BENNETT G A, SHOTWELL O L, KWOLEK W F (1985), 'Liquid chromatographic determination of α-zearalenol and zearalenone in corn: Collaborative study', *J. Ass. Off. Anal. Chem.*, 68.

BETINA V (1993), *Mycotoxins: chemical, biological and environmental aspects*, Elsevier, Amsterdam.

BRERA C, MIRAGLIA M, ONORI R (1996), 'HACCP and Mycotoxins: What is the Point of Interaction?', in Miraglia M, van Egmond H P, Brera C, Gilbert J (eds), *Mycotoxins and Phycotoxins Toxicology and Food Safety*, Alaken, Inc. Fort Collins, CO.

BRERA C, MIRAGLIA M, CALFAPIETRA F R, PAZZAGLINI B, GROSSI S, YAZDANPANAH H (2000), 'Ochratoxin A in human milk: Exposure assessment of babies', in De Koe W, Samson R, van Egmond H P, Gilbert J, (eds) *Mycotoxins and Phycotoxins in Perpective at the Turn of the Millennium.* Wageningen, The Netherlands

BRERA C, DEBEGNACH F, GROSSI S, MIRAGLIA M (2004), 'Effect of the industrial processing on the distribution of fumonisins B_1 in dry milling corn fractions', accepted for publication in *Journal of Food Protection* vol. 67.

CANDLISH A A G (1991), 'The Determination of Mycotoxins in Animal Feeds by Biological Methods', in Smith J E, Henderson R S (eds), *Mycotoxins and Animal Foods*, CRC Press, Boca Raton, FL.

CANTAFORA A, GROSSI M, MIRAGLIA M, BENELLI L (1983), 'Determination of ochratoxin A in coffee beans using reverse phase high performance liquid chromatography', *Riv. Soc. Ital. Sci. Alim.* 12, 103–108.

CAPPIELLO A, FAMIGLINI G, TIRILLINI B (1995), 'Determination of aflatoxins in peanut meal by LC/MS with a particle beam interface', *J. Chromatographia*, 40, 411–416.

CARAMELLI, M, DONDO A, CANTINI CORTELLAZZI G, VISCONTI A, MINERVINI F, DOKO M B AND GUARDA F (1993), 'Leukoencephalomalacia nell'equino da fumonisine: prima segnalazione in Italia', *Ippologia,* 4, 49–56.

CARLSON M A, BARGERON C B, BENSON R C, FRASER A, PHILLIPS T E, VELKY J T, GROOPMAN J D, STRICKLAND P T, KO E H W (2000), 'An automated, handheld biosensor for aflatoxin', *Biosens & Bioelectron* 14, 841–848.

CAST (2003), *Mycotoxins: Risks in Plant, Animal and Human Systems*, Task Force Report, ISSN 0194; N. 139.

COMMISSION DIRECTIVE (1998), Commission Directive 98/53/EC of 16 July 1998, laying down the sampling methods of analysis for the official control of the levels for certain contaminants in foodstuffs, OJ L 201, vol 93 17 July 1998.

COMMISSION DIRECTIVE (2002a), Commission Directive 2002/26/EC of 13 March 2002 laying down the sampling methods and the methods of analysis for the official control of the levels of ochratoxin A in foodstuffs, O J L 75 16 March 2001.

COMMISSION DIRECTIVE (2002b), Commission Directive 2002/27/EC of 13 March 2002, amending Directive 98/53/EC laying down the sampling methods and the methods of analysis for the official control of the levels for certain contaminants in foodstuffs, OJ L 75, vol 44 16 March 2002.

COMMISSION DIRECTIVE (2003), Commission Directive 2003/78/EC of 11 August 2003 laying down the sampling methods and the methods of analysis for the official control of the levels of patulin in foodstuffs, O J L 203, 12 August 2003.

COMMISSION REGULATION (2002), Commission Regulation (EC) No 472/2002 of 12 March 2002 amending Regulation (EC) No 466/2001, OJ L 75, vol 18 16 March 2002.

COMMISSION REGULATION (2003a), Commission Regulation (EC) No 2174/2003 of 12 December 2003 amending Regulation (EC) No 466/2001 as regards aflatoxins, OJ L 326, 12 December 2003.

COMMISSION REGULATION (2003b), Commission Regulation (EC) No 1425/2003 of 11 August 2003 amending Regulation (EC) No 466/2001 as regards patulin, OJ L 203, vol 46 12 August 2003.

COUNCIL DIRECTIVE (1993), 93/43/EEC June 1993 on the hygiene of foodstuffs, OJ L 175, 19 July 1993.

DE SYLOS C M, RODRIGUEZ-AMAYA D B (1999), 'Incidence of patulin in fruits and fruit juices marketed in Campinas, Brazil', *Food Addit. Contam.* 16, 71–74.

DIENER U L (1969), 'Production of aflatoxin on peanut under controlled environments', *J. Stored Prod. Res.*, 5: 251–258.

ENTWISLE A C, WILLIAMS A C, MANN P J, RUSSEL J, SLACK P T, GILBERT J (2001), 'Combined phenylsilane and immunoaffinity column clean-up with liquid chromatography for determination of ochratoxin A in roasted coffee: Collaborative study', *J. Ass. Off. Anal. Chem. Int.*, 84, 1116–1122.

FAO (1990), Food and Agricolture Organization of the United Nations, 'Training in Mycotoxins Analysis. Manual of food quality control'.

FAO (1997), Worldwide regulations for mycotoxins – A compendium. FAO, Food and Nutrition Paper No 64 FAO, Rome, Italy.

FAO/WHO (1995), 'Application of risk analysis to food standards issues. Report of the Joint FAO/WHO Expert Consultation', Geneva, 13–17 March WHO.

FINK-GREMMELS J (1998), 'Mycotoxins: Mechanism of Action at the Molecular Level', in Miraglia M, van Egmond H P, Brera C, Gilbert J, (eds) *Mycotoxins and Phycotoxins – Developments in Chemistry, Toxicology and Food Safety*, Alaken, Inc. Fort Collins, CO.

FRISVAD J C (1989), 'Terverticillate penicellia: chemotaxonomy and mycotoxin production', *J Mycologia*, 81, 837–861.

GARNER R C, WHATTMAN M M, TAYLOR P J L, STOW M W (1993), 'Analysis of United Kingdom purchased spices of aflatoxins using an immunoaffinity columns cleanup procedure followed by high performance liquid chromatography analysis and postcolumn derivatization with pyridinium bromide perbromide', *J. Chromatog.* 648, 485–490.

GELDERBLOM W C A, KRIEK N P J, MARASAS W F O, THIEL P G (1991), 'Toxicity and carcinogeniticy of the Fusarium moniliforme metabolite, fumonisin B_1, in rats', *Carcinogenesis,* 12, 1247–1251.

HARRISON L R, COLVIN B M, GREENE J T, NEWMAN L E, COLE J R (1990), 'Pulmonary edema and hydrothorax in swine produced by fumonisin B_1, a toxic metabolite of Fusarium moniliforme', *Journal of Veterinary Diagnostic Investigation,* 2, 217–221.

HARTL M, HERDERICH M, HUMPF H U (1999), 'Rapid determination of Fumonisin FB_1 in corn products by high perfomannce liquid chromatography electrospray mass spectrometry', *Eur. Food Res. Technol.,* 209, 348–351.

HEILMANN W, REHFELDT A G, ROTZOLL F (1999), 'Behaviour and reduction of ochratoxin A in green coffee beans in response to various processing methods', *Eur. Food Res.*

Technol., 209, 297–300.

HEISEL S (1986), 'Deoxinivalenol in barley and malt', *J. Am. Soc. Brew. Chem.*, 54, 268–270.

HERRY M P, LEMÉAYER N (1996), 'Liquid chromatography determination of patulin in French apple ciders', *J. Ass. Off. Anal. Chem. Int.*, 79, 1107–1110.

HINES H B, BRUEGGEMANN E E, HOLCOMB M, HOLDER C L (1995), Fumonisin B_1 analysis with capillary electrophoresis electrospray ionization mass spectrometry', *Rapid. Commun. Mass. Spectrom.*, 9,519–524.

http://europa.eu.int/comm/food/fs/sc/scf/outcome_en.htlm

http://europa.eu.int/comm/food/fs/sc/scf/reports_en.htlm

IARC (1993), 'Monograph on the evaluation of carcinogenic Risk to Human', Vol 56. http://www.iarc.uaf.edu/2002_conferences.html.

IARC (2002), 'Monograph on the evaluation of carcinogenic Risk to Human' Vol 82. http://www.iarc.uaf.edu/2002_conferences.html.

IAVICOLI I, BRERA C, CARELLI G, CAPUTI R, MARINACCIO A, MIRAGLIA M (2002), 'External and internal dose of subjects occupationally exposed to ochratoxin A', *J Int. Arch. Occup. Environ. Health.*, 75 (6), 381–6.

IPCS (1990), *Environmental health Criteria 105*, Selected mycotoxins WHO, Vammala.

ISO (1999), ISO/IEC/EN 17025, Test and Calibration Lab Requirements Sanctioned Interpretation to ISO/TS 16949. http://www.fasor.com/iso25.

ISO/IEC/EN 17025, *Formerly ISO Guide 25 & EN45001, General Requirements for the Competence of Calibration and Testing Laboratories.*

IUPAC (1997), 'Harmonized guidelines for the use of recovery information in analytical mesurement', Resulting from the Symposium on Harmonization of Internal Quality Assurance Systems for Analytical Laboratories, Orlando, USA, 4–5 September 1996, held under the sponsorship of IUPAC, ISO and AOAC Int.

JOSEPHS L (1996), 'Detection and characterization of fumonisin mycotoxins by liquid chromatography/electrospray ionisation using ion trap and triple quadrupole mass spectrometry', *Rapid Commun. Mass Spectrom.*, 10, 1333–1344.

KOK W, BRINKAM U A, FREI R W (1986a), 'Online electrochemical reagent production for detection in HPLC and continuous flow system', *Anal. Chim. Acta* 162, 19–32.

KOK W, VAN NEER C H, TRAAG V A, TUNISTRA L G M (1986b), 'Determination of aflatoxins in cattle feed by liquid chromatography and postcolumn derivatization with electrochemically generated bromine', *J. Chromatog.* 367, 231–236.

KOS G (2001), 'Entwicklung einer neuen Detektionsmethode zur Bestimmung von Fusarien Pilzen auf Mais mittels FT-IR/ATR Spektroscopie', Proceedings of the 23th Mycotoxins Workshop. Wien.

KROGH P (1987), *Mycotoxins in Food. Food Science and Tecnology*, Academic Press.

KRSKA R, BAUMGARTNER S, JOSEPHS R (2001), The state-of-the-art in the analysis of type-A and B trichothecene mycotoxins in cereals', *Fresenius J Anal. Chem.*, 371, 285–299.

LAGANÀ A, CURINI R, D'ASCENZO G, DE LEVA I, FABERI A, PASTORINI E (2003), 'Liquid chromatography/tandem mass spectrometry for the identification and determination of tricothecenes in maize', *Rapid Communications in Mass Spectrometry*, 17 (10), 1037–43.

LLOVERA M, VILADRICH R, TORRES M, CANELA R (1999), 'Analysis of underivatizated patulin by a GC-MS technique', *J. Food Prot.*, 62, 202–205.

LOPEZ-GARCIA R (2001), 'Mycotoxin management: an integrated approach', in Miraglia M, van Egmond H P, Brera C, Gilbert J, (eds) *Mycotoxins and Phycotoxins Toxicology and Food Safety*, Alaken, Inc. Fort Collins, CO.

MACDONALD S, LONG M, GILBERT J (2000), 'Liquid chromatographic method for determination of patulin in clear and cloudy apple juices and apple puree: Collaborative study', *J. Ass. Off. Anal. Chem. Int.*, 83, 1387–1394.

MANNON J (1985), 'Fungi down on the farm', *J. New Scientist*, 195:12–16, 1985

MARAGOS C M, THOMPSON V S (1999), 'Fiber-optic immunosensor for mycotoxins', *Nat Toxins* 7, 371–376.

MARAGOS C M, JOLLEY M E, NASIR M S (2002a), *Food. Addit. Contam.*, 19, 400–407.

MARAGOS C M, PLATTNER R D (2002b), *J. Agric Food Chem.*, 50, 1827–1832.

MARRAZZA G, CHIANELLA I, MASCINI M (1999), 'Disposable DNA electrochemical biosensors for environmental monitoring', *Anal. Chim. Acta.* 387, 297–307.

MCFADDEN T F, SCHUELER T A (1969), Malt beverage preservation', United States Patent, 18.

MEISTER U (2001), 'Investigations on the change of fumonisin content of maize during hidrothermal treatment of maize. Analysis by means of HPLC methods and ELISA', *Eur. Food Res. Technol.*, 213, 187–193.

MEREDITH F I, BACON C W, NORRED W P, PLATTNER R D (1996), 'Isolation and purification of fumonisin B_1 and B_2 from rice culture', in Jackson L S, DeVries J W, Bullerman L B, (eds) *Fumonisins in Food*, New York, Plenum Press.

MICCO C, AMBRUZZI M A, MIRAGLIA M, BRERA C, BENELLI L, CORNELI S (1995), 'Evaluation of ochratoxin A in human milk', *Food Addit. Contam.*, 12, 351–354.

MIRAGLIA M, DE SANTIS B, GROSSI S, BRERA CM (in press), 'Mycotoxin' in Nollet L, *Handbook of Food Analysis*, 2nd edn, accepted for publication in *Journal of Food Protection*.

MOLLER T E, GUSTAVSSON H F (2000), 'Determination of fumosins B1 and B2 in various maize products by a combined SAX + C18 column and immunoaffinity column', *J. Ass. Off. Anal. Chem. Int.*, 83, 99–103.

MORGAN M R A (1989), 'Mycotoxins immunoassays (with special reference to ELISAs)', *Tetrahedron*, 45, 2237–2249.

MULLET W, LAI E P, YEUNG J M (1998), 'Immunoassay of fumonisins by a surface plasmon resonance biosensor', *Analytical Biochem.*, 258 (2), 161–7.

MUSSER S M (1996a), 'Quantitation and identification of fumonisins by liquid chromatography/mass spectrometry', in Jackson L S, DeVries J W, Bullerman L B, (eds) *Fumonisins in Food*. New York, Plenum Press.

MUSSER S M (1996b), 'Quantitation and identification of fumonisins by liquid chromatography/mass spectrometry', *Adv. Exp. Med. Bio.*, 1392, 65–74.

NIKOLELIS D P, HIANIK T, KRULL U J (1999), 'Biosensors based on thin lipid films and liposomes' [Review], *Electroanalysis* 11, 7–15.

OMINSKI K H, FROHLICH A A, MARQURDT R R, CROW G H, ABRAMSON D (1996), 'The incidence and distribution or ochratoxin A in western Canadian swine', *Food Addit. Contam.*, 13, 185–198.

OSBORNE B G, IBE F, BROWN G L, PETAGINE F, SCUDAMORE K A, BANSK J N, HETMANSKI M T, LEONARD C T (1996), 'The effects of miling and processing on wheat contaminated with ochratoxin A, *Food Addit. Contam.*, 13 (2) 141–153.

PALLI D, MIRAGLIA M, SAPEVA C, MASSALA G, CAVA E, COLATOSTI M, CORSI A M, RUSSO A, BRERA C (1999), 'Serum levels of ochratoxin A in healthy adults in Tuscany: correlation with individual characteristic and between repeat measurements', *Cancer Epidemiol. Biomarkers Prev.* 8, 265–267.

PAPADOPOULOU-BOURAOUI A, STROKA J, ANKLAM E (2002), 'Comparison of two post-column derivatization systems, ultraviolet irradiation and electrochemical determination, for the liquid chromatographic determination of aflatoxins in food', *J. Ass. Off. Anal. Chem. Int.* 85, 411–416.

PARK J J, CHU F S (1996), 'Assessment of immunochemical methods for the analysis of trichothecene mycotoxins in naturally occurring mouldy corn', *J. Assoc. Off. Anal. Chem. Int.* 79, 465–471.

PATEL P D (2002), 'Biosensor for measurement of analytes implicated in food safety: a review', *Trends Anal. Chem.,* 21, 96–115.

PAYNE A G (1998), 'Process of Contamination by Aflatoxin-producing Fungi and their Impact on Crops', in Sinha K K S, Bhtnagar D, *Mycotoxins in Agroculture and Food Safety*, Marcel Dekker, Inc., New York.

PERAICA M, DOMIJAN A M, MATASIN M, LUCIC A, BOZICA R, DELAS F, HORVAT M, BOSANAC I, BALIJA M, GRGICEVIC D (2001), 'Variations of ochratoxin A concentration in the blood of healthy populations in some Croatian cities', *Short Communication*, Springer Verlag.

PETTERSON H (2001), Near infrared spectroscopy for screening of mycotoxins', in *Proceedings of the World Mycotoxin Forum*, Noordwijk.

PLATTNER R D (1995), 'Detection of fumonisins produced in *Fusarium moniliforme* cultures by HPLC with electrospray MS and evaporative light scattering detectors', *Nat. Toxins*, 3, 294–298.

PLATTNER R D, MARAGOS C M (2003), 'Determination of deoxynivalenol and nivalenol in corn and wheat by liquid chromatography with electrospray mass spectrometry', *J. AOAC Int.*, 86 (1), 61–5.

PLATTNER R D, WEISLEDER D, POLING S M (1996), Analytical determination of fumonisins and other metabolites produced by *Fusarium moniliforme* and related species in corn', in Jackson L S, DeVries J W, Bullerman L B (eds), *Fumonisins in Food*, New York, Plenum Press.

RAZZAZI-FAZELI E, BÖHM J, LUF W J (1999), 'Determination of nivalenol and deoxynivalenol in wheat using liquid chromatography-mass spectrometry with negative ion atmospheric pressure chemical ionisation', *J. Chromatog. A*, 854, 45–55.

Reg. (EC) 2003, N. 1425/2003 of 11 August 2003, Official Journal of European Union, L203, Vol 46, 12 August 2003.

ROACH J A, WHITE K D, TRUCKSESS M W, THOMAS F S (2000), 'Capillary gas chromatography/mass spectrometry with chemical ionization and negative ion detection for confirmation of identity of patulin in apple juice', *J. Ass. Off. Anal. Chem. Int.*, 83, 104–112.

ROSS P F, NELSON P E, RICHARD J L, OSWEILER G D, RICE L G, PLATTNER R D, WILSON T M (1990), 'Production of fumonisins by *Fusarium moniliforme* and *Fusarium proliferatum* isolates associated with equine leukoencephalomalacia and a pulmonary oedema syndrome in swine', *Appl. Env. Microbiol.,* 56, 3225–3228.

RUPP H S, TURNIPSEED S B (2000), 'Confirmation of patulin and 5–hydroxymethylfurfural in apple juice by gas chromatography/mass spectrometry', *J. Ass. Off. Anal. Chem. Int.,* 83, 612–620.

RYCHLIK M, SCHIEBERLE P (2001), 'Model studies on the diffusion behavior of the mycotoxin patulin in apples, tomates, and wheat bread', *Eur. Food Res. Technol.*, 212, 274–278.

SCF (1999), 'Opinion on Fusarium Toxins. Part1: Deoxynivalenol (DON)' SCF/CS/CNTM/MYC/19 Final, http://europa.eu.int/comm/food/fs/sc/scf/out44_en.pdf.

SCF (2000a), 'Opinion of the Scientific Committee on Food on Fusarium Toxins. Part 2: Zearalenone (ZEA).' SCF/CS/CNTM/MYC/22 Rev 3 Final, http://europa.eu.int/comm/food/fs/sc/scf/out65_en.pdf.

SCF (2000b), 'Opinion of the Scientific Committee on Food on Fusarium Toxins. Part 3: Fumonisin B1 (FB1)', SCF/CS/CNTM/MYC/24 Final, http://europa.eu.int/comm/food/fs/sc/scf/out73_en.pdf.

SCF (2000c), 'Opinion of the Scientific Committee on Food on Fusarium Toxins. Part 4: Nivalenol', SCF/CS/CNTM/MYC/26 Final http://europa.eu.int/comm/food/fs/sc/scf/out74_en.pdf.

SCF (2001), 'Opinion of the Scientific Committee on Food on Fusarium Toxins. Part 5: T-2 Toxin and HT-2 Toxin', SCF/CS/CNTM/MYC/25 Rev 6 Final, http://europa.eu.int/comm/food/fs/sc/scf/out88_en.pdf.

SCF (2002), 'Opinion of the Scientific Committee on Food on Fusarium Toxins. Part 6: Group evaluation of T-2 toxin, HT-2 toxin, nivalenol and deoxynivalenol', SCF/CS/CNTM/MYC/27 Final, http://europa.eu.int/comm/food/fs/sc/scf/out123_en.pdf.

SCHNEIDER E, USLEBER E, MARTLBAUER E, DIETRICH R, TERPLAN G (1995), 'Multimycotoxin dipstick enzyme immunoassay applied to wheat', *Food Addit. Contam.*, 12 (3), 387–93.

SCOTT P M (1996),'Effects of processing and detoxification treatments on ochratoxin A: intoduction', *Food Addit. Contam.*, 13, 19–21.

SCOTT P M, KANHERE S R, TARTER E J (1986), 'Determination of nivalenol and deoxynivalenol in cereals by electron-capture gas chromatography', *J. Ass. Off. Anal. Chem.*, 69, 889–893.

SCOTT P M, KANHERE S R, LAU B P, LEWIS D A, HAYWARD S, RYAN J J, KUIPERGOODMAN (1998), 'Survey of Canadian human blood plasma for ochratoxin A', *Food Addit and Contam.*, 15, 555–562.

SCUDAMORE K A (1996), 'Ochratoxin A in animal feed-effects of processing', *Food Addit. Contam.*, 13, 39–42.

SEO J A, KIM J C, LEE Y W (1996), 'Isolation and characterization of two new type C fumonisins produced by *Fusarium oxysporum', J. Nat. Prod.*, 59, 1003–1005.

SIEDEL V, POGLITIS E, SCHILLER K, LINDNER W (1993), 'Simultaneous determination of ochratoxin A and zearalenone in maize by reversed phase high performance liquid chromatography with fluorescence detection and β-cyclodestrin as mobile phase additive', *J. Chromatog.*, 635, 227–235.

SMITH J E, LACEY J, CUERO R, RAMAKRISHNA N, AND GQALENI N (1998), 'Storage Product Ecology and Mycotoxin Formation', in Miraglia M, van Egmond H P, Brera C, Gilbert J, (eds) *Mycotoxins and Phicotoxins Developments in Chemistry, Toxicology and Food Safety*, Alaken, Inc. Fort Collins, CO.

SOFLRIZZO M, DE GIROLAMO A, VISCONTI A, SIZOO E, VAN EGMOND H P (2000), 'Determination of fumonisins B1 and B2 in corn based foodstuffs by high performance liquid chromatography after immunoaffinity clean-up – In house and interlaboratory validation', in De Koe W, Samson R, van Egmond H P, Gilbert J, (eds) *Mycotoxins and Phycotoxins in Perspective at the Turn of the Millennium*. Wageningen, The Netherlands.

SOLEAS G J, YAN J, GOLDBERG D M (2001), Assay of ochratoxin A in wine and beer by high pressure chromatography photodiode array and gas ghromatography mass selective detection', *J. Agric. Food Chem.*, 49, 2733–2740.

STROKA J, ANKLAM E (2002a), New strategies for the screening and determination of aflatoxins and the detection of aflatoxin-producing moulds in food and feed', *Trends Anal. Chem.* 21, 90–95.

STROKA J, ANKLAM E (2002b), Determination of aflatoxin B_1 in baby food (infant formula) by immunoaffiniy column clean-up liquid chromatography with post-column bromination: Collaborative study', *J. Ass. Off. Anal. Chem. Int.*, 84, 1116–1122.

STROKA J, VAN OTTERDIJK R, ANKLAM E (2000), 'Immunoaffinity column clean up prior to thin layer choromatography for the determination of aflatoxin in various food matrices', *J Chrom. A*, 904, 251–256.

SUBIRADE I (1996), 'Fate of ochratoxin A during breadmaking', *Food Addit. Contam.*, 13, 25–26.

SYDENHAM E W, SHEPHARD G S, THIEL P G (1992), 'Liquid chromatographic determination of fumonisins B_1 B_2 and B_3 in foods and feeds', *J. Ass. Off. Anal. Chem. Int.,* 75, 313–318.

SYDENHAM E W, THIEL P G, VLEGGAR R (1996), 'Physicochemical data for some selected Fusarium toxins', *J Ass. Off. Anal. Chem. Int.* 79, 1365–1379.

SYDENHAM W E, VISMER H F, MARASAS W F O, BROWN N L, SCHLECHTER M, RHEEDER J P (1997), 'The influence of deck storage and initial processing on patulin levels in apple juice', *Food Addit. Contam.*, 14, 429–434.

TANAKA T, TESHIRNA R, IKEBUCHI H, SAWADA J, TERAO T, ICHINOE M (1993), Sensitive determination of zearalenone and α-zearalenol in bar1ey and Job's-tears by liquid chromatography with fluorescence detection', *J. Ass. Off. Anal. Chem. Int.*, 76, 1006–1009.

TASK 3.2.7 (2002), 'Assessment of Dietary Intake of Ochratoxin A by the Population of EU Member States', http://europa.eu.int/comm/food/fs/scoop/3.2.7_en.pdf.

TASK 3.2.8 (2002), 'Assessment of Dietary Intake of Patulin by the Population of EU Member States', http://europa.eu.int/comm/food/fs/scoop/3.2.8_en.pdf

TASK 3.2.10 (2003), 'Collection of Occurrence Data of Fusarium Toxins in Food and Assessment of Dietary Intake by the Population of EU Member States', http://europa.eu.int/comm/food/fs/scoop/task3210.pdf

TASK 9.1 (2002), Scientific Cooperation Task 9.1, 'Preparation of a working document in support of the uniform interpretation of legislative standards and the laboratory quality standards prescribed under directive 93/99/EEC', WPCC/%% revised ANNEX 1, January 2002.

TATEO F, MIRAGLIA M, BONONI M (1998), 'First results on the applicability of MS/DI (direct inlet sistem) for the confirmatory analysis of aflatoxins', in Miraglia M, van Egmond H P, Brera C, Gilbert J, (eds) *Mycotoxin and Phycotoxins – Developments in Chemistry, Toxicology and Food Safety*. Alaken, Inc. Fort Collins, CO.

THOMPSON, ELLISON S L, WOOD R (1999), IUPAC 'Harmonized guidelines for single laboratory validation of methods of analysis', Resulting from the Symposium on Harmonization of Quality Assurance Systems for Analytical Laboratories, Budapest, Hungary, 4–5 November 1999, held under the sponsorship of IUPAC, ISO and AOAC Int.

TIEBACH R, BLAAS W, KELLERT M, STEINMEYER S, WEBER R (1985), 'Confirmation of nivalenol and deoxynivalenol by on-line liquid chromatography-mass spectrometry. Comparison of methods', *J. Chromatog*. 318, 103–111.

TRIGO-STOCKLI D M, CORTEZ-ROCHA O, SANCHEZ-MARINEZ R I, REED C R (2002), 'Fumonisin B1 levels in 1995 and 1996 Kansas Corn', *Bull. Environ. Contam. Toxicol.*, 68, 720–724.

TRUCKSESS M W, TANG Y (1999), 'Solid-phase extraction method for patulin in apple juice and unfiltered apple juice', *J. Ass. Off. Anal. Chem. Int.*, 82, 1109–1113.

TRUCKSESS M W, READY D W R, PENDER M K, LIGMOND C A, WOOD G E, PAGE S W (1996), 'Determination and survey of deoxynivalenol in white flour, whole wheat flour, and bran', *J. Ass. Off. Anal. Chem. Int.* 79, 883–887.

TSAO R, ZHOU T (2000), 'Micellar electrokinetic capillary electrophoresis for rapid analysis of patulin in apple cider', *J. Agric. Food Chem.*, 48, 5231–5235.

TUNISTRA L G M, HAASNOOT W (1983), 'Rapid determination of aflatoxin B_1 in Dutch feeding stuffs by high performance liquid chromatography and postcolumn derivatization', *J. Chromatog.* 282, 457–462.

UCHIYAMA S, SAITO Y, VCHIYAMA M (1985), 'Protein-binding of ochratoxin A and its extractability from proteinous food', *J. Food Hygene Soc. Japan* 26, 651–657.

UENO Y, MAKI S, LIN J, FURUYA M, SUGIURA Y, KAWAMURA O (1998), 'A 4-year study of plasma ochratoxin A in a selected population in Tokyo by immunoassay and immunoaffinity column-linked HPLC', *Food Chem. Toxicol.* 36: 445–449.

US NTP (1999), NTP Technical Report on the Toxicology and Carcinogenesis Studies of Fumonisin B1 (CAS No. 116355–83–0) in F344/N Rats and B6C3F1 Mice (Feed Studies). NTP TR 496, NIH Publication No. 99–3955 (Research Triangle Park, NC: US Departments of Health and Human Services), pp. 123–131, Appendix A, Appendix D.

VAHL M, JØRGENSEN K (1998), Determination of aflatoxin in food using LC/MS/MS', *Z Lebensm Unters Forsch A.*, 206, 243–245.

VAN DER GAAG B, SPATH S, DIETRICH H, STIGTER E, BOONZAAIJER G, VAN OSENBRUGGEN T, KOOPAL K (2003), 'Biosensor and multiple mycotoxin analysis', *Food Control*, 14 (4), 251–254.

WARE J M, CARMAN A, FRANCIS O, KUAN S (1984), 'Gas chromatographic determination of deoxynivalenol in wheat with electron capture detection', *J. Ass. Off. Anal. Chem.*, 67, 731–734.

WHITAKER T, HAGLER JR. W H, JOHANSSON A S, GIESBRECHT F G, TRUKSESS M W (2001), 'Sampling shelled corn for fumonisins', in in De Koe W, Samson R, van Egmond H P, Gilbert J, (eds) *Mycotoxins and Phycotoxins in Perpective at the Turn of the Millenium.* Wageningen, The Netherlands.

WHITAKER T B, DICKENS J W, SLATE A B (1990), 'Computerized system to quantify aflatoxin using thin-layer chromatography', *J Peanut Sci.* 17, 96–100.

WHO (1980), 'Requirements for kits for immunoassay and other protein binding systems', document number: WHO/BS/80.1270/HRP/80.1, Geneva, CH.

WHO (1990), *Selected Mycotoxins: Ochratoxins, Trichothecenes, Ergot (Environmental Health Criteria 105)*, Geneva.

WHO (2002), WHO Technical Report Series 906, 'Evaluation of certain mycotoxins in food', Fifty-sixth report of the joint FAO/WHO Expert Committee on Food Additives, Geneva.

WILD C P (1998), 'The molecular epidemiology of mycotoxin-related disease', in Miraglia M, van Egmond H P, Brera C, Gilbert J, (eds) *Mycotoxins and Phycotoxins – Developments in Chemistry, Toxicology and Food Safety*, Alaken, Inc. Fort Collins, CO.

WILKES J G, SUTHERLAND J B, CHURCHWELL M I, WILLIAMS A L, (1995) 'Determination of fumonisins B_1, B_2, B_3 and B_4 by high-performance liquid chromatography with evaporative light-scattering detection', *J. Chromatog.*, 69, 319–323.

WILSON T M, ROSS P E, OWENS D L, RICE L G, GREEN S A, JENKINS S J AND NELSON H A (1992), 'Experimental reproduction of ELEM a study to determine the minimum toxic dose in ponies', *Mycopathologia,* 117, 115–120.

YOUNG J C (1992), 'Supercritical fluid chromatography of *fusarium* mycotoxins', *J. Chromatog.*, 627, 247–254.

Index